Rational Use of Intravenous Fluids in Critically Ill Patients

Manu L. N. G. Malbrain
Adrian Wong • Prashant Nasa
Supradip Ghosh
Editors

Rational Use of Intravenous Fluids in Critically Ill Patients

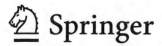 Springer

Editors
Manu L. N. G. Malbrain
First Department of Anaesthesiology and
Intensive Therapy
Medical University of Lublin
Lublin, Poland

Prashant Nasa
Critical Care Medicine, Chairperson,
Prevention and Infection Control
NMC Specialty Hospital, Dubai,
Dubai, United Arab Emirates

Adrian Wong
Intensive Care and Anaesthesia
King's College Hospital NHS Foundation Trust
London, UK

Supradip Ghosh
Department of Critical Care Medicine
Fortis - Escort Hospital
Faridabad, Haryana, India

ISBN 978-3-031-42207-2   ISBN 978-3-031-42205-8   (eBook)
https://doi.org/10.1007/978-3-031-42205-8

This book is an open access publication.

International Fluid Academy (IFA)

This Springer imprint is published by the registered company Springer Nature Switzerland AG
The registered company address is: Gewerbestrasse 11, 6330 Cham, Switzerland

Paper in this product is recyclable.

Contents

Part I Fundamentals of Intravenous Fluid Therapy

1 Terms and Definitions of Fluid Therapy 3
Manu L. N. G. Malbrain, Adrian Wong, Luca Malbrain, Prashant Nasa,
and Jonny Wilkinson
Introduction... 4
Terms and Definitions... 5
Conclusions.. 42
References... 43

**2 Fluid Physiology Part 1: Volume and Distribution of Water
and Its Major Solutes Between Plasma, the Interstitium
and Intracellular Fluid** 47
Thomas Woodcock
Introduction... 50
Total Body Water 50
Clinical Use of Total Body Water Estimation and Modified Body Weights.... 51
Water Absorption 52
Plasma Volume 53
The Starling Principle and Microvessel Heterogeneity 54
    Exceptions to the No-Absorption Rule............................. 55
    The Current Understanding of Starling Forces..................... 56
    Starling Forces; Steady State Variations Versus Abrupt Disequilibrium 57
Interstitium and Lymphatics 57
    The Triphasic Interstitium; Collagen Phase 58
    The Triphasic Interstitium; Hyaluronan Gel Phase................. 59
    The Triphasic Interstitium; Aqueous Phase 59
    Gel Swelling Pressure... 60
    Interstitial Starling Forces...................................... 60
Lymphatic Vascular System 61
Interstitial Fluid Dynamics 62

Lymphatics and the Interstitial Storage of Sodium...................... 64
   Interstitial Fluid and Lymph in Critical Illness........................ 65
Pulmonary Starling Forces and the Extravascular Lung Water 67
Cell Fluid and Extracellular Fluid..................................... 67
   Starling Forces Between Extracellular and Intracellular Fluids........... 67
   Maintenance of the Extracellular-Intracellular Solute
   Balance is Energy-Dependent....................................... 68
   Potassium and Magnesium Ions 69
   Cell Volume Regulation and Intracranial Pressure 69
   Cell Volume Regulation beyond the Brain 70
   Hessels' Alternative Model of Water, Sodium and
   Potassium Distribution 71
Water Excretion.. 71
References.. 72

**3 Fluid Physiology Part 2: Regulation of Body Fluids
and the Distribution of Infusion Fluids** 75
Robert G. Hahn
Introduction.. 77
Fluid Balance 78
   Fluid Intake... 78
   Fluid Losses 78
Fluid Movement and Edema Formation 79
   Cell Membrane 79
   Capillary Membrane 80
   The Starling Equation 81
   Edema Formation 81
The Importance of Organ Function..................................... 82
   The Kidneys 82
   Nervous Control 82
   Hormones 83
Cardiac Response to Fluid 83
Electrolytes 84
Crystalloid Fluid Solutions.. 85
   Ringer's Solution 85
   Other Crystalloid Fluids 86
Colloid Fluid Solutions.. 87
Measurement of Body Fluid Volumes................................... 87
Fluid Efficiency... 88
Volume Kinetics, Basic Concepts...................................... 89
Crystalloids Versus Colloids... 92
Goals of Fluid Therapy 93
References.. 94

4   Fluid Dynamics During Resuscitation: From Frank–Starling
      to the Reappraisal of Guyton   97
      Supradip Ghosh
      Introduction.   101
      What Are the Factors That Determine Flow of Blood from
      Peripheral Circulation to Heart?.   102
      What Are the Factors That Determine Mean Systemic Pressure?   103
      Guyton's Experiment and Venous Return Curve   103
      Starling's Experiment   104
      Effect of Fluid Bolus on Venous Return Curve.   105
      Cardiac Function Curve   106
      Integrating the Return Function with Cardiac Function   107
      Overall Effect of Fluid Bolus on Circulation 108
      Validation of Guytonian Model in Human Studies.   109
      Conclusion   110
      References.   111

5   Understanding Heart-Lung Interactions: Concepts of
      Fluid Responsiveness   113
      Ajeet Singh and Shrikanth Srinivasan
      Introduction.   118
      Basics of Respiratory and Cardio-Circulatory Physiology. 119
      Effects of Mechanical Ventilation on Intrathoracic Pressure   120
      The Pump   121
          Venous Return and Ventricular Preload   121
          Ventricular Afterload.   123
          Left Ventricular Afterload   123
          Right Ventricular Afterload.   123
      Ventricular Interdependence   124
      Heart-Lung Interactions: Clinical Application   124
          Functional Hemodynamic Monitoring   124
      Dynamic Indicators for Fluid Responsiveness   126
          Invasive Assessment of Respiratory Changes in LV Stroke Volume 126
      Pulse Pressure Variation   127
          Non-invasive Assessment of Respiratory Changes in LV Stroke Volume . . .   130
      Other Clinically Significant Clinical Interactions.   131
      Cardiopulmonary Changes in Prone Positioning   132
      Conclusions.   133
      References.   134

6   Acid-Base Homeostasis: Traditional Approach   139
      Supradip Ghosh
      Introduction.   142
      Definitions. 142

Acid-Base Homeostasis   143
High AG Metabolic Acidosis   146
Normal AG Metabolic Acidosis   147
Metabolic Alkalosis   148
Some More Illustrative Cases   150
Conclusion   151
Reference   152

7   Acid Base Homeostasis: Stewart Approach at the Bedside 153
Supradip Ghosh
Introduction.   156
Physicochemical Perspective   157
SID and Acid Base Balance   158
Total Nonvolatile Acid Anion (A_{tot}) and Acid Base Balance   158
Total CO_2.   158
Stewart at Bedside: Fencl-Stewart Approach   159
Fencl-Stewart: Putting It All Together   159
Stewart at Bedside: Using Standard Base Excess.   160
Effect of Different IV Fluids on Acid-Base Balance   161
Some More Illustrative Case.   163
Conclusion   164
References.   164

8   The 4-indications of Fluid Therapy: Resuscitation, Replacement,
Maintenance and Nutrition Fluids, and Beyond 167
Manu L. N. G. Malbrain, Michaël Mekeirele, Matthias Raes,
Steven Hendrickx, Idris Ghijselings, Luca Malbrain, and Adrian Wong
Introduction.   171
The Four Indications   172
    Resuscitation Fluids   172
    Maintenance Fluids.   172
    Replacement Fluids.   177
    Nutrition Fluids.   177
The Four Questions.   178
    When to Start IV Fluids?   178
    When to Stop IV Fluids?.   179
    When to Start Fluid Removal?   179
    When to Stop Fluid Removal?   179
The Four (or Six) D's   180
    Diagnosis.   180
    Drug   180
    Dose   181
    Duration   188

De-escalation.   188
Discharge   189
The Four Hits   189
First Hit: Initial Insult   189
Second Hit: Ischemia-Reperfusion   189
Third Hit: Global Increased Permeability Syndrome   189
Fourth Hit: Hypoperfusion   190
The Four Phases (ROSE Concept)   191
Resuscitation.   192
Optimization   193
Stabilization   193
Evacuation.   193
The Other Fours   196
The Four Compartments   196
The Four Spaces   196
The Four Losses   196
Conclusions.   197
References.   199

Part II   Available Intravenous Fluids

9   The Place of Crystalloids. 205
Amandeep Singh and Aayush Chawla
Introduction.   208
Fluid Physiology.   208
Types of Crystalloids   210
Isotonic Crystalloids   212
Isotonic Saline or 0.9% Saline   213
Balanced Crystalloids   214
Clinical Evidence: 0.9% Saline Vs Balanced   215
Observational Studies   215
Randomized Controlled Studies   216
Hypotonic Crystalloids   218
Hypertonic Crystalloids   220
Hypertonic Saline   220
Sodium Bicarbonate Solution   221
Conclusion   223
References.   224

10   The Case for Albumin as Volume Expander and beyond. 227
Prashant Nasa, Rajesh Kumar, Deven Juneja, and Supradip Gosh
Introduction.   230
Albumin in Health.   231

Albumin in Critical Illness 232
Evidence on Albumin as a Plasma Expander 232
Timing of Albumin Administration during Resuscitation. 234
Comparison of Different Strengths of Albumin 234
Albumin beyond Resuscitation 235
    Patients with Liver Disease. 235
    Treatment of Hypoalbuminemia with Peripheral Oedema 235
    Deresuscitation 236
    Other Indications. 236
Caution with the Use of Albumin 236
Conclusion 238
References. 239

11   The Place for Starches and Other Colloids 243
Ripenmeet Salhotra, Adrian Wong, and Manu L. N. G. Malbrain
Introduction. 245
Hydroxyethyl Starch 246
    Pharmacology 246
    Is Hydroxyethyl Starch Beneficial? 248
    Evidence in Critically Ill Patients 248
    Perioperative Use of HES 253
    Controversies and Restrictions on HES 254
Gelatins 254
Dextrans 255
Conclusion 256
References. 256

12   How to Use Blood and Blood Products 259
Kapil Dev Soni and Rahul Chaurasia
Introduction. 261
Anemia and Red Cell Administration. 262
Age of RBC and Transfusion Outcomes. 265
Thrombocytopenia and Platelet Transfusion 266
Coagulopathy and Plasma Transfusion. 267
Adverse Transfusion Reactions in Critical Care. 269
Alternatives to Transfusion 270
Conclusion 271
References. 272

13   Nutrition Delivery in Critically Ill Patients 275
Ranajit Chatterjee and Ashutosh Kumar Garg
Introduction. 281
Goals of Nutrition in the ICU 282
Nutrition Assessment 282

Assessment of Energy Needs 283
Initiate Early EN 283
Dosing of EN 284
Monitoring Tolerance and Adequacy of EN 285
Selection of Appropriate Enteral Formulation 285
When to Use PN 285
When Indicated, Maximize Efficacy of PN 286
Special Situations 286
    Pulmonary Failure. 286
    Renal Failure. 286
    Hepatic Failure 287
    Acute Pancreatitis 287
    Trauma 287
    Burns. 288
    Sepsis 288
    Postoperative Major Surgery. 288
    Obese Patients. 288
Fluid Therapy and Nutrition 289
Conclusion 290
References. 292

Part III   Fluid Therapy in Special Conditions

14   Fluid Management in Septic Shock 295
Supradip Ghosh and Garima Arora
Introduction. 300
Septic Shock: Pathophysiology. 300
Septic Shock: Diagnosis 301
Septic Shock: Management. 302
Resuscitation. 303
Which Fluid?. 303
Dose of Fluid. 306
Interaction with Vasopressors 306
Septic Shock: Monitoring. 307
Limiting Cumulative Fluid Balance 308
Conclusion 309
References. 310

15   Fluid Management in Cardiogenic Shock 315
Shrikanth Srinivasan and Riddhi Kundu
Introduction. 316
Fluid Management of Left-Ventricular Failure. 317
How Should Fluid Responsiveness Be Assessed and Fluid
Therapy Titrated in these Patients?. 318

Fluid Management in Right-Ventricular Failure........................ 321
How to Assess Fluid Responsiveness and Titrate Fluids in RV Failure? 324
Conclusion 327
References.. 327

16 **Fluid Management in Trauma** 329
Kapil Dev Soni and Basant Gauli
Introduction.. 332
Goals of Early Resuscitation... 332
Initial Choice of Fluid for Trauma Resuscitation 335
Crystalloids.. 335
Colloids.. 336
Hypertonic Solutions 337
Penetrating Versus Blunt Injury Versus Head Injuries 337
Initial Trauma Resuscitation Fluid Volume............................ 338
Practical Approach to Initial Fluid Resuscitation and Pattern of Responses ... 339
Completion of Resuscitation... 339
Post-Resuscitation Fluid Management 340
Deresuscitation 340
Conclusion 341
References.. 342

17 **Fluid Management in Neurocritical Care** 345
Roop Kishen
Introduction.. 348
Physiological Considerations 348
What Kind of Fluid Is Appropriate in NIC Patients? 350
Does Tonicity of the IV Fluids Matter in NIC Patients?................. 351
Hyperosmolar Therapy in NIC Patients 352
End Points of Fluid Therapy Management in Neurocritical Care:
How Much Fluid Is Enough? 352
Monitoring Fluid Therapy in NIC Patients............................ 353
A Note on Common Electrolyte Disturbances in NIC Patients 353
    General Considerations... 353
    Hyponatraemia 354
    Hypernatremia... 356
    Hyperchloraemia.. 356
    Other Electrolyte Disturbances................................... 356
Fluid Therapy Management in Neurocritical Care: Clinical Practice
Recommendations... 357
Conclusion 358
References.. 359

18 Perioperative Fluid Manangement................................. 363

Anirban Hom Choudhuri and Kiranlata Kiro

Introduction... 365

Types Fluid 366

Calculation of Third-Space Loss......................... 366

Monitoring Intravascular Volume Status During the Perioperative Period..... 367

Choosing Between Crystalloids and Colloids.............. 368

'Restrictive' Versus 'Liberal' Strategy 369

Fluid Requirements in Special Situations................. 371

    Neurosurgery....................................... 371

    Open-Heart Surgery 372

    Kidney and Liver Transplant Surgery................. 372

    Obstetric Surgery 373

    Pediatric Surgery.................................. 373

Outpatient and Day-Care Surgery....................... 375

Conclusion 376

References.. 376

19 Fluid Management in Major Burns......................... 379

Aditya Lyall and Abhay Singh Bhadauria

Introduction... 386

Pathophysiology 387

Fluid Estimation and Administration 388

Choice of Fluid and Monitoring 389

Conclusion 391

References.. 392

20 Fluid Management in Paediatric Patients................... 395

Sonali Ghosh

Introduction... 399

Physiology of Body Fluid in Children 399

    Fluids for the Paediatric Population: Resuscitation,

    Replacement and Maintenance........................ 400

Individual Clinical Scenarios 403

    Children with Dehydration 403

Sepsis and Septic Shock 405

Diabetic Ketoacidosis 406

Conclusion 408

References.. 408

21 Fluid Management in Liver Failure......................... 411

Michaël Mekeirele and Alexander Wilmer

Introduction... 413

Acute-On-Chronic Liver Failure (ACLF)................. 414

Pathophysiology of Circulatory Dysfunction in Patients with Cirrhosis 414
Hemodynamic Approach During Decompensation 415
Acute Liver Failure (ALF) 419
Conclusion 421
References. 423

22 Fluid Management in Intra-abdominal Hypertension 427
Manu L. N. G. Malbrain, Prashant Nasa, Inneke De laet, Jan De Waele,
Rita Jacobs, Robert Wise, Luca Malbrain, Wojciech Dabrowski,
and Adrian Wong
Introduction. 430
Definitions. 431
Intra-abdominal Pressure 431
Intra-abdominal Hypertension and Abdominal Compartment Syndrome . . . 431
Hemodynamic Effects and Impact on End-Organ Function. 432
Globally Increased Permeability Syndrome 432
Fluids and IAH 433
Why Do We Like Fluids in IAH? 433
Understanding the Linkage Between Over Fluids and IAH? 434
Do Patients with IAH Have a More Positive Fluid Balance? 436
Does IAP Improve with Interventions Acting on Reducing Fluid Balance? . 442
Conclusion 451
References. 452

23 Sodium and Chloride Balance in Critically Ill Patients 459
Ranajit Chatterjee and Ashutosh Kumar Garg
Introduction. 461
Water and Sodium Balance. 462
Management of Hyponatremia 466
Management of Hypernatremia 470
Chloride Balance. 471
Introduction. 471
Chloride Distribution and Measurement. 472
Chloride Physiology 473
Chloride and the Stewart Approach 473
Disorders of Chloraemia and Manipulation of Chloride in the ICU 474
Clinical Approach to Dyschloremia 475
Critical Analysis of Crystalloids on the Basis of above Discussion 477
Chloride in the ICU: The Research Agenda 478
Conclusions. 479
References. 479

24 Balanced Solutions: Choice of Buffer 481

Suneel Kumar Garg

Introduction... 483

Buffered/Balanced Crystalloids 483

Sodium Lactate *Vs* Sodium Acetate Solution...................... 485

Acetate and Gluconate Buffered Solutions......................... 487

Acetate and Malate Buffered Solutions 489

Conclusion.. 490

References.. 490

25 Fluid Accumulation and Deresuscitation...................... 495

Manu L. N. G. Malbrain, Jonny Wilkinson, Luca Malbrain,
Prashant Nasa, and Adrian Wong

Introduction.. 502

Definitions... 504

Pathophysiology 506

Liberal Versus Restrictive Fluid Regimens........................ 508

Monitoring Hypervolemia and Guiding Deresuscitation 511

    Clinical Signs of Hypervolemia 511

    Laboratory Signs and Biomarkers 513

    Radiological and Imaging Signs.............................. 515

    Advanced Hemodynamic Monitoring......................... 517

How to Perform Deresuscitation?................................ 518

Conclusions... 521

References.. 523

26 Fluid Management in COVID-19 527

Manu L. N. G. Malbrain, Serene Ho, Prashant Nasa, and Adrian Wong

Introduction.. 530

What Do We Know?... 530

What Guidelines Are Available?.................................. 531

    Surviving Sepsis Campaign 531

    World Health Organization.................................. 532

    UK Joint Anaesthetic and Intensive Care Guidelines............ 532

Guidance and Recommendations from the International Fluid Academy 533

    Assessment and Monitoring 533

    Resuscitation... 534

    Maintenance Fluids.. 534

    Fluid Creep 535

The Role of Ultrasound... 535

Fluid Stewardship: Knowing What We Are Doing................... 536

Conclusion 538

References.. 540

Part IV   Concepts of Fluid Stewardship and Appropriate Fluid Prescription

27   Introduction to Fluid Stewardship 545
Adrian Wong, Jonny Wilkinson, Prashant Nasa, Luca Malbrain,
and Manu L. N. G. Malbrain
Introduction   547
Definitions   548
   Appropriate Fluid Prescription   548
   The 5 P's of Fluid Prescription   548
Fluid Management in the ICU as a Quality Improvement Project   548
Quality Improvement in Healthcare   549
Stewardship (or Champions in Healthcare)   551
   How to Mandate Change?   551
   Strategy and Policy Development   551
   Designing Overarching Systems   551
   Encouraging Collaboration   552
   Ensuring Robust Governance and Accountability Process   552
Fluid Stewardship   553
   Goals   553
   The 4 Questions of Fluid Therapy   554
   The 7 D's of Fluid Therapy   556
Different Phases During Implementation of Fluid Stewardship   558
   Start-up Phase   558
   Knowledge Phase   560
   Strategy Phase   560
   Preparation Phase   561
   Education Phase   561
   Implementation Phase   562
   Post-Implementation Phase   562
Conclusion   563
References   564

28   A Logical Prescription of Intravenous Fluids 567
Jonny Wilkinson, Lisa Yates, Prashant Nasa, Manu L. N. G. Malbrain,
and Ashley Miller
Introduction   570
The Problem   570
Application of these Clinical Guidelines   573
   Target Group   573
   Exclusions   573
   Professional Groups   574
Clarification of Terms   574
   Dehydration   574

Background Clinical Physiology 574
Considerations Prior to All IV Fluid Prescriptions..................... 576
Assessment 576
General Principles... 576
Step 1: Assess Fluid Status 576
Step 2: Check Body Weight 578
Step 3: Check U&E Levels in the Last 24 h........................ 578
Step 4: Calculate Fluid Balance in the Last 24 h 578
Step 5: Prescribe the Appropriate IV Fluid on a Daily Basis 579
Fluid Prescription: Work Out What You Need!........................ 580
Maintenance Fluid 580
Replacement Solutions 582
Resuscitation Fluid 583
Appropriateness of IV Fluid Therapy................................ 585
Which IV Fluid?... 587
Difficult Situations and Tips 588
Conclusion 592
References... 593

Contributors

Garima Arora Department of Critical Care Medicine, Werribee Mercy Hospital, Werribee, VIC, Australia

Abhay Singh Bhadauria Department of Critical Care Medicine, Apollomedics Hospital, Lucknow, UP, India

Ranajit Chatterjee Intensive Care Unit and Accident and Emergency Swami Dayanand Hospital, New Delhi, India

Critical Care, Swami Dayanand Hospital, Delhi, India

Rahul Chaurasia Department of Transfusion Medicine, All India Institute of Medical Sciences, New Delhi, India

Aayush Chawla Amrita Hospital, Faridabad, India

Anirban Hom Choudhuri Department of Anesthesiology and Intensive Care, GB Pant Institute of Postgraduate Medical Education and Research, New Delhi, India

Wojciech Dabrowski First Department of Anaesthesiology and Intensive Therapy, Medical University Lublin, Lublin, Poland

Inneke De laet Intensive Care Unit, Ziekenhuis Netwerk Antwerpen, ZNA Stuivenberg, Antwerp, Belgium

Jan De Waele Intensive Care Unit, Universitair Ziekenhuis Gent, Ghent, Belgium

Ashutosh Garg Kailash Deepak Hospital, Karkardooma, New Delhi, India

Suneel Kumar Garg Saiman Healthcare, Delhi, India

Basant Gauli Department of Anaesthesia and Critical Care Medicine, Chitwan Medical College, Bharatpur, Nepal

Idris Ghijselings Intensive Care Department, University Hospital Brussels (UZB), Jette, Belgium

Sonali Ghosh PICU, MarengoAsia Hospital, Faridabad, Haryana, India

Supradip Ghosh Department of Critical Care Medicine, Fortis - Escorts Hospital, Faridabad, Haryana, India

Robert G. Hahn Anaesthesia and Intensive Care, Karolinska Institutet, Stockholm, Sweden

Steven Hendrickx Intensive Care Department, University Hospital Brussels (UZB), Jette, Belgium

Serene Ho Cavendish Clinic, London, UK

Rita Jacobs Intensive Care Unit, Universitair Ziekenhuis Antwerpen, Antwerp, Belgium

Deven Juneja Institute of Critical Care Medicine, Max Super Specialty Hospital, Saket, New Delhi, India

Kiranlata Kiro Department of Anesthesiology and Intensive Care, GB Pant Institute of Postgraduate Medical Education and Research, New Delhi, India

Roop Kishen Retired Consultant, Intensive Care Medicine & Anaesthesia, Hope Hospital, Salford Royal NHS Foundation Trust, Salford, Manchester, UK

Anaesthesia, Translational Medicine and Neurosciences, Victoria University of Manchester, Manchester, UK

Rajesh Kumar Department of Critical Care Medicine, NMC Specialty Hospital, Dubai, UAE

Riddhi Kundu Critical Care Medicine, Ruby Hall Clinic, Pune, India

Aditya Lyall Department of Critical Care Medicine, Fortis-Escorts Hospital, Faridabad, Haryana, India

Luca Malbrain University School of Medicine, Katholieke Universiteit Leuven (KUL), Leuven, Belgium

Manu L. N. G. Malbrain First Department of Anaesthesiology and Intensive Therapy, Medical University of Lublin, Lublin, Poland

International Fluid Academy, Lovenjoel, Belgium

Medical Data Management, Medaman, Geel, Belgium

Michaël Mekeirele Intensive Care Department, University Hospital Brussels (UZB), Jette, Belgium

Department of Critical Care, Vrije Universiteit Brussel (VUB), Universitair Ziekenhuis Brussel (UZB), Jette, Belgium

Ashley Miller Department of Intensive Care and Anaesthesia, Shrewsbury, UK

Prashant Nasa Critical Care Medicine, Prevention and Infection Control, NMC Specialty Hospital, Dubai, United Arab Emirates

Internal Medicine, College of Medicine and Health Sciences, Al Ain, UAE

Matthias Raes Intensive Care Department, University Hospital Brussels (UZB), Jette, Belgium

Ripenmeet Salhotra Department of Anaesthesiology and Critical Care, Amrita Hospital, Faridabad, India

Ajeet Singh Critical Care Medicine, Manipal Hospital, Dwarka, New Delhi, India

Amandeep Singh, MD, IDCCM Department of Critical Cate Medicine, Fortis Escorts Hospital, Faridabad, Haryana, India

Kapil Dev Soni Critical and Intensive Care, JPN Apex Trauma Center, All India Institute of Medical Sciences, New Delhi, India

Shrikanth Srinivasan Critical Care Medicine, Manipal Hospital, Dwarka, New Delhi, India

Jonny Wilkinson ITU and Anaesthesia and NICE IV Fluid Lead, Northampton, UK

Department of Intensive Care and Anaesthesia, Critical Care Northampton, Northampton, UK

Alexander Wilmer Medical Intensive Care Unit, Katholieke Universiteit Leuven (KUL), Universitair Ziekenhuis Gasthuisberg, Leuven, Belgium

Robert Wise Discipline of Anaesthesia and Critical Care, School of Clinical Medicine, University of KwaZulu-Natal, Durban, South Africa

Intensive Care Department, Oxford University Trust Hospitals, John Radcliffe Hospital, Oxford, UK

Adrian Wong Intensive Care and Anaesthesia, King's College Hospital NHS Foundation Trust, London, UK

Intensive Care Unit, King's College Hospital, London, UK

Thomas Woodcock Department of Critical Care, University Hospital Southampton, Southampton, UK

Lisa Yates Department of Intensive Care and Anaesthesia, Critical Care, Northampton, UK

Part I

Fundamentals of Intravenous Fluid Therapy

Terms and Definitions of Fluid Therapy

Manu L. N. G. Malbrain (iD), Adrian Wong, Luca Malbrain,
Prashant Nasa, and Jonny Wilkinson

Contents

Introduction 4
Terms and Definitions 5
Conclusions 42
References 43

Manu L. N. G. Malbrain (✉)
First Department of Anaesthesiology and Intensive Therapy, Medical University of Lublin, Lublin, Poland

A. Wong
Intensive Care and Anaesthesia, King's College Hospital NHS Foundation Trust, London, UK
e-mail: adrian.wong@nhs.net

L. Malbrain
University School of Medicine, Katholieke Universiteit Leuven (KUL), Leuven, Belgium

P. Nasa
Critical Care Medicine, NMC Specialty Hospital, Dubai, United Arab Emirates
e-mail: dr.prashantnasa@hotmail.com

J. Wilkinson
ITU and Anaesthesia and NICE IV Fluid Lead, Northampton, UK

© The Author(s) 2024
M. L. N. G. Malbrain et al. (eds.), *Rational Use of Intravenous Fluids in Critically Ill Patients*, https://doi.org/10.1007/978-3-031-42205-8_1

IFA Commentary

The chapter on terms and definitions of fluid therapy and monitoring in the book "Rational Fluid Use in the Critically Ill" provides an essential foundation for understanding the importance of intravenous (IV) fluid therapy in critically ill patients. The authors effectively highlight the need to view IV fluids as drugs and not simply as a routine treatment option. The chapter's approach is practical, providing clear definitions of essential and common terms used in fluid therapy and organ function monitoring, emphasizing the significance of appropriate fluid therapy such as volume status, resuscitation, maintenance fluids, colloids and crystalloids. This practical approach is critical for clinicians as it provides them with a clear understanding of what they are administering and how to administer it appropriately.

Introduction

This introductory chapter will list the common terms and definitions used throughout this book. Intravenous fluid (IV) therapy is a cornerstone to treating shock status and providing water, electrolytes and glucose needs. Worldwide thousands of litres of IV fluids are administered every day. However, IV fluids are not yet treated in the same way as other medications given to our patients. We need to see them as drugs, and they come with a dose, duration and de-escalation, and they need to be given in a timely manner, but only when needed and when the patient cannot have oral fluid intake. They have indications, contra-indications and potential adverse effects. Inappropriate fluid therapy is one of the main concerns.

Thus, the appropriate use of IV fluids is an essential part of patient safety and deserves careful oversight and guidance, given the association between fluid (mis)use and the deleterious effects causing patient morbidity and mortality [1]. Correct definitions, implementation of a fluid stewardship and organ function monitoring may limit the deleterious effects of inappropriate fluid prescription and fluid overload [2]. The literature on fluid therapy in the critically ill is continuously expanding, however, sometimes, different definitions are used. For example, fluid overload, fluid accumulation, hypervolemia and hyperhydration are often used interchangeably, while, they may indicate different clinical situations [3]. Using wrong definitions can lead to misunderstandings, misinterpretations and inappropriate therapeutic decisions regarding fluid administration or fluid removal.

In this chapter, we provide definitions of the different terms important in the context of fluid therapy in hospitalized patients, and intensive care units [4–10]. These definitions will be repeated throughout the different chapters when these conditions are discussed in more detail.

Terms and Definitions

4 compartments: This can be dealt with in different ways, classically you have fat–water–protein–and minerals while water on its own is also distributed into four compartments: intracellular water (ICW), interstitial water, intravascular water and transcellular, with extracellular water (ECW) calculated as the sum of interstitial + intravascular + transcellular water content.

4 D's: Fluids are medications in which one should take into account the 4D's in analogy to antimicrobial stewardship: Drug–Dose–Duration–De-escalation.

4 hits: The four hits are:

first hit = initial insult,
second hit = ischemia reperfusion,
third hit = global increased permeability syndrome (GIPS).
fourth hit = potential risk of hypoperfusion during de-resuscitation.

4 indications: Fluids can be given for four reasons: resuscitation, maintenance, replacement and nutrition.

4 fluid losses: Traditionally four ways can be taken into account with regard to fluid losses: insensible loss, urine output, gastrointestinal losses and third space. Additional losses can occur in trauma with overt bleeding or in severely burned patients.

4 phases: The four dynamic fluid phases are: resuscitation, optimization, stabilization and evacuation.

4 questions: The four main questions surrounding fluid therapy that need to be solved are:

when to start IV fluids?
when to stop IV fluids?
when to start fluid removal?
when to stop fluid removal?

4 spaces: There are traditionally four fluid spaces:

first space = intravascular.
second space = interstitial.
third space = pleural or peritoneal space.
fourth space = transcellular fluid, and not to forget the lymphatic system.

Abdominal compartment syndrome (ACS): Abdominal compartment syndrome (ACS) is defined as a sustained intra–abdominal pressure (IAP) >20 mmHg (with or without an abdominal perfusion perfusion (APP) <60 mmHg) that is associated with new organ dysfunction/failure. Primary ACS is a condition associated with injury or disease in the abdomino-pelvic region that frequently requires early surgical or interventional radiological intervention. Secondary ACS refers to conditions that do not originate from the abdomino-pelvic region. Recurrent ACS refers to the condition in which ACS redevelops following previous surgical or medical treatment of primary or secondary ACS [11].

Abdominal perfusion pressure (APP): Abdominal perfusion pressure (APP) = mean arterial pressure (MAP) − IAP. The Filtration Gradient (FG) = glomerular filtration pressure (GFP) − proximal tubular pressure (PTP) = MAP − 2 × IAP [11].

Abdominal West zones: West zones describe areas of the abdomen based upon variations in IAP, central venous pressure (CVP) and inferior vena cava pressure (IVCP). These differences result from vascular flow, gravity and pressure transmission from the abdominal to the thoracic compartment. The concept of abdominal vascular zones may be present in the patient with IAH, analogous to the pulmonary vascular zone conditions described by West. In this concept, an increased IAP increases venous return when the transmural IVCP (defined as IVCP minus IAP) at the thoracic inlet significantly exceeds the critical closing transmural pressure (= zone 3 abdomen). This is most often the case in hypervolemic patients with a high IVCP. In zone 3 conditions, the abdominal venous compartment functions as a capacitor. In contrast, when the transmural IVCP at the thoracic inlet is below the critical closure transmural pressure (= zone 2 abdomen), venous return is significantly decreased. This is most often the case in hypovolemic patients and by extension in most non-cardiogenic shock patients. In zone 2 conditions, the abdominal venous compartment functions as a collapsible starling transistor [12] (Fig. 1.1). This model clearly illustrates why hypovolemia (and especially in combination with positive pressure

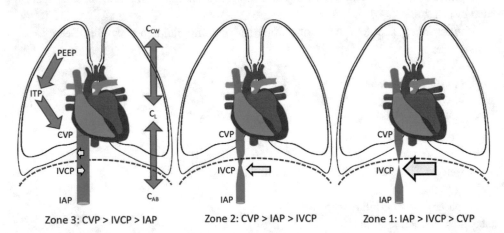

Fig. 1.1 Abdominal West zones. The abdomen can be divided into discrete regions according to the interplay between IAP, CVP and IVCP. These regions are zone 1, where IAP is higher than IVCP or CVP; zone 2, where the IAP is lower than the CVP but higher than the IVCP and zone 3, where both CVP and IVCP are higher than IAP. Other contributing factors (but more difficult to assess) are the compliance of the lungs (C_L), chest wall (C_{CW}) and abdominal wall (C_{AB}) as well as the use of positive pressure ventilation with PEEP and intrathoracic pressure. *CVP* central venous pressure, *IAP* intra-abdominal pressure, *ITP* intrathoracic pressure, *IVCP* inferior vena cava pressure, *PEEP* positive end-expiratory pressure

Table 1.1 AKI criteria according to different guidelines (with KDIGO being most commonly used)

Stage	RIFLE	AKIN	KDIGO
Stage 1/ risk	sCr 1.5 × baseline (within 7 days) Or GFR decrease >25%	sCr 1.5–2.0 × baseline (within 7 days) Or ≥0.3 mg/dL increase (within 48 h)	sCr 1.5–1.9 × baseline (within 7 days) Or ≥0.3 mg/dL increase (within 48 h)
Urine output <0.5 mL/kg/h × 6 h			
Stage 2/ injury	sCr 2 × baseline Or GFR decrease >50%	sCr 2–3 × baseline	sCr 2–2.9 × baseline
Urine output <0.5 mL/kg/h × 12 h			
Stage 3/ failure	sCr 3 × baseline Or GFR decrease >75% Or sCr ≥4 (with acute rise ≥0.5 mg/dL)	sCr 3 × baseline Or sCr ≥4 (with acute rise ≥0.5 mg/dL) Or Initiation of kidney replacement therapy	sCr 3 × baseline Or sCr ≥4 (with ≥0.3 mg/dL increase within 48 h or 1.5 × baseline) Or Initiation of kidney replacement therapy
Urine output <0.3 mL/kg/h × 24 h Or Anuria × 12 h			
Loss	Complete loss of kidney function >4 weeks		
ESRD	End-stage kidney disease (>3 months)		

AKIN acute kidney injury network, *ESRD* end-stage renal disease, *KDIGO* kidney disease: improving global outcomes, *RIFLE* risk failure loss end-stage renal disease, *sCr* serum creatinine

ventilation and high levels of PEEP) predisposes patients to lower cardiac output (CO) in response to elevated IAP than normovolemia. In real life, the model may be more complex and should also take into account, volemia status, compliance and positive pressure ventilation with PEEP settings.

Acid: A molecule or substance that is able to increase the concentration of hydrogen ions (H+) when dissolved in water or an aqueous solution.

Acidemia: A blood pH that is lower than the normal physiologic range.

Acidosis: A process in the body in which there is a net accumulation of acid.

Acute kidney injury (AKI): According to the KDIGO guidelines [13], acute kidney injury is defined by either an increase in serum creatinine ≥0.3 mg/dL within 48 h or an increase in serum creatinine ≥1.5 times baseline or a urine output ≤0.5 mL/kg/h for 6 h (Table 1.1).

Albumin leak index: Laboratory index correlated with ongoing infection or poor source control, can be calculated by dividing the urine albumin by the urine creatinine level.

Alkalemia: A blood pH that is greater than the normal physiologic range.

Alkalosis: A process in the body in which there is a net accumulation of base.

Anion: A negatively charged atom or molecule, such as chloride (Cl^-) and bicarbonate (HCO_3^-).

Anion Gap (AG): The calculated difference between the major cations and anions in plasma. The anion gap is calculated by the following formula: $AG = (Na^+ + K^+) - (Cl^- + HCO_3^-)$. Anion gap is useful to help narrow down the potential causes of metabolic acidosis.

Autotransfusion: A blood conservation strategy used during haemorrhage or surgery where blood is collected, filtered and reinfused into the patient. This process is also referred to as blood salvage or cell salvage. The passive leg raising test can be seen as a sort of autotransfusion with 300 mL blood coming from the legs and mesenteric venous pool increasing venous return into the central circulation. Another example of autotransfusion is the use of vasopressors in vasoplegia with relative hypovolemia, increased unstressed volume and a decreased stressed volume. See also under vasoplegia.

Balanced solution: An intravenous crystalloid fluid that contains an electrolyte composition similar to normal plasma. An iso-osmotic and isotonic balanced solution maintains the acid–base status and does not induce inappropriate fluid shifts. Recently, fluids with low chloride content are also labelled as "balanced" solutions. Hence, a balanced solution can be categorized into (1) IV fluids with strong ion difference (SID) close to that of plasma, i.e. 24–29 mEq/L, causing a minimal effect on the acid–base equilibrium and (2) IV fluids containing normal or sub-normal chloride content (i.e. serum chloride ≤110 mEq/L).

Base: A molecule or substance that is able to increase the concentration of hydroxyl ions (OH^-) when dissolved in water or an aqueous solution. The hydroxyl ions (OH^-) will interact with hydrogen ions (H^+) to form water molecules ($OH^- + H^+ = H_2O$), so said in other words a base is a substance or molecule that combines with hydrogen ions (H^+) already present in the solution.

Base deficit: The amount of a strong base that must be added in vitro to 1 L of oxygenated blood to return the pH to 7.40, at a partial pressure of carbon dioxide of 40 mmHg, and temperature of 37 °C, in the presence of metabolic acidosis.

Base excess: The amount of a strong acid in mmol/L that must be added in vitro to 1 L of oxygenated blood to return the pH to 7.40, at a partial pressure of carbon dioxide of 40 mmHg, and temperature of 37 °C, in the presence of metabolic alkalosis.

Breathing ongoing loss: As we breathe, we exhale moisture in the form of water vapour. This is particularly noticeable in cold weather, when our breath may condense and form visible clouds. This is a form of ongoing fluid loss. See also replacement fluids.

Buffered solution: An intravenous crystalloid fluid that contains an acid–base buffer in order to help maintain the SID. The most common buffers are bicarbonate or organic anions (e.g. lactate, acetate, gluconate).

Capillary leak index: This index is correlated with ongoing infection or poor source control, and can be calculated by dividing the serum C-reactive protein (CRP) by the

Fig. 1.2 The main drivers of cardiac output are preload, afterload and contractility and they affect oxygen delivery and mean arterial pressure. *CO* cardiac output, *CVP* central venous pressure, *DO₂* oxygen delivery, *MAP* mean arterial pressure, *MSFP* mean systemic filling pressure, *RVR* resistance to venous return, *VR* venous return

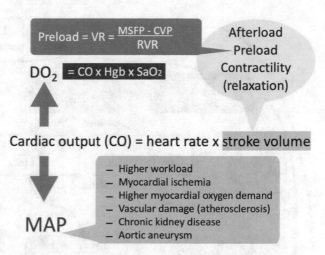

serum albumin level, the higher the CRP, the more the inflammation and the lower the albumin, the more the leak to the interstitium.

Cardiac output (CO): The amount of volume that is present at the end of the diastole and that is ejected from the left ventricle (stroke volume) multiplied by the number of heartbeats per minute, usually around 5–6 L/min. The cardiac index is CO normalized per body surface area (in m²). The main drivers of cardiac output are preload, afterload and contractility (Fig. 1.2).

Cardio-abdominal-renal syndrome (CARS): An organ–organ interaction between heart, kidney and abdomen through elevated IAP has been proposed. Therefore, the traditional perception of worsening renal failure secondary to hypoperfusion of the kidneys through low-flow states in critically ill patients, especially those with advanced decompensated heart failure, has been challenged. The low cardiac output with venous congestion of heart failure is proposed to cause elevated CVP, IAP, sodium and water retention, and decreased renal perfusion pressure, leading to the concept of "Congestive Kidney Failure" or "Cardio-Abdomino-Renal Syndrome (CARS)" (Fig. 1.3) [14].

Cation: A positively charged atom or molecule, such as chloride (Cl⁺), sodium (Na⁺), potassium (K⁺), calcium (Ca²⁺) and bicarbonate (NH₄⁺).

Classification of fluid dynamics: With respect to the different phases of fluid resuscitation (early vs. late) one can classify the dynamics of fluid management by combining early adequate (EA) or early conservative (EC) and late conservative (LC) or late liberal (LL) fluid management. Based on this theoretical concept, four distinct strategies can be defined: EALC, EALL, ECLC and ECLL. The EALC and ECLC groups carry the best prognosis (Fig. 1.4).

Circulating blood volume (CBV): The total (intravascular) volume of blood contained within the circulatory system.

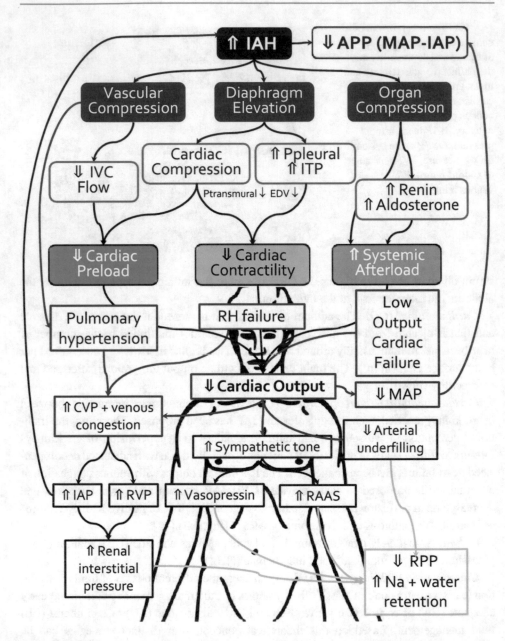

Fig. 1.3 Pathophysiological effect of heart failure (in RED forward failure) related venous congestion (in BLUE backward failure) on organ function and net effects on salt and water homeostasis (in ORANGE). *CVP* central venous pressure, *EDV* end-diastolic volume, *IAH* intra-abdominal hypertension, *IAP* intra-abdominal pressure, *ITP* intra-thoracic pressure, *IVC* inferior vena cava, *MAP* mean arterial pressure, *Na* sodium, *RAAS* renin–angiotensin–aldosterone system, *RH* right heart, *RPP* renal perfusion pressure, *RVP* renal venous pressure. (Adapted with permission from Dabrowski et al. according to the Open Access CC BY License 4.0 [15])

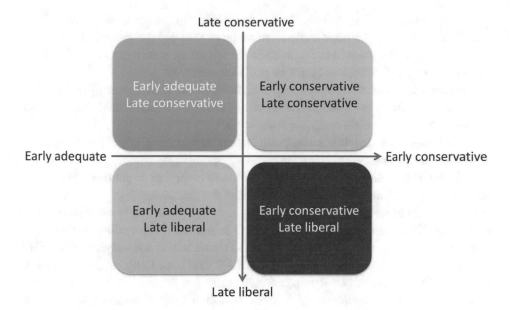

Fig. 1.4 Different phases and types of fluid resuscitation

Coherence: Coherence between microcirculation and macrocirculation in order to obtain adequate regional and tissue oxygen delivery [16]. The hemodynamic coherence depends on the type of the shock state and can be either: hypovolemic, cardiogenic, distributive or obstructive. Four different types of microcirculatory alterations have been described: heterogeneity, hemodilution, hyperpermeability and vasoconstriction [17].

Colloid solution: Solutions constituted of macromolecules (with a molecular weight >30 kDa) that are preferentially retained in the intravascular space following intravenous administration. There are natural colloids (e.g. plasma and albumin) and synthetic colloids (e.g. hydroxyethyl starches, dextrans and gelatins).

Colloid osmotic pressure (COP): The osmotic force exerted by large molecules (colloids) in a solution when separated by a semipermeable membrane from a region with a different colloid concentration. The colloid osmotic pressure provided by plasma proteins is also referred to as oncotic pressure. The normal value for COP is around 20 mmHg and should be at least maintained above 16 mmHg.

Crystalloid: A solution that contains electrolytes and other small water-soluble molecules, and/or dextrose or glucose. Crystalloids are categorized by their tonicity relative to plasma: isotonic, hypotonic and hypertonic.

Cumulative fluid balance: The cumulative fluid balance is the amount of fluid accumulated by calculating the sum of daily fluid balances over a set period of time. Usually, the first week of ICU stay is taken into account for prognostication. A positive cumulative fluid balance is a state where cumulative fluid intakes exceed cumulative fluid outputs.

Daily fluid balance: Daily fluid balance is the difference between all fluids given to a patient during a 24-h period and combined output. As a consequence, daily fluid balance can be negative, neutral or positive. The daily fluid balance does not usually include insensible losses unless the patient is being cared for on an ICU bed that can weigh the patient. Caution should be exercised when using daily weight as a surrogate of fluid balance because muscle and tissue loss cannot be easily measured.

De-escalation: Refers to not initiating extra fluids (withhold) or lowering of the dose or speed of administration (withdraw/reduction) of previously started fluid therapy due to improvement in the clinical condition of the patient.

Dehydration (see also fluid underload): Defined as excessive loss of body water, with or without salt, at a rate greater than the body can replace it. Dehydration has a wide range of aetiologies, including gastrointestinal loss of fluid (vomiting or diarrhoea), heat exposure, prolonged vigorous exercise, kidney disease and medication (e.g. diuretics). A drop in weight might be an indication of dehydration, though regular weight monitoring is often difficult in ICU. The percentage of fluid loss is defined by dividing the cumulative fluid balance in litres by the patient's baseline body weight and multiplying it by 100%. Dehydration is defined by a minimum value of 5% fluid loss. Dehydration is considered mild (5–7.5%), moderate (7.5–10%), or severe (>10%).

De-resuscitation: Correction of fluid accumulation or fluid overload by the active removal of the excess fluids using non-pharmacological (e.g. dialysis with net ultrafiltration) or pharmacological (e.g. diuretics) methods.

Diffusion: See osmosis.

Digestive processes ongoing loss: The digestive system processes food and drink, absorbing nutrients and water from the food and excreting waste products. The amount of fluid lost through digestion can vary depending on the type and amount of food consumed, as well as individual digestive function. See also replacement fluids.

Drug: A medical substance or therapeutic that comes with indications, contraindications and potential adverse effects. It should be given judiciously and its effect should be monitored. The dose must be appropriate as well as the duration. The drug should be stopped when no longer needed.

Early adequate goal-directed fluid management (EAFM): EAFM is the initial hemodynamic resuscitation of patients with septic shock by administering fluids within the first 6 h of the initiation of therapy. Most studies looking at the treatment of septic shock define the early goal as giving 25–50 mL/kg (on average around 30 mL/kg) of fluids within the first 6 h. The recent update of the surviving sepsis campaign guidelines defines EAFM as the administration of 30 mL/kg of IV fluids within the first 1–3 h. However, it has been suggested that fluid resuscitation using such large volumes of fluid in all patients may cause "iatrogenic salt water drowning" and a more conservative strategy for fluid resuscitation might be warranted.

Early goal directed (fluid) therapy (EGDT): A protocol-driven treatment algorithm introduced by Rivers et al. aiming to guide fluids, vasopressors, inotropes, blood products and other resuscitation therapy towards specific hemodynamic end-points, with the goal of maintaining and improving hemodynamic stability, adequate tissue perfusion and optimizing oxygen delivery [18]. See also EAFM.

Ebb phase: This refers to the initial phase of septic shock when the patient shows hyperdynamic circulatory shock with decreased systemic vascular resistance due to vaso-dilation, increased capillary permeability, and severe absolute or relative intravascular hypovolemia. Fluids are mandatory and lifesaving in this phase. The patient in this stage needs EAFM.

Edema: Peripheral and generalized oedema (anasarca) is not only of cosmetic concern, as believed by some, but is harmful to the patient, as it can cause organ oedema and dys-function. Oedema mirrors fluid overload that has potential harmful consequences on dif-ferent end-organ systems, with consequential effects on patient morbidity and mortality. As such, fluid therapy can be considered a double-edged sword.

Effective osmole: An electrolyte (ion) that exerts an osmotic force across a semi-permeable membrane and determines a solution's tonicity. Sodium ion is the predominant effective osmole in the body. See also under tonicity.

E:I ratio: The ratio of extracellular water to intracellular water (ECW/ICW) is nor-mally below 1 (0.7–0.8). An increase in ICW will result in a decrease in the *E:I* ratio and is seen in patients with heart failure, liver cirrhosis or renal failure, especially in early stage. A decrease in ICW will result in a increase in the *E:I* ratio and is generally due to osmotic leakage. Finally, an increase in ECW will also increase the *E:I* ratio and occurs due to shift from intra to extracellular space or capillary leak and resulting second (inter-stitial) and third space fluid accumulation and/or oedema.

Electrolyte: Dissolved anions and cations in solution carrying a positive or negative electric charge, such as sodium, potassium, chloride and calcium amongst others.

End-expiratory occlusion test: This is a test of fluid responsiveness that consists of pausing the flow of mechanical ventilation at end-expiration for 15 s and measuring the resultant changes in cardiac output. The test increases cardiac preload by stopping the cyclic impediment of venous return that occurs at each insufflation of the ventilator. An increase in cardiac output above the threshold of 5% indicates preload/fluid responsive-ness. A continuous monitoring of cardiac output is recommended for an accurate measure-ment of the change. When the test is performed with echocardiography, it is better to add the effects of an end-inspiratory occlusion and if the combined change in velocity-time integral is greater than or equal to 13% in total, fluid responsiveness is accurately pre-dicted. This threshold is more compatible with the precision of echocardiography than that obtained by end-expiratory occlusion alone, because the diagnostic threshold of changes in stroke volume may vary with precision of echocardiography.

Endothelial glycocalyx (EG): The EG is a thin negatively charged proteinaceous mesh-like layer, a gel-like matrix that surrounds all vascular endothelium on the luminal surface. The endothelial glycocalyx (EG) is easy to imagine. It is like sea grass, a virtual structure that lies flat on the ground where the river or sea is shallow (during low tide). Seagrass stands tall when the river or sea is flooded (Fig. 1.5). It is composed of membrane-bound glycoproteins and proteoglycans. The EG was previously thought to be inert but plays a key role in vascular integrity and function; regulation of vascular permeability, endothelial anticoagulation and modulation of interactions between the endothelium and the vascular

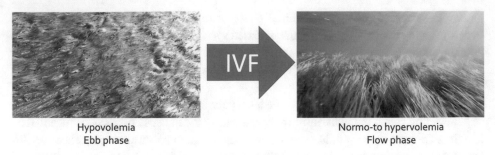

Hypovolemia   Normo-to hypervolemia
Ebb phase   Flow phase

Fig. 1.5 Seagrass analogy to illustrate the endothelial glycocalyx. Administration of intravenous fluids (IVF) will result in the seagrass to change from the flat to the standing position

environment. Thus, the EG prevents free movement of water and electrolytes. Disruption or degradation of the glycocalyx may be an important mediator of inflammation, oedema, sepsis syndromes and capillary leak syndromes. Hence, in various surgical and disease states the glycocalyx has the potential to be a novel therapeutic target.

Euvolemia: Normal circulating blood volume.

Evacuation phase: A phase during fluid therapy in critically ill patients with a focus on organ recovery and resolving fluid overload (in case of no flow state), characterized by active late goal-directed fluid removal (LGFR) by means of either diuretics or renal replacement therapy with net ultrafiltration. The fluid removal may be performed in combination with hypertonic solutions (hypertonic saline 3% or 7.2% or albumin 20%) in order to obtain a negative fluid balance. See also under, late conservative fluid management, late goal-directed fluid removal and de-resuscitation.

Extracellular water (ECW): Extracellular water is the body water that exists outside of the cell membrane (like blood, interstitial fluid, etc.). The extracellular water can be further subdivided into interstitial, lymphatic fluid, trans-cellular water and blood. This accounts for up to 40% of total body water.

Extravascular fluid (EVF): Fluids that exist or accumulate outside the intravascular space. This accounts for up to 75% of ECW.

Flow phase: This refers to the phase of septic shock after initial stabilization where the patient will mobilize the excess fluid spontaneously, a classic example is when a patient enters a polyuric phase recovering from acute kidney injury (AKI). In contrast to the "ebb" phase, the "flow" phase refers to the time period after the acute circulatory shock has been resolved. In this post-shock phase, the metabolic turnover is increased, the innate immune system is activated, and a hepatic acute-phase response is induced. This hypercatabolic metabolic state is characterized by an increase in oxygen consumption and energy expenditure.

Fluid accumulation: An increase in net fluid balance resulting in the accumulation of excess fluids in body tissues and weight gain and in some cases, peripheral oedema. This results from pathophysiological processes of renal fluid and salt reabsorption. The term fluid accumulation is preferred over fluid overload and describes a pathologic state of overhydration associated with a clinical impact which may vary by age, comorbidity and

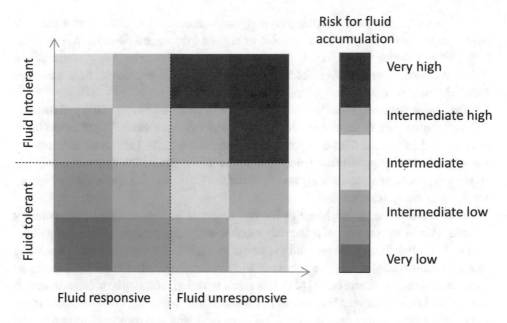

Fig. 1.6 Relationship between fluid responsiveness and fluid tolerance and the risk of fluid accumulation. (Adapted with permission from Monnet et al. [19])

phase of illness. It may occur with concomitant intravascular hypovolemia, euvolemia and hypervolemia and may or may not be associated with clinical or imaging signs of oedema. It describes a continuum. No specific threshold of fluid balance alone can define fluid accumulation across all individuals. Fluid overload, volume overload and fluid accumulation generally refer to the expansion of the extracellular fluid volume and usually indicate water and sodium retention. The risk for fluid accumulation is dependent on the presence of fluid unresponsiveness in combination with fluid intolerance (Fig. 1.6).

Fluid accumulation syndrome: The term to describe the presence of any degree of fluid accumulation or fluid overload with a negative impact on end-organ function which may or may not be associated with global increased permeability syndrome.

Fluid administration: The administration of fluids (or infusion) to a (critically ill) patient either via the oral, enteral or parenteral route. The rate or speed of fluid administration is usually described in mL/kg/min (for fluid bolus or fluid challenge) or mL/kg/h (for maintenance or nutrition solutions). Fluid rates described in mL/h or mL/min are meaningless unless they are referenced to body weight. The dose, duration and de-escalation of fluid administration should be stated and prescribed.

Fluid balance: See under daily and cumulative fluid balance.

Fluid bolus: A fluid bolus is the rapid infusion of fluids over a short period of time. In clinical practice, a fluid bolus is usually given to correct hypovolemia, hypotension, inadequate blood flow or impaired microcirculatory perfusion. A fluid bolus typically includes the infusion of 4–6 mL/kg of IV fluid over a maximum of 10–20 min.

Fluid challenge: A fluid challenge is a dynamic functional test to assess a patient's fluid responsiveness by giving a fluid bolus of at least 4 mL/kg over 5–10 min and simultaneously monitoring the evolution of the hemodynamic status to be able to identify fluid responsive state. Recently, it has been shown that in clinical practice there is a marked variability in how fluid challenge tests are performed [20].

Fluid compartments: Describes the distribution of total body water (TBW) within several well-defined spaces separated from each other by cell membranes. Together, the intravascular and interstitial fluid compartments comprise the ECW (see under extracellular water), and contain approximately one-third of the TBW, while ICW (see under intracellular water) contains approximately two-thirds of the TBW. See also under the four spaces and the four compartments.

Fluid creep: A term that refers to the unintentional and unmeasured fluid volumes administered in the process of delivering medication (antibiotics, sedatives, painkillers, etc.) and nutrition through enteral and parenteral routes. Fluid creep can also be described as the administration of fluids in excess of the requirements calculated by the Parkland Formula [not only in severe burns] [21]. It is also a term that refers to the unintentional and unmeasured fluid volumes administered in the process of delivering medication (antibiotics, sedatives, painkillers, etc.) and nutrition through enteral and parenteral routes. It may sum up to 33% of all fluids administered, compared to maintenance (25%), nutrition (33%) and resuscitation (6%) type of fluids [22].

Fluid infusion: See fluid administration.

Fluid loss and gain: Fluid loss is defined as a negative fluid balance, regardless of intravascular status. Fluid gain is the opposite of fluid loss (Table 1.2).

Fluid overload (see overhydration): An increase in total body fluid (both water and electrolytes) in excess of physiologic requirements. Traditionally it is defined as excess fluid buildup in the body and has a negative impact on end-organ function. Some publications identify a threshold of 10% or more cumulative fluid balance for increased risk of

Table 1.2 Effect of fluid loss and gain on interstitial, plasma and intracellular volume and plasma tonicity

Conditions	Interstitial fluid volume	Plasma volume (volemia)	Intracellular volume	Plasma tonicity
Isotonic fluid loss	↓ (dehydration)	↓ (hypovolemia)	= (normal)	= (plasma isotonicity)
Hypotonic fluid loss	↓ (dehydration)	=/ ↓ (normo- or hypovolemia)	↓ (dehydration)	↑ (plasma hypertonicity)
Isotonic fluid gain	↑ (hyperhydration)	↑ (hypervolemia)	= (normal)	= (plasma isotonicity)
Hypotonic fluid gain	↑ (hyperhydration)	=/↑ (normo- or hypervolemia)	↑ (hyperhydration)	↓ (plasma hypotonicity)
Hypertonic fluid gain	↑ (hyperhydration)	↑ (hypervolemia)	↓ (dehydration)	↑ (plasma hypertonicity)

↑ Increased, = No change, ↓ Decreased

adverse effects. There is an ambiguity in this term, as it is interchangeably used in situations of volume overload, which refers to excess fluid in the intravascular fluid compartment, and overhydration, which describes increased total body water but does not necessarily reflect intravascular volume overload. While volume overload usually leads to hypervolemia and hyperhydration resulting in peripheral oedema, the opposite is not always true as oedema can be present in the absence of volume overload. Therefore, some colleagues suggest avoiding the misleading term fluid overload (all or nothing) and using fluid accumulation (graded phenomenon) instead [3].

Fluid refill rate: In stable patients undergoing intermittent haemodialysis, the fluid refill rate is 2–6 mL/kg/h but may exceed 10 mL/kg/h at high rates of ultrafiltration [23]. Since transcapillary refill rate depends on oncotic pressure, vascular integrity and blood pressure, it is reduced during critical illness [24]. A recent study showed that in critically ill adults receiving continuous venovenous hemodiafiltration for acute kidney injury, the rate of net ultrafiltration (UF) at which mortality is increased seemed to be from 1.75 mL/kg/h and certainly from 2.8 mL/kg/h upwards [25].

Fluid responsiveness: Fluid responsiveness indicates a condition in which a patient will respond to fluid administration by a significant increase in stroke volume and/or cardiac output or their surrogates. A threshold of 15% is commonly used for this definition. Physiologically, fluid responsiveness means that a linear relationship exists between cardiac output and cardiac preload, i.e. the steep portion of the slope on the Frank–Starling relationship. However, this may not be true at all times (in euvolemia or hypervolemia) and in all patients (pre-existing cardiac dysfunction). Many studies have shown that fluid responsiveness, which is a normal physiologic condition, exists in only half of the patients receiving a fluid challenge in intensive care units. Different techniques for assessing fluid responsiveness and the thresholds used are shown in Fig. 1.7.

Fluid resuscitation: See under resuscitation solutions and resuscitation phase.

Fluid or water retention: Non-specific term used for describing the accumulation of excess fluid in body tissues resulting in clinical oedema. See under fluid accumulation.

Fluid space: See under four spaces.

Fluid stewardship: Fluid stewardship is a series of coordinated interventions, introduced to select the optimal fluid, dose and duration of therapy that results in the best clinical outcome, prevention of adverse events and cost reduction with a focus on value-based healthcare.

Fluid therapy: The process of administering fluids as a medical treatment or preventative measure to maintain or restore normal body fluid balance. There are four indications for fluid therapy: resuscitation, maintenance, replacement, and nutrition.

Fluid titration: Adjustment of IV fluid based on choice, type, rate, speed, dose, volume and timing in order to improve hemodynamic stability and optimize tissue perfusion (microcirculation), oxygen delivery and uptake.

Fluid tolerance: Can be defined as the degree to which a patient can tolerate the administration of fluids without causation of organ dysfunction [26]. Fluid tolerance comes to fill in the continuum between fluid responsiveness and fluid overload or accumulation and

Fig. 1.7 Illustration of the concept of preload dependence. (**a**) Fluid responsiveness illustrated by a greater increase in mean systemic filling pressure with 7 mmHg (from 22 to 29 mmHg) compared to the 2 mmHg increase in CVP (from 6 to 8 mmHg) resulting in a 15% increase in cardiac output from 5.4 to 6.2 L/min. (**b**) Fluid unresponsiveness illustrated by an equal increase in mean systemic filling pressure with 4 mmHg (from 24 to 28 mmHg) and a 3 mmHg increase in CVP (from 8 to 11 mmHg) not resulting in a significant increase in cardiac output (from 5.9 to 6.0 L/min)

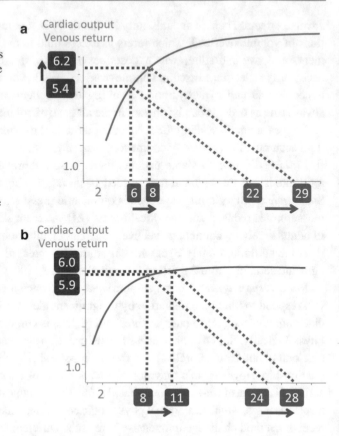

overcome their inherent limitations (Table 1.3). It balances the impact of fluids during the resuscitation phase from downstream (i.e. organ perfusion) to upstream (i.e. venous congestion). This may allow clinicians to potentially modify their strategy and provide a more harmonic resuscitation.

Fluid underload: Decrease in total body fluid, resulting in a fluid deficit of the extracellular and/or intracellular fluid. Similar to dehydration and the opposite of fluid overload.

Global increased permeability syndrome (GIPS): The term used to describe the ongoing fluid accumulation due to increased vascular permeability; often referred to as "the third hit of shock". Some patients will not transgress to the "flow" phase spontaneously and will remain in a persistent state of global increased permeability syndrome (GIPS) and ongoing fluid accumulation. It typically has a positive cumulative fluid balance with ongoing capillary leak and organ failure.

Goal-directed therapy (GDT): See under early goal-directed (fluid) therapy (EGDT).

Hyperchloremic metabolic acidosis: Metabolic acidosis caused by hyperchloremia, accompanied by a decrease in bicarbonate levels. Bicarbonate loss or dilution is a possible explanation (Henderson–Hasselbalch approach) for metabolic acidosis. However, according to Stewart's approach, a decrease in SID caused by an increase in chloride (e.g. after

Table 1.3 Key characteristics of fluid responsiveness, fluid tolerance and fluid overload concepts (adapted from [26]). *CO* cardiac output, *IAP* intraabdominal pressure, *PEEP* positive end-expiratory pressure, *PPV* pulse pressure variation, *SVV* stroke volume variation.

Characteristic	Fluid responsiveness	Fluid tolerance	Fluid overload/ accumulation
Definition	Increase in cardiac output after preload incrementation by manipulation of venous return in a dynamic test context; increase in CO $\geq$15% after fluid challenge; increase in CO $\geq$10% after passive leg raising test or increase in CO $\geq$5% after end-expiratory occlusion test	Fluid tolerance is the degree to which a patient can tolerate the administration of fluids without causing organ dysfunction or failure	A state of global body accumulation of fluids after resuscitation with a deleterious impact on end-organ function
When to use	During resuscitation phase	During resuscitation phase	After resuscitation and during de-resuscitation phase
Adequate use	Increase CO through a fluid challenge in fluid responsive patients to resolve hypoperfusion	Modify resuscitation strategy (vasopressors, other types of fluids, etc.)	Prompt de-resuscitation when present
Inadequate use	Consider fluid responsiveness as a mandatory trigger for fluid administration, irrespective of tissue perfusion status. Presence of fluid responsiveness does not mean that fluids need to be given at all times	Assume that fluid intolerance only occurs in fluid unresponsive patients	Inadequate timing or intensity of de-resuscitation (too late, too little, too long)
Limitations	Not assessable in all patients and technical challenges; take into account heart–lung interactions; functional hemodynamics (PPV and SVV) trustworthy if and tidal volume >8 mL/kg, IAP normal, no right heart failure, no excessive PEEP/auto PEEP, no arrythmias	Theoretical construct, not clinically validated yet	Retrospective diagnosis; still lack of evidence on how to best de-resuscitate

infusion of large amounts of (ab)normal saline 0.9% NaCl) is responsible for metabolic acidosis. Synonym: normal anion gap acidosis.

Hyperdynamic state: Hemodynamic status characterized by supraphysiologic blood flow and cardiac output to the tissues (e.g. thyrotoxicosis, liver cirrhosis, severe burns, severe pancreatitis, morbus Paget, thiamine deficiency (Beri-Beri), multiple myeloma and plasmocytoma, chronic anaemia or polycythemia, AV fistula. Synonym: hyperperfusion.

Hyperhydration (see overhydration).

Hyperoncotic solution: A colloid solution with an oncotic pressure above that of plasma (e.g. 10% hydroxyethyl starch, 20% human albumin).

Hypertonicity: Plasma hypertonicity is accompanied by cell shrinkage (dehydration). The water balance is regulated via antidiuretic hormone (ADH), thirst and the renin–angiotensin–aldosterone system (RAAS).

Hypertonic solution: An IV crystalloid solution with a higher effective osmolality than plasma (e.g. 3% sodium chloride has an osmolality of 1027 mOsm/L). Hypertonic saline is a sterile hypertonic intravenous crystalloid composed of water, sodium and chloride. Available in multiple concentrations including 3%, 5% and 7.2%.

Hypertonic–hyperoncotic solution: A solution containing a hypertonic crystalloid (>310 mOsm/L) in combination with a hyperoncotic (>5%) colloid that is used as an alternative strategy during small-volume fluid resuscitation (e.g. 7.5% saline and 6% Dextran-70, however this solution is no longer available).

Hypervolemia: Hypervolemia is the opposite of hypovolemia and is defined by intravascular overfilling. This can be monitored in different ways: the absence of fluid responsiveness, increased barometric or volumetric preload indicators, and ultrasound findings.

Hypo-oncotic solution: A colloid solution with an oncotic pressure below that of plasma (e.g. 4% human albumin).

Hypoperfusion: Inadequate blood flow to the tissues, resulting in decreased oxygen delivery. End-organ hypoperfusion can clinically manifest as cool extremities, reduced pulse quality (pulsus filiformis), increased capillary refill time, tachycardia and oliguria [27].

Hypotonicity: Plasma hypotonicity is accompanied by cellular oedema (hyperhydration). The water balance is regulated via antidiuretic hormone (ADH) and thirst and the renin–angiotensin–aldosterone system (RAAS).

Hypotonic solution: An IV solution with a lower effective osmolality than plasma (e.g. 0.45% sodium chloride: 154 mOsm/L). It has to be noted that glucose-containing solutions like 5% dextrose in water is also classified as hypotonic solution despite having a normal osmolality (278 mOsm/L) since the dextrose is rapidly taken up into cells and metabolized following infusion, leaving water behind.

Hypovolemia: Hypovolemia is the term used to describe a patient with insufficient total intravascular circulating blood volume. It does not refer to total body fluid but rather refers solely to the intravascular compartment. Absolute hypovolemia can be caused by dehydration (i.e. water and electrolyte loss) or the loss of blood from the body or into a body cavity (e.g. abdomen) [6]. Total body fluid comprises approximately 60% of the body weight of men and 50% of women. Blood volume can be estimated according to Gilcher's rule of fives at 70 mL/kg for men and 65 mL/kg for women. Blood loss is frequently followed by the recruitment of interstitial fluid and the movement of fluid from the interstitium to the intravascular compartment. Vasoconstriction of the splanchnic mesenteric vasculature is one of the first physiologic responses. Sodium and water retention results from the activation of the RAAS which replenishes the interstitial reserves and maintains trans-capillary perfusion. As a result, the body may lose up to 30% of blood volume before hypovolemia becomes clinically apparent. Therefore, undiagnosed hypovolemia may be present long before clinical signs and symptoms occur. Hypovolemia can also occur in oedematous patients, where total body water is increased, but intravascular volume is reduced (e.g. eclamptic patients). Finally, some patients are fluid responsive but not necessarily hypovolemic. Even the most basic of paradigms, such as the description of early sepsis and distributive shock being a hypovolemic state needing aggressive fluid resuscitation, has recently been called into question, with data suggesting improved outcomes with less or even no administered intravenous fluid. Greater focus on the health and function of the microcirculation and the endothelial glycocalyx, potential new treatment paradigms calling for less fluids and earlier vasopressor use has become the focus. These elements make an accurate assessment of fluid status in the critically ill a challenging task.

Ineffective osmoles: Small dissolved particles in solution that contribute to total osmolality but do not exert an osmotic pressure because they freely cross and equilibrate across cell membranes (e.g. urea, dextrose).

Insensible water loss: Body fluid losses that cannot be easily measured, such as evaporative losses from the skin and respiratory tract, and the water content of the stool. The daily amount of insensible losses can be calculated with Dubois' formula: 550 mL/body surface area, where body surface area $= 71.84 \times$ (body weight in kg)$^{0.425} \times$ (height in cm)$^{0.725}$. In the case of mechanical ventilation or active humidification, this value can be divided by 2. Temperature corrections can also be made (for each 1 °C increase of temperature above 37 °C, a 13% increase in insensible losses).

Interstitial dehydration: A negative sodium balance leads to a decrease in extracellular volume.

Interstitial fluid: The total volume of extracellular water contained within the interstitial tissues surrounding cells (12–15% of total body weight), or thus the fluid in which cells are bathed.

Interstitial hyperhydration: A positive sodium balance leads to an increase in extracellular volume (interstitial fluid overload).

Intra-abdominal hypertension (IAH): IAH is defined by a sustained or repeated pathologic elevation of IAP $\geq$12 mmHg. IAH is graded as follows: Grade I: IAP 12–15 mmHg, Grade II: IAP 16–20 mmHg, Grade III: IAP 21–25 mmHg and Grade IV: IAP >25 mmHg [11]. IAH has a tremendous impact on organ function within and outside the abdominal cavity (Fig. 1.8) [28].

Intra-abdominal pressure (IAP): Intra-abdominal pressure (IAP) is the pressure concealed within the abdominal cavity. IAP should be expressed in mmHg and measured at end-expiration in the complete supine position after ensuring that abdominal muscle contractions are absent and with the transducer zeroed at the level of the mid-axillary line. The reference standard for intermittent IAP measurement is via the bladder with a maximal instillation volume of 20–25 mL of sterile saline. Normal IAP is approximately 5–7 mmHg and around 10 mmHg in critically ill adults [11].

Intracellular volume (ICV): See intracellular water.

Intracellular water (ICW): Intracellular water is the body water that exists inside the cell membrane, or thus the fluid of all body cells, and comprises 60% of total body water or 40% of total body weight. Water balance is regulated via ADH, thirst and the RAAS.

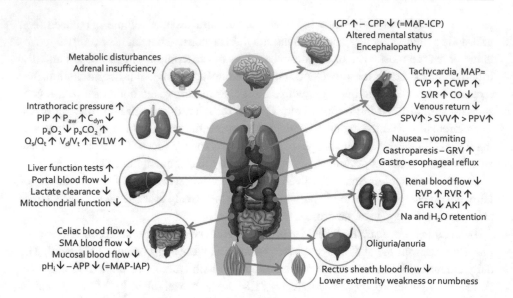

Fig. 1.8 Summary of the most important pathophysiologic effects of increased intra-abdominal pressure on end-organ function within and outside the abdominal cavity. *AKI* acute kidney injury, *APP* abdominal perfusion pressure, *Cdyn* dynamic respiratory compliance, *CO* cardiac output, *CPP* cerebral perfusion pressure, *CVP* central venous pressure, *EVLW* extravascular lung water, *GFR* glomerular filtration rate, *GRV* gastric residual volume, *HR* heart rate, *IAP* intra-abdominal pressure, *ICP* intra-cranial pressure, *ITP* intra-thoracic pressure, *MAP* mean arterial pressure, *PIP* peak inspiratory pressure, *Paw* airway pressures, *PCWP* pulmonary capillary wedge pressure, *pHi* intramucosal gastric pH, *PPV* pulse pressure variation, *Qs/Qt* shunt fraction, *RVP* renal venous pressure, *RVR* renal vascular resistance, *SMA* superior mesenteric artery, *SPV* systolic pressure variation, *SVR* systemic vascular resistance, *SVV* stroke volume variation, *Vd/Vt* dead-space ventilation

Intravascular fluid (IVF): Fluids that exist inside the intravascular space (arteries, veins and capillaries) and account for up to 6–8% of total body weight.

Isooncotic solution: A colloid solution with an oncotic pressure similar to that of plasma (e.g. 6% hydroxyethyl starch, 5% human albumin).

Isotonic solution: An IV solution with an effective osmolality close to that of normal plasma (278 mOsm/L). The osmolality of intravenous solutions containing sodium (the main driver for osmolality) is approximately 0.93 × the osmolarity, due to the fact that sodium chloride is not 100% disassociated in solution and plasma (but rather 93%). Therefore, the osmolality of both plasma and 0.9% saline is approximately 287 mOsm/kg (308 mOsm/L × 0.93) [29].

Late conservative fluid management (LCFM): LCFM describes a moderate fluid management strategy following the initial EAFM in order to avoid (or reverse) fluid overload. Recent studies showed that LCFM, defined as two consecutive days of negative fluid balance within the first week of the ICU stay is a strong and independent predictor of survival [30]. LCFM must be adapted according to the variable clinical course of septic shock during the first days of ICU treatment, e.g. patients with persistent systemic inflammation maintain trans-capillary albumin leakage and do not reach the flow phase mounting up positive fluid balances.

Late goal-directed fluid removal (LGFR): LGFR describes that in some patients more aggressive and active fluid removal by means of diuretics or renal replacement therapy with net ultrafiltration being needed either or not in combination with hypertonic solutions to mobilize the excess interstitial oedema. This is referred to as de-resuscitation, a term that was coined for the first time in 2014 [1].

Liberal vs. *restrictive fluid therapy*: Term applied to studies looking at the effect on morbidity and mortality of a conservative (restrictive) fluid strategy, compared to a standard (liberal) fluid regimen [31, 32]. Most standard and liberal fluid regimens are more likely to result in a positive fluid balance [33, 34]. The fluid strategy is probably more important than the fluid itself (Fig. 1.9).

Macrocirculation: Large and medium-sized arteries and veins that serve as conduit vessels, transporting blood and oxygen to and from organs.

Maintenance solutions: These IV fluids are given to cover the daily needs for water (1 mL/kg/h), glucose (1–1.5 g/kg/day) and electrolytes, mainly potassium (0.75–1.25 mmol/kg/day), sodium (1–1.5 mmol/kg/day), phosphate (0.1–0.5 mmol/kg/day), chloride (1 mmol/kg/day), calcium (0.1–0.2 mmol/kg/day) and magnesium (0.1–0.2 mmol/kg/day).

Mean systemic or circulatory filling pressure (Pmsf): Pmsf is the blood pressure throughout the vascular system at zero flow and offers information on vascular

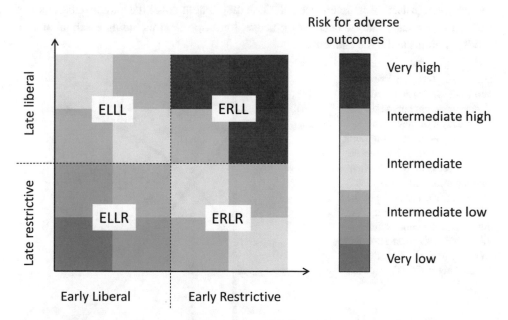

Fig. 1.9 The fluid strategy, protocol or guidelines are more important than the type of fluid itself in relation to morbidity and mortality. In view of some recent results and insights, early liberal should probably be replaced by early adequate fluid management. *EL* early liberal, *ER* early restrictive, *LL* late liberal, *LR* late restrictive

compliance, volume responsiveness and it allows the calculation of (un)stressed volume. For the determination of mean circulatory filling pressure, two bedside methods are available, either based on inspiratory hold-derived venous return curves (Pmsf hold) or on arterial and venous pressure equilibration (Pmsf arm) [35]. Pmsf hold is based on the linear relation between CVP and venous return (VR): $VR = (Pmsf-CVP)/RVR$, where RVR is the resistance to VR. Hereby, the CVP is increased by performing a series of end-inspiratory hold manoeuvres and CO is measured in the last 3 s of the 12 s inspiratory hold. After 7–10 s, a steady state occurs when VR = CO. By plotting the CVP and CO values, a VR curve is constructed and the zero-flow pressure (Pmsf) is extrapolated (Fig. 1.10). As Pmsf is defined as the steady-state blood pressure during no-flow conditions, the arm is used to estimate the Pmsf arm. The upper arm is occluded to 50 mmHg above systolic blood pressure, using a rapid cuff inflator or a pneumatic tourniquet. Measurements of arterial and venous pressures through a radial artery catheter and a peripheral venous cannula in the forearm are performed. When these two pressures equalize, Pmsf arm values are obtained.

Microcirculation: Blood vessels <200–300 μm in diameter, consisting of small arteries, arterioles, capillaries and venules where oxygen diffuses to the tissues.

Mini fluid challenge: A mini fluid challenge is a dynamic functional test to assess a patient's fluid responsiveness by giving a fluid bolus of 1 mL/kg over 1–5 min to predict the fluid responsiveness (10% increase in VTI) of a full fluid challenge.

Nutrition solutions: These solutions come in different types and can be given either orally (total enteral nutrition, TEN) or intravenously (total parenteral nutrition, TPN). When given instead of maintenance solutions they should cover the daily needs for water as well as the daily caloric needs for glucose, lipids, protein, including essential amino-acids, vitamins and trace elements.

Fig. 1.10 Integrated venous return curve (**a**) and cardiac function/output curve (**b**). The intersection of these two curves (**c**) is the working point of the circulation. The central venous pressure (CVP) when venous return equals zero is the Pmsf (**d**). The slope of the VR is determined by the resistance to venous return. (Adapted with permission from Wijnberge et al. under the Open Access CC BY License 4.0 [35])

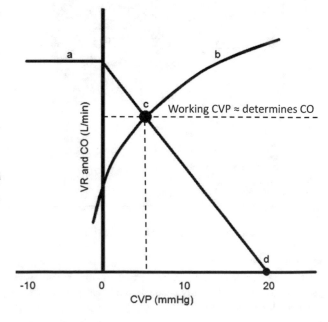

Oncoticity: Refers to the oncotic pressure, also called the colloid osmotic pressure (COP), which is a form of osmotic pressure (see tonicity) exerted by the amount of proteins in the intravascular space. Oncotic pressure shifts fluids from the extravascular space, or interstitial tissues, into the intravascular space. Hence, depleted COP increases the risk of interstitial and generalized oedema. A higher COP of a fluid prolongs the intravascular half-life and consequently results in prolonged effects on blood pressure and perfusion. When given 1 L of fluids, the intravascular volume will be increased after 1 h with 83 mL for dextrose 5% in water, 250 mL for saline or balanced crystalloids and 1000 mL for a colloid solution.

Ongoing fluid losses: See replacement fluids.

Optimization phase: The optimization phase focuses on organ rescue (maintenance) and avoiding fluid overload (fluid creep). Aiming for neutral fluid balance.

Osmolality: A measure of the concentration of osmotically active particles per unit volume of solution, measured in milliosmoles per litre of solution (mOsm/L). In clinical practice, osmolarity and osmolality are similar enough to be used interchangeably. It determines the tolerability of a solution. Serum osmolality can be calculated by the simplified formula: $2 \times$ serum sodium (mmol/l) + BUN (blood urea nitrogen)/2.8 (mg/dL) + glucose/18 (mg/dL) or $2 \times$ Na + BUN + glucose (all in mmol/L) [36].

Osmolal gap (serum): measured serum osmolality—calculated serum osmolality.

Osmolarity: A measure of the concentration of osmotically active particles per unit mass of solution, measured in milliosmoles per kilogram of solution (mOsm/kg). Figure 1.11 shows the regulation of vasopressin secretion by plasma osmolarity.

Osmosis: Osmosis or diffusion is the movement of water across a semi-permeable membrane from a less concentrated solution into a more concentrated solution.

Overhydration (see also fluid overload and fluid accumulation): A state of having a positive fluid balance or description of a state where there is excess water in the body. Dividing the cumulative fluid balance in litres by the patient's baseline body weight and multiplying by 100 defines the percentage of fluid accumulation. Overhydration at any stage is the opposite of dehydration and can be classified as mild (5%), moderate (5–10%) or severe (>10%) fluid accumulation. Overhydration is also associated with worse outcomes. Fluid administration potentially induces a vicious cycle, where interstitial oedema induces organ dysfunction that contributes to fluid accumulation.

Oxygen consumption (VO_2): The amount of oxygen consumed by the cells. Can be calculated as the difference between oxygen delivery (DO_2) measured at the arterial side versus the mixed venous side. Simplified formula: $VO_2 = (SaO_2 - SvO_2) \times CO \times Hgb$; with SaO_2: arterial oxygen satuation, SvO_2: mixed venous oxygen saturation, Hgb: Haemoglobin.

Oxygen delivery (DO_2): The amount of oxygen delivered to the cells can be calculated as follows: cardiac output × total arterial oxygen content. With cardiac output equal to heart rate multiplied by stroke volume. And total oxygen content is defined by the oxygen bound to haemoglobin (Hgb × Sat × 1.36) plus the oxygen freely dissolved in the plasma ($pO_2 \times 0.0036$). Simplified formula: $DO_2 = SaO_2 \times CO \times Hgb$. The DO_2 vs VO_2 relationship is illustrated in Fig. 1.12.

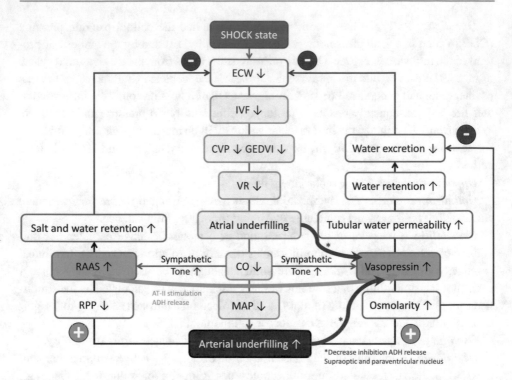

Fig. 1.11 Control of vasopressin (ADH) secretion by plasma osmolarity and circulating blood volume in a shock state. Hypovolemia results in increased plasma osmolarity and decreased arterial pressure that both will increase vasopressin release. Negative and positive feedback loops are indicated with (−) and (+), respectively. *ADH* antidiuretic hormone, *AT-II* angiotensin II, *CO* cardiac output, *CVP* central venous pressure, *ECW* extracellular water, *GEDVI* global end-diastolic volume index, *IVF* intravascular fluid, *MAP* mean arterial pressure, *RAAS* renin–angiotensin–aldosterone system, *RPP* renal perfusion pressure, *VR* venous return

Fig. 1.12 Simplified oxygen delivery and oxygen consumption (DO$_2$-VO$_2$) relationship in normal conditions (black line) and sepsis (red line). The initial part shows supply dependency from the critical DO$_2$ (red dot) value onwards. At this point ScvO$_2$ (mixed venous oxygen saturation) will drop and lactate will increase illustrating DO$_2$-VO$_2$ imbalance and anaerobic metabolism

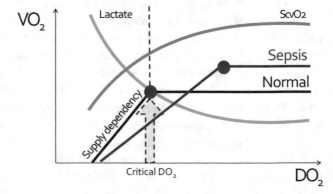

Parenteral: Administration of food or medication through a non-enteral (e.g. non-oral) route, such as intravenous, subcutaneous, intramuscular and intradermal.

Parkland formula: A fluid resuscitation protocol for burn patients which suggests administration of a balanced crystalloid solution (e.g. Ringer's lactate) dosed at 4 mL/kg/% of the total body surface area burned (TBSA) [37, 38]. Half of the volume is then delivered over the first 8 h and the remainder over the next 16 h.

Passive leg raising test: The passive leg raising test is aimed at evidencing fluid responsiveness. It consists of moving a patient from the semi-recumbent position to a position where the legs are lifted at 45° and the trunk is horizontal. The transfer of venous blood from the inferior limbs and the splanchnic compartment towards the cardiac cavities mimics the increase in cardiac preload induced by fluid [39]. In general, the threshold to define fluid responsiveness with the passive leg raising test is a threshold of 10% increase in stroke volume and/or cardiac output.

Perfusion: The passage of fluid through the circulatory system to organs and tissues.

Permissive hypotension: Permissive hypotension involves keeping the blood pressure low enough (systolic pressures <90 mmHg) to avoid exacerbating uncontrolled haemorrhage while maintaining perfusion to vital end-organs. The potential detrimental mechanisms of early, aggressive crystalloid resuscitation are well known and the limitation of fluid intake by using colloids, hypertonic saline or hyperoncotic albumin solutions has been associated with favourable effects [40]. Hypertonic saline allows not only for rapid restoration of circulating intravascular volume with less administered fluid but also attenuates post-injury oedema at the microcirculatory level and may improve microvascular perfusion.

Pharmacodynamics: Pharmacodynamics relates the drug concentrations to its specific effect. For fluids, the Frank–Starling relationship between cardiac output and cardiac preload is the equivalent of the dose–effect curve for standard medications. Because of the shape of the Frank–Starling relationship, the response of cardiac output to the fluid-induced increase in cardiac preload is not constant (Fig. 1.13).

Pharmacokinetics: Describes how the body affects a drug resulting in a particular plasma and effect site concentration. Pharmacokinetics of intravenous fluids depend on distribution volume, osmolality, tonicity, oncoticity and kidney function. Eventually, the half-time depends on the type of fluid and also on the patient's condition and the clinical context.

Plasma: The portion of blood that remains after the cells are removed. Plasma is retrieved by centrifugation of an anticoagulated blood sample, and unlike serum, it contains fibrinogen and clotting factors.

Prediction of fluid responsiveness: A process that consists of predicting before fluid administration whether or not fluid administration will increase cardiac output. It avoids unnecessary fluid administration and contributes to reduce the cumulative fluid balance. It also allows one to undertake fluid removal being sure that it will not result in a hemodynamic impairment. Prediction of fluid responsiveness cannot be achieved with static markers of cardiac preload, such as the central venous pressure, the pulmonary artery occlusion

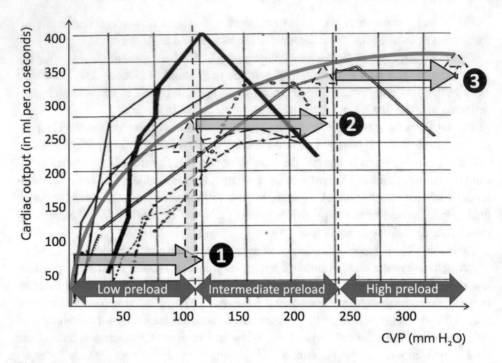

Fig. 1.13 Frank–Starling curve adapted from the original paper by Patterson and Starling where central venous pressure (CVP) was on the Y-axis and cardiac output on the X-axis [41]. The dark lines represent the individual curves obtained per dog in the experiment. The blue line is the mean interpolation. The light blue arrows indicate fluid loading: (1) great increase in stroke volume (SV) in a state of low preload; (2) moderate increase in SV in case of intermediate preload and (3) absent increase in SV after fluid bolus in case of high preload. This reflects the dose–response or dose–effect curve or thus the pharmacodynamics for fluids. The dotted red lines indicate the separation between low–intermediate–high preload

pressure and its echocardiographic estimates or the left ventricular end-diastolic dimensions. It is based on a dynamic assessment of the cardiac output/preload relationship. The classic fluid challenge predicts fluid responsiveness but is inherently associated with fluid boluses that do not increase cardiac output. The respiratory variations of stroke volume and its surrogates (arterial pulse pressure, aortic blood flow, maximal velocity in the left ventricular outflow tract, amplitude of the plethysmographic signal) in patients under mechanical ventilation are reliable predictors of fluid responsiveness but are not reliable in some conditions, the most common being spontaneous breathing, cardiac arrhythmias, ventilation at low tidal volume and low lung compliance. The respiratory variation in the diameter of the inferior and superior venae cavae shares the same limitations, except cardiac arrhythmias. The passive leg raising (see below) and the end-expiratory occlusion test are reliable in these circumstances. The threshold to define fluid responsiveness depends on the change in cardiac preload induced by the test (e.g. 15% for the fluid challenge, 10% for the PLR test and 5% for the end-expiratory occlusion test) (Fig. 1.14).

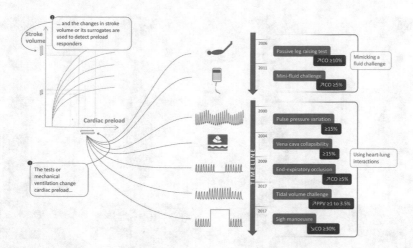

Fig. 1.14 Tests and indices of preload responsiveness with proposed timeline. The principle of the dynamic assessment of preload responsiveness is to observe spontaneous or induced changes in cardiac preload, and the resulting change in cardiac output, stroke volume or their surrogates. Some tests or indices use heart–lung interactions in mechanically ventilated patients, while some others mimic a classical fluid challenge. Diagnostic threshold and year of description are indicated. *CO* cardiac output, *PPV* pulse pressure variation. (Adapted with permission from Monnet et al. [19])

Plasma volume: See volemia.

Preload: From a theoretical point of view preload is the initial stretch on a single myocyte prior to contraction. From a practical point, preload is the LVEDV and corresponding LVEDP that stretches the left ventricle to its greatest dimensions under variable physiologic demand. Ideally, preload is a (combination of) parameter(s) that tell(s) the clinician if fluids are needed and can be given safely. In real life, preload is also affected by the afterload and contractility as illustrated schematically in Fig. 1.15.

Pulmonary West zones: West zones describe areas of the lung based upon variations in pulmonary arterial pressure (p_a), pulmonary venous pressure (p_v) and alveolar pressure (p_A). These differences result from a 20 mmHg increase in blood flow found in the base of the lung relative to the apex as a result of gravity in an upright patient. The lung can be divided into discrete regions according to the interplay between p_A, p_a and p_v. These regions are zone 1, where alveolar pressure is higher than arterial or venous pressure; zone 2, where the alveolar pressure is lower than the arterial but higher than the venous pressure and zone 3, where both arterial pressure and venous pressure are higher than alveolar. This is illustrated in Fig. 1.16.

Pulse pressure (PP): The difference between arterial systolic and diastolic blood pressure measured in millimetres of mercury (mmHg) as illustrated in Fig. 1.17.

Pulse pressure variation (PPV): The mean difference between the maximum (PP_{max}) and minimum (PP_{min}) arterial pulse pressures during a series of respiratory cycles, expressed as a percentage [42]. PPV is a functional hemodynamic parameter that predicts fluid responsiveness in mechanically ventilated patients.

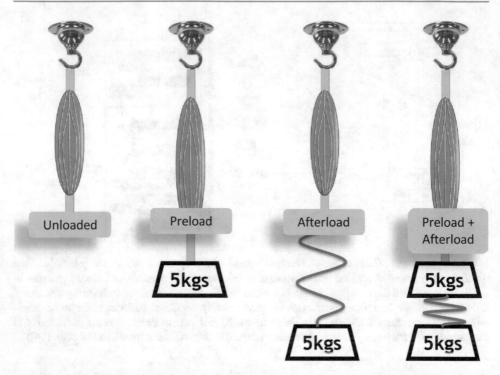

Fig. 1.15 Schematic representation of preload (initial stretch at the end of diastole on a single actin–myosin complex in the cardiac myocyte prior to contraction) and afterload

Redistribution: When a fluid is infused into the body via an intravenous (IV) route, it is introduced directly into the bloodstream. As a result, there can be an initial change in the volume and distribution of body fluids as the body responds to the extra influx of fluids. Intravenous infusion can cause a temporary increase in the volume of fluid in the circulatory system, which can result in an increase in blood pressure and/or stroke volume. This can trigger a response from the kidneys, which attempt to compensate by excreting more fluid and electrolytes. The net result of this process is a redistribution of fluid from the circulatory system to other body compartments, such as the interstitial spaces (the spaces between cells) and the intracellular spaces (the fluid within cells). The speed and extent of fluid redistribution can be influenced by a variety of factors, including the rate of infusion, the characteristics of the fluid being infused, and the overall health status and comorbidities of the patient receiving the infusion. In some cases, fluid redistribution can lead to unwanted side effects, such as swelling, oedema or electrolyte imbalances. However, in many cases, the body is able to adjust to the changes in fluid volume and distribution and return to a state of equilibrium relatively quickly. One must bear in mind that every ml of fluid that is infused will be lost at some point to the extravascular space (Fig. 1.18).

Relative hypovolemia: See vasoplegia.

Replacement solutions: These IV fluids are given to replace ongoing fluid losses (insensible losses, diarrhoea, vomiting, during fever, burns, etc.). As such they must resemble as close as possible to the fluid that is lost. Ongoing fluid losses refer to the

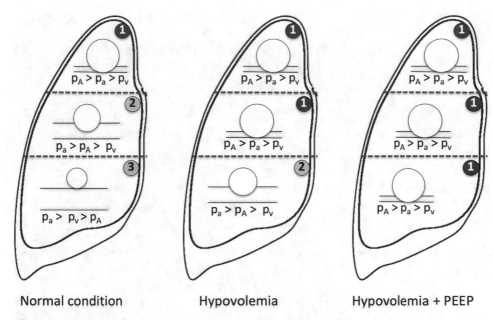

Fig. 1.16 Evolution of West zones during hypovolemia and PEEP. Left panel shows normal West zone distribution. The middle panel shows the situation in a patient under mechanical ventilation and hypovolemia where zone 1 conditions ($p_A > p_a > p_v$) expand to zone 2 ($p_a > p_A > p_v$) and zone 2 conditions to zone 3 ($p_a > p_v > p_A$). With p_a arterial capillary pressure, p_A > alveolar pressure and p_v venous capillary pressure. The right panel shows the situation in a hypovolemic patient with excessive PEEP causing further excursion of zone 1 conditions to zone 3 resulting in a right-to-left shunt explaining the premature hump seen on the transpulmonary thermodilution curve. (Adapted with permission from Hofkens et al. [42])

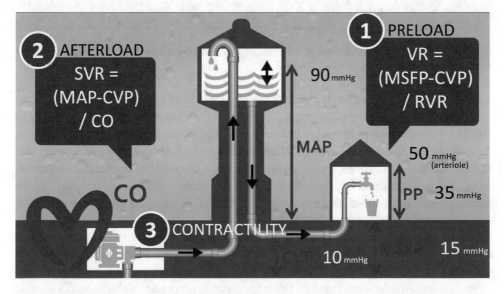

Fig. 1.17 Schematic representation of the waterfall-effect. *CO* cardiac output, represented by the pump. *CVP* central venous pressure, *MAP* mean arterial pressure, represented by the height of the water tower, *MSFP* mean systemic filling pressure, *PP* pulse pressure, *RVR* resistance to venous return, *SVR* systemic vascular resistance, *VR* venous return

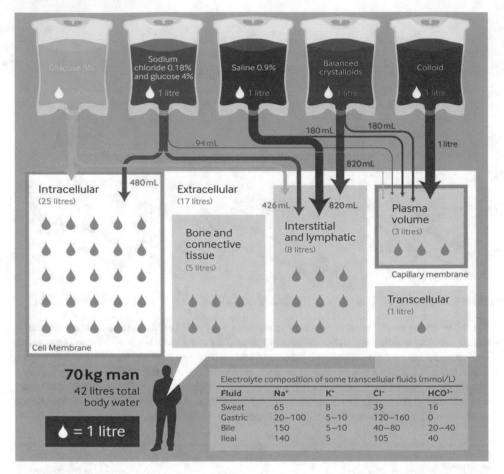

Fig. 1.18 Theoretical redistribution of intravenous fluids after infusion for a 70 kg man. (Adapted with permission from Frost [43])

continuous loss of fluids from the body over time. Fluid losses can occur through a variety of mechanisms, including urine output, sweating, breathing and digestive processes. In order to maintain proper hydration and prevent dehydration, it is important to replenish fluid losses through drinking fluids and consuming foods that contain water. The amount of fluids needed will vary depending on factors such as age, activity level and environmental conditions. In cases of excessive fluid loss, such as due to illness or exercise, it may be necessary to increase fluid intake to avoid dehydration. Figure 1.19 gives an overview of the different potential ongoing fluid losses per day.

Resuscitation phase: Life-saving resuscitation phase with focus on patient rescue and early adequate fluid management (EAFM), e.g. 30 mL/kg/1 h according to surviving sepsis campaign guidelines or a fluid challenge/bolus of 4 mL/kg given in 5–10 min.

Resuscitation solutions: These IV fluids are given to restore and stabilize hemodynamic status in order to save lives in patients with shock and imbalance between oxygen delivery and oxygen consumption illustrated by an increase in serum lactate levels beyond 3 mmol/L.

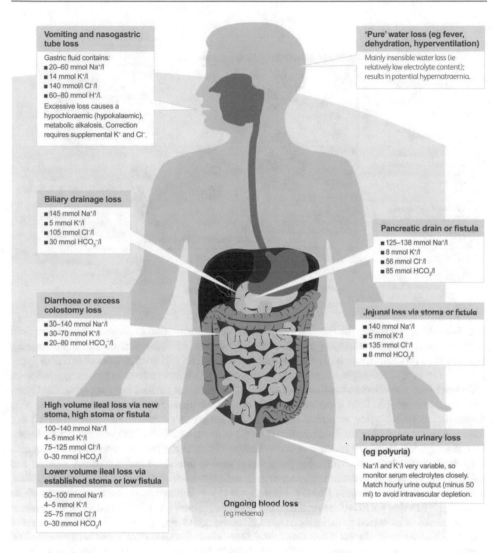

Vomiting and nasogastric tube loss

Gastric fluid contains:
- 20–60 mmol Na⁺/l
- 14 mmol K⁺/l
- 140 mmol/l Cl⁻/l
- 60–80 mmol H⁺/l.

Excessive loss causes a hypochloraemic (hypokalaemic), metabolic alkalosis. Correction requires supplemental K⁺ and Cl⁻.

'Pure' water loss (eg fever, dehydration, hyperventilation)

Mainly insensible water loss (ie relatively low electrolyte content); results in potential hypernatraemia.

Biliary drainage loss
- 145 mmol Na⁺/l
- 5 mmol K⁺/l
- 105 mmol Cl⁻/l
- 30 mmol HCO₃⁻/l

Pancreatic drain or fistula
- 125–138 mmol Na⁺/l
- 8 mmol K⁺/l
- 56 mmol Cl⁻/l
- 85 mmol HCO₃/l

Diarrhoea or excess colostomy loss
- 30–140 mmol Na⁺/l
- 30–70 mmol K⁺/l
- 20–80 mmol HCO₃⁻/l

Jejunal loss via stoma or fistula
- 140 mmol Na⁺/l
- 5 mmol K⁺/l
- 135 mmol Cl⁻/l
- 8 mmol HCO₃/l

High volume ileal loss via new stoma, high stoma or fistula
100–140 mmol Na⁺/l
4–5 mmol K⁺/l
75–125 mmol Cl⁻/l
0–30 mmol HCO₃/l

Lower volume ileal loss via established stoma or low fistula
50–100 mmol Na⁺/l
4–5 mmol K⁺/l
25–75 mmol Cl⁻/l
0–30 mmol HCO₃/l

Inappropriate urinary loss (eg polyuria)
Na⁺/l and K⁺/l very variable, so monitor serum electrolytes closely. Match hourly urine output (minus 50 ml) to avoid intravascular depletion.

Ongoing blood loss
(eg melaena)

Fig. 1.19 Diagram of ongoing losses. (Adapted from National Clinical Guideline Centre "Intravenous fluid therapy in adults in hospital", NICE clinical guideline 174 (December 2013) © National Institute for Health and Care Excellence 2013. All rights reserved. https://www.nice.org.uk/guidance/cg174/resources/diagram-of-ongoing-losses-pdf-191664109)

Revised Starling equation: An updated version of the traditional Starling equation that incorporates current understanding of the role of the endothelial glycocalyx in transvascular fluid filtration, also known as the Starling Principle.

ROSE: A conceptual framework that describes four different stages of fluid resuscitation, beginning with initial rapid fluid administration to treat life-threatening shock (Rescue), continued fluid therapy until adequate perfusion is restored (Optimization), followed by ongoing maintenance fluids (Stabilization) and gradual discontinuation of fluid support (i.e. evacuation or de-escalation) [1, 5, 44, 45]. This is illustrated in Fig. 1.20.

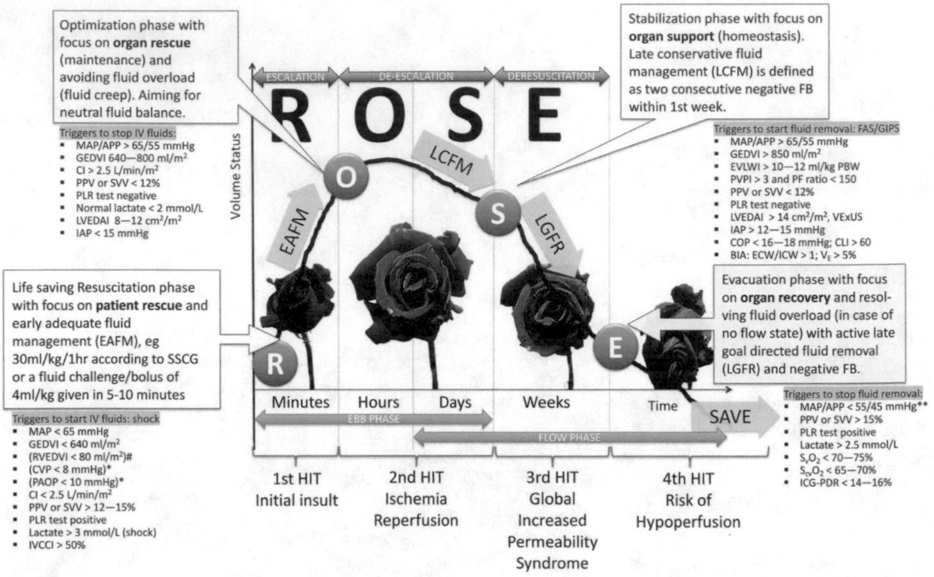
Optimization phase with focus on organ rescue (maintenance) and avoiding fluid overload (fluid creep). Aiming for neutral fluid balance.
Triggers to stop IV fluids:
MAP/APP > 65/55 mmHg
GEDVI 640—800 ml/m²
CI > 2.5 L/min/m²
PPV or SVV < 12%
PLR test negative
Normal lactate < 2 mmol/L
LVEDAI 8—12 cm²/m²
IAP < 15 mmHg
Volume Status
ESCALATION
DE-ESCALATION
DERESUSCITATION
R O S E
EAFM
LCFM
LGFR
Stabilization phase with focus on organ support (homeostasis). Late conservative fluid management (LCFM) is defined as two consecutive negative FB within 1st week.
Triggers to start fluid removal: FAS/GIPS
MAP/APP > 65/55 mmHg
GEDVI > 850 ml/m²
EVLWI > 10—12 ml/kg PBW
PVPI > 3 and PF ratio < 150
PPV or SVV < 12%
PLR test negative
LVEDAI > 14 cm²/m², VExUS
IAP > 12—15 mmHg
COP < 16—18 mmHg; CLI > 60
BIA: ECW/ICW > 1; V_E > 5%
Life saving Resuscitation phase with focus on patient rescue and early adequate fluid management (EAFM), eg 30ml/kg/1hr according to SSCG or a fluid challenge/bolus of 4ml/kg given in 5-10 minutes
Evacuation phase with focus on organ recovery and resolving fluid overload (in case of no flow state) with active late goal directed fluid removal (LGFR) and negative FB.
Minutes
Hours
Days
Weeks
Time
SAVE
EBB PHASE
FLOW PHASE
Triggers to start IV fluids: shock
MAP < 65 mmHg
GEDVI < 640 ml/m²
(RVEDVI < 80 ml/m²)#
(CVP < 8 mmHg)*
(PAOP < 10 mmHg)*
CI < 2.5 L/min/m²
PPV or SVV > 12—15%
PLR test positive
Lactate > 3 mmol/L (shock)
IVCCI > 50%
1st HIT Initial insult
2nd HIT Ischemia Reperfusion
3rd HIT Global Increased Permeability Syndrome
4th HIT Risk of Hypoperfusion
Triggers to stop fluid removal:
MAP/APP < 55/45 mmHg**
PPV or SVV > 15%
PLR test positive
Lactate > 2.5 mmol/L
SvO2 < 70—75%
ScvO2 < 65—70%
ICG-PDR < 14—16%

Fig. 1.20 Graph showing the four-hit model of shock with evolution of patients' cumulative fluid volume status over time during the five distinct phases of resuscitation: Resuscitation (R), Optimization (O), Stabilization (S) and Evacuation (E) (ROSE), followed by a possible risk of hypoperfusion in case of too aggressive de-resuscitation. On admission patients are often hypovolemic, followed by normovolemia after fluid resuscitation (escalation or EAFM, early adequate fluid management), and possible fluid overload, again followed by a phase returning to normovolemia with de-escalation via achieving zero fluid balance or late conservative fluid management (LCFM) and followed by late goal directed fluid removal (LGFR) or de-resuscitation. In the case of hypovolemia, O_2 cannot get into the tissue because of convective problems, in the case of hypervolemia O_2 cannot get into the tissue because of diffusion problems related to interstitial and pulmonary oedema and gut oedema (ileus and abdominal hypertension). Adapted from Malbrain et al. with permission, according to the Open Access CC BY License 4.0 [5]. * Volumetric preload indicators such as GEDVI, LVEDAI or RVEDVI are preferred over barometric ones like CVP or PAOP. ** Vasopressor can be started or increased to maintain MAP/APP above 55/45 during the de-resuscitation phase. # can only be measured via the Swan-Ganz pulmonary artery catheter (PAC) and became obsolete. *APP* abdominal perfusion pressure (APP = MAP-IAP), *BIA* bio-electrical impedance analysis, *CI* cardiac index, *CLI* capillary leak index (serum CRP divided by serum albumin), *COP* colloid oncotic pressure, *CVP* central venous pressure, *EAFM* early adequate fluid management, *ECW/ICW* extracellular/intracellular water, *EVLWI* extravascular lung water index, *FAS* fluid accumulation syndrome, *GEDVI* global end-diastolic volume index, *GIPS* global increased permeability syndrome, *IAP* intra-abdominal pressure, *ICG-PDR* indocyanine green plasma disappearance rate, *IVCCI* inferior vena cava collapsibility index, *LCFM* late conservative fluid management, *LGFR* late goal-directed fluid removal, *LVEDAI* left ventricular end-diastolic area index, *MAP* mean arterial pressure, *PAOP* pulmonary artery occlusion pressure, *PF* P_aO_2 over F_iO_2 ratio, *PLR* passive leg raising, *PPV* pulse pressure variation, *PVPI* pulmonary vascular permeability index, *RVEDVI* right ventricular end-diastolic volume index, $S_{cv}O_2$ central venous oxygen saturation, *SSCG* surviving sepsis campaign guidelines, S_vO_2 mixed venous oxygen saturation, *SVV* stroke volume variation, V_E volume excess (from baseline body weight), *VExUS* venous congestion by ultrasound

Saline: Normal saline, also known as 0.9% sodium chloride (NaCl) solution, is a type of intravenous infusion fluid that is commonly used in medical settings. It is a sterile solution of water and sodium chloride, with a concentration of 9 g of salt per litre of water and 3.5 g of sodium (the daily dietary requirement being 2.3 g). Normal saline is used for a variety of purposes, including to restore fluid and electrolyte balance, to flush intravenous lines, to dilute medications or to maintain intravenous access. Normal saline is generally considered safe and well-tolerated, however there are substantial side effects. Excessive infusion of normal saline can lead to salt and fluid accumulation, electrolyte (increased sodium, chloride and potassium levels) and acid–base disturbances (hyperchloremic metabolic acidosis), increased vasopressor and RRT need and AKI (Fig. 1.21). A recent meta-analysis showed that normal saline should also be used with caution in patients with sepsis, burns or diabetic ketoacidosis as well as those with heart failure, kidney disease or other conditions that can affect fluid and electrolyte balance [46]. The only indications for abnormal saline left are patients with traumatic brain injury and those with excessive gastro-intestinal losses.

Sensible water loss: Measurable macroscopic body fluid losses, such as urine production, vomiting and diarrhoea.

Serum: The portion of plasma that does not contain fibrinogen and clotting factors.

Shock state: A life-threatening, generalized form of acute circulatory failure associated with imbalance between oxygen delivery and oxygen consumption, resulting in inadequate anaerobic oxygen metabolism by the cells. Shock can be classified into four major classifications: hypovolemic shock refers to reduced effective circulating volume, from

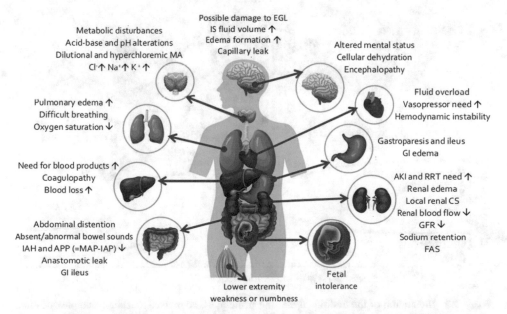

Fig. 1.21 Deleterious effects of excessive intravenous abnormal saline infusion. *AKI* acute kidney injury, *APP* abdominal perfusion pressure, *Cl-* chloride, *CS* compartment syndrome, *EGL* endothelial glycocalix layer, *FAS* fluid accumulation syndrome, *GFR* glomerular filtration rate, *GI* gastrointestinal, *IAH* intra-abdominal hypertension, *IAP* intra-abdominal pressure, *IS* interstitial, *K+* potassium, *MAP* mean arterial pressure, *Na+* sodium, *RRT* renal replacement therapy

internal or external intravascular fluid loss; obstructive shock results from physical impairment to blood flow, such as from thromboembolic disease; distributive shock is caused by maldistribution of blood flow due to loss of vasomotor tone, such as during sepsis or anaphylaxis and cardiogenic shock describes cardiac pump dysfunction resulting in decreased forward flow.

Stabilization phase: Stabilization phase with focus on organ support (homeostasis). Late conservative fluid management (LCFM) is defined as two consecutive days of negative fluid balance within the first week.

Standard base excess (SBE): Standard base excess or the base excess of the extracellular fluid is the amount of strong acid (millimoles per litre) that needs to be added in vitro to 1 L of fully oxygenated whole blood to return the sample to standard conditions (pH of 7.40, PCO_2 of 40 mmHg, and temperature of 37 °C), at a haemoglobin concentration of ~50 g/L. Standard base excess has been adjusted to reflect the extracellular fluid buffering capacity of haemoglobin in vivo, which is not the case for traditional base excess. It is used clinically to determine the degree of metabolic acidosis.

Starling principle: Traditional principle describing the fluid passage across the semipermeable capillary membrane, which is determined by the net result between hydrostatic and oncotic pressures such that fluid leaves the capillary at the arterial end of the capillary and is absorbed at the venous end of capillary (Fig. 1.22).

Stewart's approach to acid–base: In the late 1970s Peter Stewart, a Canadian biophysicist, described a quantitative approach to acid–base disorder. His approach was based upon fundamental physicochemical properties of a solution that include principles of

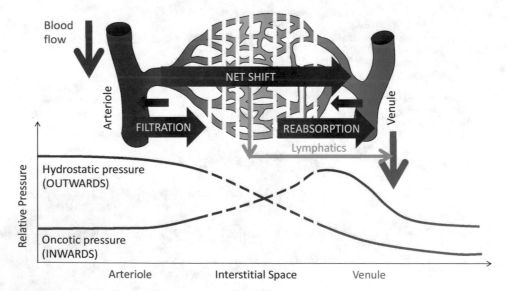

Fig. 1.22 Illustration of the traditional Starling principle. The revised Starling principle questions the proposed filtration and re-absorption mechanisms and points towards the importance of the role of the endothelial glycocalyx and the lymphatics

electroneutrality, law of conservation of mass and dissociation equilibrium of all incompletely dissociated substances in a solution.

Stressed volume: The circulating blood volume that creates positive transmural pressure via the elastic recoil of the vessel wall is termed "stressed volume". See also under vasoplegia.

Stroke volume variation (SVV): The mean difference between the maximum (SV_{max}) and minimum (SV_{min}) stroke volume during a series of respiratory cycles, expressed as a percentage [42]. SVV is a functional hemodynamic parameter that predicts fluid responsiveness in mechanically ventilated patients.

Strong ion: An anion or cation that is considered to be fully dissociated at physiologic pH. The major strong anions are sulphate, chloride and lactate, while the major strong cations in plasma are calcium, sodium and magnesium.

Strong ion difference (SID): The difference between the concentrations of strong cations and strong anions in plasma.

Strong ion gap (SIG): SIG is a predictor of morbidity and mortality and quantifies [unmeasured anions] − [unmeasured cations] of both strong and weak ions. It reflects the difference between the activity of all common cations (Na^+, K^+, Mg^{2+}, Ca^{2+}) and the common anions (Cl^-, lactate, urate) and other measured non-volatile weak acids (A^-). SIG is calculated as SIDa − SIDe, or more specifically, as $[Na^+] + [K^+] + [Mg^{2+}] + [Ca^{2+}] − [Cl^-$ corrected] − [lactate] − $[A^-] − [HCO_3^-]$, in milli-equivalents per litre; where SIDa is the apparent strong ion difference and SIDe is the effective strong ion difference.

Surviving sepsis campaign guidelines (SSCG): Sepsis and septic shock are leading causes of death worldwide. The international Surviving Sepsis Campaign (SSC) is a joint initiative of the European Society of Intensive Care Medicine (ESICM) and the Society of Critical Care Medicine (SCCM). The SSC is led by multidisciplinary international experts committed to improving time to recognition and treatment of sepsis and septic shock. Initiated in 2002 at the ESICM's annual meeting with the Barcelona Declaration, the campaign progressed has several aims, including the development of guidelines for diagnosis, treatment and post-ICU care of sepsis and a reduction of mortality from sepsis. The latest update was done in 2021 [47, 48].

Sweating ongoing loss: Sweat is produced by the sweat glands in response to heat or exercise, and helps to regulate body temperature. The amount of sweat produced can vary depending on environmental conditions, activity level and individual factors such as age and fitness level. See also replacement fluids.

Therapeutic dilemma: A therapeutic conflict is a situation where each of the possible therapeutic decisions carries some potential harm. In high-risk patients, the decision about fluid administration should be made within the context of a therapeutic conflict. Therapeutic conflicts are the biggest challenge for protocolized cardiovascular management in anaesthetized and critically ill patients. A therapeutic conflict is where our decisions can make the most difference (Fig. 1.23).

Third space fluid: Fluid without a physiological function confined in a body fluid compartments or spaces that is anatomically separated from other compartments. Fluid

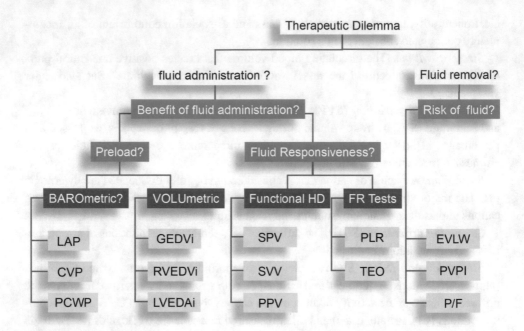

Fig. 1.23 Diagnostic and therapeutic options when confronted with a therapeutic dilemma: one must always outweigh the potential risks and benefits of fluid administration versus fluid removal. *CVP* central venous pressure, *EVLW* extravascular lung water, *GEDVI* global end-diastolic volume index, *LAP* left atrial pressure, *LVEDAI* left ventricular end-diastolic area index, *PCWP* pulmonary capillary wedge pressure, *P/F PaO$_2$* over FiO$_2$ ratio, *PLR* passive leg raising test, *PPV* pulse pressure variation, *PVPI* pulmonary vascular permeability index, *RVEDVI* right ventricular end-diastolic volume index, *SPV* systolic pressure variation, *SVV* stroke volume variation, *TEO* tele-expirtatory occlusion test

movement to these spaces may occur following overzealous intravenous fluid administration, but need probably to be included in the interstitial fluids. Because third space fluids are reabsorbed into the central fluid compartment some consider them to be a myth.

Tonicity: The measurement of the effective osmolality of a solution (also referred to as osmotic pressure) is the concentration of a solution as described by total solutes per volume which corresponds to its ability to cause water to diffuse across a semi-permeable membrane, such as the cell membrane. The tonicity determines the distribution of the given solution. The cell will shrink when placed in a hypertonic solution, swell when placed in a hypotonic solution and the cell volume will remain unchanged when placed in an isotonic solution. Serum osmolality can be calculated by the simplified formula: 2 × serum sodium (in mmol/L).

Total body water (TBW): Total body water is the body water that exists in- and outside of the cell membrane: TBW = ICW + ECW. Accounts for 55% (female) up to 65% (man) of total body weight (Fig. 1.24).

Unstressed volume: The volume inside a vessel at near zero transmural pressure is termed " unstressed volume" . This volume fills the system without exerting tension on the

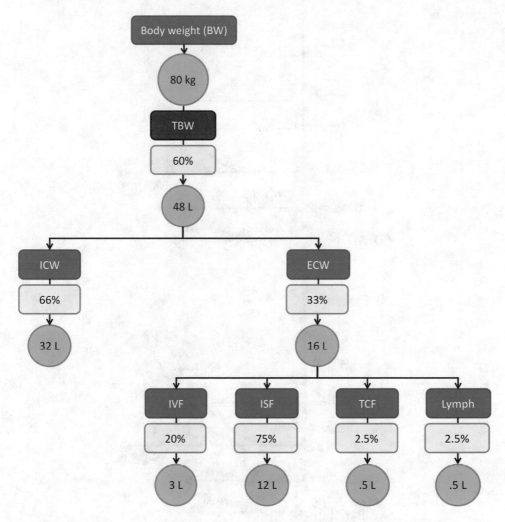

Fig. 1.24 Body water composition for an adult 80 kg male. *ECW* extracellular water, *ICW* intracellular water, *ISF* interstitial fluid, *IVF* intravascular fluid, *TBW* total body water, *TCF* transcellular fluid. These fluids are contained within epithelial lined spaces. Examples of this fluid are cerebrospinal fluid, pleural fluid, pericardial fluid, peritoneal fluid, bladder urine, eye fluid, joint fluid, etc.

vessel wall. The sum of the stressed (~30% of total volume) and unstressed (~70% of total volume) volumes is the total blood volume within the venous system. More than 70% of total circulating blood volume (CBV) is located in the large veins, and increased vascular compliance (vasoplegia) like in sepsis or induced by anesthesia can cause a substantial increase in CBV (with up to 80%). This increased venous compliance and increased CBV in early sepsis may represent a recruitable source of preload, as veins are very sensitive to low doses of vasopressor. These drugs directly convert unstressed blood volume to stressed blood volume while maintaining nearly normal venous elastance (Fig. 1.25).

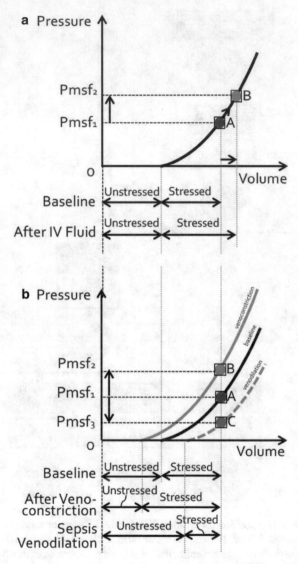

Fig. 1.25 Effect of fluid loading and venoconstriction on volume. (**a**) Effect of volume loading on mean systemic filling pressure (*P*msf) and (un)stressed volume. Administration of a fluid bolus increases *P*msf (from *P*msf1 to *P*msf2, indicated respectively by position A (red dot) to B (green dot) on the pressure/volume curve). *Unstressed* volume remains constant while *stressed* volume increases. Total volume = unstressed + stressed increases, carrying a risk for fluid overload. (**b**) Effect of venoconstriction and venodilation on mean systemic filling pressure (*P*msf) and (un) stressed volume. Venoconstriction increases *P*msf (from *P*msf1 to *P*msf2, indicated respectively by position A (red dot) to B (green dot) on the pressure/volume curve). *Unstressed* volume decreases while *stressed* volume increases. Total volume = unstressed + stressed remains constant, resulting in an auto-transfusion effect. Venodilation as seen in sepsis (vasoplegia) decreases *P*msf (from *P*msf1 to *P*msf3, indicated respectively by position A (red dot) to C (blue dot) on the pressure/volume curve). *Unstressed* volume increases while *stressed* volume decreases. Total volume = unstressed + stressed remains constant, resulting in an intravascular underfilling effect. (Adapted according to the Open Access CC BY License 4.0 with permission from Jacobs et al. [49])

Urine output: The kidneys filter waste products and excess fluids from the blood, and these are excreted from the body as urine. The amount of urine produced can be affected by factors such as hydration status, medications and underlying medical conditions. Urine output is normally between 1 and 2 mL/kg/h and is sometimes used as a resuscitation target in severely burned patients. Oliguria <0.3–0.5 mL/kg/h and anuria are part of the KDGO definition of AKI. See also replacement fluids.

Vascular volume: See circulating blood volume.

Vasoplegia: Condition characterized by a low systemic vascular resistance in conjunction with profound hypotension and a normal to increased cardiac output. Also known as vasoplegic, distributive or hyperdynamic shock. Results in relative hypovolemia with a reduction in the effective circulating blood volume due to venodilation and increased venous capacitance. The early use of vasopressors may cause an autotransfusion effect with an increase in mean systemic filling pressure and redistribution and recruitment of preload from the venous side, thereby increasing the stressed volume towards the central circulation [49].

Volemia (plasma volume): Anatomically defined as the volume limited by the vascular endothelium. The effective arterial blood volume that really perfuses organs; cannot be really measured. Interstitial and plasma volume can be uncoupled = most frequently interstitial fluid accumulation associated with hypovolemia (plasma dehydration). *Euvolema* normal volemia, *hypovolemia* low volemia, *hypervolemia* high volemia.

Volume depletion: The loss of water and electrolytes from the extracellular fluid compartment.

Volume kinetics: This is an adaptation of pharmacokinetic theory that makes it possible to analyse and simulate the distribution and elimination following an infusion of intravenous fluids. Applying this concept, it is possible, by simulation, to determine the infusion rate that is required to reach a predetermined plasma volume expansion.

Volume overload: See fluid overload and fluid accumulation.

Water: Because water contains a lot of small water molecules (with a molar mass of 18 Da and a molecular weight of 18 g/mol), the molar concentration of water is about 55.3 mol/L at 37 °C. There are much less hydrogen ions than there are water molecules in a glass of water. In reality water is only slightly dissociated and a virtually inexhaustible source of protons (H+). The concentration of $[H^+]$ is therefore solely determined by the dissociation of water and not by the amount of $[H^+]$ that is added or removed. According to Stewart's approach, the three independent variables that determine the dissociation of water and hence the amount of $[H^+]$ are the strong ion difference (SID), the amount of weak acids and the partial pressure of carbon dioxide (pCO_2).

Weak ion: An anion or cation that is not fully dissociated at physiologic pH.

West zones (abdominal): See abdominal West zones.

West zones (pulmonary): See pulmonary West zones.

Worsening renal function (WRF): Recent interest has focused on worsening renal function (WRF), a situation strongly related to mortality, but seemingly only when heart failure status deteriorates [50]. Worsening renal function (WRF) is defined as a 0.3–0.5 mg/

Fig. 1.26 Statistical model of nonparametric logistic regression showing the relationship between mean central venous pressure during the first 24 h after admission and the probability of new or persistent acute kidney injury. Note the plateau for the incidence of acute kidney injury (AKI) when the lower limit of central venous pressure (CVP) was between 8 and 12 mmHg. Over this limit, the rise in CVP was associated with a sharp increase in new or persistent AKI incidence. (Adapted from Legrand et al. [53])

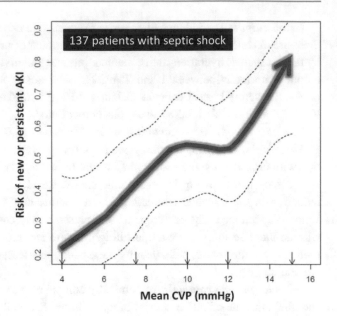

dL rise in serum creatinine or a decrease in glomerular filtration rate (GFR) of 9–15 mL/ min during hospitalization for acute decompensated heart failure. From the patients with acute decompensated heart failure who develop WRF, 66% die within 1 year [51]. Previous data have shown that CVP may even be more important than CO to predict WRF especially in patients with ADHF as well as sepsis [52, 53] (Fig. 1.26).

Conclusions

We hereby would like to quote and thank Rosalind S. Chow [6]: "Despite the frequency with which fluids are administered to critically ill patients, developing an effective fluid management plan and strategy may at times be surprisingly complex. A thorough understanding of the physiology of body fluids, fluid administration routes, therapeutic delivery strategies, risks, and complications will help to optimize patient outcomes. National and multinational organizations, such as the International Fluid Academy (IFA, www.fluid-academy.org), provide opportunities for clinicians and researchers to promote research and education in the practice of fluid therapy. The use of clear and consistent terminology is a key component to fostering effective communication and collaboration within the veterinary and human healthcare fields."

Acknowledgements The definitions presented herein have been adapted from a number of recent papers with permission according to the Open Access CC BY License 4.0 [1, 2, 4–10].

References

1. Malbrain ML, Marik PE, Witters I, Cordemans C, Kirkpatrick AW, Roberts DJ, Van Regenmortel N. Fluid overload, de-resuscitation, and outcomes in critically ill or injured patients: a systematic review with suggestions for clinical practice. Anaesthesiol Intensive Ther. 2014;46(5):361–80.
2. Malbrain ML, Mythen M, Rice TW, Wuyts S. It is time for improved fluid stewardship. ICU Manag Pract. 2018;18(3):158–62.
3. Vincent JL, Pinsky MR. We should avoid the term "fluid overload". Crit Care. 2018;22(1):214.
4. Malbrain M, Van Regenmortel N, Owczuk R. It is time to consider the four D's of fluid management. Anaesthesiol Intensive Ther. 2015;47:S1–5.
5. Malbrain M, Van Regenmortel N, Saugel B, De Tavernier B, Van Gaal PJ, Joannes-Boyau O, Teboul JL, Rice TW, Mythen M, Monnet X. Principles of fluid management and stewardship in septic shock: it is time to consider the four D's and the four phases of fluid therapy. Ann Intensive Care. 2018;8(1):66.
6. Chow RS. Terms, definitions, nomenclature, and routes of fluid administration. Front Vet Sci. 2020;7:591218.
7. Malbrain M, Langer T, Annane D, Gattinoni L, Elbers P, Hahn RG, De Laet I, Minini A, Wong A, Ince C, et al. Intravenous fluid therapy in the perioperative and critical care setting: executive summary of the International Fluid Academy (IFA). Ann Intensive Care. 2020;10(1):64.
8. Hawkins WA, Smith SE, Newsome AS, Carr JR, Bland CM, Branan TN. Fluid stewardship during critical illness: a call to action. J Pharm Pract. 2020;33(6):863–73.
9. Benes J, Kirov M, Kuzkov V, Lainscak M, Molnar Z, Voga G, Monnet X. Fluid therapy: double-edged sword during critical care? Biomed Res Int. 2015;2015:729075.
10. Malbrain ML, Van Regenmortel N, Owczuk R. The debate on fluid management and haemodynamic monitoring continues: between Scylla and Charybdis, or faith and evidence. Anaesthesiol Intensive Ther. 2014;46(5):313–8.
11. Kirkpatrick AW, Roberts DJ, De Waele J, Jaeschke R, Malbrain ML, De Keulenaer B, Duchesne J, Bjorck M, Leppaniemi A, Ejike JC, et al. Intra-abdominal hypertension and the abdominal compartment syndrome: updated consensus definitions and clinical practice guidelines from the World Society of the Abdominal Compartment Syndrome. Intensive Care Med. 2013;39(7):1190–206.
12. Takata M, Wise RA, Robotham JL. Effects of abdominal pressure on venous return: abdominal vascular zone conditions. J Appl Physiol (1985). 1990;69(6):1961–72.
13. Kellum JA, Lameire N. Diagnosis, evaluation, and management of acute kidney injury: a KDIGO summary (Part 1). Crit Care. 2013;17(1):204.
14. Minini A, Rola P, Malbrain MLNG. Kidney failure associated with polycompartment syndrome. In: Coccolini F, Malbrain ML, Kirkpatrick AW, Gamberini E, editors. Compartment syndrome hot topics in acute care surgery and trauma. Cham: Springer; 2021.
15. Dabrowski W, Rola P, Malbrain M. Intra-abdominal pressure monitoring in cardiac surgery: is this the canary in the coalmine for kidney injury? J Clin Monit Comput. 2022;37(2):351–8.
16. Ince C. Hemodynamic coherence and the rationale for monitoring the microcirculation. Crit Care. 2015;19(Suppl 3):S8.
17. Ince C, Boerma EC, Cecconi M, De Backer D, Shapiro NI, Duranteau J, Pinsky MR, Artigas A, Teboul JL, Reiss IKM, et al. Second consensus on the assessment of sublingual microcirculation in critically ill patients: results from a task force of the European Society of Intensive Care Medicine. Intensive Care Med. 2018;44(3):281–99.
18. Rivers E, Nguyen B, Havstad S, Ressler J, Muzzin A, Knoblich B, Peterson E, Tomlanovich M. Early goal-directed therapy in the treatment of severe sepsis and septic shock. N Engl J Med. 2001;345(19):1368–77.

19. Monnet X, Malbrain M, Pinsky MR. The prediction of fluid responsiveness. Intensive Care Med. 2022;49(1):83–6.
20. Toscani L, Aya HD, Antonakaki D, Bastoni D, Watson X, Arulkumaran N, Rhodes A, Cecconi M. What is the impact of the fluid challenge technique on diagnosis of fluid responsiveness? A systematic review and meta-analysis. Crit Care. 2017;21(1):207.
21. Cartotto R, Zhou A. Fluid creep: the pendulum hasn't swung back yet! J Burn Care Res. 2010;31(4):551–8.
22. Van Regenmortel N, Verbrugghe W, Roelant E, Van den Wyngaert T, Jorens PG. Maintenance fluid therapy and fluid creep impose more significant fluid, sodium, and chloride burdens than resuscitation fluids in critically ill patients: a retrospective study in a tertiary mixed ICU population. Intensive Care Med. 2018;44(4):409–17.
23. Mitsides N, Pietribiasi M, Waniewski J, Brenchley P, Mitra S. Transcapillary refilling rate and its determinants during haemodialysis with standard and high ultrafiltration rates. Am J Nephrol. 2019;50(2):133–43.
24. Dull RO, Hahn RG. Transcapillary refill: The physiology underlying fluid reabsorption. J Trauma Acute Care Surg. 2021;90(2):e31–9.
25. Murugan R, Kerti SJ, Chang CH, Gallagher M, Clermont G, Palevsky PM, Kellum JA, Bellomo R. Association of net ultrafiltration rate with mortality among critically ill adults with acute kidney injury receiving continuous venovenous hemodiafiltration: a secondary analysis of the randomized evaluation of normal vs augmented level (RENAL) of renal replacement therapy trial. JAMA Netw Open. 2019;2(6):e195418.
26. Kattan E, Castro R, Miralles-Aguiar F, Hernandez G, Rola P. The emerging concept of fluid tolerance: a position paper. J Crit Care. 2022;71:154070.
27. Van der Mullen J, Wise R, Vermeulen G, Moonen PJ, Malbrain M. Assessment of hypovolaemia in the critically ill. Anaesthesiol Intensive Ther. 2018;50(2):141–9.
28. Regli A, Pelosi P, Malbrain M. Ventilation in patients with intra-abdominal hypertension: what every critical care physician needs to know. Ann Intensive Care. 2019;9(1):52.
29. Moritz ML. Why 0.9% saline is isotonic: understanding the aqueous phase of plasma and the difference between osmolarity and osmolality. Pediatr Nephrol. 2019;34(7):1299–300.
30. Murphy CV, Schramm GE, Doherty JA, Reichley RM, Gajic O, Afessa B, Micek ST, Kollef MH. The importance of fluid management in acute lung injury secondary to septic shock. Chest. 2009;136(1):102–9.
31. Silversides JA, Major E, Ferguson AJ, Mann EE, McAuley DF, Marshall JC, Blackwood B, Fan E. Conservative fluid management or deresuscitation for patients with sepsis or acute respiratory distress syndrome following the resuscitation phase of critical illness: a systematic review and meta-analysis. Intensive Care Med. 2017;43(2):155–70.
32. Silversides JA, Perner A, Malbrain M. Liberal versus restrictive fluid therapy in critically ill patients. Intensive Care Med. 2019;45(10):1440–2.
33. Meyhoff TS, Hjortrup PB, Wetterslev J, Sivapalan P, Laake JH, Cronhjort M, Jakob SM, Cecconi M, Nalos M, Ostermann M, et al. Restriction of intravenous fluid in ICU patients with septic shock. N Engl J Med. 2022;386(26):2459–70.
34. Silversides JA, McMullan R, Emerson LM, Bradbury I, Bannard-Smith J, Szakmany T, Trinder J, Rostron AJ, Johnston P, Ferguson AJ, et al. Feasibility of conservative fluid administration and deresuscitation compared with usual care in critical illness: the Role of Active Deresuscitation After Resuscitation-2 (RADAR-2) randomised clinical trial. Intensive Care Med. 2022;48(2):190–200.
35. Wijnberge M, Sindhunata DP, Pinsky MR, Vlaar AP, Ouweneel E, Jansen JR, Veelo DP, Geerts BF. Estimating mean circulatory filling pressure in clinical practice: a systematic review comparing three bedside methods in the critically ill. Ann Intensive Care. 2018;8(1):73.

36. Faria DK, Mendes ME, Sumita NM. The measurement of serum osmolality and itsapplication to clinical practice and laboratory:literature review. J Bras Patol Med Lab. 2017;53(1):38–45.

37. Peeters Y, Lebeer M, Wise R, Malbrain M. An overview on fluid resuscitation and resuscitation endpoints in burns: past, present and future. Part 2—avoiding complications by using the right endpoints with a new personalized protocolized approach. Anaesthesiol Intensive Ther. 2015;47:S15–26.

38. Peeters Y, Vandervelden S, Wise R, Malbrain M. An overview on fluid resuscitation and resuscitation endpoints in burns: past, present and future. Part 1—historical background, resuscitation fluid and adjunctive treatment. Anaesthesiol Intensive Ther. 2015;47:S6–S14.

39. Monnet X, Teboul JL. Passive leg raising: five rules, not a drop of fluid! Crit Care. 2015;19:18.

40. Duchesne JC, Kaplan LJ, Balogh ZJ, Malbrain M. Role of permissive hypotension, hypertonic resuscitation and the global increased permeability syndrome in patients with severe haemorrhage: adjuncts to damage control resuscitation to prevent intra-abdominal hypertension. Anaesthesiol Intensive Ther. 2015;47(2):143–55.

41. Patterson SW, Starling EH. On the mechanical factors which determine the output of the ventricles. J Physiol. 1914;48(5):357–79.

42. Hofkens PJ, Verrijcken A, Merveille K, Neirynck S, Van Regenmortel N, De Laet I, Schoonheydt K, Dits H, Bein B, Huber W, et al. Common pitfalls and tips and tricks to get the most out of your transpulmonary thermodilution device: results of a survey and state-of-the-art review. Anaesthesiol Intensive Ther. 2015;47(2):89–116.

43. Frost P. Intravenous fluid therapy in adult inpatients. BMJ. 2015;350:g7620.

44. Hoste EA, Maitland K, Brudney CS, Mehta R, Vincent JL, Yates D, Kellum JA, Mythen MG, Shaw AD, Group AXI. Four phases of intravenous fluid therapy: a conceptual model. Br J Anaesth. 2014;113(5):740–7.

45. Vincent JL, De Backer D. Circulatory shock. N Engl J Med. 2013;369(18):1726–34.

46. Hammond NE, Zampieri FG, Tanna GLD, Garside T, Adigbli D, Cavalcanti AB, Machado FR, Micallef S, Myburgh J, Ramanan M, et al. Balanced crystalloids versus saline in critically ill adults: a systematic review with meta-analysis. NEJM Evid. 2022;1(2):EVIDoa2100010.

47. Evans L, Rhodes A, Alhazzani W, Antonelli M, Coopersmith CM, French C, Machado FR, McIntyre L, Ostermann M, Prescott HC, et al. Executive summary: surviving sepsis campaign: international guidelines for the management of sepsis and septic shock 2021. Crit Care Med. 2021;49(11):1974–82.

48. Evans L, Rhodes A, Alhazzani W, Antonelli M, Coopersmith CM, French C, Machado FR, McIntyre L, Ostermann M, Prescott HC, et al. Surviving sepsis campaign: international guidelines for management of sepsis and septic shock 2021. Crit Care Med. 2021;49(11):e1063–143.

49. Jacobs R, Lochy S, Malbrain M. Phenylephrine-induced recruitable preload from the venous side. J Clin Monit Comput. 2019;33(3):373–6.

50. Damman K, Testani JM. The kidney in heart failure: an update. Eur Heart J. 2015;36(23):1437–44.

51. Metra M, Ponikowski P, Dickstein K, McMurray JJ, Gavazzi A, Bergh CH, Fraser AG, Jaarsma T, Pitsis A, Mohacsi P, et al. Advanced chronic heart failure: a position statement from the Study Group on Advanced Heart Failure of the Heart Failure Association of the European Society of Cardiology. Eur J Heart Fail. 2007;9(6-7):684–94.

52. Verbrugge FH, Dupont M, Steels P, Grieten L, Malbrain M, Tang WH, Mullens W. Abdominal contributions to cardiorenal dysfunction in congestive heart failure. J Am Coll Cardiol. 2013;62(6):485–95.

53. Legrand M, Dupuis C, Simon C, Gayat E, Mateo J, Lukaszewicz AC, Payen D. Association between systemic hemodynamics and septic acute kidney injury in critically ill patients: a retrospective observational study. Crit Care. 2013;17(6):R278.

Fluid Physiology Part 1: Volume and Distribution of Water and Its Major Solutes Between Plasma, the Interstitium and Intracellular Fluid

Thomas Woodcock

Contents

Introduction 50
Total Body Water 50
Clinical Use of Total Body Water Estimation and Modified Body Weights 51
Water Absorption 52
Plasma Volume 53
The Starling Principle and Microvessel Heterogeneity 54
   Exceptions to the No-Absorption Rule 55
   The Current Understanding of Starling Forces 56
   Starling Forces; Steady State Variations Versus Abrupt Disequilibrium 57
Interstitium and Lymphatics 57
   The Triphasic Interstitium; Collagen Phase 58
   The Triphasic Interstitium; Hyaluronan Gel Phase 59
   The Triphasic Interstitium; Aqueous Phase 59
   Gel Swelling Pressure 60
   Interstitial Starling Forces 60
Lymphatic Vascular System 61
Interstitial Fluid Dynamics 62
Lymphatics and the Interstitial Storage of Sodium 64
   Interstitial Fluid and Lymph in Critical Illness 65
Pulmonary Starling Forces and the Extravascular Lung Water 67
Cell Fluid and Extracellular Fluid 67
   Starling Forces Between Extracellular and Intracellular Fluids 67
   Maintenance of the Extracellular-Intracellular Solute Balance is Energy-Dependent 68
      Double Donnan Effect 68

T. Woodcock (✉)
Department of Critical Care, University Hospital Southampton, Southampton, UK

© The Author(s) 2024   47
M. L. N. G. Malbrain et al. (eds.), *Rational Use of Intravenous Fluids in Critically Ill Patients*, https://doi.org/10.1007/978-3-031-42205-8_2

Potassium and Magnesium Ions 69
Cell Volume Regulation and Intracranial Pressure 69
Cell Volume Regulation beyond the Brain 70
Hessels' Alternative Model of Water, Sodium and Potassium Distribution 71
Water Excretion 71
References 72

IFA Commentary (MLNGM)

In this chapter, we undertake a deep dive into the secrets of the different fluid spaces and learn about body composition. How many body compartments exist? This question can be dealt with in different ways, classically there are fat tissue—water—proteins—and minerals while water on its own is also distributed into four compartments: intracellular water—interstitial water—intravascular water—and transcellular, with extracellular water calculated as the sum of interstitial plus intravascular plus transcellular water content (Fig. 2.1). There is ongoing discussion about the different fluid spaces and there are traditionally four: the first or intravascular space—the second or interstitial space—the third or pleural and peritoneal space—and the fourth space or the transcellular fluid. And not to forget the lymphatic system. Each compartment or space is separated from each other and the surrounding fluids by specific cells and membranes and an endothelial glycocalyx layer surrounding the vascular space, which regulates fluid and electrolyte shifts and transport between different compartments, spaces and cells. The endothelial glycocalyx is a thin negatively charged proteinaceous mesh-like layer, a gel-like matrix that surrounds all vascular endothelium on the luminal surface. It is composed of membrane-bound glycoproteins and proteoglycans. It was previously thought to be inert but plays a key role in vascular integrity and function: the regulation of vascular permeability, endothelial anticoagulation and modulation of interactions between the endothelium and the vascular environment. Thus, it prevents the free movement of water and electrolytes. Disruption or degradation of the glycocalyx may be an important mediator of inflammation, oedema, sepsis syndromes and capillary leak syndromes. Therefore, in various surgical and disease states, the glycocalyx has the potential as a novel therapeutic target. These new insights gave birth to an updated version of the traditional Starling equation that incorporates the current understanding of the role of the endothelial glycocalyx in transvascular fluid filtration, also known as the Starling Principle. The traditional principle describes the fluid passage across the semipermeable capillary membrane, which is determined by the net result between hydrostatic and oncotic pressures such that the fluid leaves the capillary at the

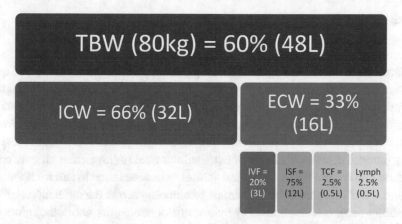

Fig. 2.1 Body water composition for an adult 80 kg male. *ECW* extracellular water, *ICW* intracellular water, *ISF* interstitial fluid, *IVF* intravascular fluid, *TBW* total body water, *TCF* transcellular fluid

arterial end of the capillary and is absorbed at the venous end of the capillary. The Revised or extended Starling Principle recognises that, because microvessels are permeable to macromolecules, a balance of pressures cannot halt fluid exchange. In most tissues, steady oncotic pressure differences between plasma and interstitial fluid depend on low levels of steady filtration from plasma to tissues for which the Revised Principle provides the theory [1].

Learning Objectives

After reading this chapter, you will:

1. Learn about interstitial fluid dynamics in order to manage clinical problems of fluid and albumin maldistribution.
2. Understand that lymphangions propel lymph flow, an active and vital part of the circulation of extracellular fluid and soluble proteins including albumin from capillary beds to the great veins.
3. Learn that the lymphatic and immune cell systems have an important role in the storage and release of sodium ions.
4. Understand that the relationship between intravenous sodium dose and oedema is not as clear cut as previously believed.
5. Comprehend that the separation of cytosol from extracellular fluid includes volume-regulated anion channels within cell membranes, enabling intracellular fluid volume to be maintained in the face of wide variations in extracellular fluid composition.
6. Know that the prescription of adequate amounts of potassium to patients is important.

Introduction

An appreciation of the distribution of water (the aqueous biological solvent) and its solutes is fundamental to understanding the physiology of body fluid spaces. The normal compartmentalisation of body water has been measured in various ways, and the decompartmentalisation seen in many critical illnesses is held to be an important pathophysiological phenomenon. Traditionally blood has been treated as an intravascular fluid circulation, while the lymphatic vessels have been called a drainage system. The modern view is of an actively pumped double circulation of extracellular fluid (intravascular plasma, and interstitial fluid and lymph) that enables vital solutes to be transferred to and from the intracellular fluid. Fluid flux across cell membrane barriers and across the different microvascular permeability barriers is determined by hydrostatic pressure differences and solute concentration gradients. Total body water volume is largely regulated by the pituitary hormonal effect of arginine vasopressin acting on vasopressin type 2 receptors in renal collecting ducts to retain or release water. In critical illness, arginine vasopressin deficiency predisposes patients to dilutional hyponatremia if the infused volume is larger than necessary or excessively prescribed as 'electrolyte-free water'. Body sodium is conserved by the renin–angiotensin–aldosterone axis regulating the degree of sodium reabsorption in renal distal tubules. Body sodium largely determines the proportion of body water that comprises extracellular fluid volume, but there is significant non-osmotic sodium storage capacity in the interstitium, particularly in the interstitium of the skin, which may have clinical relevance. In addition, volume-regulated anion channels enable cells to discharge osmotic molecules to the interstitium to protect intracellular fluid volume when body water tonicity is low. Balancing the body's potassium (mostly intracellular) with sodium (mostly extracellular) depends on an adequate availability of magnesium. Rapid extracellular fluid osmolality changes can dangerously disturb the intracellular–extracellular fluid equilibrium, so awareness of the major contributors to plasma osmolality is essential. However, evidence from surgical practice suggests that adaptive mechanisms exist to stabilise the intracellular volume in the face of excessive intravenous fluid infusions, and an alternative model of body water response to intravenous infusions is proposed. See also Chap. 3 for the second part on fluid physiology.

Total Body Water

The deuterium nuclear magnetic resonance (^{2}H NMR) is a modern method that has been validated for the determination of total body water in humans. The ^{2}H NMR method has advantages over other techniques based on ^{2}H$_2$O dilution. It is fast, accurate, needs only a small dose of ^{2}H$_2$O, and can be done using any body fluid [2]. Total body water data from the Fels Longitudinal Study (1999) suggest that the average white American woman has around 30 kg of total body water contributing to her body weight of 65–75 kg, while the average white American man has around 42–44 kg of total body water contributing to his body weight of 75–93 kg [3]. Bioimpedance spectroscopy (BIS) and multifrequency bio-impedance analysis (MFBIA) are alternative research technologies [4]. Direct measurement of body water has yet to find a role in the clinical diagnosis of dehydration [5].

Most tissues contain 70–80% water, the exceptions being bone and adipose tissue at 10–20%. The major contributors to variation in an individual's total body water to weight are muscle mass (high in water content) and adiposity (fat is low in water content). This explains why females and older individuals typically have a lower percentage of total body water to body weight and may be more prone to disorders of tonicity. As a rule of thumb, the total body water can be estimated as 50% of body weight. In very muscular adults, total body water may be greater than the average. For greater precision, there are a number of anthropomorphic equations for the calculation of total body water. The Watson formula for total body water was derived from and validated on several hundreds of patients. It uses height, weight, age and gender:

- Women Total body water = −2.097 + 0.1069 × Height + 0.2466 × Weight.
- Men Total body water = 2.447 − 0.09156 × Age + 0.1074 × Height + 0.3362 × Weight

.

Clinical Use of Total Body Water Estimation and Modified Body Weights

The rational fluid prescriber is greatly assisted by an estimate of the patient's total body water to make measured decisions about solvent/solute imbalances and the doses of fluid and/or electrolytes needed to correct them. Total body water estimates are also needed to decide the appropriate doses of hydrophilic drugs. For non-obese patients, total body water is proportionate to body weight, but with increasing obesity the utility of body weight as a scalar of total body water and cardiac output diminishes; the excess weight is predominantly fat rather than water and takes little of the cardiac output. Anaesthetic muscle relaxant drugs and antibiotics are hydrophilic and the preferred scalar of dose should logically be total body water. In anaesthetic practice, the recommended dose of hydrophilic drugs such as non-depolarising muscle relaxants is usually scaled to body weight for the non-obese, and to the ideal body weight for obese patients. The Devine formula is widely used:

- Women: Ideal Body Weight (in kilograms) = 45.5 + 2.3 kg/in. over 5 ft.
- Men: Ideal Body Weight (in kilograms) = 50 + 2.3 kg/in. over 5 ft.

Ideal body weight is the best-adjusted weight for following total body water. It is reasonable to presume that the volume of distribution of urea is the total body water and thereby be able to titrate haemofiltration or haemodialysis prescription by ideal body weight to the desired rate of change of urea concentration or to clear other toxins.

An **estimated lean body mass** formula (eLBM) for the normalisation of body fluid volumes was proposed in 1984, the Boer formula [6].

- Women: eLBM = 0.252W + 0.473H − 48.3.
- Men: eLBM = 0.407W + 0.267H − 19.2.

The Peters formula has been proposed for use in anaesthesia and critical care of boys and girls 14 years or younger. The formula first calculates the estimated extracellular fluid volume and then derives the eLBM [7].

- Estimated extracellular fluid volume (eECV) = $0.0215 \times W^{0.6469} \times H^{0.7236}$.
- eLBM = 3.8 × eECV.

Estimated lean body mass is the best scalar of cardiac output in obese patients and is therefore the preferred scalar of the induction dose of hypnotic agents such as di-isopropyl phenol or thiopentone sodium and for the initial dosing of intravenous opiates such as fentanyl and remifentanil. Notice however that these agents are lipophilic and so the measured body weight is the appropriate scalar for setting the steady-state rate of maintenance infusion, even in obese patients.

Tidal volume recommendations for pulmonary ventilation are given in mL/kg **predicted body weight** (PBW), a parameter calculated from height and gender as height most closely predicts normal lung volumes in men and women [8]. In emergency situations when body weight has not been measured or recorded, predicted body weight can rapidly be estimated from height and gender to guide fluid therapy and drug dosing.

Water Absorption

Water is absorbed into the body from the intestinal lumen across the intestinal epithelial membrane and absorption is influenced by luminal osmolality, solute absorption and the anatomical structures of the intestine [9]. Epithelial cells pump intracellular sodium via membrane-bound sodium potassium ATP-ase into the mucosal interstitium, enabling an isosmotic diffusion of water from the lumen into the epithelial cell and thence into the mucosal interstitial fluid. For as long as the epithelium is secreting salt and water to the interstitium, the mucosal capillaries and venules can continue in a steady state of fluid absorption to the plasma. These are diaphragm-fenestrated capillaries, specialised to permit high transendothelial absorption rates. The fenestrations are 10–30 nm wide and formed by the condensation of the luminal and abluminal endothelial cell membranes. They support a diaphragm that functions as a low-resistance filtration/absorption barrier.

Figure 2.2 illustrates the absorption pathway from the intestinal lumen to the plasma. Some interstitial fluid is also removed by lymphatic pumping. Should intestinal water absorption dry up, the epithelial secretion of solvent and small solutes that provides an

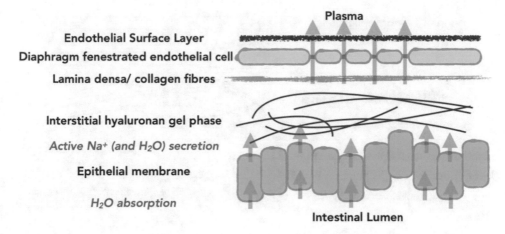

Fig. 2.2 The absorption pathway from intestinal lumen to plasma

exception to the Michel–Weinbaum model of steady-state fluid filtration also ceases, so that microvascular steady-state filtration of plasma solvent to the tissues without reabsorption is restored and gastro-intestinal fluid loss is prevented.

The other tissue microvascular beds in which we find diaphragm-fenestrated capillaries for the absorption of interstitial fluid include exocrine glands, renal peritubular, endocrine glands, peripheral ganglia, nerve epineurium, circumventricular organs, choroid plexus and the ciliary process of the eye.

Plasma Volume

Plasma volume is a critical care concept rather than an anatomic entity. It is often measured as the volume of distribution of an indicator dye such as Evans Blue or radio-labelled albumin, spaces which are substantially larger than the calculated intravascular erythrocyte dilution volume. When reading clinical studies that report plasma volume, it is helpful to bear in mind what has actually been measured or calculated. Broadly, the normal circulating plasma volume is around 2.5–3.0 L at sea level in men and falls by 15–20% with a sojourn to high-altitude living. The circulating plasma contains around 2 L of blood cells (mostly erythrocytes), giving a circulating blood volume at sea level of about 4.5 L [10]. The third contributor to the total intravascular volume is the slower-moving fluid within the endothelial glycocalyx layer, which has been estimated to be as much as 1.5 L in healthy adults or as little as a few hundred milli litres in a variety of cardiovascular disease states [11, 12]. For our approximation we can call it 0.5 L, giving a total intravascular volume of about 5 L at sea level.

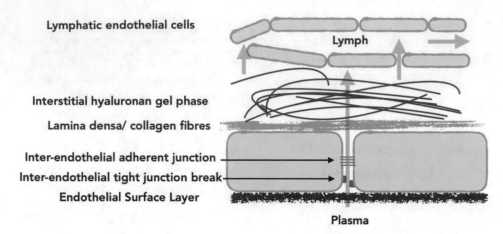

Fig. 2.3 The paracellular (inter endothelial cleft) fluid filtration pathway of continuous capillaries

The circulatory flow rate of blood (Q_t) is supported by the elastic recoil of venules and small veins on the post-capillary blood volume. The venular filling pressure of around 18 mmHg provides a gradient down to the central venous pressure, which is kept close to zero by the healthy heart. The ventricles fill during diastole from the venous excess volume, and the flow to the ventricle is kept nearly constant by the contraction of the atrium. The ventricles eject blood against an afterload that raises the pressure of blood within pulmonary and systemic arteries for distribution to the tissues [13].

Critical care practitioners fear reduced plasma volume with consequent reduced Q_t. They place wide-bore catheters within large veins for 'access' by which to administer vital medicines, and to allow the infusion of 'resuscitation' fluids. In most critical care patients, the intravenous route is the predominant source of fluid input.

The fluid leaves the circulating plasma volume by transendothelial microvascular filtration to the extravascular extracellular fluid of the perfused tissue or organ [14]. Figure 2.3 illustrates the paracellular (inter endothelial cleft) fluid filtration pathway of continuous capillaries.

Traditional clinical teaching has too often ignored the Starling principle and the heterogeneity of the permeability barriers in tissues and organs, which we consider next.

The Starling Principle and Microvessel Heterogeneity

The idea that a single capillary could simultaneously filter fluid from plasma to the interstitial fluid and absorb it back again was always difficult to believe and had never been seen in laboratory experiments. The diagram showing a declining sum of hydrostatic and osmotic pressure differences from the arteriolar entry to the venular exit of a capillary, with flow reversal as the osmotic pressure difference exceeds the hydrostatic pressure difference, has been called The Diagram to Forget. The capillaries of sinusoidal organs such as liver, spleen and bone marrow receive 25–30% of the left ventricular output via the hepatic artery and portal vein. The splanchnic microvessels are very 'leaky' indeed. They have a discontinuous endothelial surface layer that allows proteins to pass freely in either direction through transendothelial fenestrae and through interendothelial junction gaps so that no osmotic pressure gradient can occur. In such tissues, the unopposed hydrostatic pressure difference ensures that only transendothelial fluid filtration occurs.

In non-sinusoidal tissues, the endothelial surface layer is continuous and largely impermeable to proteins. The paracellular endothelial barrier here presents a layered structure that depends on a continuous activation of signalling pathways regulated by sphingosine-1-phosphate (S1P) and intracellular cAMP. The layers are

- The glycocalyx and its endothelial surface layer
- The junction breaks (or gaps) of the tight junction strand
- The adherens junction

Solvent and small solutes first pass through the resistance of the endothelial surface layer. The greater resistance occurs where fluid is jetted though infrequent slit-like interendothelial tight junction breaks to the interendothelial cleft. The adherens junction provides a third, variable resistance to the paracellular flow of filtrate [15].

Plasma proteins are concentrated on the intravascular aspect of the endothelial surface layer and the filtrate entering the interendothelial cleft is almost protein-free. Soluble interstitial proteins diffuse into the post-glycocalyx solvent filtrate, and the protein concentration in the fluid of the interendothelial clefts will therefore depend on the rates at which the solvent from the plasma filtrate and protein from the interstitium enter the cleft. At high filtration rates, the protein concentration (and colloid osmotic pressure) in the cleft is low, but as the transendothelial filtration rate falls the protein concentration (and colloid osmotic pressure) in the interendothelial cleft rises. The dependence of the colloid osmotic pressure Starling force on the solvent filtration rate within a subglycocalyx 'protected region' of the general interstitial fluid thus ensures that the osmotic forces oppose but, at steady state, do not reverse the flow of the filtrate. This is the Michel–Weinbaum Model, confirmed by experiments published in 2004.

Exceptions to the No-Absorption Rule

We have, however, already mentioned an exception to the steady-state filtration rule in the intestinal mucosal microvasculature. A supply of protein-free solvent to the interstitium by an adjacent secreting epithelium keeps the interstitial colloid osmotic pressure low so that the colloid osmotic pressure difference that drives fluid absorption can be sustained. Similar conditions are found in the peritubular capillaries of the renal cortex and the ascending vasa recta of the renal medulla, which are in a continuous state of absorption of interstitial fluid because it is continuously secreted by the renal tubular epithelium. In lymph nodes, the interstitial fluid is continuously replenished by the flow of the prenodal lymph with a low protein concentration.

We know that fluids (and water-soluble medicines) injected into the subcutaneous tissue or muscle are rapidly absorbed because the injected volume creates a local exception to the Michel–Weinbaum Model. If Starling's nineteenth century experiments on the absorption of infused fluids from a dog's leg are to be criticised, we can point to his failure to notice that he was creating an artefactual exception, a low-protein lacuna of injected fluid within the interstitium.

Such exceptions aside, in the microcirculation of most tissues the reabsorption of filtered fluid occurs only transiently and only after a substantial disequilibrium of the Starling forces. Tissue fluid balance thus depends critically on the circulation of extracellular fluid through the interstitium and the efficiency of lymphatic pumping in most tissues. Herein, the clinician finds rational approaches to manipulating the distribution of extracellular fluid. Plasma volume can be preserved, and interstitial fluid volume reduced, by reducing the transendothelial solvent filtration rate and by enhancing lymphatic pumping of high protein fluid to the great veins. Biophysical colloid osmotic pressure therapy was once liberally used to support the plasma volume, but advances in physiology and pathophysiology now explain the limitations of that approach.

The Current Understanding of Starling Forces

Capillary hydrostatic pressure P_c is the main driving force of transendothelial solvent filtration (J_v) from plasma to the interstitium. In congestive states elevated P_c increases J_v and oedema ensues if it is not matched by increased lymph flow. Hypovolaemia reduces P_c so that J_v approaches zero; or put another way, fluid cannot leave the hypovolaemic circulation. The clinician can protect the plasma volume by avoiding transient peaks of high P_c by using smaller bolus doses of intravenous fluid. An infusion of the arteriolar constrictor norepinephrine will also protect against increased P_c and J_v. The optimal norepinephrine dose for the arteriolar effect on P_c is less than the dose that raises arterial pressure [11].

Interstitial hydrostatic pressure P_i falls in the first stages of inflammation because of molecular conformational changes in the biomatrix and enhanced lymphatic pumping, and greatly increases J_v before there is any change in capillary permeability.

Plasma colloid osmotic pressure Π_p is by far the largest Starling force at play, but its influence on J_v is modified by the dependence of the subglycocalyx colloid osmotic pressure Π_g on J_v. As J_v falls, Π_g rises and the colloid osmotic pressure difference ($\Pi_p - \Pi_g$) cannot sustain negative J_v (absorption) for more than about 30 min.

The general interstitial fluid colloid osmotic pressure Π_i is now known to have no direct effect on J_v. Interstitial proteins play their part in regulating J_v by diffusing into interendothelial clefts and varying Π_g.

The net rate of solvent filtration from the plasma to interstitium (excluding the glomerular filtration of more than 100 mL/min) is normally just a few mL/min, averaging 0.3–0.4 L/h or 8 L/day. Evidence from the data of Robert Hahn's fluid kinetic studies suggests that under the extreme disequilibrium of rapid isotonic salt solution infusion (50 mL/min), J_v in patients can transiently approach 25–30 mL/min [16].

Starling Forces; Steady State Variations Versus Abrupt Disequilibrium

Clinical researchers who claim to have discredited the Michel–Weinbaum account of the steady-state Starling principle fail to understand that an abrupt change in a Starling force can, if large enough, result in a transient reversal of transendothelial solvent flow. Acute reduction in capillary hydrostatic pressure or acute elevation of plasma colloid osmotic pressure can result in the absorption of interstitial fluid into the plasma. The well-recognised phenomenon is called autotransfusion, and in adults could be as much as 0.5 L. It is, however, soon followed by a return to steady-state filtration. Pulmonary microcirculation is an obvious example for the clinician of steady-state filtration sustained even at low capillary pressures.

Interstitium and Lymphatics

It has long been appreciated that, at a steady state, the quantity and pressure of the extracellular fluid are just as important in determining plasma volume as is the quantity of plasma protein. A decrease in the volume of the circulating red blood cells is normally compensated by an increase in plasma volume, and an increase in the volume of the circulating red cells is compensated by a decrease in plasma volume. The infusion of hyperosmotic albumin solution causes a transient rise in plasma volume, and the removal of plasma protein causes a temporary decrease in plasma volume. The changes in plasma volume produced by varying the amount of circulating plasma protein are not permanent in normal subjects because the body is able to add protein to the bloodstream or remove it. When the blood volume is raised by the addition of protein, the body withdraws protein from the circulation. When the volume is decreased by lowering the quantity of the circulating protein, the body adds protein to the bloodstream. In conditions of increased body water, the plasma volume rises while plasma protein concentration falls [17].

Extracellular fluid circulates. In health the skeletal muscles (female or male) account for 2.2 or 3.5 L, connective tissues 2.4 or 3.0 L, skin 2.0 or 3.0 L, adipose tissue 2.0 or 1.6 L and nervous system 1.4 and 1.5 L. In either sex, there is roughly a litre of fluid in each of the bone, bone marrow and transcellular spaces. The water in the adipose tissue is predominantly extracellular, so the proportion of total body water that is extracellular tends to be higher in women and in the obese. In morbid obesity, 50–60% of the total body water may be extracellular.

The basement membrane, where it exists, is a specialised part of the extracellular matrix 60–100 nm in thickness, composed of type IV collagen and laminin and closely adherent to the cell membrane. It imposes some resistance to the circulation of extracellular fluid as it leaves the interendothelial cleft and enters the interstitium.

The interstitium is the extracellular matrix within which reside tissue parenchymal cells. It accounts for about one-sixth of the total body volume. The perivascular extracellular matrix forms an organ-specific vascular niche that orchestrates mechano-, growth factor and angiocrine signalling required for tissue homeostasis and organ repair. The composition of the interstitium is controlled by the regulation of synthesis and turnover of each of its individual components, driven by cytokines and growth factors [18]. Around half of the total body albumin is circulating through the interstitium at any one time, and this proportion increases in critical illness as the transendothelial albumin transfer rate from plasma to interstitium increases. This accelerated transfer of albumin is the major cause of post-surgical or post-traumatic hypoalbuminaemia.

Interstitial fluid traverses three 'phases' of the interstitium. The fact of an extravascular circulation of extracellular fluid draws our attention to the way interstitium channels the flow. The major structural elements of the interstitium are collagen fibre bundles, which are visible to light microscopy and can extend for long distances. Probe-based confocal laser endomicroscopy (pCLE) is an in vivo imaging technology that provides real-time histologic assessment of tissue structures in patients. The technology has recently been used to visualise the interstitium of the gastrointestinal tract and urinary bladder submucosae, the dermis, peri-bronchial and peri-arterial soft tissues and fascia. The interstitial space is generally defined by a complex lattice of thick collagen bundles that are intermittently lined on one side by fibroblast-like cells that can be stained with endothelial cell markers. These cell-lined collagen bundles channel the circulation of interstitial fluid.

The Triphasic Interstitium; Collagen Phase

For the purposes of understanding interstitial water disposition, the interstitium has been described as triphasic [19]. The collagen triple helix consists of three intertwined polypeptide chains that entangle water molecules, a property called collagen hydration. Collagen fibre bundles can therefore be considered one of the interstitial aqueous phases. Collagen bundles of several interstitial spaces have been reported to be associated with thin, flat cells (spindle-shaped in cross section) that have scant cytoplasm and an oblong nucleus, and express the transmembrane phosphoglycoprotein CD34. These cells lack the ultrastructural features of endothelial differentiation yet appear to channel the flow of interstitial fluid [20]. Endothelial cell membrane-bound integrins can act upon collagen fibrils in the adjacent (perivascular) extracellular matrix, exposing glycosaminoglycans (GAGs) to take up water and thereby lower the interstitial pressure.

The Triphasic Interstitium; Hyaluronan Gel Phase

The interstitial gel phase is largely composed of coiled and twisted proteoglycan filaments, barely visible on electron microscopy but holding 99% of the interstitial water in association with glycosaminoglycans, mostly hyaluronan. Hyaluronan restricts the movement of water and forms a diffusion barrier that regulates the transport of substances through intercellular spaces. Hyaluronan takes part in the partitioning of plasma proteins between vascular and extravascular spaces, and creates the excluded volume phenomenon that affects the solubility of macromolecules in the interstitium, changes chemical equilibria, and stabilises the structure of collagen fibres. Interstitial water and solutes of the gel phase occupy the spaces within the proteoglycan/ hyaluronan matrix. The effective radius of these spaces, known as their hydraulic radius, is as small as 3 nm in cartilage and up to 300 nm in the vitreous body of the eye. The hydraulic radius of a matrix determines its resistance to the flow of solvent and solutes through that part of the interstitium. The Wharton's Jelly of the umbilical cord is an open and loosely organised matrix with a hydraulic radius of about 30 nm and is a good example of the gel nature of the interstitium. The interstitial gel restricts water mobility and so stabilises tissue shape. It also prevents interstitial fluid displacement by gravity and slows the spread of organisms such as bacteria. Interstitial hyaluronan washout when lymph flow is raised during systemic inflammation could well contribute to elevated plasma hyaluronan concentrations which are most commonly attributed to disturbance of the endothelial glycocalyx.

Toll-like receptors are found within the extracellular matrix and are believed to have a pivotal role in the early development of systemic inflammatory response and ventilator-induced lung injury. Integrins and their receptors modulate cell locomotion through the extracellular matrix, and can also modulate the interstitial pressure.

The Triphasic Interstitium; Aqueous Phase

Around 1% of interstitial water is normally within a gel-free phase through which water can flow alongside collagen fibre bundles with their associated CD34+ interstitial cells. This space appears microscopically as fluid vesicles and rivulets. The proportion of the gel-free water phase is increased in interstitial oedema, and in the most severe cases up to 50%. Interstitial gel-free solvents and solutes are drawn into collecting lymphatics in order to complete the circulation of interstitial fluid.

Gel Swelling Pressure

GAGs attract water molecules and confer the ability of the interstitial gel phase to swell by taking up water. The gel swelling pressure is defined as the subatmospheric pressure that precisely balances the suction effect of the interstitial GAGs, and is an osmotic pressure largely due to sodium ions attracted by the fixed negative charges—the Gibbs–Donnan effect. Many tissues maintain a subatmospheric interstitial fluid pressure in health because the GAGs are normally under-saturated with water. The lymphatic system maintains this state of under-saturation by pumping fluid away from the gel phase of the interstitium into the aqueous lymph. Reduction of the pumping capacity of the lymphatic system therefore predisposes to fluid retention and oedema.

In collagen-rich tissues such as the skin, the swelling tendency of the interstitial matrix is further counteracted by tissue fibroblasts which tension the collagen fibrils under the regulation of collagen-binding integrins at the cell membrane contact points. The tension of collagen fibres restricts the swelling of GAGs. Collagen-binding integrins only have a limited role in adult connective tissue homeostasis because of the relative paucity of cell-binding sites in the mature fibrillar collagen matrices. Their importance may be greater in connective tissue remodelling, such as wound healing. The skin has been recognised to hold a substantial non-osmotic store of sodium within its interstitium, with a regulatory role in salt and water homeostasis.

Interstitial Starling Forces

Aqueous interstitial fluid can be harvested from nylon wicks implanted subcutaneously, for instance in the arm and leg. In a study of anaesthetised children, the mean plasma colloid osmotic pressure was 26 mmHg while the sampled interstitial fluid colloid osmotic pressure was about 14 mmHg. Albumin is largely excluded from the interstitial gel phase and the collagen phase but is present in the free-flowing interstitial aqueous phase and in the lymph within lymphatic vessels. Water and small solutes (Na^+, Cl^-, and urea) move easily between aqueous and gel phases, and between intracellular fluid and extracellular fluid according to prevailing osmotic, hydrostatic and electrochemical forces. The presence of proteins will affect the viscosity of the flow and accumulation of water in hypoproteinaemic oedematous conditions. As interstitial fluid accumulates and the aqueous phase expands relative to the gel phase, this mechanism becomes increasingly relevant.

Interstitial fluid volume, and so pressure, varies from tissue to tissue and with the rate of fluid exchange. Integrin activation and subsequent conformational changes to collagen allow the GAGs to become hydrated. This brings about an acute reduction in interstitial fluid pressure in inflammatory conditions, increasing the transendothelial pressure difference and thereby increasing J_v by as much as 20-fold independently of other causes of capillary leak.

Water absorption from the gut lumen is associated with the increased mucosal intersti-tial fluid pressure that promotes water transfer to the plasma by fenestrated mucosal capil-laries. Fluid secretion, for instance by endocrine and salivary glands, reduces their interstitial pressure and so increases transendothelial filtration to supply the water needed to continue the secretion. The matrix compressive effect of fibroblasts via collagen-binding integrins has only a limited effect on the regulation of interstitial fluid pressure.

Lymphatic Vascular System

St George's Hospital surgeon William Hunter demonstrated the role of lymphatics in absorbing tissue fluids to the bloodstream in the mid-eighteenth century, yet in clinical teaching today the role of the lymphatic vascular system is often misrepresented by calling it a drainage system. The lymphatic system pumps fluid from tissues and returns it to blood vessels. Lymphatics also transport lymphocytes and dendritic cells to the lymphoid organs. The lymphatic system vasculature consists of thin-walled capillaries and larger vessels that are lined by endothelial cells [21]. There are unique lymphatic markers that differentiate lymph vessels from blood vessels. These include Prox1, a transcription factor required for programming the phenotype of the lymphatic endothelial cell, and LYVE-1, a CD44 homologue. Vascular endothelial growth factor receptor 3 is a receptor for vascular endothelial growth factors (VEGF) C and D, and is not detected in blood vascular endo-thelial cells. VEGF-C and VEGF-D regulate lymphangiogenesis by activating VEGFR-3, a cell-surface tyrosine kinase receptor, leading to the initiation of a downstream signalling cascade.

The afferent lymphatic vessels are of two types, initial and collecting. They differ ana-tomically (i.e. the presence or absence of surrounding smooth muscle cells and semilunar lymphatic valves), in their expression pattern of adhesion molecules and in their permis-siveness to fluid and cell entry. A lymphangion is defined as the functional unit of a lymph vessel that lies between two lymphatic valves.

The afferent lymphatics deliver around 8 L of lymph to lymph nodes per day. The col-loid osmotic pressure of lymph is substantially lower than Π_p and its continuous delivery to the lymph node creates a Starling principle exception, allowing the absorption of sol-vent to the plasma, about 4 L/day, to be sustained. The remaining 4 L/day of lymph pro-ceed to the efferent system.

Efferent lymphatic vessels conduct lymph away from lymph nodes, to further lymph nodes or the lymphatic trunks. They also feature semilunar valves to ensure one-way flow and an investment of smooth muscle to pump the contained fluid. The right and left lumbar trunks and the intestinal trunk constitute the cisterna chyli. The left lymphatic duct, more often called the thoracic duct when seen in the chest, originates on the 12th thoracic ver-tebra from the confluence of the right and left lumbar trunks, then traverses the diaphragm at the aortic aperture and ascends the superior and posterior mediastinum between the descending thoracic aorta and the azygos vein. The left lymphatic duct averages about

5 mm diameter as it passes behind the left carotid artery and left internal jugular vein at the fifth thoracic vertebral level and drains into the venous angle of the left subclavian and internal jugular veins. There are two valves at the junction of the duct with the left subclavian vein that prevent the flow of venous blood into the duct when central venous pressure exceeds thoracic duct lymph pressure. Efferent lymph from the right thorax, right arm, head and neck is conducted by the smaller right lymphatic duct.

The terminal section of the thoracic duct can be examined at the bedside by 2D ultrasound using high-resolution linear probes (7–12 MHz). Anatomic variations were noted in 27% of subjects in a clinical series of several hundred patients. The normal thoracic duct diameter is about 2.5 mm, independent of the subjects' age. The diameter is substantially increased in subjects with congestive heart failure and liver cirrhosis. Dynamic imaging of the chyle flow and valve function was possible. This technology holds promise for future clinical research [22].

A non-muscular lymphatic endothelial vessel network in the dura mater of the mouse brain was discovered by researchers in Helsinki. The dural lymphatic vessels absorb cerebrospinal fluid from the adjacent subarachnoid space and brain interstitial fluid via the glymphatic system described by Iliff [23]. The traditional view of cerebrospinal fluid (CSF) circulation is that it is produced in the choroid plexus, flows slowly through the subarachnoid space, and is reabsorbed by arachnoid villi or around spinal nerves. In the new paradigm, CSF is a fluid with tightly controlled chemical constituents that flows rapidly around the subarachnoid space and through the brain and spinal cord tissue, fulfilling a role similar to the lymphatic system in other organs. A significant portion of CSF enters the brain via para-vascular spaces (Virchow–Robin spaces) that surround penetrating arteries and arterioles (periarterial spaces). The fluid then leaves the brain via peri-venular spaces. This fluid flow is facilitated at least in part by aquaporins in the end feet of astrocytes, which surround the brain vasculature and form a key component of the blood–brain barrier. Functional lymphatic tissue has been found lining the dural sinuses, which conduct fluid into deep cervical lymph nodes via foramina at the base of the skull, where solvent and small solutes can be absorbed to lymph node venules while efferent lymph flows to the right thoracic duct.

The renal medulla has no lymphatic vessels. Fluid that is absorbed from the collecting ducts into the renal medullary interstitium must therefore be continuously absorbed into the bloodstream by the ascending vasa recta capillaries. It has been demonstrated that labelled albumin is cleared from the medullary interstitium directly into the blood, and it has been calculated that the convective flow of large solutes can account for this efficient clearance.

Interstitial Fluid Dynamics

Intrinsic lymphatic pumping is regulated by four major factors: preload, afterload, spontaneous contraction frequency and contractility. The similarity to the Frank–Starling relationship for the heart is obvious.

- **Preload** is the end-diastolic pressure (or volume) within the valved muscular lymphangion. Increasing the 'filling pressure' over a physiologic range increases the **amplitude of contraction** and so enhances pump output.
- **Afterload**: The lymphatic pump must adapt to elevated outflow pressures resulting from partial outflow obstruction, increased central venous pressure and/or gravitational shifts. Lymphangions in series can propel lymph against higher pressures than individual lymphangions.
- **Contraction frequency** of collecting lymphatics is exquisitely sensitive to pressure, and changes as small as 0.5 cm H_2O can double the contraction frequency.
- **Contractility** is often used in the lymphatic context to describe the enhancement of amplitude or frequency of contraction in response to a pressure increase or agonist activation. The cardiac parallel is the concept of inotropy and inotropic agents.

There are of course extrinsic pump mechanisms operative in vivo. Leg muscles, for example, contribute significantly to the energy expended on pumping lymph to the inguinal, femoral and iliac lymph nodes. Lymph flow in the thoracic duct is supported by the cycle of breathing. The thoracic duct smooth muscle is capable of contracting with sufficient force to propel lymph towards the jugular venous junction at 1–3 mL/min which is just about sufficient to move the normal daily efferent lymph volume of around 4 L.

Lymphatic muscle contractions, like cardiac muscle contractions, can occur spontaneously, but in health, they are subject to neural modulation. Sympathetic adrenergic nerve fibres appear to be the dominant neural innervation of the lymphatic vasculature. α-adrenergic stimulation of contractile lymphatic vessels consistently increases tone, amplitude and frequency, while β-adrenergic receptor activation decreases them. Substance P, commonly associated with afferent nerve endings, augments tone and increases frequency. Muscarinic receptors promote an increase in frequency, but the inhibitory effect of endothelial nitric oxide synthase (eNOS) activation seems to be predominant. Mu receptor agonists such as endorphins and morphine reduce the spontaneous contractility of smooth muscle everywhere. Serotonin (5-HT) can either inhibit or increase spontaneous lymphatic contractions depending on the species and the state of serotonin receptor expression. Other inhibitory factors include vasoactive intestinal peptides and calcitonin gene-related peptides.

Contraction synchrony within a lymphangion generates a systolic pressure pulse that can open the outflow valve and eject lymph. Lymphatic contractions are triggered by an action potential achieved in a pacemaker lymphatic microvascular cell, and the action potential propagates rapidly from cell to cell over the length of the lymphangion. Electrical coupling between the cells is presumably through connexins that form intercellular gap junctions. Application of gap-junction blockers in mesenteric lymphatic vessel segments leads to uncoordinated contractions.

Valve function is critical. Collecting lymphatics contain bicuspid (semilunar) valves whose leaflets extend from a ring-shaped base and insert into the vessel wall. The valve opening is a tapered funnel. A dilated sinus downstream from the valve facilitates valve opening and partially balances the high resistance of the narrow orifice created by the valve leaflets. Valves are spaced at semi-regular intervals, and the factors that control their spacing are not known.

Barrier function of lymphatic vessels was once disregarded, presuming they were impermeable to fluid and solute. More recent analyses of collecting lymphatic endothelial junction proteins reveal no major differences from those of blood vessels. Collecting lymphatics are not only permeable to solute and fluid, their albumin permeability is comparable to that of post-capillary venules. Like venules, lymphatic permeability is actively regulated because it can be modified by several signalling pathways, including nitric oxide. Lymphatic capillaries are an order of magnitude more permeable than collecting lymphatic microvessels, most likely due to their discontinuous pattern of junctional adhesion proteins, facilitating fluid and solute absorption from the interstitium.

Lymphatic contractile dysfunction is often contingent on inflammatory states such as trauma, sepsis, burns and even major surgery. It is a likely contributor to the accumulation of interstitial fluid or oedema seen in these conditions.

Lymphatics and the Interstitial Storage of Sodium

It has long been taught that body sodium content directly determines the extracellular fluid volume and therefore the effective circulating fluid volume. Long-term blood pressure regulation, it was taught, relies on renal mechanisms to retain or excrete sodium in order to keep the effective circulating fluid volume within very narrow margins of equilibrium. Clinicians therefore use isotonic salt solutions to resuscitate patients with reduced effective circulating fluid volume (hypovolaemia) and are cautioned that excessive sodium administration must cause oedema. Recent investigations in humans confirm animal laboratory evidence that some sodium is in fact stored within the body without commensurate water. This phenomenon was observed with salt solution infusions in surgical patients as long ago as 1986. Indeed, it appears that electrolyte homeostasis in the body cannot be achieved by renal excretion alone, and involves extrarenal regulatory mechanisms such as this. The sodium store is now shown to be an interstitial reservoir that buffers the free extracellular sodium and is regulated by extrarenal, tissue-specific mechanisms for the release and storage of sodium. Immune cells from the mononuclear phagocyte system, including macrophages and dendritic cells, are the local sensors of interstitial electrolyte concentration. The major anatomic site of this sodium regulation is the interstitium of the skin, with its substantial volume of interstitial fluid and lymphatic vasculature forming a vessel network that can be expanded or reduced according to long-term sodium intake. Skin macrophages and lymphatics are now known to act in concert as systemic regulators of body fluid volume and long-term blood pressure. Interstitial electrolyte concentrations are higher than in blood, and macrophages regulate local interstitial electrolyte composition via a tonicity-responsive enhancer-binding protein which induces vascular endothelial growth factor (VEGF-C) production as tonicity rises. Acting on VEGF Receptor 3, VEGF-C stimulates lymphangiogenesis to extend the capillary network and enhance the capacity for interstitial fluid clearance. At the same time, VEGF-C stimulates VEGF Receptor 2 on blood capillaries promoting endogenous nitric oxide synthesis and increasing local blood flow. Free sodium ions are thus presented via the bloodstream for renal excretion and the extracellular space is protected from major sodium-induced fluid volume fluctuations [24].

A recent study has shown that fluid leaving the skin as lymph is isosmotic to plasma, even after a high sodium intake, but raises the possibility that the skin can differentially control its electrolyte microenvironment by creating local gradients that may be functionally important [25].

To investigate the effects of sodium intake on the endothelial surface layer, 12 healthy male volunteers were randomised to low sodium (less than 50 mmol/day) or high sodium (more than 200 mmol/day) diets for 8 days. There was no measurable effect on arterial pressure, perfused boundary region (endothelial surface layer thickness) or glycosaminoglycan excretion. Body weight increased by around 2.5 kg with high salt intake, suggesting an extracellular volume expansion. Plasma volume measured by the central volume of distribution of radiolabelled albumin was unaffected. Subjects who had followed a low sodium diet were then given 540 mL of 2.4% (hypertonic) sodium chloride as an acute sodium load. This challenge increased the volume of distribution of albumin by 250 mL and increased the transcapillary escape rate of albumin from 7% to 10% per hour. There was no acute effect on arterial pressure or perfused boundary region. The authors' interpretation of their data was that acute intravenous sodium loading was associated with increased microvascular permeability, suggesting functional damage to the endothelial surface layer, but there are other plausible interpretations, including a natriuretic peptide effect. In the same experiment plasma sodium concentration at the end of hypertonic saline infusion was as predicted by standard sodium kinetics, but 4 h later had decreased by 1.8 mmol/L against a predicted fall of less than 1 mmol/L. The authors therefore concluded that healthy individuals are able to osmotically inactivate significant amounts of sodium after hypertonic saline infusion.

Interstitial Fluid and Lymph in Critical Illness

Cope and Litwin (1962) were perhaps the first to demonstrate that fluid absorption to the plasma after acute haemorrhage (reduced capillary pressure) did not fully explain the observed restoration of plasma volume [26]. That volume largely came from a rise in thoracic duct lymph flow, and over the following 24 h lymph flow had returned about twice the amount of protein that had been lost by haemorrhage. They called this phenomenon 'the essentiality of the lymphatic system to the recovery from shock'. Plasma volume refill after blood loss was measured in the 1960s, but is rarely considered in current teaching. Values of 1 mL/min or more imply that the efferent lymph flow is at least doubled during plasma volume refill. Robert Demling in Boston made important contributions to the pathophysiology of oedema [27]. We see in his work an appreciation of the abrupt disequilibrium of Starling forces moving to a steady state. His laboratory demonstrated that a marked increase in fluid flux after sustained protein depletion is unrelated to colloid osmotic pressure. They drew attention to the possible contribution of decreasing viscosity of the interstitial matrix leading to a more rapid interstitial fluid accumulation. The surgical research team in Denver, Colorado, have developed a hypothesis that mesenteric ischaemia/reperfusion primes polymorphonuclear leucocytes which can then be provoked, for example by endotoxin, to cause distant organ injury by migrating across the endothelium cell and releasing reactive oxygen species [28]. The gut-lymph hypothesis is a variant; the shock-injured gut releases biologically active factors into mesenteric lymph, and these factors activate circulating neutrophils to injure distant endothelial cells.

We now have a dynamic model of an extracellular fluid circulation of solvent, small solutes and albumin in various tissue beds, driven by the lymphatic pump, contributing to the supply and removal of larger, less diffusible molecules to the cells and their intracellular fluid compartment. I summarise this in Fig. 2.4. The relative sizes of the fluid compartments as illustrated here are not to scale with actual volumes.

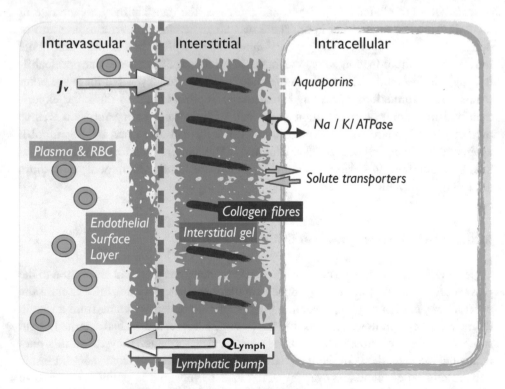

Fig. 2.4 Dynamic model of an extracellular fluid circulation of solvent, small solutes and albumin in various tissue beds

Pulmonary Starling Forces and the Extravascular Lung Water

The pulmonary circulation operates at much lower hydrostatic capillary pressure than the various systemic loops but sustains steady-state solvent filtration to the pulmonary interstitium. As the lungs reside in a sub-atmospheric pressured body space, the interstitial fluid pressure there is lower than that in subcutaneous tissue and fluid from pulmonary capillaries is primarily drawn into the perivascular interstitial space by virtue of the sub-pleural pressure there. Fluids and solutes are largely excluded from the alveoli by the tight junctions of the alveolar epithelium.

In the progression of pulmonary oedema, fluid accumulates first in the interstitial space around the airways forming 'peribronchial cuffs'. The Staverman reflection co-efficient sigma for albumin in pulmonary capillaries is, on average, around 0.7. There is thus more interstitial protein in the lung than in other tissues with continuous capillaries, and the colloid osmotic pressure difference only weakly opposes steady-state filtration at low capillary pressure. Bronchial artery-supplied capillaries also filter fluid to the pulmonary interstitium and so contribute to the interstitial fluid volume and pulmonary lymph flow.

The volume of pulmonary interstitial fluid is strictly controlled by the lymphatic system. Extravascular lung water can be measured at the bedside by double indicator dilution or by thermodilution alone but includes intracellular fluid. The normal value is about 0.5 L. In severe pulmonary oedema values of more than 1.5 L are recorded, almost all of the excess being extracellular fluid in the interstitium or alveoli.

Cell Fluid and Extracellular Fluid

There are of course cellular elements in the blood which, in females or males, account for 1.0–1.4 L of the intracellular fluid. Skeletal muscle intracellular water varies greatly with muscle mass, but we may nominally expect 11.5 or 18.2 L. The nervous system accounts for 2.5 or 2.8 L. Bone and bone marrow have barely 0.5 L of intracellular fluid, similar to the adipose tissue. Connective tissues and transcellular fluid have very few cells and so very little intracellular water.

Starling Forces Between Extracellular and Intracellular Fluids

Body water distribution between the extracellular and intracellular compartments in each tissue reflects a steady state of hydrostatic pressure and osmosis. At equilibrium, the difference between the intracellular pressure and extracellular pressure is equal and opposite to the osmotic pressure difference across the cell membrane. The magnitude of diffusive water flux due to the osmotic pressure difference of an impermeable solute across an ideal membrane is proportional to the solute's concentration difference and the membrane's hydraulic conductance (L_p). In reality, the cell membranes are less than ideal barriers, and most solutes are not fully impermeable. A fraction of the partially impermeable solute molecules will therefore be washed through the permeability barrier with solvent flux; this is the convective transport of solutes. In the 1950s Staverman proposed the reflection coefficient sigma (σ) to account for the observed osmotic pressure gradient relative to the ideal osmotic pressure gradient for an impermeable solute. A solute whose sigma approaches zero exerts almost no osmotic pressure (an ineffective osmol), and a solute whose sigma approaches 1 is almost fully effective. Albumin and urea are examples of important solutes whose σ for cell membranes approaches 1 in health, and Staverman's reflection coefficient σ for a solute can be thought of as the fraction of molecules that are reflected by the membrane. When almost all the molecules are reflected σ approaches 1.0. When half of the molecules are reflected, σ is 0.5, and when only one in ten molecules is reflected σ is 0.1.

Maintenance of the Extracellular-Intracellular Solute Balance is Energy-Dependent

Cells need a near-continuous supply of adenosine tri-phosphate (ATP) to extrude permeable Na^+ ions (via membrane channels) which are then balanced by an influx of permeable K^+ ions; sodium and potassium therefore behave like impermeable effective osmoles sequestered in the ECF and ICF. Magnesium is an important co-factor. The sodium-potassium pump was discovered in 1957 by the Danish scientist Jens Christian Skou, a Nobel Prize winner in 1997. For every ATP molecule consumed, three sodium ions leave the cell and two potassium ions enter; there is thus a net export of a positive charge per cycle creating a membrane potential. Chloride (Cl^-) concentrates in the ECF, while fixed anions predominate in the ICF. The fixed intracellular anions include;

- Metabolites such as ATP, phosphocreatine and sulphate
- Nucleotides
- Proteins, which provide most of the intracellular anionic equivalence

Along with potassium they create the Donnan effect osmotic gradient which would draw water into the cell were it not for the **double Donnan effect** of sodium potassium ATP-ase.

Double Donnan Effect
- The intracellular protein concentration (non-diffusible anion) is higher than extracellular, bringing about the first Gibbs–Donnan equilibrium. With unequal distribution of diffusible ions and electric charge, water tends to move into cells.

- Active extrusion of sodium by Na-K pump makes sodium the major extracellular cation, and it has low membrane permeability. This brings about a second Gibbs–Donnan equilibrium that tends to move water out of cells.
- At steady state the two effects balance out and cell volume remains stable, but if sodium potassium ATP-ase is inhibited cells will swell and rupture due to the first Gibbs–Donnan equilibrium. Water is therefore passively distributed between intracellular and extracellular compartments in proportion to the effective Na^+ and K^+ contents to reach effective osmotic equilibrium (tonicity) and establish cell volume.

Potassium and Magnesium Ions

Potassium is the major intracellular cation and 98% of the total body potassium is intracellular. The plasma levels of potassium and magnesium are generally poor indicators of the whole-body content of these electrolytes which are the major intracellular cations, but deficiency does eventually manifest as reduced plasma concentrations. It is a common clinical experience that hypomagnesaemia limits the ability to normalise plasma potassium by giving potassium supplements. Sometimes hypokalaemia only improves after magnesium has been given. The predominant factor seems to be magnesium's part in the working of several weak inward-rectifier potassium channels found in various isoforms along the renal tubular epithelium. The renal outer medullary potassium channel (ROMK) is the prototypic member of this family, and it plays a central role in the regulation of salt and potassium homeostasis [29]. Intracellular magnesium and poly-amines enter the inward-rectifier potassium channel cytoplasmic pore and plug the potassium permeation pathway, giving rise to the phenomenon of 'inward rectification'. In simple terms, intracellular magnesium blocks what would otherwise be the inward flow of potassium and so the recovery of potassium from the lumen of the distal tubule. When intracellular magnesium is depleted, the block is lifted allowing potassium to be conserved.

Cell Volume Regulation and Intracranial Pressure

The principle that cell volume is closely linked to plasma tonicity is particularly important in the nervous system; as plasma tonicity falls, cells swell. An acute onset (usually in <24 h) of hyponatremia causes severe, and sometimes fatal, cerebral oedema. It takes just a 3% fall in plasma osmolality (from 288 to 280 mosmol^{-1}) to bring about a 3% increase in brain cell volume, around 40 mL. As the cranial cavity is a rigid box, the same volume (40 mL) of blood and cerebrospinal fluid must be displaced, and this represents 30% of the normal intracranial fluid volume. When intracranial pressure is raised, or intracranial compliance is low, a rapid fall in plasma tonicity can have grave consequences for cerebral perfusion. Hypertonic salt solution boluses (e.g. 3% sodium chloride or 8.4% sodium bicarbonate) acutely raise plasma tonicity and thus draw water out of brain cells, allowing the intracranial blood volume and perfusion to increase.

With slower tonicity changes, the brain is protected by adaptive steady-state mechanisms, permitting survival at very low serum sodium concentrations. Adaptation to severe hyponatremia is critically dependent on the loss of organic osmolytes from brain cells. These intracellular, osmotically active solutes contribute substantially to the osmolality of cell water and do not adversely affect cell functions when their concentration changes. The volume-regulated anion channels (VRAC) are members of the superfamily of chloride/anion channels. VRAC are activated by cell swelling and restore cell volume by discharging anionic osmoles to the interstitium. VRAC also play a role in cell proliferation, apoptosis, cell migration and the release of various mediators. They could prove to have an important role in central nervous system pathophysiology.

The adaptation that permits survival in patients with severe, chronic (>48 h' duration) hyponatremia also makes the brain vulnerable to injury (osmotic demyelination) if the electrolyte disturbance is corrected too rapidly. The reuptake of organic osmolytes after correction of hyponatremia is slower than the loss of organic osmolytes during the adaptation to hyponatremia. Areas of the brain that remain most depleted of organic osmolytes are the most severely injured by rapid correction. The brain's reuptake of myoinositol, one of the most abundant osmolytes, occurs much more rapidly in a uremic environment, and patients with uraemia are less susceptible to osmotic demyelination. Cerebral demyelination is a rare complication of overly rapid correction of hyponatremia. The principal risk factors for cerebral demyelination are correction of the serum sodium of more than 25 mEq/L in the first 48 h of therapy, correction past the point of 140 mEq/L, chronic liver disease and prior hypoxic/anoxic episode.

Cell Volume Regulation beyond the Brain

Volume-regulated anion channels (VRAC) are not unique to the central nervous system and may prove to have a pivotal role in cell volume regulation in all cell types. Research into the therapeutic potential of hypertonic saline led to the observation that variations in cell volume have quite profound effects on cellular metabolism and gene expression and could, for example, protect against lung injury in a haemorrhagic shock model. Meta-analysis of human studies confirms the expectation of lower-volume resuscitation from sepsis with hypertonic saline, but with no signal of outcome advantage. Hypertonic sodium is also effective as chloride-free sodium lactate. VRAC activity could explain the finding from clinical experience that neither electrolyte-free water nor potassium solution infusions increase the steady-state intracellular fluid volume. Total body water expansion by intravenous fluid infusions of any tonicity appears to be limited to the extracellular fluid volume. Hessels and her colleagues at Groningen have therefore proposed an 'alternative model' of water, sodium and potassium distribution.

Hessels' Alternative Model of Water, Sodium and Potassium Distribution

It has been taught that an infusion of electrolyte-free water will increase the volume of all compartments of the total body water and reduce osmolarity. In a cohort study of post-surgical patients treated in an Intensive Care Unit with conventional intravenous fluids for 4 days, Hessels and colleagues found that there was a strongly positive accumulation of sodium and total fluid, but a negative balance of electrolyte-free water and potassium [30]. In a sub-study comparing the effects of prescribing potassium to a target of 4.0 mmol/L or 4.5 mmol/L they found that all the excess potassium of the second group was renally excreted. They interpreted these observations as showing that excess fluid in clinical practice results in interstitial expansion (extracellular oedema) while the intracellular volume, where potassium is the dominant osmolar cation, is regulated close to its healthy normal. They speculate that the cytosol is able to clear alternative osmolytes when there is a volume increase by electrolyte-free water infusion, and generate alternative osmolytes when hypertonic saline infusion reduces cell volume. Intracellular volume is thereby conserved in the face of changing body water tonicity. Further research including a broader population of critically ill patients would be interesting. Hessels and colleagues have considered the possibility that excess infused sodium is stored non-osmotically in the skin of patients. Their data confirmed 'Missing extracellular sodium' ions, and 'missing extracellular chloride' too [31].

Studies to identify whether the missing ions are held non-osmotically or shifted to the intracellular fluid are warranted.

Water Excretion

There are of course a number of insensible losses, but the major route of water excretion is renal. The glomerular capillaries operate at a high P_c driving a very high filtration rate (the glomerular filtration rate) of solvent and small solutes from the plasma to the renal tubules. The glomerular capillaries feature open (that is, non-diaphragm) fenestrations that have just enough glycocalyx overhanging the edge to retain albumin in the bloodstream. Of the 120 mL/min that are filtered, barely 1 mL/min leaves the collecting ducts to enter the renal pelvis, ureter and urinary bladder for micturition. The filtration capacity of the glomerular capillaries is therefore nearly matched by the absorptive capacity of the peritubular capillaries of the renal cortex and the ascending vasa recta of the renal medulla. The renal tubules and collecting ducts are the secreting epithelia that provide an independent supply of low-protein solvent to the renal interstitium that creates an exception to the no-absorption rule and allows the diaphragm-fenestrated peritubular capillaries and ascending vasa recta to sustain a high absorption rate. Aldosterone adjusts sodium and potassium secretion/absorption in the tubular fluid emerging from the loops of Henle into the distal convoluted tubules. Arginine vasopressin is the hormone that makes final adjustments to the water conductance of the collecting ducts.

Take Home Messages
- Quantitative consideration of the patient's body water volumes is essential to the prescription of an appropriate rate and total dose of fluid infusion.
- The distribution of extracellular fluid between plasma and the interstitium is most effectively managed by consideration of capillary pressure P_c, or perhaps more specifically of the venular filling pressure.
- While the colloid osmotic pressure of plasma Π_p has historically been considered to be important, we now know that the colloid osmotic pressure difference that opposes filtration varies substantially with the filtration rate J_v and cannot create a sustained (steady state) absorption of interstitial fluid to the plasma.
- While the healthy blood–brain barrier is close to impermeable, all other capillaries are to a greater or lesser extent leaky to solvents and solutes.
- The sinusoidal tissue capillaries take a quarter of the left ventricular output and are totally leaky, so we must dismiss the oft-taught shibboleth that albumin and plasma proteins are confined to the intravascular space.

References

1. Michel CC, Woodcock TE, Curry FE. Understanding and extending the Starling principle. Acta Anaesthesiol Scand. 2020;64(8):1032–7.
2. Khaled MA, Lukaski HC, Watkins CL. Determination of total body water by deuterium NMR. Am J Clin Nutr. 1987;45:1–6.
3. Chumlea WC, Guo SS, Zeller CM, Reo NV, Siervogel RM. Total body water data for white adults 18 to 64 years of age: the Fels Longitudinal Study. Kidney Int. 1999;56:244–52.
4. Ellegård L, Bertz F, Winkvist A, Bosaeus I, Brekke HK. Body composition in overweight and obese women postpartum: bioimpedance methods validated by dual energy X-ray absorptiometry and doubly labeled water. Eur J Clin Nutr. 2016;70:1181–8.
5. Lacey J, Corbett J, Forni L, et al. A multidisciplinary consensus on dehydration: definitions, diagnostic methods and clinical implications. Ann Med. 2019;51:232–51.
6. Boer P. Estimated lean body mass as an index for normalization of body fluid volumes in humans. Am J Physiol. 1984;247:F632–6.
7. Peters AM, Snelling HL, Glass DM, Bird NJ. Estimation of lean body mass in children. Br J Anaesth. 2011;106:719–23.
8. Brower RG, Lanken PN, MacIntyre N, et al. Higher versus lower positive end-expiratory pressures in patients with the acute respiratory distress syndrome. N Engl J Med. 2004;351:327–36.
9. Shi X, Passe DH. Water and solute absorption from carbohydrate-electrolyte solutions in the human proximal small intestine: a review and statistical analysis. Int J Sport Nutr Exerc Metab. 2010;20:427–42.
10. Young AJ, Karl JP, Berryman CE, Montain SJ, Beidleman BA, Pasiakos SM. Variability in human plasma volume responses during high-altitude sojourn. Physiol Rep. 2019;7:e14051.

11. Woodcock TE, Woodcock TM. Revised Starling equation and the glycocalyx model of transvascular fluid exchange: an improved paradigm for prescribing intravenous fluid therapy. Br J Anaesth. 2012;108:384–94.
12. Woodcock TE. Plasma volume, tissue oedema, and the steady-state Starling principle. BJA Educ. 2017;17:74–8.
13. Woodcock T. Fluid physiology: a handbook for anaesthesia and critical care practice. Cambridge Scholars Publishing; 2019.
14. Levick JR, Michel CC. Microvascular fluid exchange and the revised Starling principle. Cardiovasc Res. 2010;87:198–210.
15. Curry FR, Adamson RH. Tonic regulation of vascular permeability. Acta Physiol (Oxf). 2013;207:628–49.
16. Hahn RG. Volume kinetics for infusion fluids. Anesthesiology. 2010;113:470–81.
17. Warren JV, Merrill AJ, Stead EA. The role of the extracellular fluid in the maintenance of a normal plasma volume. J Clin Invest. 1943;22:635–41.
18. Wiig H, Swartz MA. Interstitial fluid and lymph formation and transport: physiological regulation and roles in inflammation and cancer. Physiol Rev. 2012;92:1005–60.
19. Bhave G, Neilson EG. Body fluid dynamics: back to the future. J Am Soc Nephrol. 2011;22:2166–81.
20. Benias PC, Wells RG, Sackey-Aboagye B, et al. Structure and distribution of an unrecognized interstitium in human tissues. Sci Rep. 2018;8:4947.
21. Scallan JP, Zawieja SD, Castorena-Gonzalez JA, Davis MJ. Lymphatic pumping: mechanics, mechanisms and malfunction. J Physiol. 2016;594:5749–68.
22. Seeger M, Bewig B, Günther R, et al. Terminal part of thoracic duct: high-resolution US imaging. Radiology. 2009;252(3):897–904.
23. Iliff JJ, Goldman SA, Nedergaard M. Implications of the discovery of brain lymphatic pathways. Lancet Neurol. 2015;14:977–9.
24. Wiig H, Luft FC, Titze JM. The interstitium conducts extrarenal storage of sodium and represents a third compartment essential for extracellular volume and blood pressure homeostasis. Acta Physiol (Oxf). 2018;222
25. Nikpey E, Karlsen TV, Rakova N, Titze JM, Tenstad O, Wiig H. High-salt diet causes osmotic gradients and hypcrosmolality in skin without affecting interstitial fluid and lymph. Hypertension. 2017;69:660–8.
26. Cope O, Litwin SB. Contribution of the lymphatic system to the replenishment of the plasma volume following a hemorrhage. Ann Surg. 1962;156:655–67.
27. Demling RH, Kramer GC, Gunther R, Nerlich M. Effect of nonprotein colloid on postburn edema formation in soft tissues and lung. Surgery. 1984;95:593–602.
28. Dzieciatkowska M, D'Alessandro A, Moore EE, et al. Lymph is not a plasma ultrafiltrate: a proteomic analysis of injured patients. Shock. 2014;42:485–98.
29. Hadchouel J, Ellison DH, Gamba G. Regulation of renal electrolyte transport by WNK and SPAK-OSR1 kinases. Annu Rev Physiol. 2016;78:367–89.
30. Hessels L, Oude Lansink A, Renes MH, et al. Postoperative fluid retention after heart surgery is accompanied by a strongly positive sodium balance and a negative potassium balance. Physiol Rep. 2016;4
31. Hessels L, Oude Lansink-Hartgring A, Zeillemaker-Hoekstra M, Nijsten MW. Estimation of sodium and chloride storage in critically ill patients: a balance study. Ann Intensive Care. 2018;8:97.

Fluid Physiology Part 2: Regulation of Body Fluids and the Distribution of Infusion Fluids

3

Robert G. Hahn

Contents

Introduction 77
Fluid Balance 78
   Fluid Intake 78
   Fluid Losses 78
Fluid Movement and Edema Formation 79
   Cell Membrane 79
   Capillary Membrane 80
   The Starling Equation 81
   Edema Formation 81
The Importance of Organ Function 82
   The Kidneys 82
   Nervous Control 82
   Hormones 83
Cardiac Response to Fluid 83
Electrolytes 84
Crystalloid Fluid Solutions 85
   Ringer's Solution 85
   Other Crystalloid Fluids 86
Colloid Fluid Solutions 87
Measurement of Body Fluid Volumes 87
Fluid Efficiency 88
Volume Kinetics, Basic Concepts 89
Crystalloids Versus Colloids 92
Goals of Fluid Therapy 93
References 94

R. G. Hahn (✉)
Anaesthesia and Intensive Care, Karolinska Institutet, Stockholm, Sweden
e-mail: r.hahn@telia.com; robert.hahn@sll.se

© The Author(s) 2024
M. L. N. G. Malbrain et al. (eds.), *Rational Use of Intravenous Fluids in Critically Ill Patients*, https://doi.org/10.1007/978-3-031-42205-8_3

IFA Commentary (MLNGM)

We continue a similar but also different deep dive in the second part on fluid physiology. Are colloids and crystalloids really different with respect to their plasma volume-increasing or volume-expanding effects? In conditions of low blood pressure and hypoperfusion (e.g., postoperative or shock state, after anesthesia induction, and trauma), it seems that as long as they are infused crystalloids and colloids have similar effects compared to healthy volunteers where colloids have a greater effect on effective plasma volume. Can we talk about the pharmacokinetics and pharmacodynamics of fluids in analogy to antibiotics or other drugs? Volume kinetics is an adaptation of the pharmacokinetic theory that makes it possible to analyze and simulate the distribution and elimination following an infusion of intravenous fluids. Applying this concept, it is possible, by simulation, to determine the infusion rate that is required to reach a predetermined plasma volume expansion. Fluid pharmacokinetics describes how the body affects a drug, resulting in a particular plasma and effect site concentration. The pharmacokinetics of intravenous fluids depends on distribution volume, osmolality, tonicity, oncoticity, and kidney function. Eventually, the half-time depends not only on the type of fluid, but also on the patient's condition, comorbidities, and the clinical context. Fluid pharmacodynamics relates drug concentrations to their specific effect. For fluids, the Frank–Starling relationship between cardiac output and cardiac preload is the equivalent of the dose–effect curve for standard medications. Because of the shape of the Frank–Starling relationship, the response of cardiac output to the fluid-induced increase in cardiac preload is not constant. This chapter will give a concise overview of fluid kinetics and dynamics with a focus on fluid intake and fluid loss and the important role of the cell and capillary membrane. It will discuss the Starling equation and edema formation and how organ dysfunction (e.g., kidney, neurologic, cardiovascular, and endocrine) may alter fluid homeostasis. An overview will be given on daily electrolyte needs (Table 3.1) the different crystalloid and colloid solutions and how they may have different impacts on fluid efficiency (Fig. 3.1).

Table 3.1 Daily electrolyte requirements

Electrolyte	Function	mmol/kg/day	mmol/day (80 kg)
Sodium	Main extracellular cation	1–1.5	80–120
Potassium	Main intracellular cation, acid–base regulation, neuromuscular contractility	0.75–1.25	60–100
Chloride	Extracellular anion, acid–base regulation	0.75–1.25	60–100
Phosphate	Main intracellular anion, acid–base regulation, energy source (ATP)	0.2–0.5	20–45
Magnesium	Co-factor in enzyme systems, neuromuscular contractility	0.1–0.2	5–10
Calcium	Bone mineralization, neuromuscular contractility	0.1–0.2	5–10

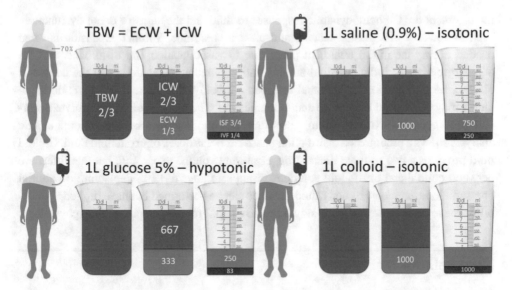

Fig. 3.1 Different volume expansion effects in stable (not critically ill) conditions after 1 h of administration of 1 L of IV solution

Learning Objectives

After reading this chapter, you will:
1. Know what the normal need for fluid is in a human and what might cause this need to change.
2. Understand how osmotic and colloid osmotic pressure in an infusion fluid alters its distribution between body fluid compartments.
3. Comprehend the traditional Starling equation.
4. Identify how fast glucose can be administered by intravenous infusion without causing harm and how this can be monitored.
5. Learn the cardiac and renal responses to dehydration and fluid loading.

Introduction

The turnover of fluid is fairly slow in humans, with a basic need of 1.0 mL/kg/h. The body has limited tolerance for losses of body fluid, so the intensivist has to deal with derangements such as hypovolemia, volume depletion, and dehydration. An infusion fluid can be tailored to distribute into any of the body fluid spaces, including the plasma, the extracellular fluid space, or the total body water. The fluid balance is controlled by the kidneys, the nervous system, and hormones; however, these control systems may be dysfunctional during intensive care due to the disease and the medical treatment. The key clinical guides to fluid management are the hemodynamic responses to fluid and the signs of organ dysfunction, such as lowered pH, plasma lactate, and plasma creatinine. Volume expansion is often needed during the initial treatment phase due to vasodilatation and disturbances of the adrenergic system. Judicious fluid administration is recommended later in the course of disease, because fluid underload and overload are both problematic. Electrolyte derangements may be induced by disease and/or medication. The most essential electrolyte disturbances to consider involve sodium, potassium, calcium, and bicarbonate. Volume kinetic analysis shows a pronounced distribution phase for bolus doses of crystalloid fluid. Colloid fluid provides a two to three times stronger plasma volume expansion, but the difference between colloid and crystalloid solutions disappears after 6–12 h, depending on arterial pressure. Measurements of body fluid volumes can be performed but have limited applicability due to the complex methodology. See also Chap. 2 for the first part on fluid physiology.

Fluid Balance

Fluid Intake

Water constitutes between 50% and 60% of the body weight in adult females and males, respectively, with some decrease over the lifespan. The water volume is distributed over two compartments, the intra- and extracellular fluid spaces (ICF and ECF, respectively); the ECF is further divided into plasma and interstitial fluid. These volumes are tightly controlled by hormonal, neurological, and cardiovascular mechanisms.

The turnover of fluid in the body is fairly slow. The basic need for fluid is 1.0 mL/kg/h, i.e., 1.2 L/day in a patient weighing 50 kg and 2.4 L in a patient weighing 100 kg. To obtain a reasonable margin, the basic need is usually set 25% higher.

The so-called 4/2/1 rule provides a recommendation for suitable water intake for children. This rule suggests 4 mL/kg/h for infants weighing 3–10 kg; 40 mL/kg plus 2 mL/kg/h for each kg over 10 kg for children weighing 10–20 kg; and 60 mL/h plus 1 mL/kg/h for each kg over 20 kg in children weighing >20 kg.

Fluid Losses

Fluid losses from the body consist primarily of insensible water losses (i.e., evaporation, which is mostly derived from the airways) and baseline diuresis. These two sources each account for half of the water loss in a fasting individual. A small amount of water, approximately 300 mL/day, is created in the body as a result of the metabolism of glucose. Water losses by sweating are normally quite small, but these increase in fever conditions and during physical exercise.

The body has a limited tolerance for losses of body fluid. The blood volume, which is a part of both the ICF and ECF, is particularly sensitive. A loss of blood volume below

Table 3.2 Effect of fluid loss and gain on interstitial, plasma, and intracellular volume and plasma tonicity

Conditions	Interstitial fluid volume	Plasma volume (volemia)	Intracellular volume	Plasma tonicity
Isotonic fluid loss	↓ (dehydration)	↓ (hypovolemia)	= (normal)	= (plasma isotonicity)
Hypotonic fluid loss	↓ (dehydration)	=/ ↓ (normo- or hypovolemia)	↓ (dehydration)	↑ (plasma hypertonicity)
Isotonic fluid gain	↑ (hyperhydration)	↑ (hypervolemia)	= (normal)	= (plasma isotonicity)
Hypotonic fluid gain	↑ (hyperhydration)	=/↑ (normo- or hypervolemia)	↑ (hyperhydration)	↓ (plasma hypotonicity)
Hypertonic fluid gain	↑ (hyperhydration)	↑ (hypervolemia)	↓ (dehydration)	↑ (plasma hypertonicity)

↑ increased, = no change, ↓ decreased

normal is called *hypovolemia*. The arterial pressure is maintained by catecholamine release during blood losses of up to 20% of the blood volume (approximately 1 L in the adult) although cardiac output falls. The body then changes strategy to vasodilatation, which creates an abrupt drop in pressure. The reason for this changeover is unclear from a physiological point of view; however, a low flow and low blood pressure more effectively allow blood clots to form, which is beneficial in uncontrolled hemorrhage.

Loss of extracellular fluid is called *volume depletion* and occurs in patients experiencing diarrhea and vomiting. Finally, loss of total body water is due to insufficient intake of water and is common in the elderly. The hallmark of insufficient water intake is a rise in serum osmolality to 300 mosmol/kg or more. This condition is often called *dehydration* in daily language, but it is more specifically *hyperosmotic dehydration* or else *intracellular volume depletion* and occurs in patients experiencing diarrhea and vomiting. Finally, loss of total body water is due to insufficient intake of water and is common in the elderly. The hallmark of insufficient water intake is a rise in serum osmolality *dehydration*. In conscious humans, dehydration quickly leads to poor mental and physical performance.

Table 3.2 shows the effect of fluid loss and gain on interstitial, plasma, and intracellular volume and plasma tonicity.

Fluid Movement and Edema Formation

Cell Membrane

Movements of fluid between the body fluid volumes are determined by specific factors. The distribution across the *cell membrane*, i.e., the separation between the ICF and ECF, is governed by osmolality and the permeability of the cell membrane for the molecules that contribute to the osmolality. For example, sodium is important for fluid distribution because only small amounts of this ion enter the cells, and whatever amount enters is quickly expelled via the sodium–potassium pump. By contrast, ethanol markedly raises the osmolality but does not redistribute water because ethanol easily passes through the cell membrane. Many molecules, such as amino acids, have intermediate characteristics and may, like glucose, be actively pumped into the cells, and water then follows by virtue of osmosis. Therefore, the influence of a glucose solution on the fluid distribution is time-dependent. The ability of a solution to redistribute water across the cell membrane is called its *tonicity*. A saline solution with a concentration higher than 0.9% withdraws fluid from the ICF to the ECF and is therefore called *hypertonic*. By contrast, pure water is strongly *hypotonic*, as it distributes across the cell membrane in proportion to the sizes of the ICF and ECF. An ethanol solution can be hyperosmotic while still being hypotonic.

Capillary Membrane

The *capillary membrane* separates the blood from the interstitial fluid. This membrane allows the filtration of fluid from the plasma to the interstitium through pores and fenestrations over a very short distance of the length of the capillary. The pores are either small (40–45 Å) and allow small ions to pass with ease, or they are large (250 Å) and allow proteins to pass. The proteins follow the flow of fluid through the large pores, in a process called *convection*, and leave the plasma at a rate of 5–8% per hour. This means that small molecules, such as electrolytes and glucose, are filtered freely in both the small and large pores, while macromolecules (such as albumin) pass slowly through the large ones only. Filtered fluid is mostly returned to the plasma by lymphatic flow, while absorption from the interstitium to the plasma occurs in the gastrointestinal canal and lymphatic glands. Absorption also occurs from other body areas in hypovolemic states.

In healthy humans, the hydrostatic pressure in the capillaries is 17–25 mmHg, whereas it is slightly negative, at about −3 mmHg, in the interstitial fluid. The interstitial fluid space is filled with proteoglycan filaments and collagen fibrils that bind the tissues together. The connective tissue has an initial low compliance for volume expansion, which counteracts fluid accumulation. The jelly-like consistency of the interstitium restricts the rapid movement of fluid, whereas electrolytes and metabolic products diffuse almost freely.

The interstitial fluid volume corresponds to 15% of the body weight; of this, only two-thirds becomes expanded by an infusion of crystalloid fluid. Very dense areas of the interstitial fluid space, such as bone tissue, might even be difficult to expand by fluid at all.

The osmolality created by the macromolecules is called the *colloid osmotic pressure*. It accounts for only a small fraction of the total osmolality in the body fluids but is still, together with the hydrostatic pressure, the pressure that determines the distribution of fluid between the plasma and the interstitium. A colloid infusion fluid that expands the plasma volume by its own volume is considered *iso-oncotic*.

The difficulty for macromolecules to pass the endothelium is partly explained by the existence of a layer on the luminal side of the endothelium called the *glycocalyx*. This layer might be degraded in inflammatory states and ischemia, which then accelerates the passage of macromolecules. The functions of the glycocalyx layer have been mostly disclosed during the past 25 years, and many details of its physiological role probably remain to be established.

The integrity of the glycocalyx layer in living humans can be explored by filming the microcirculation with a camera placed on the nail bed or below the tongue. Alternatively, molecular constituents of the glycocalyx layer, such as syndecan-1, heparan sulfate, and hyaluronic acid, are found in increasing concentrations in plasma and urine. However, so far, linking increasing plasma levels to a physiological effect in humans has been challenging.

The Starling Equation

Fluid exchange across the capillary membrane was investigated by the English physiologist Ernest Starling (1866–1927) who, in 1896, formulated his *Starling Equation*, which is still considered to be valid. The "traditional" equation summarizes the factors that determine the transcapillary exchange in the following way:

$$\text{Fluid exchange} = K_f \left[\left(P_c - P_i \right) - \sigma \left(\pi_p - \pi_i \right) \right]$$

where K_f is a proportionality constant, P_c and P_i are the hydrostatic fluid pressure in the capillary and interstitium, respectively, and π_p and π_i are the colloid osmotic pressure in the plasma and interstitial fluid, respectively. The symbol σ is the reflection coefficient, which explains how easily macromolecules pass through the capillary wall. A reflection coefficient of 1.0 means that the membrane is impermeable, and 0 means that the molecule passes without any difficulty. The value of σ greatly varies between vascular beds.

Recent microcirculatory research suggests that the principles behind the Starling equation need to be revised due to the active role played by the endothelial glycocalyx layer in forming the transcapillary fluid equilibrium. These alternations are discussed in detail by Tom Woodcock in the first chapter of this book.

Edema Formation

Edema develops in response to the rapid infusion of crystalloid fluid, which overwhelms the capacity of the lymphatic system to return the infused volume. Edema can also occur due to the blunted return of fluid from the interstitial fluid space to the plasma, as in the case of acute burns, toxicosis of pregnancy, and sepsis. A gradual loss of the elastic properties of the interstitial meshwork of proteoglycans occurs if volume expansion progresses. Massive expansion of the interstitial fluid space, corresponding to a crystalloid fluid infusion of approximately 7–8 L, finally overcomes the negative pressure. The tissue then breaks up, and fluid accumulates in small pools or *lacunae* in the skin and certain organs, such as the heart.

The brain is not subject to edema by fluid overload with isotonic fluid. Instead, brain edema arises due to metabolic or physical damage or reductions in serum osmolality. Edema is particularly critical in this organ as the skull provides the brain with only a limited capacity to swell.

The Importance of Organ Function

The Kidneys

Approximately 20% of the renal plasma flow is filtered in the glomeruli and creates the *primary urine*. The renal blood flow and the glomerular filtration rate are affected by the arterial pressure, but they are autoregulated between 80 and 160 mmHg. The primary urine is refined within the kidneys with regard to volume and the composition of small molecules. The kidneys have a remarkable capacity to match variability in the intake of water with urinary excretion. Proteins are not excreted in healthy humans.

Normal urinary excretion in an adult is 1.0–1.5 L per 24 h. Excretion of less than 400 mL is called *oliguria* and less than 100 mL is called *anuria*. The reasons for anuria can be pre-renal (low arterial pressure), intra-renal (kidney injury), or post-renal (renal stones and outflow obstruction).

Poor urinary excretion is often treated with a bolus infusion of 500 mL of crystalloid fluid in case the patient is hypovolemic. A second treatment is an injection of loop diuretics, which increase sodium excretion and urine volume. A third method is to boost urinary excretion with 100–200 mL of hyperosmotic 10–20% mannitol, which is not metabolized and only eliminated by osmotic diuresis.

Nervous Control

The autonomic nervous system maintains a balance between parasympathetic and sympathetic nervous impulses. The sympathetic impulses are of particular interest for fluid balance, as they constrict arterioles, which raises peripheral resistance. Sympathetic impulses also constrict large veins, which increases cardiac output, and stimulates the release of *noradrenaline* and *adrenaline* from the adrenals into the blood. These are short-acting hormones that cause vasoconstriction, although adrenaline causes vasodilatation in muscle tissue.

Urinary excretion is reduced by beta-1-receptor stimulation, which can be created by providing the drug isoprenaline, while diuresis is increased by alpha-1-stimulation, which is achieved by phenylephrine.

Hormones

Besides the two hormones excreted from the adrenal medulla, which are under the control of sympathetic nerves, a number of other agents also affect the fluid balance. *Cortisol* is excreted from the adrenal cortex. This stress hormone has profound effects on metabolism, but it also promotes fluid retention by increasing the reabsorption of sodium in the kidneys. Cortisol excretion is elevated by surgical stress.

Renin is excreted by the kidneys in response to low arterial pressure. Renin activates a vasoconstrictor and *angiotensin* and further stimulates the secretion of *aldosterone*, which is another hormone that reduces sodium excretion and thereby promotes water retention in the body.

Vasopressin (antidiuretic hormone) is excreted from the brain in response to high serum osmolality. This hormone acts on the kidneys to increase the reabsorption of water. Vasopressin is important for the long-term correction of the body's fluid balance in plasma concentrations between 1 and 6 pg/mL. Very high plasma concentrations, up to several hundred pg/mL, occur in response to any short period of hemorrhagic hypotension. In this range, the hormone also has a vasoconstrictive effect. Despite the short half-life of vasopressin, the elevation of its plasma concentration is sufficient to cause renal fluid retention that lasts for several hours.

Atrial natriuretic peptide (ANP) is excreted in response to the distention of the atrial muscle cells of the heart. The key effect of ANP is to decrease the blood volume by increasing sodium excretion and capillary leakage of proteins. A structurally similar hormone, *brain natriuretic peptide (BNP)*, is released from the cardiac ventricles in response to distention. These hormones act on the same receptors, but ANP exerts a stronger effect.

Vasopressin, ANP, noradrenaline, and adrenaline exert immediate effects and have short half-lives, whereas the steroid hormones cortisol and aldosterone act more slowly.

Cardiac Response to Fluid

The typical hemodynamic response to volume loading with an infusion fluid is an increase in cardiac output, with no change in arterial pressure, while peripheral resistance decreases. The rise in cardiac output requires a sufficient venous return and the ability of the heart to pump more fluid. Cardiac output does not increase if the vascular system is already adequately filled with volume. The ability of the heart to pump more volume in response to fluid loading is called *fluid responsiveness*. This can be tested in many ways, both by infusing a bolus volume of fluid (during general anesthesia) or by recording the response in cardiac stroke volume to leg lifting ("passive leg raising test" in the conscious patient). Providing infusion fluid to a patient who is not fluid-responsive is hardly meaningful, as it impairs oxygen delivery and raises the central venous pressure. However, a patient can be made more fluid-responsive by the administration of adrenergic drugs.

Monitoring of the central hemodynamic response to volume loading has a key role in guiding fluid therapy and will be reviewed in greater detail elsewhere in this book.

Electrolytes

Sodium This ion is essential to nerve function and is the most abundant positively charged ion in the ECF. Sodium is essential for maintaining fluid balance across the cell membrane. Sodium enters the cells, but, as already mentioned, intracellular sodium is actively pumped out to the ECF again. The normal plasma sodium concentration is 133–146 mmol/L. A drop in concentration below 130 mmol/L triggers the appearance of nervous system symptoms, consisting of confusion and various degrees of muscular weakness and depressed consciousness [1, 2]. Severe forms of hyponatremia, involving brain damage, correspond to plasma concentrations below 120 mmol/L.

Hyponatremia can be acute (excessive water ingestion), subacute (2–3 days after surgery), or chronic (unhealthy diet, kidney injury, and diuretics). The chronic form is most commonly seen in intensive care. The speed at which hyponatremia is restored must match the rate at which it has developed because the brain adapts slowly to a new ionic environment [3]. Hypernatremia also blurs consciousness, and the cause is usually iatrogenic.

Chloride This is the negatively charged ion that balances the sodium ion in the ECF. Elevated concentrations, which are usually iatrogenic, reduce urinary excretion by local vasoconstriction and are associated with acidosis. Hypochloremia arises as a result of vomiting and causes metabolic alkalosis.

Calcium Half of the calcium in plasma is abound to albumin and the other half is the biologically active free ionized fraction, which is important for muscle and nerve function and serves as a co-factor for coagulation proteins.

Infusion of approximately 4 L of fluid that lacks calcium (0.9% saline and PlasmaLyte) dilutes the calcium concentration enough to impair muscle function. The deterioration also includes the heart, whereby cardiac output decreases. Blood transfusions having citrate as a preservative have the same effect, but they work by binding calcium rather than diluting the concentration. Intravenous calcium is an effective treatment.

Injections of large amounts of calcium stop the heart in systole; however, in a clinical setting, plasma calcium is rarely high enough to disturb heart function.

Bicarbonate This ion has a profound importance for the acid–base balance due to its capacity to buffer hydrogen ions; however, perhaps even more importantly, it increases the strong ion difference to create a neutral blood pH. Sodium bicarbonate is marketed as a hypertonic infusion fluid and might be considered for temporary relief in severe metabolic acidosis (pH < 7.0). Instead, the chief therapeutic effort should be directed toward treating the cause of the acidosis.

Potassium This is the most abundant positively charged ion within the cells, whereas its concentration in the ECF is quite low (3.6–5.1 mmol/L). A deviation of 50% from the upper or lower border of the normal range may have a fatal outcome on the heart. The effect of potassium on the heart is opposite that of potassium, but arrhythmia is the most typical sign of abnormal values.

Acute stress causes a temporary shift of potassium from the ECF to the ICF and is often seen after trauma and surgery. The mechanism is adrenergic beta-2-receptor stimulation. Therefore, hyperkalemia can be treated with adrenaline. Chronic hypokalemia is usually the result of diuretic therapy or an aberrant diet.

Potassium should be added to infusion fluids used for maintenance therapy (20–40 mmol/L). Due to the risk of cardiac arrhythmias, it should be provided no faster than 10 mmol//h unless the electrocardiograph is monitored continuously. Hence, infusions with a higher potassium concentration than the plasma cannot be administered at a high rate.

Crystalloid Fluid Solutions

Ringer's Solution

Ringer's solutions are aimed to resemble the composition of the ECF fluid. However, the sodium concentration is 130 mmol/L, which is lower than in the plasma (mean 138 mmol/L). A buffer (*lactate* or *acetate*) is usually added to maintain a normal pH. These fluids still exert a slight acidifying effect. Both lactate and acetate also have some vasodilating properties. These solutions are slightly hypotonic (270 mosmol/kg).

Ringer's solutions are distributed from the plasma across the ECF volume in a process that requires approximately 30 min for completion. However, very small amounts (5 mL/kg) undergo barely any distribution and almost exclusively fill up the plasma volume [4]. Larger volumes infused over 30 min expand the plasma volume by approximately half its volume. When the infusion is turned off, the plasma volume expansion rapidly falls until full equilibration in the ECF volume has been achieved. Thereafter, the fluid is eliminated by voiding with a half-life of between 20 and 40 min (volunteers) to several hundred minutes (arterial hypotension, anesthetized patients).

The suitable rates of infusion of Ringer's solutions are often said to be limited only by the patient's hemodynamic capacity. However, large-scale infusions (75–100 mL/kg over 30 min) change the integrity of the interstitial meshwork of the interstitial fluid space and thereby promote edema [4]. Body areas that are particularly susceptible to crystalloid fluid overload, such as the skin, lungs, and gastrointestinal wall, have a high compliance for volume expansion. Volume loading might also cause degradation of the endothelial glycocalyx layer. However, infusing 25 mL/kg seems to be innocuous in this respect [5].

Ringer's solutions are used to expand the ECF volume, which is needed to combat fluid and blood losses during surgery and intensive care. ECF volume expansion also compensates the blood flow for disturbances of the autonomic nervous system, which occur due to general anesthesia and severe disease.

Other Crystalloid Fluids

Normal (0.9%) saline is an isotonic fluid that contains only sodium and chloride in equal amounts. The fluid causes slight metabolic acidosis when the infused volume is 2 L or more. The half-life in volunteers is twice as long as for Ringer's solutions and amounts to approximately 90 min [6]. The indication for isotonic saline is restricted to hyponatremia and volume replacement after vomiting.

Saline may also be used in a 3% or 7.5% solution to combat brain edema or severe hyponatremia, and for fluid resuscitation in acute trauma care. These hypertonic fluids should not be infused together with erythrocytes.

Mannitol is a sugar isomer that can only be eliminated by urinary excretion. The half-life is almost the same as for isotonic saline. Mannitol is iso-osmotic in a 5% concentration but is used in a 10–20% preparation to treat brain edema and to stimulate diuresis. Hypertonic mannitol contains no electrolytes, which are therefore excreted along with the osmotic diuresis. The resulting decrease in the electrolyte concentrations in the ECF causes post-infusion cellular swelling (rebound effect).

Glucose (dextrose) fluids are maintenance solutions. They cannot be infused as liberally as the previous crystalloid solutions due to an accompanying rise in plasma glucose. A glucose solution is iso-osmotic at a 5% concentration, which only contains 200 kcal/L. This small amount of calories can only prevent starvation and does not provide adequate nutrition. The chief indication for its use is to prevent hypoglycemia and severe muscle wasting and to provide water for hydration of the ICF space.

The main problem with glucose solutions is that intravenous administration trespasses the gastrointestinal hormones that aid the glucose metabolism. Hence, the hyperglycemic effect of an intravenous infusion is much greater when compared to oral intake of glucose. Even worse, the trauma associated with intensive care causes resistance to the effects of insulin. Therefore, plasma glucose should be measured often and not allowed to rise above 9–10 mmol/L. This is usually achieved by not allowing 1 L of glucose 5% to be infused over a shorter time period than 6 h [7].

The use of glucose solutions of concentrations higher than 5% should be monitored carefully with measurements of plasma glucose. Insulin administration is often needed. The aim is then to increase the administration of calories and/or to restrict the administration of fluid volume.

Allowing very high plasma concentrations of glucose (>12 mmol/L) is discouraged, not only because they promote bacterial growth, but also because osmotic diuresis develops. If cardiac arrest develops, any brain damage will be greater in the hyperglycemic compared to the normoglycemic patient [8].

Colloid Fluid Solutions

Colloid fluids contain water, electrolytes, and a macromolecule that contributes to the intravascular colloid osmotic pressure. Large volumes improve the microcirculation and slightly impair coagulation. In contrast to crystalloids, colloids all share an allergic potential. Hence, colloid fluids should only be given if drugs to combat allergic reactions are at hand.

Albumin is the chief plasma protein and is marketed for plasma volume expansion in iso-oncotic or nearly iso-oncotic preparations (3–5%) and in a hyper-oncotic concentration (20%). Albumin also serves as an antioxidant.

The 4% albumin preparation expands the plasma volume by approximately the same amount as the infused volume. The half-life of its plasma volume expansion is several hours, which is closely related to the intravascular persistence of the albumin [9]. The intravascular persistence is probably shorter in septic patients due to increased capillary leakage of albumin [10].

The 20% preparation increases the circulating plasma volume by twice the infused volume [11].

Repeated infusions of large amounts of albumin put a burden on protein metabolism and urea excretion, which can be an issue in intensive care patient.

There is no evidence that albumin promotes kidney injury in septic patients [12].

Hydroxyethyl starch (HES) is a colloid solution prepared from plants. HES preparations are colloids intended for plasma volume expansion. The most widely used, Voluven (Fresenius Kabi), expands the plasma volume by as much as the infused amount. The elimination is complex and involves a mixture of urinary excretion, molecular cleavage, and phagocytosis.

Impairment of kidney function has been associated with the use of HES in septic patients. Therefore, HES has only limited importance as a plasma volume expander in intensive care.

Gelatin contains small colloid molecules prepared from animals. Elimination is by renal excretion. Therefore, the volume expansion is claimed to be short-lived (2 h). Allergic reactions are fairly common but are mostly limited to fever reactions.

Plasma expands the plasma volume by as much as is observed with 5% albumin [9]. However, plasma should not be used for volume expansion because plasma contains coagulation proteins and has a greater allergic potential than 5% albumin.

Measurement of Body Fluid Volumes

Many techniques can be used to assess the body fluid volumes. These were of greatest importance in the 1950s and 1960s but are considered too cumbersome for clinical use today. However, these methods are still used in research and have contributed much knowledge about macroscopic fluid physiology.

The leading principle is the *dilution concept*. A substance that distributes in one body fluid space only is injected and allowed to equilibrate. A blood sample is taken, and the volume occupied by the injected substance is calculated as the dose divided by the plasma concentration. This principle is most attractive if the turnover of the injected substance is slow. If not, several samples must be taken into account for substance elimination.

Tracers for the measurement of the ECF volume include *bromide*, which has a slow turnover, and *iohexol*, which also yields the glomerular filtration rate. To use iohexol, several samples must be taken into account for urinary excretion of the tracer [13].

Tracers for the measurement of total body water are *tritium* (radioactive) and *deuterium* (not radioactive). Several hours are required for equilibration. *Ethanol* has been proposed for this purpose, as ethanol is a solvent and distributes evenly in water alone [14].

The *plasma volume* has frequently been measured with *radioiodinated albumin*, which is radioactive. Several blood samples are usually taken. *Evans blue* is a dye that colors albumin in the plasma. Plasma tracers overestimate the plasma volume by almost 10% [15]. *Indocyanine green* (ICG) is also a dye that binds to plasma albumin. The half-life is only 3 min, due to rapid uptake by the liver [16]. The transit time from injection in the central circulation to the liver is approximately 1 min. Whether ICG overestimates the plasma volume is not known.

The red cell mass can be measured with labeling techniques, such as *chromium, technetium, and carbon monoxide.*

Bioimpedance (BIA) uses the fact that water volumes oppose electrical currents and that the opposition is different inside and outside the cells. BIA is measured by running a series of electrical currents through the body, usually from the arm to one leg, and then evaluating the impedance pattern in relationship with the quantification of the body fluid volumes by tracer techniques [17]. The measurement requires about 1 min to complete and is painless, but it is disturbed by body movements.

Anthropometric equations are created based on tracer measurements. They point out typical correlations between body fluid volumes and characteristics of the individual, such as gender, height, and weight [18, 19]. The most common assumptions are that the blood volume constitutes 7%, the interstitial fluid 15%, the ECF volume 20%, the ICF volume 35–40%, and the total body water 55–60% of the body weight. Albeit crude, these assumptions are quite useful in everyday clinical work.

Fluid Efficiency

The intravascular volume expansion resulting from infusing a fluid is often related to the amount infused. The concept of *fluid efficiency* has two characteristics: the degree and the duration of volume expansion relative to the infused volume. Tracer methods have been used to assess fluid efficiency, and physiological endpoints are also useful.

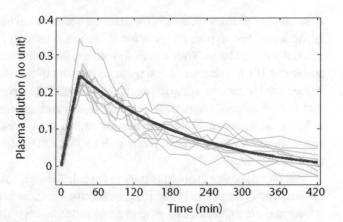

Fig. 3.2 Plasma dilution in ten volunteers (thin lines) and the simulated average (thick) during and after a 30-min infusion of 10 mL/kg hydroxyethyl starch (Voluven). (From Ref. 22)

A widely used approach is to use hemodilution for this purpose. The hemodilution tells us over how large a space the infused fluid volume has distributed. The hemodilution will be quite large if a colloid fluid distributes only over the plasma volume (Fig. 3.2).

The volume of distribution of a fluid that spreads across the total body of water can also be estimated using the dilution concept, although the hemodilution will be much smaller. If we specifically want to estimate how much the blood volume has increased, we must assume a blood volume at baseline, which may or may not be correct.

Commonly used equations assume that the hemoglobin concentration is measured before (Hb) and after (Hb(*t*)) the infusion. Here, BV denotes the blood volume at baseline.

$$\Delta BV = BV\left(Hb / Hb(t)\right) - BV$$

$$\text{Fluid efficiency} = \Delta BV / \text{infused volume}$$

These relationships assume that no bleeding occurs. If this is the case, then the intensivist can estimate the total hemoglobin mass as BV × Hb, from which losses of Hb are subtracted. The new Hb mass is then divided by Hb(*t*) to yield the new BV [20]. This calculation is very useful clinically.

A key insight is that hemodilution should ideally parallel the relationship between bleeding and BV. The patient is hypervolemic if the hemodilution is greater than the blood loss divided by BV, whereas the patient is hypovolemic if the hemodilution is small in relation to the bled volume.

Volume Kinetics, Basic Concepts

The hemodilution concept can be elaborated upon to capture flows of fluid between body fluid compartments over time. This approach is called *volume kinetics* and has similarities to pharmacokinetics. One important difference is that the walls of the body fluid compartments are expandable [21]. Another difference is the choice of input variable. In conventional pharmacokinetics, the plasma concentration of the drug to be studied serves as the input. For volume kinetics, hemodilution is used to capture the distribution of the infused water volume. With regard to volume, the blood contains almost exclusively Hb and water. If Hb is decreased, the water component of the blood is increased. The increase in the blood water concentration then seems to yield the same concept as a drug concentration in conventional pharmacokinetics. Sadly, though, this is an illusion, because the rise in blood water concentration that occurs when a fluid is infused represents a dilution of administered water in a much larger water volume. This fact adds some requirements to the calculations.

The blood volume is not important to the calculations, but volume kinetics is still based on serial analysis of the blood Hb concentration and, at best, the urine volume as well, during and after infusion of a fluid in a controlled setting. The results have shown that the interstitial fluid space after expansion by a crystalloid fluid is only twice as large as the plasma volume, i.e., less than commonly assumed. The distribution of crystalloid fluid occurs with a half-life of 8 min, except in association with an abrupt drop in arterial pressure, when distribution is temporarily arrested. Hence, when the blood pressure drops, it does not matter if one infuses a crystalloid or a colloid fluid.

The simple experiment shown in Fig. 3.2 illustrates the basic thoughts on volume kinetics. Serial measurements of Hb in ten volunteers are performed during and after a 30-min infusion of 10 mL/kg of hydroxyethyl starch in ten male volunteers weighing 80 kg. The hemodilution is corrected for baseline hematocrit to express the plasma dilution. Extrapolation to time 0 of the exponential elimination curve yields a plasma dilution of 0.3. If we divide the infused volume (800 mL) by the plasma dilution at time 0 (i.e., 0.3), we obtain the volume of distribution for the infused starch volume. This is almost precisely 3.0 L, which is the expected plasma volume in these volunteers [22]. From this estimation, we can conclude that the starch preparation only distributes in the plasma volume.

We can also obtain the half-life of the intravascular persistence from Fig. 3.2. By plotting the curve on a logarithmic paper, it becomes apparent to the naked eye that half of the plasma volume expansion has subsided after 120 min. The volume expansion of the starch preparation lasts for 4 half-lives, i.e., 480 min.

The volume kinetic calculations become more complicated, necessitating the use of a computer, when crystalloid electrolyte fluids and glucose solutions are studied. Here, the infused fluid is assumed to distribute between a central fluid space, which is the plasma, and a peripheral fluid space, which is the interstitial fluid. Fluid distributed from the plasma to the interstitium is governed by a rate parameter k_{12} and the return of fluid by another rate parameter k_{21}. The elimination of fluid, mostly by urinary excretion, is determined by a rate parameter k_{10}. Figure 3.3 shows how volume kinetics can reveal that the edema and hypovolemia in toxicosis of pregnancy are due to poor return of distributed fluid, whereas the diuretic response to infused fluid is well maintained [21].

Fig. 3.3 Output of volume kinetic analysis of an infusion of 10 mL/kg Ringer's acetate in eight women with mild–moderate degree of toxicosis of pregnant and eight pregnant controls matched for a gestational week. Three rate parameters determine the distribution of infusion fluid. Edema is caused by poor return of fluid after distribution to interstitial fluid space (low k_{21}). (From Ref. 21)

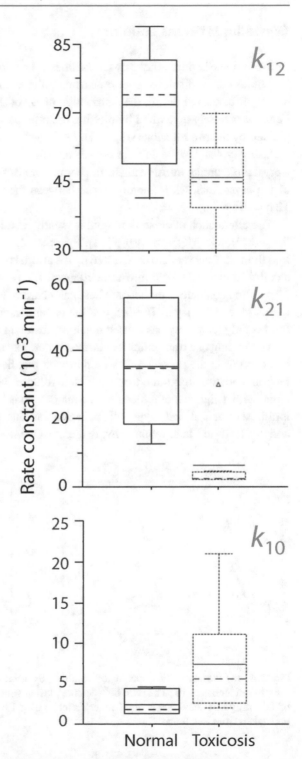

Crystalloids Versus Colloids

The difference in fluid efficiency (sometimes called *potency*) between crystalloid and colloid fluids can be disclosed over time using volume kinetics. The colloid is more efficient during infusion and during the distribution phase of the crystalloid (Fig. 3.3), which can be more precisely quantified by plotting the ratio between the plasma volume expansion yielded by the two infusions (Fig. 3.4).

Using typical kinetic data for conscious volunteers, the colloid is twice as effective as a crystalloid during infusion and is three times more effective during the distribution phase of the crystalloid, while the difference between the two types of infusion disappears at 12 h (ratio = 1.0).

The elimination of crystalloid fluid is greatly retarded during general anesthesia due to the reduction in arterial pressure [21]. By contrast, the intravascular persistence of a colloid fluid does not seem to be affected by the arterial pressure. Therefore, the ratio between a colloid and a crystalloid infusion will reach 1.0 by 5–6 h after a 60-min infusion and by 10 h during continuous infusions. These calculations do not assume any injury to the endothelial glycocalyx layer. The fact that the better plasma volume expansion from a colloid fluid is only temporary has caused much confusion in intensive care [23].

The finding of a transient 50% plasma volume expansion of crystalloid electrolyte fluid is worrying in the presence of a hemorrhage that has not been stopped surgically. The recommendation that three times the bled volume should be infused leads to hypervolemia, with a high risk of rebleeding if a major vein is injured. Moreover, urinary excretion is almost normal, despite hypovolemia, at least as long as the arterial pressure is unchanged, and this leads to a later rebound hypovolemia. One would think that the body would retain

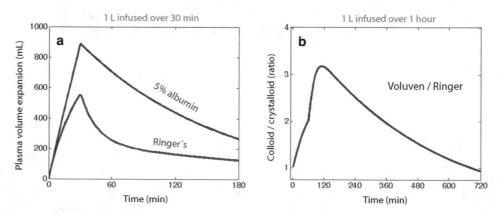

Fig. 3.4 (**a**) Plasma volume expansion resulting from infusing 1 L of 5% albumin and Ringer's acetate in volunteers. (**b**) The ratio between the plasma volume expansion during and after infusion of 1 L of hydroxyethyl starch and Ringer's acetate over 1 h. (Simulations based on volume kinetic data taken from Ref. 9 and 22)

a sufficient amount of the infused fluid to restore and maintain normovolemia, but this is not the case. Therefore, optimal handling is to infuse 1.5 times the bled volume over 30 min and not to stop the infusion, but to gradually reduce the rate of infusion by 50% every 30 min. This practice restores the blood volume while avoiding both hyper- and hypovolemia [24].

Goals of Fluid Therapy

A primary goal of fluid therapy in intensive care is to safeguard cardiovascular sufficiency to ensure normal tissue perfusion and oxygenation of the body organs. For this purpose, the response of cardiac output to fluid administration is a useful guide. However, it might be questioned whether striving toward a high cardiac output is needed in the absence of signs of organ dysfunction (normal plasma lactate, creatinine, low pH, etc.). Using repeated fluid boluses to achieve this goal might lead to overhydration and problems with edema later in the disease process.

Both fluid underload and overload are problematic; hypovolemia causes a *convection limitation* because too little blood and oxygen reach the capillaries. Fluid overload creates another problem, *diffusion limitation*, because interstitial edema increases the distance that oxygen and metabolic products must travel between the capillaries and the cells [25]. To avoid mistakes, combinations of fluids and vasopressors/inotropes are titrated carefully to find an optimal fluid balance situation where organ function is preserved.

Systemic vasodilatation and disturbance of adrenergic function are the main reasons why fluid therapy should be aggressive in the early stages of severe disease. To avoid fluid-associated complications, early deliberate fluid overload must later be reversed by applying a dehydrating strategy (*de-escalation*). More about fluid management during these stages is discussed in other chapters of this book.

Arterial pressure, central venous pressure, and urinary excretion only give vague signals about inappropriate fluid therapy. Central venous pressure rises when the volume of administered fluid has passed the flat portion of the Frank–Starling curve, but this pressure might be affected by other stimuli as well. Arterial pressure and urinary excretion do indicate underhydration, but only at a very late stage. Clinical judgment is blurred by the release of a host of hormones and cytokines, as well as drug effects and therapeutic interventions, such as mechanical ventilation, which affect fluid physiology.

The management of fluid therapy during intensive care is a difficult task that requires skill, knowledge, and good clinical judgment to ensure normal tissue perfusion and oxygenation of the body organs. The tools are given in this book, but it takes a good doctor to use them successfully.

Take Home Messages

- Plasma volume expansion is needed during the initial treatment phase of acute disease due to vasodilatation and disturbances of the adrenergic system.
- The "traditional Starling equation" summarizes the factors that determine the transcapillary exchange in a way that is sufficient in most practical settings.
- Fluid accumulation and fluid overload cause edema by, in part, a gradual loss of the elastic properties of the interstitial meshwork of proteoglycans.
- A drop in plasma sodium to below 130 mmol/L triggers the appearance of nervous system symptoms, consisting of confusion and various degrees of muscular weakness and depressed consciousness.
- Infusion of approximately 4 L of fluid that lacks calcium (0.9% saline and PlasmaLyte) dilutes the calcium concentration enough to impair muscle function. The deterioration also includes the heart, whereby cardiac output decreases.
- The *fluid efficiency* is the plasma volume expansion divided by the infused fluid volume. This is 0.5 for a crystalloid fluid infused over 30 min, approximately 0.8 for 5% albumin, 1.0 for hydroxyethyl starch 130/0.4, and 2.0 for 20% albumin.
- The blood volume expansion during infusion of crystalloid fluid is at least 50% as long as the **infusion** is continued. The reason for this is the slow distribution. After infusion this fraction drops to 20% within 30 min.
- If mean arterial pressure decreases by 20% (e.g., after induction of anesthesia, during surgery, in case of hypovolemic shock), crystalloid **distribution** stops and 100% of the infused fluid then remains in the blood. The explanation for this is the Starling mechanism.
- **Excretion** of a crystalloid fluid is very slow during anesthesia. The reason for this observation is mainly the reduced arterial pressure, while the pressure hardly affects the intravascular persistence of colloid fluids. This helps us to understand why crystalloids and colloids in this setting may have similar volume expansion effects.

References

1. Arieff AI. Hyponatremia, convulsions, respiratory arrest, and permanent brain damage after elective surgery in healthy women. N Engl J Med. 1986;314:1529–35.
2. Häggström J, Hedlund M, Hahn RG. Subacute hyponatraemia after transurethral resection of the prostate. Scand J Urol Nephrol. 2001;35:250–1.
3. Arieff AI. Treatment of symptomatic hyponatremia: neither haste nor waste. Crit Care Med. 1991;19:748–51.
4. Hahn RG, Drobin D, Zdolsek J. Distribution of crystalloid fluid changes with the rate of infusion: a population-based study. Acta Anaesthesiol Scand. 2016;60:569–78.
5. Nemme J, Krizhanovskii C, Ntikia S, Sabelnikovs O, Vanags I, Hahn RG. Hypervolaemia does not cause shedding of the endothelial glycocalyx layer during hysterectomy; a randomised

clinical trial comparing sevoflurane and propofol anaesthesia. Acta Anaesthesiol Scand. 2019; https://doi.org/10.1111/aas.13511.

6. Hahn RG. Influences of the red blood cell count on the distribution and elimination of crystalloid fluid. Medicina. 2017;53:233–41.

7. Hahn RG. How fast can glucose be infused in the perioperative setting? Perioper Med. 2016;5:1.

8. Siemkowicz E. The effect of glucose upon restitution after transient cerebral ischemia: a summary. Acta Neurol Scand. 1985;71:417–27.

9. Hedin A, Hahn RG. Volume expansion and plasma protein clearance during intravenous infusion of 5% albumin and autologous plasma. Clin Sci. 2005;106:217–24.

10. Fleck A, Raines G, Hawker F, Trotter J, Wallace PI, Ledingham IM, Calman KC. Increased vascular permeability: a major cause of hypoalbuminaemia in disease and injury. Lancet. 1985;325:781–4.

11. Hasselgren E, Zdolsek M, Zdolsek JH, Björne H, Krizhanovskii C, Ntika S, Hahn RG. Long intravascular persistence of 20% albumin in postoperative patients. Anesth Analg. 2019;129:1232–9.

12. Caironi P, Tognoni G, Masson S, Fumagalli R, Pesenti A, Romero M, Fanizza C, Caspani L, Faenza S, Grasselli G, Iapichino G, Antonelli M, Parrini V, Fiore G, Latini R, Gattinoni L, ALBIOS Study Investigators. Albumin replacement in patients with severe sepsis or septic shock. N Engl J Med. 2014;370:1412–21.

13. Zdolsek J, Lisander B, Hahn RG. Measuring the size of the extracellular space using bromide, iohexol and sodium dilution. Anest Analg. 2005;101:1770–7.

14. Norberg Å, Sandhagen B, Bratteby L-E, Gabrielsson J, Jones AW, Fan H, Hahn RG. Do ethanol and deuterium oxide distribute into the same water space in healthy volunteers? Alcohol Clin Exp Res. 2001;25:1423–30.

15. Chaplin H Jr, Mollison PL, Vetter H. The body/venous hematocrit ratio: its constancy over a wide hematocrit range. J Clin Invest. 1953;32:1309–16.

16. Jacob M, Conzen P, Finsterer U, Krafft A, Becker BF, Rehm M. Technical and physiological background of plasma volume measurement with indocyanine green: a clarification of misunderstandings. J Appl Physiol. 2007;102:1235–342.

17. Johnson HL, Virk SP, Mayclin P, Barbieri T. Predicting total body water and extracellular fluid volumes from bioelectrical measurements of the human body. J Am Coll Nutr. 1992;11:539–47.

18. Nadler SB, Hidalgo JU, Bloch UT. Prediction of blood volume in normal human adults. Surgery. 1962;51:224–32.

19. Retzlaff JA, Tauxe WN, Kiely JM, Stroebel CF. Erythrocyte volume, plasma volume, and lean body mass in adult men and women. Blood. 1969;33:649–61.

20. Hahn RG. Blood volume at the onset of hypotension in TURP performed during epidural anaesthesia. Eur J Anaesthesiol. 1993;10:219–25.

21. Hahn RG. Understanding volume kinetics. Acta Anaesthesiol Scand. 2019; https://doi.org/10.1111/aas.1353.

22. Hahn RG, Bergek C, Gebäck T, Zdolsek J. Interactions between the volume effects of hydroxyethyl starch 130/0.4 and Ringer's acetate. Crit Care. 2013;17:R104.

23. Hahn RG. Why are crystalloid and colloid fluid requirements similar during surgery and intensive care? Eur J Anaesthesiol. 2013;30:515–8.

24. Hahn RG, Drobin D, Li Y, Zdolsek J. Kinetics of Ringer's solution in extracellular dehydration and hemorrhage. Shock. 2019; https://doi.org/10.1097/SHK.0000000000001422.

25. Kara A, Akin S, Ince C. Monitoring of the microcirculation. In: Hahn RG, editor. Clinical fluid therapy in the perioperative setting. 2nd ed. Cambridge: Cambridge University Press; 2016. p. 82–91.

Fluid Dynamics During Resuscitation: From Frank–Starling to the Reappraisal of Guyton

4

Supradip Ghosh

Contents

Introduction 101
What Are the Factors That Determine Flow of Blood from Peripheral Circulation to Heart? ... 102
What Are the Factors That Determine Mean Systemic Pressure? 103
Guyton's Experiment and Venous Return Curve 103
Starling's Experiment 104
Effect of Fluid Bolus on Venous Return Curve 105
Cardiac Function Curve 106
Integrating the Return Function with Cardiac Function 107
Overall Effect of Fluid Bolus on Circulation 108
Validation of Guytonian Model in Human Studies 109
Conclusion 110
References 111

S. Ghosh (✉)
Department of Critical Care Medicine, Fortis - Escorts Hospital, Faridabad, Haryana, India

© The Author(s) 2024
M. L. N. G. Malbrain et al. (eds.), *Rational Use of Intravenous Fluids in Critically Ill Patients*, https://doi.org/10.1007/978-3-031-42205-8_4

97

IFA Commentary (MLNGM)

In this chapter, the different hemodynamic principles from Frank–Starling to Guyton–Hall will be discussed. However, it were Sydney Patterson (1882–1960) and Ernest Starling (1866–1927) that first described the mechanical factors that determine the output of both ventricles [1]. Before Patterson, it was Otto Frank (1865–1944) who continued the experiments at Carl Ludwig's Physiological Institute. He looked at an improved frog heart preparation from the viewpoint of skeletal muscle mechanics, substituting volume and pressure for length and tension, which enabled him to measure isovolumetric and isotonic contractions. With increasing filling of the frog ventricle, diastolic pressure was elevated at each step. However, beyond a certain filling pressure, it decreased. Otto Frank compiled all of the data in the famous pressure–volume diagram [2]. Afterwards, Arthur Guyton (1919–2003) credited Ernest Starling for appreciating that output from the heart is dependent upon the return of venous blood and that venous return is dependent upon the pressure upstream to the heart in the systemic circulation, which Starling called mean systemic pressure. Starling had not dealt with the mechanics of the systemic circulation or the factors that determine flow back to the heart; the concept of venous return and its determinants awaited Guyton: "When a change occurs in the hemodynamics of the circulatory system one cannot predict what will happen to the cardiac output unless he takes into consideration both the effect of this change on the ability of the heart to pump blood and also the tendency for blood to return to the heart from the blood vessels" [3]. Together with John Hall, he wrote the famous Guyton and Hall Textbook of Medical Physiology. Going further back in time, William Harvey (1578–1657) was an English physician who made seminal contributions to anatomy and physiology. He was the first known physician to describe completely and in detail the systemic circulation and properties of blood being pumped to the brain and body by the heart. Stephen Hales (1677–1761) was an English clergyman who made major contributions to a range of scientific fields including botany, pneumatic chemistry and physiology. He was the first person to measure blood pressure and he invented several devices, including a ventilator. We need to understand that pulse pressure is more important than mean arterial pressure (MAP) as flow needs to bring oxygen to the tissues. On the other hand, in patients with advanced decompensated heart failure (but also in sepsis) we already know that central venous pressure (CVP) is more important than cardiac output (CO) in explaining worsening renal function (WRF) (Fig. 4.1) [4, 5].

However, the microcirculation is equally important as it manages bodily fluids. The endothelial glycocalyx (EG) is a thin-walled layer that keeps fluids in place and only limited filtration occurs (at the venous side). The revised Starling principle developed by Charles Michel and Sheldon Weinbaum has gained importance, and we know that diffusion and convection are two different things as are coherence and heterogeneity [6, 7]. The physiological compartment that manages fluids in the body is the microcirculation. That is why titrating IV fluids based on macrocirculatory parameters can lead to inappropriate administration of fluids leading to overload and organ dysfunction. In order to preserve organ and microcirculatory function, we should therefore limit fluid intake and avoid fluid accumulation. Besides giving a fluid bolus to increase circulating volume and to improve CO, the use of early vaso-pressors can help to convert unstressed to stressed volume, but this may not be suf-ficient in patients with profound capillary leak and vasodilation. A rapid fluid bolus can potentially improve hemodynamic parameters during shock states; however, too rapid infusion may cause harm to the EG layer and too much fluid may cause venous congestion and significant morbidity and mortality as previously stated. Fluids are drugs and should only be given when the patient is a fluid responder (i.e. both ven-tricles acting on the steep part of Frank–Starling curve) and when needed (i.e. shock state with increased lactate). They should never be used to treat or improve the "numbers" (e.g. low MAP, CO, CVP or urine output) (Fig. 4.2).

Suggested Reading

1. Patterson SW, Starling EH. On the mechanical factors which determine the output of the ventricles. J Physiol 1914;48(5): 357–79.
2. Zimmer HG. Who discovered the Frank-Starling mechanism? News Physiol Sci 2002;17:181-84.
3. Guyton AC, Lindsey AW, Abernathy B, Richardson T. Venous return at vari-ous right atrial pressures and the normal venous return curve. Am J Physiol 1957;189(3):609-15.
4. Verbrugge FH, Dupont M, Steels P, Grieten L, Malbrain M, Tang WH, Mullens W. Abdominal contributions to cardiorenal dysfunction in conges-tive heart failure. J Am Coll Cardiol 2013;62(6):485-95.
5. Legrand M, Dupuis C, Simon C, Gayat E, Mateo J, Lukaszewicz AC, Payen D. Association between systemic hemodynamics and septic acute kidney injury in critically ill patients: a retrospective observational study. Critical Care 2013;17(6):R278.
6. Michel CC, Woodcock TE, Curry FE: Understanding and extending the Starling principle. Acta Anaesthesiol Scand 2020;64(8):1032-7.
7. Adamson RH, Lenz JF, Zhang X, Adamson GN, Weinbaum S, Curry FE. Oncotic pressures opposing filtration across non-fenestrated rat microves-sels. J Physiol 2004;557(Pt 3):889-907.

Fig. 4.1 Statistical model of nonparametric logistic regression showing the relationship between mean central venous pressure during the first 24 h after admission and the probability of new or persistent acute kidney injury. Note the plateau for the incidence of acute kidney injury (AKI) when the lower limit of central venous pressure (CVP) was between 8 and 12 mmHg. Over this limit, the rise in CVP was associated with a sharp increase in new or persistent AKI incidence. Adapted from Legrand et al. [5]

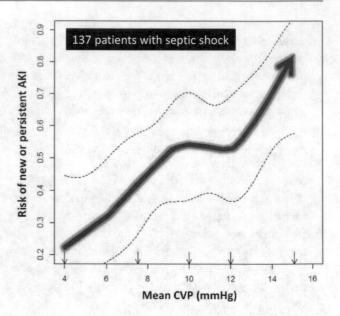

Fig. 4.2 Illustration of the concept of preload dependence. (**a**) Fluid responsiveness illustrated by a greater increase in mean systemic filling pressure with 7 mmHg (from 22 to 29 mmHg) compared to the 2 mmHg increase in CVP (from 6 to 8 mmHg) resulting in a 15% increase in cardiac output from 5.4 to 6.2 L/min. (**b**) Fluid unresponsiveness illustrated by an equal increase in mean systemic filling pressure with 4 mmHg (from 24 to 28 mmHg) and a 3 mmHg increase in CVP (from 8 to 11 mmHg) not resulting in a significant increase in cardiac output (from 5.9 to 6.0 L/min)

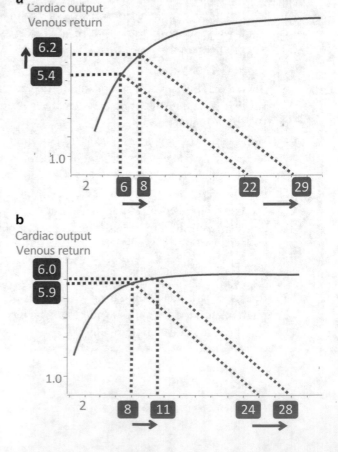

Case Vignette

Mr. X, a 67-year-old gentleman with a history of long-standing diabetes mellitus and benign prostatic hypertrophy, presented to the emergency department (ED) with fever and dysuria for the past 3 days. His wife noticed him to be disoriented since morning and decided to bring him to the ED. On examination, he was drowsy but rousable. His extremities were cold to touch. He had a heart rate of 116/min, blood pressure of 70 mmHg systolic and respiratory rate of 24/min. Pulse oximetry reading showed 95% while breathing room air. Capillary refill time was 6 seconds. Systemic examination findings were unremarkable except for some tenderness on deep palpation of the right flank. The emergency physician decided to infuse him rapidly with 500 ml of Ringer's lactate.

Questions

Q1. What are the possible hemodynamic effects of this fluid bolus on Mr. X?

Learning Objectives

The learning objectives of this chapter are:

1. To learn about various factors regulating venous return.
2. To understand the possible effects of fluid boluses and vasoactive drugs on venous return.
3. To learn about cardiac function curve and factors contributing to the shape of the curve.
4. To understand the effects of fluid boluses and vasoactive drugs on cardiac function curves and cardiac output.
5. To understand the framework provided by Guyton in understanding the circulation of blood and the effects (and possible harmful effects) of fluid boluses on the macro-hemodynamic parameters.

Introduction

The purpose of resuscitation in a shocked patient is to maintain the perfusion of tissues and organs. Options available for resuscitation are basically limited to intravenous fluids, vasoactive agents (vasopressors and inotropes) and blood transfusion (in specific situations). A detailed understanding of the effects of these agents on circulation is important for their appropriate use. Numerous scientists have contributed to our current understanding of circulatory physiology [1]. Prominent among them were the German physiologist Otto Frank and British physiologist Earnest Henry Starling. They are credited with describing the relationship between the length of cardiac muscle just before cardiac contraction and the strength of the contraction itself (Frank–Starling law). American physiologist, Arthur C Guyton, went a step further and described the dynamics of blood in circulatory physiology. His model of circulation integrated two different functions "the return function" and "the cardiac function" previously described separately by various researchers. The Guytonian model of circulation is now the most widely followed model of circulatory physiology and is described in detail in Guyton and Hall's Textbook of Physiology [2]. In this chapter, we shall reappraise the circulatory physiology as proposed by Guyton and understand the possible effects of fluid and vasoactive agents on circulation. See also Chap. 5 to understand heart-lung interactions and fluid responsiveness.

What Are the Factors That Determine Flow of Blood from Peripheral Circulation to Heart?

Hagen–Poiseuille's law states that the flow of fluid through a system is related to the pressure gradient between two parts of the system (difference between upstream pressure and downstream pressure) divided by the resistance to flow (analogous to Ohm's law of electrical current flow).

$$\text{FLOW}(F) = \frac{\text{Upstream Pressure}(P1) - \text{Downstream Pressure}(P2)}{\text{Resistance to Flow}(R)}$$

Bayliss and Starling first proposed the role of peripheral circulation in determining the return of blood to the heart ("venous return"). They coined the term mean circulatory filling pressure (P_{mcf}), described as the average pressure in the circulation when the heart is stopped momentarily and the pressure in the entire circulatory system equilibrates, for example after administration of the cardioplegic solution. [3] A closely related and more widely used term is mean systemic pressure (P_{ms}) defined as the equilibrium pressure only in the systemic circulation in the absence of any flow, ignoring the heart and pulmonary circulation (e.g. by clamping the aorta and venae cavae). Bayliss and Starling also realized that during active flow, P_{ms} (or P_{mcf}) is determined primarily by the pressure in the venous side of the circulation as the larger volume of blood is stored in the high-capacitance venous system. Years later, Guyton proposed P_{ms} as the upstream pressure for the venous return [4]. He described the right atrial pressure (RAP) as the downstream pressure with the difference between P_{ms} and RAP as the net driving pressure for venous return to the heart. Following the Hagen–Poiseuille's law, the relationship between VR, P_{ms}, RAP and RVR can be plotted as follows:

$$VR = \frac{(Pms - RAP)}{RVR}$$

VR venous return, P_{ms} mean systemic pressure, *RAP* right atrial pressure, *RVR* resistance to venous return

What Are the Factors That Determine Mean Systemic Pressure?

P_{ms} is the result of elastic recoil potential, stored in the walls of the components of the circulatory system and is determined by the volume of blood that stretches the vessels further beyond their normal shape (so-called stressed volume). Stressed volume, in turn, depends on two factors—total circulatory volume and the capacitance of the circulatory system. Normally, only 30% of the blood volume (mostly in the venous circulation) contributes to the stressed volume. The rest of the blood volume (so-called unstressed volume) does not contribute to the circulation but acts only as a reserve. There can be only two ways to increase "stressed volume" (and P_{ms} in this process), either by increasing circulatory volume (e.g. by fluid loading) or by decreasing venous capacitance (e.g. by increasing sympathetic tone with norepinephrine or other vasopressors).

Under normal circumstances, the blood volume remains near constant. Thus, the major factor that determines the return of blood to the heart is resistance to venous return, produced as a result of changes in resistance of blood vessels at the level of organs [2]. The change in resistance and venous capacitance is determined by local factors. For example, during states of high oxygen demand at the organ level, local vasodilator substances are released, decreasing the overall resistance to venous return. Another important factor that determines venous return in the physiological state is RAP, the downstream pressure for VR. Appropriate gradient to VR is maintained by keeping the RAP closer to 0 mmHg by cardiac action [2].

Guyton's Experiment and Venous Return Curve

In the classical animal experiment, Guyton and colleagues cannulated the right atrium and pulmonary artery of anaesthetized dogs and drained the right atrial blood directly to the pulmonary artery via a horizontal thin rubber tubing bypassing the right ventricle [5]. Blood was pumped from the right atrium to the pulmonary artery by using an artificial pump. The pump speed was maintained sufficiently to keep the rubber tubing in a semi-closed state. Pressure at the beginning of the perfusion circuit (reflecting right atrial pressure) was varied by adjusting the height of the horizontal rubber tubing. From this model, they could demonstrate the effects of varying right atrial pressure (from very high positive to very low negative) on venous return (quantified by the amount of blood flowing to the pulmonary artery). They graphically represented their findings with RAP plotted on the *x*-axis and VR on the *y*-axis as shown in Fig. 4.3

As can be seen from the extreme left curve in Fig. 4.3, with progressive lowering of RAP, VR increases until a point beyond which it remains in a plateau state at all RAP values more negative than −2 to −4 mmHg. Guyton demonstrated that this plateau is produced because of the progressive collapse of great veins, due to higher surrounding pressure. In the intersection between VR curve with X-axis, the RAP

Fig. 4.3 Venous return curves. Relationship between right atrial pressure and venous return (left curve). Change in the shape of the curve with a decrease in resistance to venous return (middle blue curve) and with an increase in P_{ms} or mean systemic pressure (right curve)

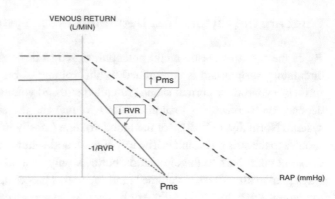

reaches the value of P_{ms} and the VR becomes zero (thankfully only in theory!). The slope of the curve is related to $-1/RVR$, i.e. steeper venous return curve means a decrease in resistance to VR.

Starling's Experiment

In anaesthetized dogs, Starling and his colleagues ligated the inferior vena cava, distal aorta and branches of the aortic arch, keeping the pulmonary circulation and blood flow to the heart itself intact [6]. Through an aortic cannula, systemic blood flow was diverted via the extracorporeal circuit into an elevated reservoir. Blood was returned back to the right atrium through a cannula placed in the superior vena cava. The rate of blood flow from the reservoir into the right atrium was adjusted using a resistor. Over a wide range, the heart could eject whatever volume of blood the system returned to the right atrium. With the increasing the return of blood into the right atrium (by adjusting the Starling resistor), there was a slow rise in right atrial pressure up to a certain limit. Beyond that limit, the rise in RAP was abrupt, limiting the further return of blood to the right atrium. Starling graphically displayed RAP on the y-axis and the return of blood to the right atrium (VR) on the x-axis [6]. Starling's original series of curves are shown in Fig. 4.4.

Cardiac Preload (RAP)

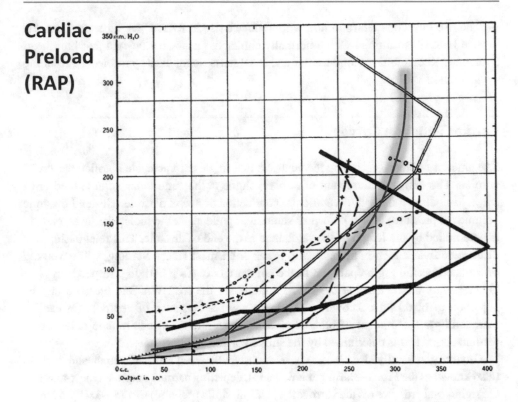

Venous Return

Fig. 4.4 Original starling curve. Relationship between right atrial pressure and venous return in different animals. Permission required [6]

Effect of Fluid Bolus on Venous Return Curve

A fluid bolus can have three potential effects on VR.

1. Fluid bolus is expected to shift the VR curve to the right by increasing the "stressed volume" (and P_{ms}) (as can be seen in the extreme right curve in Fig. 4.3). The increase in P_{ms} in turn is expected to increase the gradient (P_{ms}–RAP) for VR. In reality, the relationship between fluid bolus and an increase in P_{ms} is not as simple and depends on venous capacitance. Another factor that plays a significant role in determining the rise in P_{ms} after fluid bolus is the extent of capillary leak in various disease states. In cases of profound vasoplegia (as in septic shock), venous capacitance and capillary leak increase significantly and fluid bolus may fail to increase "stressed volume".
2. The increase in circulatory volume is also expected to shift the VR curve clockwise, resulting in a decrease in RVR. This drop in RVR can also facilitate venous return (as seen in the middle curve in Fig. 4.3).

3. The rise in venous return in turn will produce a rise in RAP. Up to a certain limit, the rise in RAP is minimal with a normally contractile heart, but beyond that limit heart cannot accommodate blood further and RAP starts rising disproportionately, resulting in a fall in VR [6].

Cardiac Function Curve

The amount of blood ejected by the ventricle in a single cardiac cycle is called the stroke volume. The critical determinant of stroke volume is the ventricular volume (and pressure), just before the onset of ventricular contraction or at end diastole. This end-diastolic volume (or pressure) is also known as ventricular preload. At the molecular level, preload is determined by the length of the sarcomere at the end of diastole. This relationship was discovered independently by both Otto Frank and Ernest Henry Starling, while working on isolated heart–lung preparation in the animal model (frog and dog, respectively) [1]. Other factors that determine the stroke volume are the load ventricle faces during the lejection of blood (also known as afterload) and the elastance of ventricle (or cardiac contractility). The amount of blood ejected by the ventricle in one minute is known as cardiac output and is determined by the stroke volume and heart rate.

Guyton graphically described this relationship between cardiac output and preload (also known as the Frank–Starling relationship), depicting cardiac output on the x-axis and the right atrial pressure (as the surrogate of end-diastolic pressure) on the y-axis producing a curvilinear pattern (cardiac function curve). Figure 4.5 below shows a series of cardiac function curves.

As can be seen in Fig. 4.5, the cardiac function curve reaches a plateau beyond a certain point (curve 1). Another important point to note is that the cardiac function curve is not a single curve but a series of curves and depends on the afterload and contractility of the ventricle. With a decrease in afterload or an increase in contractility, the cardiac function curve is shifted upwards and towards the left (curve 2 in Fig. 4.5). On the contrary, an

Fig. 4.5 Cardiac function curves. Curve 1 describes the relationship between normal cardiac contractility and afterload. Curve 2 describes the same with increased cardiac contractility and low afterload. Curve 3 with poor contractility and higher afterload. *RAP* right atrial pressure

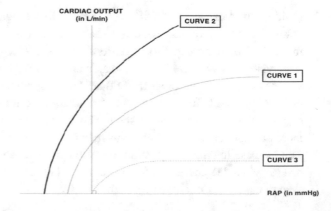

increase in afterload and a decrease in contractility shift the curve towards the right and downwards (curve 3 in Fig. 4.5).

Integrating the Return Function with Cardiac Function

Guyton and colleague proposed a framework to show how the return function of the circulation and cardiac function operate together in the overall circulatory system [7]. Two basic functions of the heart play a significant role in the circulatory dynamics. Firstly, in the steady state, the heart pumps out whatever comes in, i.e. VR must be equal to cardiac output (CO). Secondly, VR is facilitated by the constant pumping of blood from the right heart that keeps the RAP low. As VR and CO must be equal in steady state and both VR curve and cardiac function curve use RAP as the independent variable, the two curves can be superimposed, as seen in Fig. 4.6. Intersection of these two curves is the equilibrium point where VR is equal to CO. This equilibrium point defines the VR/CO in different clinical situations and will be discussed further in the next section.

Fig. 4.6 Integrated venous return and cardiac function curve. *CO* cardiac output, *VR* venous return, *RAP* right atrial pressure

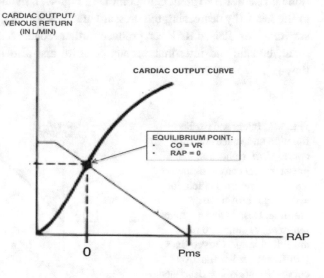

Overall Effect of Fluid Bolus on Circulation

Figure 4.7 graphically displays the overall effects of fluid bolus and vasoactive drugs.

As discussed earlier, intravenous fluid infusion raises the P_{ms} by increasing stressed volume (unless there is an extreme vasoplegia or capillary leak) and shifts the VR curve to the right. This produces a new equilibrium point in the integrated venous return and cardiac function curve. As can be seen in Fig. 4.7, following a fluid bolus, the venous return curve is shifted from the baseline (dotted line) towards the right (dashed line). This results in a shifting of the equilibrium point from point A to point B with a corresponding increase in cardiac output, provided that the new equilibrium point (point B) is in the steep part of the cardiac function curve (permissive heart; middle cardiac function curve). Fluid bolus may also increase the venous return by shifting the curve clockwise (by reducing the resistance to venous return; not shown in Fig. 4.7) [8]. Another relatively less important effect of fluid bolus is a decrease in afterload by haemodilution (and reduction in viscosity of the blood). A decrease in afterload shifts the cardiac function curve towards the left (not shown in Fig. 4.7) [6].

In cases of a poorly contractile heart (when the cardiac function curve is shifted rightward), with similar change in VR, there is minimal or no change in CO and a disproportionate rise in RAP (point C to point D in Fig. 4.7). In addition to the impediment of VR to the heart (by decreasing the pressure gradient for VR), high RAP produces back pressure changes. Raised RAP can produce further reduction in organ perfusion by increasing renal, hepatic and intestinal venous pressure and also impairment in microcirculatory flow [9].

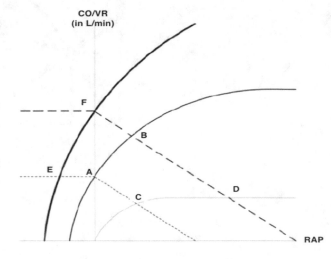

Fig. 4.7 Integrated cardiac function and venous return curves. *RAP* right atrial pressure, *CO* cardiac output, *VR* venous return. Dotted line = venous return curve at baseline. Dashed line = venous return curve shifted to right after fluid bolus. Curved lines = different cardiac function curves. Points A–F = described in detail in the text

Inotropic infusion or a decrease in afterload can shift the cardiac function curve to the left. With this changed cardiac function curve, an increase in P_{ms} (and VR) will increase CO further (point E to point F in Fig. 4.7).

Validation of Guytonian Model in Human Studies

Maas and colleagues tested the feasibility of measuring P_{ms} in intact circulation and tested the effects of hypo- and hypervolemia on P_{ms} [10]. In a study on postoperative cardiac surgery patients, they estimated the VR curve by constructing a regression line between pairs of cardiac output (as surrogate of VR) and central venous pressure (CVP as a surrogate of RAP). CVP and CO values are measured during 12-second inspiratory hold manoeuvre at four different levels of plateau pressure (5, 15, 25 and 35 cm H2O). CO was measured using pulse contour analysis. The intercept of the regression line at the x-axis was taken as P_{ms} (as discussed in an earlier section). VR curves were constructed at baseline (in resting state), during relative hypovolemia (by raising the head of the bed at 30°) and after hypervolemia (by infusion of 500 ml colloids). The study could confirm that P_{ms} decreases with hypovolemia and increases with hypervolemia [10].

In another study on postoperative cardiac surgery patients, the same group tested the effects of norepinephrine on CO and VR curves [11]. In all patients, norepinephrine caused an increase in P_{ms}, resistance to VR and systemic vascular resistance (SVR). However, the effect of norepinephrine on cardiac output was variable. Patients who had a decrease in CO on norepinephrine also had a significantly higher rise in CVP, RVR and SVR compared to those who had an increase in CO on norepinephrine [11]. Persichini and colleagues observed similar effects of norepinephrine on P_{ms} and VR in human septic shock patients [12].

Cecconi and colleagues tested the effects of fluid challenge on P_{msa} (a Pms analogue) and VR gradient (dVR = P_{msa} – CVP) using Navigator™ technology [13]. Studying postoperative patients, they found that the increase in cardiac output by >10% ("responders") with fluid challenge was associated with the corresponding increase in dVR. In "nonresponders", in turn, dVR did not increase despite the consistent increase in P_{ms}, because of a disproportionate rise in CVP [13]. These findings validate the Guytonian model of circulation.

Case Vignette

Mr. X, the patient in the vignette, has clinical evidence of septic shock and the purpose of administering a fluid bolus (500 ml Ringer's lactate in this vignette) is to improve tissue perfusion by increasing the cardiac output.

However, the effects of fluid boluses on cardiac output are variable based on the underlying pre-dominant macro-hemodynamic state. Three possible hemodynamic effects of this fluid bolus on Mr X are as follows:

- **Scenario 1:** P_{ms} may actually rise with minimal rise in RAP, thus increasing VR and CO and in turn improving the organ perfusion (desirable effect).
- **Scenario 2:** In patients with extreme vasoplegia, stressed volume and P_{ms} may not increase and both venous return and cardiac output remain unchanged. This will harm Mr. X in the long run by producing a positive cumulative fluid balance.
- **Scenario 3:** There may be a minimal rise in P_{ms} with a disproportionate increase in RAP and no change in VR or CO. The rise in RAP may in turn reduce organ perfusion further (undesirable effect).

Patients who increase their cardiac output by at least 10% after a rapid bolus of intravenous fluid are described as fluid responders (as in scenario 1). Patients who fall in scenarios 2 and 3 are called fluid non-responders. Fluid responsiveness can be detected by actually challenging the patient with a defined fluid bolus quickly or by performing certain clinical manoeuvres to look for it without actually giving fluid.

Conclusion

The effects of fluid on hemodynamic parameters are not straightforward and depend on various underlying patient-related factors. To obtain a desirable outcome of fluid bolus, it is important for the clinician to be reasonably confident about possible increase in stroke volume (and cardiac output) post-bolus administration. The later can be achieved by careful clinical examination supported by appropriate tests of fluid responsiveness or a carefully performed fluid challenge. While administering fluid boluses, one also should not forget the possible harmful consequences of a fluid bolus, especially when there is no improvement in stroke volume (or cardiac output).

Take-Home Messages
- Rapid fluid bolus can potentially improve hemodynamic parameters in a shock state provided several patient-related conditions are fulfilled.
- For an increase in stroke volume (or cardiac output), stressed volume (and mean systemic pressure) should increase significantly with only minimal change in right atrial pressure. Also, both ventricles must be working in the steep portion of the cardiac function curve.
- The increase in stressed volume may not be sufficient in profound vasodilatory state and in the presence of leaky capillaries.
- When it does not produce improvement in macro-hemodynamic parameters, fluid boluses can only contribute to fluid overload and potential harm associated with the same.
- Potential harms associated with fluid bolus cannot be ignored and need to be considered before prescription.

References

1. Katz AM. Ernest Henry Starling, his predecessors, and the "law of the heart". Circulation. 2002;106:2986–92.
2. Hall JE. Guyton and Hall textbook of medical physiology. 13th ed. Philadelphia: Elsevier; 2016.
3. Bayliss WM, Starling EH. Observations on venous pressures and their relationship to capillary pressures. J Physiol. 1894;16:159–318.
4. Guyton AC, Lindsey AW, Kaufmann BN. Effect of mean circulatory filling pressure and other peripheral circulatory factors on cardiac output. Am J Phys. 1955;180:463–8.
5. Guyton AC, Lindsey AW, Abernathy B, Richardson T. Venous return at various right atrial pressures and the normal venous return curve. Am J Phys. 1957;189:609–15.
6. Patterson SW, Starling EH. On the mechanical factors which determine the output of the ventricles. J Physiol. 1914;48:357–79.
7. Guyton AC, Coleman TG, Granger HJ. Circulation: overall regulation. Annu Rev Physiol. 1972;34:13–46.
8. Funk DJ, Jacobsohn E, Kumar A. The role of venous return in critical illness and shock—part I: physiology. Crit Care Med. 2013;41:255–62.
9. Marik PE. Iatrogenic salt water drowning and the hazards of a high central venous pressure. Ann Intensive Care. 2014;4:21.
10. Maas JJ, Geerts BF, van den Berg PC, Pinsky MR, Jansen JR. Assessment of venous return curve and mean systemic filling pressure in postoperative cardiac surgery patients. Crit Care Med. 2009;37:912–8.
11. Maas JJ, Pinsky MR, de Wilde RB, de Jonge E, Jansen JR. Cardiac output response to norepinephrine in postoperative cardiac surgery patients: interpretation with venous return and cardiac function curves. Crit Care Med. 2013;41:143–50.
12. Persichini R, Silva S, Teboul JL, Jozwiak M, Chemla D, Richard C, Monnet X. Effects of norepinephrine on mean systemic pressure and venous return in human septic shock. Crit Care Med. 2012;40:3146–53.
13. Cecconi M, Aya HD, Geisen M, Ebm C, Fletcher N, Grounds RM, Rhodes A. Changes in the mean systemic filling pressure during a fluid challenge in postsurgical intensive care patients. Intensive Care Med. 2013;39:1299–305.

Understanding Heart-Lung Interactions: Concepts of Fluid Responsiveness

5

Ajeet Singh and Shrikanth Srinivasan

Contents

Introduction 118
Basics of Respiratory and Cardio-Circulatory Physiology 119
Effects of Mechanical Ventilation on Intrathoracic Pressure 120
The Pump 121
   Venous Return and Ventricular Preload 121
   Ventricular Afterload 123
   Left Ventricular Afterload 123
   Right Ventricular Afterload 123
Ventricular Interdependence 124
Heart-Lung Interactions: Clinical Application 124
   Functional Hemodynamic Monitoring 124
      Concept of Fluid Responsiveness 124
Dynamic Indicators for Fluid Responsiveness 126
   Invasive Assessment of Respiratory Changes in LV Stroke Volume 126
Pulse Pressure Variation 127
   Non-invasive Assessment of Respiratory Changes in LV Stroke Volume 130
Other Clinically Significant Clinical Interactions 131
Cardiopulmonary Changes in Prone Positioning 132
Conclusions 133
References 134

A. Singh · S. Srinivasan (✉)
Critical Care Medicine, Manipal Hospital, Dwarka, New Delhi, India

© The Author(s) 2024
M. L. N. G. Malbrain et al. (eds.), *Rational Use of Intravenous Fluids in Critically Ill Patients*, https://doi.org/10.1007/978-3-031-42205-8_5

113

IFA Commentary (MLNGM)

This chapter will explore a variety of different methods for determining fluid responsiveness, many of which are based on heart-lung interactions. A recent review paper provides a comprehensive overview of the various monitoring tools available, including arterial waveform variations and the passive leg raising test, as well as several other approaches [1]. It is noteworthy that any test, in order to be able to predict fluid responsiveness, should monitor cardiac output (CO) continuously.

Arterial waveform analysis. The first method to be discussed involves taking advantage of heart-lung interactions, specifically the respiratory variations in arterial pressure that are seen in ventilated patients. These variations have been shown to be related to central blood volume, diastolic function, and cardiac contractility. In 2000, Michard and colleagues demonstrated that the respiratory variation in pulse pressure, or pulse pressure variation (PPV), which reflects stroke volume variation (SVV), can detect fluid responsiveness when it is increased above 12–15% during controlled mechanical ventilation [2].

Since then, numerous studies have confirmed the validity of this index, while others have described various surrogates for stroke volume whose respiratory variability predicts response to fluid, such as systolic pressure variation (SPV) with the separation of deltaUp and deltaDown phenomena [3]. Only the deltaDown is an indicator for fluid responsiveness whereas deltaUp can be increased in patients with heart failure and situations of increased intrathoracic pressure (e.g., with high PEEP, autoPEEP, or abdominal hypertension). However, the limitations of these functional hemodynamic parameters soon became apparent, as to be accurate, PPV and SVV require a fixed heart rate and a significant positive-pressure-induced increase in intrathoracic pressure.

Other factors, such as spontaneous respiratory activity, cardiac arrhythmias, lower tidal volumes used in the management of acute respiratory distress syndrome, as well as low pulmonary compliance, increased intra-abdominal pressure [4], and right heart failure, may generate false positives and false negatives [5], making neither PPV nor SVV usable across all patients with cardiovascular insufficiency.

Although a little bit counterintuitive, PPV has a better overall area under the receiver operating characteristic curve (AUROC) to predict fluid responsiveness compared to SVV, and thus is preferred. In 2004, two articles in the same issue of the journal reported the ability of changes in the inferior vena cava diameter to predict fluid responsiveness [6, 7]. Unfortunately, vena cava distensibility shares many limitations with PPV and SVV and has limited predictive value [8].

The passive leg raising test. To circumvent the limits of PPV, the passive leg raising (PLR) test has been developed. The postural change, which was used for years by rescuers in patients falling in collapse, induces a significant though transient blood transfer from the lower extremities and the splanchnic territory that increases cardiac preload. The PLR test is considered positive if the cardiac output (CO) increases with 10%.

In 2006, the ability of the PLR test to detect preload responsiveness was demonstrated, including in conditions in which PPV is invalid [9]. It has been widely validated and integrated into international recommendations [10].

The end expiratory occlusion test. In 2009, heart-lung interactions during mechanical ventilation were explored again, and the end-expiratory occlusion test was developed, consisting of temporarily stopping the cyclical drop in preload caused by insufflation. This test was shown to indicate preload responsiveness if CO increased with 5% [11].

The respiratory systolic variation test. The respiratory systolic variation test (RSVT) was developed in 2005, consisting of four incremental, successive, pressure-controlled breaths [12], and the slope of the RSVT decreased significantly after intravascular fluid administration and correlated with the end-diastolic area and with changes in cardiac output better than filling pressure. Later, in 2017, the tidal volume challenge was developed to use PPV despite low tidal volume ventilation [13]. It simply consists of transiently increasing the tidal volume from 6 to 8 mL/kg and detecting a PPV increase in preload-responsive patients. The haemodynamic effects of recruitment manoeuvres also use heart-lung interactions (Fig. 5.1).

The mini-fluid challenge test. Finally, since the "classical" fluid challenge (4 ml/kg/5–15 min) inherently induces fluid overload (when continued until the patient becomes no longer fluid responsive), a "mini-fluid challenge" made up of only 100–150 mL (1–2 ml/kg/1–5 min) of fluid was demonstrated to also predict volume responsiveness but with less inherent fluid accumulation (14). It has already received a reasonable validation.

Suggested Reading

1. Monnet X, Malbrain M, Pinsky MR. The prediction of fluid responsiveness. Ann Intensive Care. 2022;12:46.
2. Michard F, Boussat S, Chemla D, Anguel N, Mercat A, Lecarpentier Y, et al. Relation between respiratory changes in arterial pulse pressure and fluid responsiveness in septic patients with acute circulatory failure. Am J Respir Crit Care Med. 2000;162(1):134–8.
3. Perel A, Pizov R, Cotev S. Systolic blood pressure variation is a sensitive indicator of hypovolemia in ventilated dogs subjected to graded hemorrhage. Anesthesiology. 1987;67(4):498–502.
4. Malbrain MLNG, De Keulenaer BL, Khanna AK. Continuous intra-abdominal pressure: is it ready for prime time? Intensive Care Med. 2022;48(10):1501–4.

5. Monnet X, Shi R, Teboul JL. Prediction of fluid responsiveness. What's new? Ann Intensive Care. 2022;12(1):46.

6. Barbier C, Loubieres Y, Schmit C, Hayon J, Ricome JL, Jardin F, et al. Respiratory changes in inferior vena cava diameter are helpful in predicting fluid responsiveness in ventilated septic patients. Intensive Care Med. 2004;30(9):1740–6.

7. Feissel M, Michard F, Faller JP, Teboul JL. The respiratory variation in inferior vena cava diameter as a guide to fluid therapy. Intensive Care Med. 2004;30(9):1834–7.

8. Vignon P, Repesse X, Begot E, Leger J, Jacob C, Bouferrache K, et al. Comparison of Echocardiographic Indices Used to Predict Fluid Responsiveness in Ventilated Patients. Am J Respir Crit Care Med. 2017;195(8):1022–32.

9. Monnet X, Rienzo M, Osman D, Anguel N, Richard C, Pinsky MR, et al. Passive leg raising predicts fluid responsiveness in the critically ill. Crit Care Med. 2006;34(5):1402–7.

10. Evans L, Rhodes A, Alhazzani W, Antonelli M, Coopersmith CM, French C, et al. Executive Summary: Surviving sepsis campaign: international guidelines for the management of sepsis and septic shock 2021. Crit Care Med. 2021;49(11):1974–82.

11. Gavelli F, Shi R, Teboul JL, Azzolina D, Monnet X. The end-expiratory occlusion test for detecting preload responsiveness: a systematic review and meta-analysis. Ann Intensive Care. 2020;10(1):65.

12. Perel A, Minkovich L, Preisman S, Abiad M, Segal E, Coriat P. Assessing fluid-responsiveness by a standardized ventilatory maneuver: the respiratory systolic variation test. Anesth Analg. 2005;100(4):942–5.

13. Myatra SN, Prabu NR, Divatia JV, Monnet X, Kulkarni AP, Teboul JL. The changes in pulse pressure variation or stroke volume variation after a "tidal volume challenge" reliably predict fluid responsiveness during low tidal volume ventilation. Crit Care Med. 2017;45(3):415–21.

14. Muller L, Toumi M, Bousquet PJ, Riu-Poulenc B, Louart G, Candela D, et al. An increase in aortic blood flow after an infusion of 100 ml colloid over 1 minute can predict fluid responsiveness: the mini-fluid challenge study. Anesthesiology. 2011;115(3):541–7.

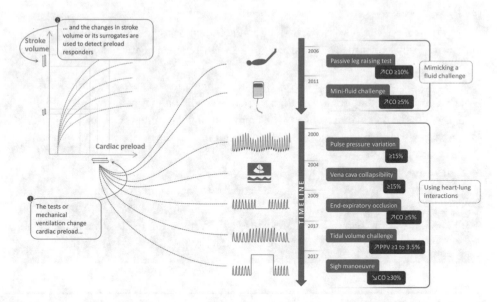

Fig. 5.1 Tests and indices of preload responsiveness with proposed timeline. The principle of the dynamic assessment of preload responsiveness is to observe spontaneous or induced changes in cardiac preload, and the resulting change in cardiac output, stroke volume or their surrogates. Some tests or indices use heart–lung interactions in mechanically ventilated patients, while some others mimic a classical fluid challenge. Diagnostic threshold and the year of description are indicated. *CO* cardiac output, *PPV* pulse pressure variation. Adapted with permission from Monnet et al. [1]

Learning Objectives

The learning objectives of this chapter are:
1. Physiology of heart-lung interactions and their effect on hemodynamics
2. Identify fluid responsiveness using heart-lung interactions
3. Physiology, techniques, and evidence of various dynamic measures of fluid responsiveness based on heart-lung interactions
4. Clinical implication of fluid responsiveness and consideration for fluid accumulation with injudicious fluid administration

Case Vignette

Mr. J, a 62-year-old male with a history of hypertension, presented to the ICU with septic shock secondary to a urinary tract infection. The patient was intubated and mechanically ventilated, and initial resuscitation with fluids and vasopressors was initiated. The patient remained hypotensive despite ongoing vasopressor support. The critical care team suspected that the patient might be volume depleted, and they wanted to assess his fluid responsiveness.

The team decided to use heart-lung interactions to assess fluid responsiveness in Mr. J. They performed a passive leg raise (PLR) maneuver and monitored the patient's hemodynamic response.

During the PLR, the team observed an increase in the stroke volume (SV) by 20%, indicating that Mr. J was fluid responsive. The patient received a fluid bolus, and his blood pressure improved. The team continued to monitor the patient closely and adjusted his fluid management accordingly.

Questions

Q1. Why did the critical care team decide to use heart-lung interactions to assess fluid responsiveness in Mr. J?

Q2. What was the hemodynamic response observed during the PLR maneuver, and what does it indicate and what are its limitations?

Introduction

A thorough understanding of ventilation and its effects on the hemodynamics of critically ill patients constitutes an integral part of managing patients in intensive care units. Cardiopulmonary interactions in ventilated and non-ventilated patients may affect the hemodynamics, which can lead to diminished tissue oxygen delivery and organ dysfunctions, thereby contributing to morbidity and mortality. Therefore, a thorough understanding of the effects of spontaneous and positive pressure ventilation on the cardiovascular system helps us to understand hemodynamic perturbations better and manage them appropriately.

The main goal of fluid administration is to increase the preload and ultimately to improve cardiac output and oxygen delivery. While consensus exists on the use of fluid challenge to assess preload responsiveness, the type of fluid, extent and rate of administration, and hemodynamic targets need to be standardized in clinical practice [1]. At times, the fluid challenge is unsafe and leads to volume overload in non-responders [2].

Increasing evidence suggests that excessive fluid administration is associated with increased mortality [3]. Fluid need and responsiveness should be assessed before fluid administration to avoid volume overload and its complications.

Differentiating fluid responders from non-responders is essential to determine the efficacy of therapy and to avoid the deleterious effects of volume overload. For this reason, various static and dynamic parameters have been used in critically ill patients to predict volume responsiveness. These parameters have varying degrees of accuracy and shortcomings in various patient groups. All these parameters are based on the impact of the cyclic variations caused by respiration on the cardiac filling and hence require a thorough understanding of heart-lung interactions. See also Chap. 4 to learn more about fluid dynamics during resuscitation according to Frank–Starling and Guyton-Hall.

Basics of Respiratory and Cardio-Circulatory Physiology

The cardiovascular system consists of mainly two components: the circuit and the pump. The circuit contains arterial resistance and venous capacitance vessels. Arteries and arterioles are the resistance vessels that have smooth muscles responsible for controlling the resistance to blood flow by changing the caliber. Venules and veins are capacitance vessels that hold at least 70% of circulating blood volume and have no major contribution to resistance. The pump is constituted of the right and left ventricles, enclosed by the pericardium. The ventricles work in parallel but pump in series and are connected to each other through pulmonary circulation. Both the heart and surrounding lungs are enclosed within the rigid chest wall, creating a chamber within a chamber effect [4]. Therefore, phasic changes in pleural pressure during the respiratory cycle will affect the pressure system of the cardiac chambers and influence the gradient for venous return, preload, and afterload [5, 6].

Transmural pressure (P_{TM}) is the difference of pressures (internal to external) across a hollow structure. In the thoracic cavity, the external pressure for the heart is pericardial pressure (P_{PER}) and for lungs, the external pressure is the pleural pressure (P_{PL}) [7, 8].

The transmural pressure (RAP_{TM}) for the right atrium can be calculated by the formula: $RAP_{TM} = RAP - P_{PL}$ [9]. However, in the clinical practice, P_{PL} and P_{PER} are assumed to be equal to intrathoracic pressure (ITP) which is the external pressure around the heart and the lungs. However, it must be noted that ITP is not homogeneously distributed throughout the thorax [10]. The P_{TM} is the actual working pressure that, together with chamber compliance, defines the venous return, cardiac filling, and hence, cardiac output. In clinical practice, P_{PL} can be estimated by measuring the esophageal pressure with an air-filled balloon in the esophagus at end-expiration [11].

The lungs are surrounded by two pleural layers and enclosed by the chest wall and the diaphragm. The two pleural layers ensure the mechanical coupling between lung and the chest wall. P_{PL} is negative in spontaneous breathing and acts as external pressure of the lung and cardiac structures. The P_{TM} for lungs or transpulmonary pressure (P_{TP}) is the difference of alveolar pressure (P_{AL}) and P_{PL}. It decides the lung volume at the end of inhalation, depending on the compliance of the lung within the chest wall [9].

Lung compliance (CL) and chest wall compliance (CCW) defines the total compliance of the respiratory system (CRS): i.e. (1/CRS = 1/CL + 1/CCW) [12].

Blood flow through the lungs depends on the driving pressure for the blood, that is (mean pulmonary artery pressure [PAPm] − mean left atrial pressure [LAPm]) and pulmonary vascular resistance (PVR) [13]. With a pulmonary artery catheter, LAPm can be estimated by measuring pulmonary artery occlusion pressure (PAOP).

The pulmonary vascular resistance is increased by vasoconstriction, hypoxic (Euler-Lilijestrand reflex [14]) or hypercapnic pulmonary vasoconstriction [15]. Pulmonary vessels are more compliant than systemic vessels, compressible by surrounding lungs and act as Starling resistors. A vessel working as a Starling resistor, can change its diameter and the related resistance to flow according to its surrounding pressure. Increased extravascular pressure (increased P_{AL} or P_{PL}) diminishes transmural pulmonary vascular pressure, resulting in an increased PVR [16]. During the respiratory cycle at end-expiration, when the lung is at its functional residual capacity (FRC) and where the resistance of interalveolar vessels equals the resistance of extra-alveolar vessels, PVR is the lowest [17].

Effects of Mechanical Ventilation on Intrathoracic Pressure

During the inspiratory phase of mechanical ventilation, the machine delivers a tidal volume through an artificial airway to the lungs leading to positive P_{AL} and P_{PL}. The transmission of airway pressure to the pleural space is lower if the CRS of the system is low, as in acute respiratory distress syndrome (ARDS), which has reduced lung compliance and therefore, has less hemodynamic effect by heart-lung interactions compare to increased compliant system as seen in chronic obstructive pulmonary disease (COPD) [18].

With the application of positive end-expiratory pressure (PEEP) and the absence of spontaneous breathing efforts, P_{PL} is positive throughout the respiratory cycle. In contrast, with unforced spontaneous breathing, P_{PL} always remains negative.

The physiological consequences of these changes in P_{PL} and P_{TP} are as follows:

1. An elevated P_{AL} combined with the supine position alters pulmonary blood flow by creating lung areas with zone 1 conditions (compression of alveolar vessels) and increasing the proportion of areas with zone 2 conditions (compression of veins), causing increased PVR and dead space ventilation.
2. An increased ITP reduces P_{TM} of large intrathoracic blood vessels as the vena cava and thoracic aorta, thereby diminishing intrathoracic blood volume.
3. The ITP is also transmitted to the pericardium, which encloses the heart.

These physiological consequences are due to respiratory swings in intrathoracic pressure, and their effects on hemodynamics are predictable; for example, as RAP increases with positive ITP, the venous return goes down [19, 20]. This could lead to profound and sometimes abrupt cardio-circulatory effects with positive pressure ventilation. This phenomenon should be expected and patients need appropriate monitoring (Fig. 5.2). The overall effect of positive pressure on preload, afterload, and pump function will be explained in detail later.

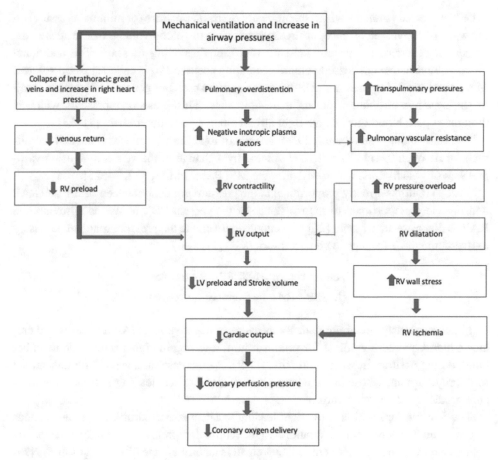

Fig. 5.2 Cardiovascular effects of mechanical ventilation

The Pump

The pumping work of the heart is to maintain adequate and optimum cardiac output. Cardiac output is determined by the heart rate and stroke volume. Stroke volume is the amount of blood expelled from the left ventricle (LV) into the systemic circulation with each heartbeat. Averaged over several seconds to minutes, LV stroke volume equals right ventricular stroke volume. The LV preload, myocardial contractility, and afterload are the main determinants of stroke volume.

Venous Return and Ventricular Preload

Cardio-circulatory physiology and heart-lung interactions can best be understood if we familiarize ourselves with determinants of venous return and the functioning of the right ventricle. Of the total blood volume, only about 15% exerts pressure, and the rest is said to be "unstressed volume", which theoretically exerts no pressure (or minimal pressure) on the walls of the vessels. Hence, unstressed volume is the blood volume that resides in the vessels at near-zero transmural pressure (P_{TM}), or distending pressure. The additional blood volume above unstressed volume generating positive P_{TM} is called stressed volume. Mean systemic filling pressure (MSFP) represents the pressure generated by elastic recoil of the systemic circulation during a no-flow state. This pressure represents which is thought to push blood towards the right atrium along a pressure gradient [21–23].

Stressed volume can be altered by a change of total intravascular volume and recruitment or de-recruitment of unstressed volume by a change in the vessel tone using vasopressors or vasodilators, which will alter the MSFP accordingly [22, 24, 25].

Venous return is directly proportional to the pressure gradient between MSFP and RAP and inversely proportional to the resistance of the vessels (Rv). MSFP as upstream and RAP as downstream pressure [26] for venous return create the pressure gradient necessary to overcome the resistance to venous return (VR) [27, 28].

$$\text{Venous return} = (\text{MSFP} - \text{RAP}) / \text{Rv}$$
$$(\text{MSFP} - \text{RAP}) = 5 \, \text{mmHg approx.}$$

In spontaneously breathing patients, because of negative P_{PL}, RAP decreases and creates a higher-pressure gradient for venous return, resulting in higher return. On the other hand, during positive pressure ventilation (PPV), P_{PL} increases and is partially transmitted to the right atrium, whose intracavitary pressure (RAP) rises, leading a decrease in pressure gradient and venous return.

The Starling curve shifts to the right leading to a decrease in cardiac output and venous return. Under mechanical ventilation, right ventricular preload is mainly affected by changes in P_{PL}, whereas left ventricular preload is mainly affected by changes in P_{TP} [29] (Fig. 5.3).

Fig. 5.3 Effects of mean intrathoracic pressure on systemic vascular return. Systemic venous return to the right atrium is passive, with blood flow occurring due to pressure gradient between the superior/inferior vena cava and the right atrium. *Psv* systemic venous pressure, *RAP* right atrial pressure, *PPV* positive pressure ventilation

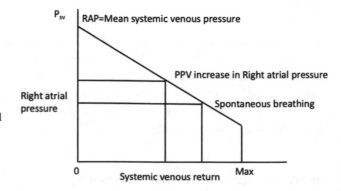

Ventricular Afterload

Afterload is defined as the force opposing ventricular ejection of blood [30]. Afterload can be approached by assessing ventricular wall tension or vascular resistance and impedance [31]. We will now discuss both ventricles separately, given their relatively different muscle mass, position, and orientation.

Left Ventricular Afterload

The work of the left ventricle depends on the aortic elastance ($\Delta P/\Delta V$) (i.e., to accommodate and release a proportion of each stroke volume temporarily) and the overall resistance of the arterial vessel tree [32]. Subtle intra-thoracic pressure swings like those during spontaneous respiration cause only minor cyclic changes in left ventricular afterload in healthy humans. However, the cardiac output can be considerably decreased by forced spontaneous inspiration or a Muller manoeuver due to an abrupt increase in transmural pressure and afterload [33].

During positive pressure ventilation or by the application of PEEP, ITP and concomitantly P_{PL} rise. P_{TM} of the LV and, to a lesser extent, of the intrathoracic part of the aorta falls, while P_{TM} in the abdominal aorta remains higher, resulting in a net afterload reduction and facilitating blood flow from the intrathoracic to the abdominal compartment. These changes seem to be mainly mediated by changes in P_{PL} [29].

With LV afterload reduction, the application of continuous positive airway pressure (CPAP) in spontaneously breathing patients or pressure support ventilation with PEEP in sedated patients can be a valuable supportive measure in the treatment of acutely decompensated left ventricular failure [34].

Right Ventricular Afterload

Blood is pumped by the right ventricle (RV) into the pulmonary vasculature, which is a highly compliant low-pressure system. Alterations in RV outflow are mainly mediated through changes in ITP [29, 35]. Changes in ITP can strongly affect transmural pulmonary vascular pressure and PVR, and thereby RV output. During spontaneous breathing, inspiration is associated with negative P_{PL}, which distend the pulmonary vasculature, reducing RV afterload and thereby increases RV output.

During mechanical ventilation, tidal breathing increases P_{PL}, thus reducing transmural pulmonary vascular pressure and consequently elevating RV afterload and decreasing RV output. In individuals with pre-existing right ventricular dysfunction, or severe hypoxic pulmonary vasoconstriction in the context of ARDS, mechanical ventilation (cyclical tidal inflation) may precipitate RV failure by increasing RV afterload [29, 35–39].

Since the RV possesses much lesser contractile reserves, acute elevations of afterload are poorly tolerated by the RV compared with the LV [39]. The lowest PVR during the respiratory cycle is seen at end-expiration at FRC. PVR rises at lung volumes both below and above the FRC [17].

Ventricular Interdependence

The LV and RV work as serial pumps connected by the pulmonary and systemic vasculature. Through their electrical and mechanical synchronization, they work in parallel within the confines of the pericardium. Due to the shared interventricular septum and the pericardial constraints, the diastolic pressure of one ventricle directly affects the diastolic filling of the other, and this phenomenon is called interventricular dependence [40, 41].

When the RV volume increases, the septum bulges to the left, leading to a decline in LV filling. This phenomenon can be seen in conditions with RV afterload elevation like pulmonary embolism, pulmonary hypertension, or mechanical ventilation. Increased RV pressure and volume leads to interventricular septum flattening or convex bowing into the LV cavity, thus decreasing the LV volume and filling. Clinically important examples of interventricular dependence are pericardial tamponade, status asthmaticus, and COPD [42].

Heart-Lung Interactions: Clinical Application

The complex cardiopulmonary physiology interplay makes heart-lung interactions in a ventilated patient, very important, as mechanical ventilation can provoke cardiovascular instability [41]. An understanding of heart-lung interactions offers possibilities to predict hemodynamic alterations and to decide appropriate treatment modalities, especially guiding volume expansion, within the framework of functional hemodynamic monitoring [42].

Functional Hemodynamic Monitoring

Concept of Fluid Responsiveness

Fluid depletion or hypovolemia is often the primary or contributory cause of acute circulatory failure, except in cases of cardiogenic shock. In intensive care units (ICUs), the decision regarding volume expansion is frequent and many a times quiet challenging. Fluid administration will lead to an increase in cardiac output only if the ventricles operate on the ascending (steep) portion of the frank starling curve (Fig. 5.4). If the preload of the

Fig. 5.4 Schematic representation of the Frank–Starling
relationship between ventricular preload and stroke volume.
A given change in preload
induces a larger change in
stroke volume when the
ventricle operates on the
ascending portion of the
relationship ((**a**) condition of
preload dependence) than
when it operates on the flat
portion of the curve ((**b**)
condition of preload
independence)

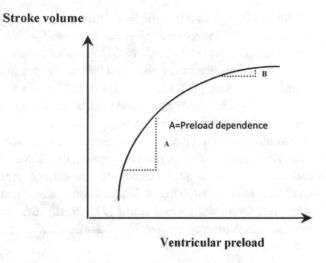

ventricles operates on the flat portion of the frank starling curve, then volume expansion
may only exert adverse effects without increasing the cardiac output or any hemodynamic
benefit [43].

Excessive fluid administration has been associated with a significant increase in mortality, acute kidney injury, and increased duration of mechanical ventilation [3]. Positive
indicators of fluid responsiveness also do not justify fluid therapy by themselves [2, 43,
44]. The literature supports that only 50% of patients are fluid-responsive in patients with
acute circulatory failure [4]. Besides, fluid responsiveness does not predict fluid tolerance.
The cardinal purpose of fluid administration in circulatory shock is to increase tissue oxygenation, not cardiac output. To achieve this goal, fluid must be administered only if
required (in circulatory shock), and are fluid responders (positive fluid responsiveness)
and fluid tolerant. Hence, the primary purpose of fluid responsiveness is to determine
which patients should not be given fluid. Several strategies have been developed to identify fluid responsiveness before fluid administration for resuscitation to avoid fluid overload and its complications. Various static and dynamic parameters have been evaluated to
identify responders to fluid therapy [2].

The static parameters are inaccurate to predict preload responsiveness [44] (Fig. 5.4).
Despite our current knowledge, there has been a continued and widespread use of static
parameters to predict fluid responsiveness. According to a recently conducted study, fluid
challenges in intensive care: the FENICE study [45], the CVP was used most often as a
predictor for fluid responsiveness. The above observation is interesting, considering that
the CVP is a poor variable to predict fluid responsiveness [46–48].

Other bedside indicators of preload, such as the RV end-diastolic volume (evaluated by
thermodilution) and the LV end-diastolic area (measured by echocardiography), have also
been tested as predictors of fluid responsiveness. Unfortunately, these parameters were
also not found accurate enough to differentiate between fluid responder and non-responders
[42, 49–53].

Studies have shown that the right atrial and pulmonary artery occlusion pressures do not always reflect transmural pressures in patients with external or intrinsic positive end-expiratory pressure (PEEP) [42, 46, 54]. In patients with decreased left ventricular compliance, the pulmonary artery occlusion pressure is not always a reliable indicator of left ventricular preload [47]. Measurement of RV end-diastolic volume by thermodilution is influenced by tricuspid regurgitation [55], which is frequently encountered in critically ill patients with pulmonary hypertension.

Studies have found that the left ventricular end-diastolic area, as measured by echocardiography, may not always accurately reflect the left ventricular end-diastolic volume and therefore may not be a reliable indicator of left ventricular preload [56]. In some cases, right ventricular dilation may offset the hemodynamic benefits of volume expansion, even when left ventricular preload is low [57]. Finally, the preload-induced changes in stroke volume also depend on contractility and afterload.

Dynamic Indicators for Fluid Responsiveness

The poor performance of static parameters has paved the way for the development of dynamic parameters based on heart-lung interaction for predicting fluid responsiveness. Dynamic indices have been shown to reduce unnecessary fluid loading and potential complications of volume overload. Dynamic indices based on heart-lung interactions are classified into two broad categories.

1. Invasive assessment of respiratory changes in LV stroke volume
   (a) Stroke volume variation with respiration
   (b) Pulse pressure variation with respiration
   (c) Systolic pressure variation with respiration
2. Non-invasive assessment of respiratory changes in LV stroke volume
   (a) Doppler echocardiography for measuring changes in LV stroke volume (VTI) with respiration
   (b) Echocardiographic assessment of the vena cava
   (c) Estimation of MSFP with ventilator maneuvers
   (d) Pulse pressure variation with respiration infrared photoplethysmography coupled with the volume clamp technique

Invasive Assessment of Respiratory Changes in LV Stroke Volume

Measurement of Stroke volume variation (SVV) and Pulse pressure variation by minimally invasive arterial pressure-based CO monitoring techniques (PiCCO, LiDCO) induced by mechanical ventilation were the first techniques used to assess fluid responsiveness. Fluid responsiveness may be assessed by calculating the variation in stroke volume (Δ SVV) with respiration which can be calculated as follow.

$$\Delta SVV\left(\%\right)=100\times\frac{\left(SV_{max}-SV_{min}\right)}{\left(SV_{max}+SV_{min}\right)/2}$$

where SV_{max} and SV_{min} are the maximal and minimal values of stroke volume over a single respiratory cycle (Fig. 5.5). The difference between the maximal and minimal values of stroke volume over a single respiratory cycle is called stroke volume variation (SVV).

The reference stroke volume is measured during an end-expiratory pause (line of reference) and is divided into two components: Delta up (Δ up) and Delta down (Δ down). Delta up is the difference between the maximal and the reference stroke volume pressure. Delta down is the difference between the reference and the minimal stroke pressure (Fig. 5.5). In mechanically ventilated patients, hypovolemia has been shown to increase SPV [58], whereas volume expansion decreases SPV [58, 59]. The threshold of SVV >12% has been shown to predict fluid responsiveness with sensitivity and specificity greater than 85%.

Interestingly, Coriat et al. [59] reported a significant relationship between Δ SV down before fluid infusion and the increase in the cardiac index in response to volume expansion in patients after aortic surgery. Therefore, Δ SV down can be considered an indicator of fluid responsiveness because the higher Δ down before volume expansion, greater the increase in the cardiac index in response to fluid infusion.

Pulse Pressure Variation

Pulse pressure is the difference between systolic and diastolic pressure. It is directly proportional to LV stroke volume and inversely related to arterial compliance [60]. An increase in pleural pressure induced by mechanical ventilation affects both systolic and diastolic pressures. Hence, the pulse pressure is not directly influenced by the cyclic changes in pleural pressure. Instead, the respiratory changes in LV stroke volume are reflected by changes in peripheral pulse pressure during the respiratory cycle [61].

The fluid responsiveness may be assessed by calculating the respiratory changes in pulse pressure (PP) as follows.

$$\Delta PP\left(\%\right)=100\times\frac{\left(PP_{max}-PP_{min}\right)}{\left(PP_{max}+PP_{min}\right)/2}$$

where PP_{max} and PP_{min} are the maximal and minimal values of pulse pressure over a single respiratory cycle, respectively. The pulse pressure (systolic minus diastolic pressure) is maximal (PP_{max}) at the end of the inspiratory period and minimal (PP_{min}) three heartbeats later (i.e., during the expiratory period) (Fig. 5.5).

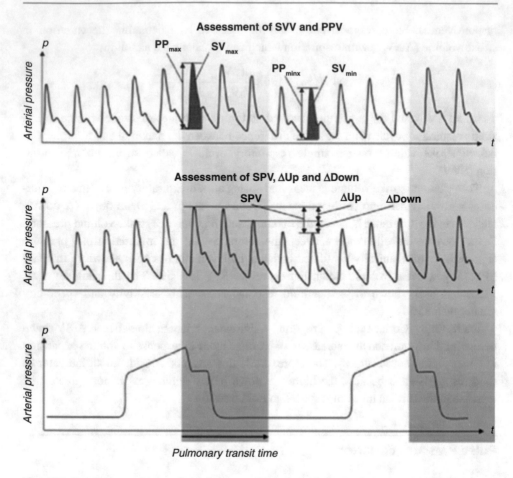

Fig. 5.5 Respiratory changes in pulse pressure and stroke volume in a mechanically ventilated patient

Michard and colleagues showed a good prediction of fluid responsiveness in septic patients with a PPV $\geq 12\%$ [62]. In recent light of the evidence, calculating PPV may be of particular help in deciding whether to institute volume expansion. Indeed, if PPV is low (<13%), then a beneficial hemodynamic effect of volume expansion is very unlikely, and inotropes or vasoactive drugs should be started in order to improve hemodynamics. In contrast, if PPV is high (>13%), then a significant increase in the cardiac index in response to the fluid infusion is very likely.

PPV of the arterial pressure is caused by preload and stroke volume changes in the right ventricle. Any factor interfering with the pulmonary vasculature or function may affect PPV [63, 64]. Its apparent simplicity may distract the clinician from several important pitfalls. PPV and SVV are influenced by any spontaneous respiratory effort [42], tidal volume (needs to be larger than 8 ml/kg, which is not current practice in lung-protective ventilation) [42], respiratory rate and pulmonary transit time [65], and the CRS [66]. The absence of sinus rhythm and frequent ectopic beats render PPV unusable. Most critically ill patients have above-mentioned limitations affecting the valid interpretation of PPV [67, 68]. The most important limitation of PPV is RV dysfunction, which also causes the arterial pressure to undulate because of smaller stroke volumes with increased afterload during mechanical inspiration.

In order to avoid deleterious volume loading, PPV should not be seen as a marker of volume responsiveness per se [35, 42, 69, 70] but rather as an indicator of LV function depending on RV stroke volume. A failure to increase cardiac output following volume expansion calls for an immediate diagnostic evaluation of the RV. If cardiac output is not augmented or vasopressors are not decreased following a volume challenge, no further volume should be applied, and careful evaluation of the RV function should be performed, if PPV is present.

If a patient's blood volume is centralized owing to adrenergic (endogenous or exogenous) vasoconstriction with concomitant insufficient tissue perfusion, a negative PPV does not exclude the need for volume infusion. Venous return is maintained by vasoconstriction that shifts volume from the pool of unstressed volume to the pool of stressed volume. In this case, volume expansion may reduce the dose of vasopressor agents and restore tissue perfusion by normalizing unstressed volume and reducing vasoconstriction.

Overall, volume administration should be done when we have critical tissue oxygenation, evidence of fluid responsiveness and a positive effect on oxygen delivery can be documented. The assessment of cardiac preload dependence is helpful in predicting volume expansion efficacy and the hemodynamic effects of any therapy that induces changes in cardiac preload conditions.

In this regard, PPV has been shown to be useful in monitoring the hemodynamic effects of PEEP in mechanically ventilated patients with acute lung injury. The negative effects of increased pleural pressure on RV filling and increased transpulmonary pressure on RV afterload lead to decreased RV stroke volume, LV preload and thus decreased mean cardiac output.

Michard et al. assessed the clinical use of respiratory changes in arterial pulse pressure to monitor the hemodynamic effects of PEEP [71].

In their study on 14 mechanically ventilated patients with acute lung injury, first, a Δ PP on zero end-expiratory pressure (ZEEP) was closely correlated with the PEEP-induced decrease in cardiac index; higher the PPV was on ZEEP, greater the decrease in cardiac index when PEEP was applied (Fig. 5.6). Also, the increase in ΔPP induced by PEEP was correlated with the decrease in cardiac index, such that changes in Δ PP from ZEEP to PEEP could be used to assess the hemodynamics effects of PEEP without the need for a pulmonary artery catheter. Finally, when cardiac index decreased with PEEP, volume expansion induced an increase in cardiac index that was proportional to PPV before fluid infusion.

Because the PP depends not only on stroke volume but also on arterial compliance, large changes in pulse pressure could theoretically be observed despite small changes in

Fig. 5.6 Relationship between the respiratory changes in pulse pressure on ZEEP (*y*-axis) and the PEEP-induced cardiac index changes (*x*-axis) in 14 ventilated patients with acute lung injury. The higher DPP is on ZEEP, the more marked the decrease in the cardiac index induced by PEEP [71]

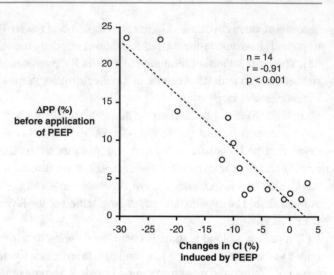

LV stroke volume if arterial compliance is low (elderly patients with peripheral vascular disease). Similarly, if arterial compliance is high (young patients without any vascular disease) despite large changes in LV stroke volume, only small changes in pulse pressure could be observed.

Non-invasive Assessment of Respiratory Changes in LV Stroke Volume

Although less invasive than pulmonary artery catheterization, femoral or radial arterial catheterization remains an invasive procedure. Infrared photoplethysmography coupled with the volume clamp technique [72] allows a non-invasive and continuous measurement of finger blood pressure, which has been shown to track changes in blood pressure accurately [73]. In mechanically ventilated patients, a close correlation and a good agreement between ΔPP measured from intra-arterial recordings and ΔPP measured noninvasively using the continuous measurement of finger blood pressure has been established [74].

Transthoracic echocardiographic measurement of variations of inferior vena cava (IVC) diameter induced by mechanical ventilation has been shown to predict preload responsiveness with reasonable sensitivity and specificity [50, 51, 75].

In a mechanically ventilated patient with no spontaneous breathing efforts, due to an increase in intrathoracic pressure, the IVC dilates during inspiration reaching maximum diameter. It collapses during expiration as the intrathoracic pressure drops, giving a minimum diameter. The percentage variation of IVC during inspiration against expiration gives the IVC distensibility index.

$$\text{Distensibility index} = \left(IVC_{max} - IVC_{min}\right) / IVC_{min} \times 100\%$$

Distensibility index >18% offers 90% sensitivity and specificity in identifying fluid responders from non-responders [53, 76].

In spontaneously breathing patients, the IVC collapses on inspiration as intrathoracic pressure becomes negative, and the degree of IVC collapsibility during inspiration can be used to predict preload responsiveness (IVC collapsibility index) [52].

$$\text{Collapsibility index} = \left(\text{IVC}_{max} - \text{IVC}_{min}\right) / \text{IVC}_{max} \times 100\%$$

IVC$_{max}$ maximum IVC diameter during expiration, IVC$_{min}$ minimum IVC diameter during inspiration.

Currently, there is insufficient evidence to support its use, but the collapsibility index of >42% may predict increase in cardiac output after fluid challenge.

The change in stroke volume over the respiratory cycle in mechanically ventilated patients assessed noninvasively by transthoracic echocardiography can be used to predict preload responsiveness. Indeed, by assuming that aortic annulus diameter is constant over the respiratory cycle, the changes in aortic blood flow should reflect changes in LV stroke volume.

Stroke volume is calculated using the velocity time integral (VTI).

$$SV = VTI \times CSA \left(\text{cross sectional area}\right)$$
$$CSA - 0.785 \times \left(\text{LVOT diameter}\right)^2$$

Cardiac output can be derived by multiplying SV to heart rate. By tracing the largest and smallest VTI over respiratory cycle, stroke volume variation (SVV) can be calculated.

$$\text{Averaged SVV} = SV_{max} - SV_{min} / \left[\left(SV_{max} + SV_{min}\right) \times 0.5\right]$$

Cardiac output measured by this method is comparable to the thermodilution method using a pulmonary artery catheter. SVV of >14% has a very high positive predictive value, and <10% has a high negative predictive value for fluid responsiveness.

Other Clinically Significant Clinical Interactions

While weaning a ventilated patient, abrupt transfer from mechanical ventilation to spontaneous breathing leads to an increase in LV preload and afterload. In a patient with compromised LV function, this might precipitate a left-side cardiac failure and cardiogenic pulmonary edema leading to weaning failure. Similarly, a patient presenting with respiratory distress due to cardiogenic pulmonary edema could greatly benefit from a trial of CPAP, because of the clear advantage of positive pressure in decreasing both preload and afterload.

In obstructive sleep apnea, patients exhibit inspiratory muscular efforts against a collapsed upper airway creating a strongly negative P_{PL}, which is transmitted to the intrathoracic large veins and the right atrium, augmenting venous return. This leads to dilation of the RV accompanied by a shift of the interventricular septum towards the LV, reducing LV compliance and stroke volume (pulsus paradoxus) [77, 78]. Chronic right heart changes (cor pulmonale) and RV dysfunction are common in patients with severe obstructive sleep apnea. Patients with an impaired RV function cannot adapt to frequent and sudden increases in venous return and are prone to RV failure. Negative P_{PL} also increases left ventricular afterload. Further arterial desaturation occurs during these apneic episodes leads to hypoxic pulmonary vasoconstriction, resulting in cor pulmonale in patients with severe obstructive sleep apnea. Nocturnal continuous positive airway pressure (CPAP) therapy helps to keep the upper airway open and prevent RV dysfunction and cor pulmonale in patients with severe OSA [77, 78].

Despite the widespread use of lung protective ventilation strategies [79], which may mitigate the mechanical effects on the right ventricle due to lower airway pressures, acute cor pulmonale in patients with ARDS is still highly prevalent. The risk of developing acute cor pulmonale becomes higher with poor oxygenation, hypercapnia, high ventilator pressures and pneumonia as the cause of ARDS [80]. In patients with ARDS, these effects are aggravated by hypoxic or hypercapnic pulmonary vasoconstriction, pulmonary microthrombosis, changes in West zones, and lung de-recruitment [81], all leading to pulmonary hypertension and a worse prognosis [82]. Thereby, RV decompensates as a result of high afterload. For the similar reasons, ARDS patients can decompensate during recruitment procedure; therefore, before recruitment, RV systolic function is to be evaluated.

In conditions like exacerbations of COPD or status asthmaticus, high lung compliance (C_L) facilitates pressure transmission from the lung to the pulmonary vasculature, so these patients are prone to develop acute cor pulmonale. The high airway resistance leads to incomplete exhalation with air trapping, dynamic over-inflation, and auto-PEEP [83, 84], resulting in elevated afterload leading to RV dysfunction.

Cardiopulmonary Changes in Prone Positioning

Prone positioning has emerged as a promising therapy for patients of ARDS with refractory hypoxemia. Placing a patient in the prone position has important implications for both venous return and RV function. During prone ventilation, there is an increase in intra-abdominal pressure which leads to increase in central blood volume due to the shift of blood from the splanchnic into the thoracic circulation, which may induce recruitment of pulmonary microvasculature, increase in pulmonary capillary wedge pressure, and reduction in PVR and RV afterload. It is to be noted that the improved venous return will only be realized in the absence of a simultaneous rise in the resistance to venous return. Therefore, careful consideration should be paid to a patient's volume status before initiating prone positioning. Additionally, the heterogeneity of lung involvement, compliance of chest wall and ventilation strategies utilized will determine to what extent the intra-thoracic milieu favours diminished RV preload, afterload, or some combination thereof [85, 86].

It follows that careful consideration should be given to the underlying cardiac function as well as the relative contributions of the pulmonary and chest wall compliance to the overall compliance of the respiratory system. Integration of these multiple, co-varying physiological elements may explain conflicting hemodynamic both in ARDS and other mechanically-ventilated patient populations.

Case Vignette

Why did the critical care team decide to use heart-lung interactions to assess fluid responsiveness in Mr. J?

– Answer: The critical care team suspected that Mr. J might be volume depleted, and they wanted to assess his fluid responsiveness. Heart-lung interactions are a useful tool for assessing fluid responsiveness in critically ill patients. The PLR maneuver is a noninvasive method that can be used to predict fluid responsiveness by observing the changes in stroke volume or cardiac output.

What was the hemodynamic response observed during the PLR maneuver, and what does it indicate?

– Answer: During the PLR maneuver, the team observed an increase in the stroke volume (SV) by 20%, indicating that Mr. J was fluid responsive. This increase in SV is a positive response to the PLR and indicates that the patient's cardiac pre-load was increased, leading to an increase in stroke volume. This response indicates that the patient may benefit from fluid administration to improve their hemodynamic status.

Limitations: Although heart-lung interactions are a useful tool for assessing fluid responsiveness, interpreting the results can be challenging. The PLR maneuver can produce false-positive results in patients with elevated intra-abdominal pressure or impaired venous return.

Lack of specificity: Heart-lung interactions are not specific to fluid responsiveness. Other factors, such as changes in vascular tone, inotropic agents, and positive pressure ventilation, can also affect the hemodynamic response to the PLR maneuver.

Conclusions

Ventilation can alter cardiovascular function by altering lung volume, intrathoracic pressure (ITP) and by increasing metabolic demands. Such cardiopulmonary interactions can have deleterious effects in critically ill patients. A thorough understanding of these interactions can help us to differentiate between fluid responders and non-responders and thus prevent the probable complications of an inappropriate fluid therapy.

Take Home Messages
- The concept of predicting fluid responsiveness emerged from a twofold observation:
  - First, the potential harm caused by fluid administration
  - Second, the variable efficacy of fluid resuscitation
- The ability to assess fluid responsiveness enables clinicians
  - To avoid administering harmful treatments to patients who do not require them
  - To provide fluids when they are needed
- Dynamic measures of fluid responsiveness allow for personalized or even individualized resuscitation strategies that can be tailored to each patient's individual needs, regardless of the type of fluid being used.
- It is important to note that these "fluid responsiveness" measures must be used carefully in the most critically ill patients, as they must balance the need for aggressive restoration of blood flow with the risk of fluid overload.
- Fluid responsive measures are an essential part of the arsenal of strategies that allow for personalized and individualized treatment of the most severe patients.
- However, as it is equally crucial to avoid fluid accumulation, and clinicians must be cautious not to administer fluids when they are not necessary.
- In the case of fluid accumulation syndrome (FAS), the presence of fluid unresponsiveness can serve as a trigger and/or safety parameter to guide fluid removal and restore euvolemia to the patient, thus ensuring optimal outcomes.

References

1. Cecconi M, De Backer D, Antonelli M, Beale R, Bakker J, Hofer C, Jaeschke R, Mebazaa A, Pinsky MR, Teboul JL, Vincent JL, Rhodes A. Consensus on circulatory shock and hemodynamic monitoring. Task force of the European Society of Intensive Care Medicine. Intensive Care Med. 2014;40(12):1795–815. https://doi.org/10.1007/s00134-014-3525-z.
2. Monnet X, Malbrain MLNG, Pinsky MR. The prediction of fluid responsiveness. Intensive Care Med. 2023;49(1):83–6. https://doi.org/10.1007/s00134-022-06900-0.
3. Messmer AS, Zingg C, Müller M, Gerber JL, Schefold JC, Pfortmueller CA. Fluid overload and mortality in adult critical care patients-a systematic review and meta-analysis of observational studies. Crit Care Med. 2020;48(12):1862–70. https://doi.org/10.1097/CCM.0000000000004617.
4. Tobin MJ. Effect of mechanical ventilation on heart-lung interactions principles and practice of mechanical ventilation. 3rd ed. New York: McGraw Hill; 2012. (Chapter 36).
5. Magder S, Verscheure S. Proper reading of pulmonary artery vascular pressure tracings. Am J Respir Crit Care Med. 2014;190(10):1196–8.
6. Marini JJ, Culver BH, Butler J. Mechanical effect of lung distention with positive pressure on cardiac function. Am Rev Respir Dis. 1981;124(4):382–6.
7. Holt JP, Rhode EA, Kines H. Pericardial and ventricular pressure. Circ Res. 1960;8(6):1171–81.
8. Tyberg JV, Smith ER. Ventricular diastole and the role of the pericardium. Herz. 1990;15(6):354–61.

9. Gubbler MR, Wigger O, Berger D. Swiss Med Wkly. 2017;147:w14491.
10. Lansdorp B, Hofhuizen C, van Lavieren M, van Swieten H, Lemson J, van Putten MJ, et al. Mechanical ventilation-induced intrathoracic pressure distribution and heart-lung interactions. Crit Care Med. 2014;42(9):1983–90.
11. Kingma I, Smiseth OA, Frais MA, Smith ER, Tyberg JV. Left ventricular external constraint: relationship between pericardial, pleural and esophageal pressures during positive end-expiratory pressure and volume loading in dogs. Ann Biomed Eng. 1987;15(3-4):331–46.
12. Rahn H, Otis AB, et al. The pressure-volume diagram of the thorax and lung. Am J Phys. 1946;146(2):161–78.
13. Naeije R. Pulmonary vascular resistance. A meaningless variable? Intensive Care Med. 2003;29(4):526–9.
14. Lumb AB, Slinger P. Hypoxic pulmonary vasoconstriction: physiology and anesthetic implications. Anesthesiology. 2015;122(4):932–46.
15. Dorrington KL, Talbot NP. Human pulmonary vascular responses to hypoxia and hypercapnia. Pflugers Arch. 2004;449(1):1–15.
16. West JB, Dollery CT, Naimark A. Distribution of blood flow in isolated lung; relation to vascular and alveolar pressures. J Appl Physiol. 1964;19:713–24.
17. Whittenberger JL, McGregor M, Berglund E, Borst HG. Influence of state of inflation of the lung on pulmonary vascular resistance. J Appl Physiol. 1960;15:878–82.
18. Jardin F, Genevray B, Brun-Ney D, Bourdarias JP. Influence of lung and chest wall compliances on transmission of airway pressure to the pleural space in critically ill patients. Chest. 1985;88(5):653–8.
19. Feihl F, Broccard AF. Interactions between respiration and systemic hemodynamics. Part I: basic concepts. Intensive Care Med. 2009;35(1):45–54.
20. Feihl F, Broccard AF. Interactions between respiration and systemic hemodynamics. Part II: practical implications in critical care. Intensive Care Med. 2009;35(2):198–205.
21. Magder S. Volume and its relationship to cardiac output and venous return. Crit Care. 2016;20(1):271. Correction in: Critical Care. 2017;21:16.
22. Magder S, De Varennes B. Clinical death and the measurement of stressed vascular volume. Crit Care Med. 1998;26(6):1061–4.
23. Berger D, Moller PW, Weber A, Bloch A, Bloechlinger S, Haenggi M, et al. Effect of PEEP, blood volume, and inspiratory hold maneuvers on venous return. Am J Physiol Heart Circ Physiol. 2016;311(3):794 806.
24. Magder S, Vanelli G. Circuit factors in the high cardiac output of sepsis. J Crit Care. 1996;11(4):155–66.
25. Bloch A, Berger D, Takala J. Understanding circulatory failure in sepsis. Intensive Care Med. 2016;42(12):2077–9.
26. Moller PW, Winkler B, Hurni S, Heinisch PP, Bloch AM, Sondergaard S, et al. Right atrial pressure and venous return during cardiopulmonary bypass. Am J Physiol Heart Circ Physiol. 2017;313(2):H408–20.
27. Berger D, Moller PW, Weber A, Bloch A, Bloechlinger S, Haenggi M, et al. Effect of PEEP, blood volume, and inspiratory hold maneuvers on venous return. Am J Physiol Heart Circ Physiol. 2016;311(3):H794–806.
28. Sondergaard S, Parkin G, Aneman A. Central venous pressure: soon an outcome-associated matter. Curr Opin Anaesthesiol. 2016;29(2):179–85.
29. Vieillard-Baron A, Matthay M, Teboul JL, Bein T, Schultz M, Magder S, et al. Experts' opinion on management of hemodynamics in ARDS patients: focus on the effects of mechanical ventilation. Intensive Care Med. 2016;42(5):739–49.

30. Reichek N, Wilson J, St John Sutton M, Plappert TA, Goldberg S, Hirshfeld JW. Noninvasive determination of left ventricular end-systolic stress: validation of the method and initial application. Circulation. 1982;65(1):99–108.
31. Borlaug BA, Kass DA. Invasive hemodynamic assessment in heart failure. Heart Fail Clin. 2009;5(2):217–28.
32. Walley KR. Left ventricular function: time-varying elastance and left ventricular aortic coupling. Crit Care. 2016;20(1):270.
33. Buda AJ, Pinsky MR, Ingels NB Jr, Daughters GT, Stinson EB, Alderman EL. Effect of intrathoracic pressure on left ventricular performance. N Engl J Med. 1979;301(9):453–9.
34. Pinsky MR. Cardiovascular issues in respiratory care. Chest. 2005;128(5):592–7.
35. Vieillard-Baron A, Loubieres Y, Schmitt JM, Page B, Dubourg O, Jardin F. Cyclic changes in right ventricular output impedance during mechanical ventilation. J Appl Physiol. 1999;87(5):1644–50.
36. Berger D, Bloechlinger S, Takala J, Sinderby C, Brander L. Heart-lung interactions during neurally adjusted ventilatory assist. Crit Care. 2014;18(5):499.
37. Mekontso Dessap A, Boissier F, Charron C, Begot E, Repesse X, Legras A, et al. Acute cor pulmonale during protective ventilation for acute respiratory distress syndrome: prevalence, predictors, and clinical impact. Intensive Care Med. 2016;42(5):862–70.
38. Jardin F, Brun-Ney D, Cazaux P, Dubourg O, Hardy A, Bourdarias JP. Relation between transpulmonary pressure and right ventricular isovolumetric pressure change during respiratory support. Catheter Cardiovasc Diagn. 1989;16(4):215–20.
39. Pinsky MR. Determinants of pulmonary arterial flow variation during respiration. J Appl Physiol. 1984;56(5):1237–45.
40. Taylor RR, Covell JW, Sonnenblick EH, Ross J Jr. Dependence of ventricular distensibility on filling of the opposite ventricle. Am J Phys. 1967;213(3):711–8.
41. Vieillard-Baron A, Schmitt JM, Augarde R, Fellahi JL, Prin S, Page B, et al. Acute cor pulmonale in acute respiratory distress syndrome submitted to protective ventilation: incidence, clinical implications, and prognosis. Crit Care Med. 2001;29(8):1551–5.
42. Michard F, Teboul JL. Using heart-lung interactions to assess fluid responsiveness during mechanical ventilation. Crit Care. 2000;4:282.
43. Pinsky MR. Functional haemodynamic monitoring. Curr Opin Crit Care. 2014;20(3):288–93.
44. Osman D, et al. Cardiac filling pressures are not appropriate to predict hemodynamic response to volume challenge. Crit Care Med. 2007;35(1):64–8.
45. Cecconi M, et al. Fluid challenges in intensive care: the FENICE study-A global inception cohort study. Intensive Care Med. 2015;41(9):1529–37.
46. Pinsky MR, Vincent JL, De Smet JM. Estimating left ventricular filling pressure during positive end-expiratory pressure in humans. Am Rev Respir Dis. 1991;143:25–31.
47. Raper R, Sibbald WJ. Misled by the wedge? The Swan-Ganz catheter and left ventricular preload. Chest. 1986;89:427–34.
48. Fessler HE, Brower RG, Wise RA, Permutt S. Mechanism of reduced LV afterload by systolic and diastolic positive pleural pressure. J Appl Physiol. 1988;65:1244–50.
49. Reuse C, Vincent JL, Pinsky MR. Measurements of right ventricular volumes during fluid challenge. Chest. 1990;98:1450–4.
50. Squara P, Journois D, Estagnasié P, Wysocki M, Brusset A, Dreyfuss D, Teboul JL. Elastic energy as an index of right ventricular filling. Chest. 1997;111:351–8.
51. Tavernier B, Makhotine O, Lebuffe G, Dupont J, Scherpereel P. Systolic pressure variation as a guide to fluid therapy in patients with sepsis-induced hypotension. Anesthesiology. 1998;89:1313–21.
52. Tousignant CP, Walsh F, Mazer CD. The use of transesophageal echocardiography for preload assessment in critically ill patients. Anesth Analg. 2000;90:351–5.

53. Wagner JG, Leatherman JW. Right ventricular end-diastolic volume as a predictor of the hemo-dynamic response to a fluid challenge. Chest. 1998;113:1048–54.
54. Teboul JL, Pinsky MR, Mercat A, Anguel N, Bernardin G, Achard JM, Boulain T, Richard C. Estimating cardiac filling pressure in mechanically ventilated patients with hyperinflation. Crit Care Med. 2000;28(11):3631–6.
55. Spinale FG, Mukherjee R, Tanaka R, Zile MR. The effects of valvular regurgitation on thermo-dilution ejection fraction measurements. Chest. 1992;101:723–31.
56. Urbanowicz JH, Shaaban J, Cohen NH, Cahalan MK, Botvinick EH, Chatterjee K, Schiller NB, Dae MW, Matthay MA. Comparison of transesophageal echocardiographic and scintigraphic estimates of left ventricular end-diastolic volume index and ejection fraction in patients follow-ing coronary artery bypass grafting. Anesthesiology. 1990;72:607–12.
57. Magder S. The cardiovascular management of the critically ill patients. In: Pinsky MR, editor. Applied cardiovascular physiology. Berlin: Springer; 1997. p. 28–35.
58. Alec Rooke G, Schwid HA, Shapira Y. The effect of graded hemorrhage and intravascular vol-ume replacement on systolic pressure variation in humans during mechanical and spontaneous ventilation. Anesth Analg. 1995;80:925–32.
59. Coriat P, Vrillon M, Perel A, Baron JF, Le Bret F, Saada M, Viars P. A comparison of systolic blood pressure variations and echocardiographic estimates of end-diastolic left ventricular size in patients after aortic surgery. Anesth Analg. 1994;78:46–53.
60. Berne RM, Levy MN. Physiology. 4th ed. St Louis: Mosby; 1998.
61. Jardin F, Farcot JC, Gueret P, Prost JF, Ozier Y, Bourdarias JP. Cyclic changes in arterial pulse during respiratory support. Circulation. 1983;68:266–74.
62. Michard F, Boussat S, Chemla D, Anguel N, Mercat A, Lecarpentier Y, et al. Relation between respiratory changes in arterial pulse pressure and fluid responsiveness in septic patients with acute circulatory failure. Am J Respir Crit Care Med. 2000;162(1):134–8.
63. Magder S. Clinical usefulness of respiratory variations in arterial pressure. Am J Respir Crit Care Med. 2004;169(2):151–5.
64. Sondergaard S. Pavane for a pulse pressure variation defunct. Crit Care. 2013;17(6):327.
65. De Backer D, Heenen S, Piagnerelli M, Koch M, Vincent JL. Pulse pressure variations to predict fluid responsiveness: influence of tidal volume. Intensive Care Med. 2005;31(4):517–23.
66. De Backer D, Taccone FS, Holsten R, Ibrahimi F, Vincent JL. Influence of respiratory rate on stroke volume variation in mechanically ventilated patients. Anesthesiology. 2009;110(5):1092–7.
67. Mesquida J, Kim HK, Pinsky MR. Effect of tidal volume, intrathoracic pressure, and cardiac contractility on variations in pulse pressure, stroke volume, and intrathoracic blood volume. Intensive Care Med. 2011;37(10):1672–9.
68. Mahjoub Y, Lejeune V, Muller L, Perbet S, Zieleskiewicz L, Bart F, et al. Evaluation of pulse pressure variation validity criteria in critically ill patients: a prospective observational multicen-tre point-prevalence study. Br J Anaesth. 2014;112(4):681–5.
69. Pinsky MR, Desmet JM, Vincent JL. Effect of positive end-expiratory pressure on right ventricu-lar function in humans. Am Rev Respir Dis. 1992;146(3):681–7.
70. Vieillard-Baron A, Chergui K, Augarde R, Prin S, Page B, Beauchet A, et al. Cyclic changes in arterial pulse during respiratory support revisited by Doppler echocardiography. Am J Respir Crit Care Med. 2003;168(6):671–6.
71. Michard F, Chemla D, Richard C, Wysocki M, Pinsky MR, Lecarpentier Y, Teboul JL. Clinical use of respiratory changes in arterial pulse pressure to monitor the hemodynamic effects of PEEP. Am J Respir Crit Care Med. 1999;159:935–9.
72. Penaz J. Criteria for set point estimation in the volume clamp method of blood pressure measure-ment. Physiol Res. 1992;41:5–10.
73. Imholz BP, Wieling W, van Montfrans GA, Wesseling KH. Fifteen years experience with finger arterial pressure monitoring: assessment of the technology. Cardiovasc Res. 1998;38:605–16.

74. Michard F, Mercat A, Chemla D, Richard C, Teboul JL. Non invasive assessment of respiratory changes in arterial pulse pressure by infrared photoplethysmography in mechanically ventilated patients. Am J Respir Crit Care Med. 1999;159:A520.
75. Michard F, Boussat S, Chemla D, Anguel N, Mercat A, Lecarpentier Y, Richard C, Pinsky MR, Teboul JL. Relation between respiratory changes in arterial pulse pressure and fluid responsiveness in septic patients with acute circulatory failure. Am J Respir Crit Care Med. 2000;162:134–8.
76. Diebel L, Wilson RF, Heins J, Larky H, Warsow K, Wilson S. Enddiastolic volume versus pulmonary artery wedge pressure in evaluating cardiac preload in trauma patients. J Trauma. 1994;37:950–5.
77. Pinsky MR. Sleeping with the enemy: the heart in obstructive sleep apnea. Chest. 2002;121(4):1022–4.
78. Chai-Coetzer CL, Antic NA, Hamilton GS, McArdle N, Wong K, Yee BJ, et al. Physician decision making and clinical outcomes with laboratory polysomnography or limited-channel sleep studies for obstructive sleep apnea: a randomized trial. Ann Intern Med. 2017;166(5):332–40.
79. Brower RG, Matthay MA, Morris A, Schoenfeld D, Thompson BT, Wheeler A, Acute Respiratory Distress Syndrome Network. Ventilation with lower tidal volumes as compared with traditional tidal volumes for acute lung injury and the acute respiratory distress syndrome. N Engl J Med. 2000;342(18):1301–8.
80. Mayo P, Mekontso Dessap A, Vieillard-Baron A. Myths about critical care echocardiography: the ten false beliefs that intensivists should understand. Intensive Care Med. 2015;41(6):1103–6.
81. Duggan M, McCaul CL, McNamara PJ, Engelberts D, Ackerley C, Kavanagh BP. Atelectasis causes vascular leak and lethal right ventricular failure in uninjured rat lungs. Am J Respir Crit Care Med. 2003,167(12):1633–40.
82. Bull TM, Clark B, McFann K, Moss M, National Institutes of Health/National Heart, Lung, and Blood Institute ARDS Network. Pulmonary vascular dysfunction is associated with poor outcomes in patients with acute lung injury. Am J Respir Crit Care Med. 2010;182(9):1123–8.
83. Pepe PE, Marini JJ. Occult positive end-expiratory pressure in mechanically ventilated patients with airflow obstruction: the auto-PEEP effect. Am Rev Respir Dis. 1982;126(1):166–70.
84. Marini JJ. Dynamic hyperinflation and auto-positive end-expiratory pressure: lessons learned over 30 years. Am J Respir Crit Care Med. 2011;184(7):756–62.
85. Vieillard-Baron A, Charron C, Caille V, et al. Prone positioning unloads the right ventricle in severe ARDS. Chest. 2007;132:1440–6.
86. Jozwiak M, Teboul JL, Anguel N, et al. Beneficial hemodynamic effects of prone positioning in patients with acute respiratory distress syndrome. Am J Respir Crit Care Med. 2013;188:1428–33.

Acid-Base Homeostasis: Traditional Approach

6

Supradip Ghosh

Contents

Introduction 142
Definitions 142
Acid-Base Homeostasis 143
High AG Metabolic Acidosis 146
Normal AG Metabolic Acidosis 147
Metabolic Alkalosis 148
Conclusion 151
Some More Illustrative Cases 150
Reference 152

S. Ghosh (✉)
Department of Critical Care Medicine, Fortis - Escort Hospital, Faridabad, Haryana, India

IFA Commentary (PN)

Acid-base disorders are a common occurrence in critically ill patients, and it is crucial to approach them systematically. There are different methods of interpreting acid-base disorders, including the traditional approach, Stewart's physiochemical approach, and Siggaard-Anderson's base excess approach, as shown in Fig. 6.1.

The traditional approach is the most commonly used method in clinical practice, based on the assumption that bicarbonate is a strong buffer and determinant of pH. It uses the Henderson-Hasselbalch equation, although it has various limitations. Despite this, it is widely used in clinical practice, and studies have not consistently shown the superiority of one approach over another.

After identifying the primary acid-base disorder, compensation formulae can be used to detect mixed disorders. It is important to note that compensation cannot normalize the pH, except in cases of chronic respiratory alkalosis. Calculating the delta anion gap (observed vs expected) is a useful tool for identifying mismatches between bicarbonate and anion gap and can help detect a third existing metabolic acid-base disorder.

It is essential to understand that the interpretation of arterial blood gas should not be done in isolation. It must be accompanied by a comprehensive patient history and physical assessment to provide a complete clinical picture.

Overall, the interpretation of acid-base disorders in critically ill patients requires a systematic approach, and understanding the various methods of interpretation is essential for clinicians. The use of compensation formulae and the calculation of the delta anion gap can help identify mixed disorders and existing third metabolic acid-base disorders. By utilizing these approaches and considering the patient's history and physical assessment, clinicians can make informed treatment decisions to optimize patient outcomes.

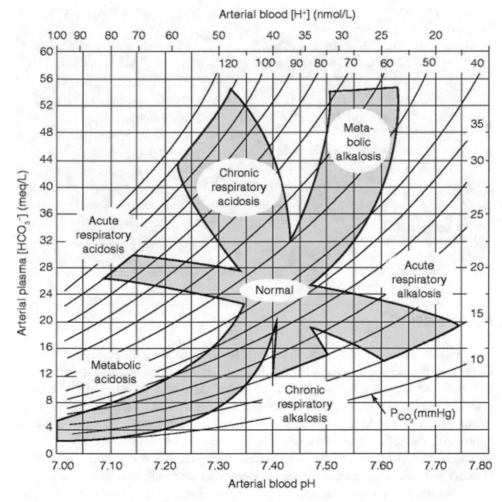

Fig. 6.1 Traditional Siggaard Anderson acid-base nomogram. Shown are the 95% confidence limits of the normal respiratory and metabolic compensations for primary acid–base disturbances (From Cogan MG (editor): Fluid and Electrolytes: Physiology and Pathophysiology. Appleton & Lange, 1991)

Learning Objectives

After reading this chapter, you will learn:

1. To understand the interpretation of acid-base disorders following the approach proposed by Henderson and Hasselbalch.
2. To interpret the presence of any primary acid-base disorder.
3. To understand and interpret the presence of any secondary disorder by applying compensatory response formulae.
4. To understand the concept of anion gap and its various application.
5. To interpret the presence of third acid-base disorder (if any) by applying the concept of delta gap.

Case Vignette

Mrs. A, a 50-year-old-woman with history of insulin-dependent diabetes mellitus (IDDM), was admitted to the ICU in semi-comatose state. She had been ill for several days. Her medications included subcutaneous insulin for managing IDDM, calcium supplement and indapamide for hypertension. On examination, she was barely rousable to verbal command, afebrile, dehydrated with a heart rate of 112/min, blood pressure of 94/60 mmHg and respiratory rate of 32/min. Systemic examination was otherwise unremarkable. Initial blood investigations showed Na-132 mmol/L, K-2.7 mmol/L, Cl-79 mmol/L, HCO_3-19 mmol/L, blood glucose-815 mg/dl, lactate 0.9 mmol/L and urine ketones 3+. Arterial blood gas analysis revealed pH 7.41, $PaCO_2$-32 mmHg, HCO_3-19 mmol/L and PaO_2-82 mmHg (in room air).

Question

Q1. How do we interpret her blood gases?

Introduction

Interpretation of acid-base disorders is critical for understanding the pathophysiology of underlying disease and making a correct diagnosis. It also helps in deciding appropriate treatment and following the progress of the patient. Acid-base disorders can be broadly classified into respiratory or metabolic disorders. There are three major approaches to the interpretation of acid-base physiology: traditional approach (or so-called physiological approach), Stewart's physicochemical approach and Siggaard-Anderson's base excess approach. All the three approaches, more or less, agree in their interpretation of respiratory disorder and differ only in their method of interpreting metabolic problems.

The traditional approach defines acid as hydrogen-ion donors and bases as hydrogen-ion acceptors (as proposed by Bronsted and Lowry) and uses the carbonic acid–bicarbonate buffer system for the interpretation of acid-base disorders. This approach suggests that a primary change in the partial pressure of carbon dioxide or $PaCO_2$ will cause secondary changes in bicarbonate and vice versa (also known as "adaptive" response). In this chapter, we shall review the traditional approach in detail. See also Chap. 7 to learn more about the Stewart's approach to acid-base.

Definitions

Following are some definitions relevant for understanding traditional approach.

- **pH:** pH is the negative logarithm of hydrogen ion concentration ($[H^+]$). Since the concentration of $[H^+]$ is normally very low (4.0×10^{-8} mol/L), the concept of pH is used in clinical medicine to describe acid-base issues. The lower the pH, the higher the $[H^+]$

concentration and vice versa. For example, a pH of 6.8 corresponds to 1.6×10^{-7} mol/L [H⁺] or pH 7.6 to 2.5×10^{-8} mol/L [H⁺]. The normal range of pH in the whole blood is between 7.35 and 7.45. However, in this chapter, we will be taking a narrower range of normal pH as 7.40 ± 0.02 (for the purpose of calculation).

- **Acidemia:** If the pH is below the physiological limit, it is called acidemia.
- **Alkalemia:** If the pH is above the physiological limit, it is known as alkalemia.
- **Acidosis:** Acidosis is defined as the clinical processes that tend to lower the pH below the physiological limit.
- **Alkalosis:** Alkalosis is defined as the clinical processes that tend to raise the pH above the physiological limit.

Acid-Base Homeostasis

Traditional approach is based on the Henderson–Hasselbalch equation, which states that: **pH = pK + log10 ([HCO₃⁻]/[0.03 × (PaCO₂)])** (pK denotes the acid dissociation constant, [HCO₃⁻] is the bicarbonate ion concentration in plasma in mmol/L and PaCO₂ is the partial pressure of CO_2 in mmHg). Simplistically, according to the traditional approach, [H⁺] concentration is proportional to [PaCO₂]/[HCO₃⁻]. An acid–base disorder is called "respiratory" when changes in [H⁺] ion concentration is primarily because of [PaCO₂] and "metabolic" when changes in [H⁺] ion concentration is attributed to variation in [HCO₃⁻].

[H⁺] ion concentration (and pH) is tightly regulated within the physiological range as virtually all human enzymes and membranes work best within this range. With any deviation of pH, the body tries to adapt and compensate, in an attempt to maintain the pH. If the primary problem is metabolic, then the compensatory mechanism is respiratory by altering the respiratory drive. Respiratory compensation is quick and activated within minutes. In cases of primary respiratory disorders, kidneys adapt and change the [HCO₃⁻] concentration. This metabolic compensation is slow and the adaptation takes up to 5 days. Compensatory responses cannot fully normalize the pH, except in cases of chronic respiratory alkalosis. Compensatory changes in PaCO₂ and [HCO₃⁻] in response to primary metabolic and respiratory disorder follows a pattern and can be predicted using empirical formulae. Traditional approach to acid-base disorders is described in a step-wise manner in subsequent paragraphs.

Step 1: Observe the pH, PaCO₂ and HCO₃.

- The purpose of this step is to look for any acid-base abnormality and to recognize a primary disorder (if any). Remember that the so-called primary disorder is solely responsible for the purpose of calculating compensatory response and not to give undue importance of one disorder over another.
- For the analysis of acid-base abnormality using the physiological approach, we shall take normal values of pH as 7.40 ± 2, [HCO₃⁻] as 24 ± 2 mmol/L and PaCO₂ as 40 ± 2 mmHg.
- Algorithm depicted in Fig. 6.2 depicts a logical step to identify any primary disorder.

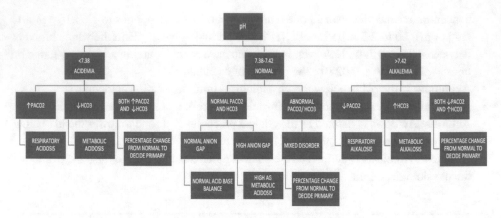

Fig. 6.2 Steps to identify primary disorder (if any)

Step 2: Look for compensatory response. Compensatory responses are calculated based on empirical formulae to identify any second disorder.

- **Metabolic Acidosis**: If the primary disorder is metabolic acidosis, then expected compensatory response is a fall in $PaCO_2$.
    - Expected $PaCO_2 = (1.5 \times [HCO_3] + 8) \pm 2$ mmHg (Winter's formula).
    - If measured $PaCO_2$ > expected $PaCO_2$ = additional respiratory acidosis.
    - If measured $PaCO_2$ < expected $PaCO_2$ = additional respiratory alkalosis.
- **Metabolic Alkalosis**: If the primary disorder is metabolic alkalosis, then expected response is an increase in $PaCO_2$.
    - Expected $PaCO_2 = (0.7 \times [HCO_3^-]) + 20 \pm 2$ mmHg.
    - If measured $PaCO_2$ > expected $PaCO_2$ = additional respiratory acidosis.
    - If measured $PaCO_2$ < expected $PaCO_2$ = additional respiratory alkalosis.
- **Respiratory Acidosis**: Expected compensatory response for primary respiratory acidosis is an increase in HCO_3. The compensation may take 2–5 days, based on that respiratory disorders may be classified as acute (without complete compensation) or chronic (with complete compensatory response).
    - For every 10 mmHg $PaCO_2$ increase above 40 mmHg, if $[HCO_3^-]$ increase by 1 mmol/L = acute respiratory acidosis.
    - For every 10 mmHg $PaCO_2$ increase above 40 mmHg, if $[HCO_3^-]$ increase by 4–5 mmol/L = chronic respiratory acidosis.
    - For every 10 mmHg $PaCO_2$ increase above 40 mmHg, if $[HCO_3^-]$ increase by <1 mmol/L = additional metabolic acidosis.
    - For every 10 mmHg $PaCO_2$ increase above 40 mmHg, if $[HCO_3^-]$ increase by >5 mmol/L = additional metabolic alkalosis.
- **Respiratory Alkalosis:** The expected compensatory response in primary respiratory alkalosis is a fall in $[HCO_3^-]$. Complete compensation takes 2–5 days.

- For every 10 mmHg $PaCO_2$ decrease below 40 mmHg, if $[HCO_3^-]$ decrease by 2 mmol/L = acute respiratory alkalosis.
- For every 10 mmHg $PaCO_2$ decrease below 40 mmHg, if $[HCO_3^-]$ decrease by 4–5 mmol/L = chronic respiratory alkalosis.
- For every 10 mmHg $PaCO_2$ decrease below 40 mmHg, if $[HCO_3^-]$ decrease by <2 mmol/L = additional metabolic alkalosis.
- For every 10 mmHg $PaCO_2$ decrease below 40 mmHg, if $[HCO_3^-]$ decrease by >5 mmol/L = additional metabolic acidosis.

Step 3: Look for anion gap.

- According to the principle of electroneutrality, the sum of cations in any body fluid (including plasma) must be equal to the sum of anions in the fluid. This can be seen from the Gamblegram (originally created by acid-base pioneer James L. Gamble to graphically represent concentrations of plasma cations (e.g., Na^+ and K^+) and plasma anions (e.g., Cl^- and HCO_3^-) (Fig. 6.3).
- That means: **$[Na^+] + [K^+]$ + Unmeasured cations = $[Cl^-] + [HCO_3^-]$ + Unmeasured anions**. To state the equation differently: **Unmeasured anions − Unmeasured cations = $[Na^+] + [K^+] − [Cl^-] − [HCO_3^-]$**.
- This difference in the concentration between plasma unmeasured anions and cations is also known as **anion gap (AG)**. Since the extracellular concentration of K^+ is low and the body needs to maintain its concentration within a narrow range, $[K^+]$ can be omitted from this equation. Thus, the anion gap can be calculated simply as = **$[Na^+] − ([Cl^-] + [HCO_3^-])$**.
- Normally, the gap between unmeasured anions and cations (or anion gap) is filled up mostly by albumin (as can be seen from the Gamblegram above) and to a lesser extent by phosphate or lactate. The albumin level is often low in critically ill patients and the calculated AG must be corrected for low albumin level.
  - Correction for albumin: For every 1 g/dl albumin decrease (normal value 4 gm/dl), increase calculated anion gap by 2.5 mmol/l.

Fig. 6.3 Gamblegram depicting the principle of electroneutrality

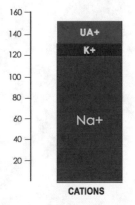 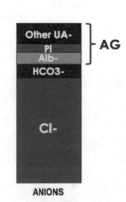

- For example: calculated AG = 5, albumin= 2 g/dl and corrected AG: 5+ [(4 − 2) × 2.5] = 10.
- For the purpose of further calculation, we shall take a normal value of AG as 12 ± 2 mmol/L.
- Calculation of AG helps in the following aspects:
  - It helps in elucidating causes of metabolic acidosis—high AG or normal AG metabolic acidosis.
  - Presence of high AG may be the sole pointer towards the presence of hidden metabolic acidosis, with multiple opposing acid-base abnormalities normalizing pH, $PaCO_2$ and [HCO_3^-].
  - Serial measurement of AG helps in following effectiveness of treatment, especially in diabetic ketoacidosis.
  - Elevated AG may be the only clue to certain clinical disorder. For example, D-lactate is not routinely measured in clinical laboratories. The presence of high AG in a patient presenting with neurological issues and past history of short bowel syndrome may be the only pointer towards D-lactic acidosis.
  - A low AG or negative AG may be a pointer towards unsuspected hypercalcemia or hypermagnesemia or other heavy metal toxicity. Other causes of negative AG include erroneous measurement of serum chloride in clinical laboratories (in the presence of bromide or iodide).

High AG Metabolic Acidosis

- Further analysis of high AG metabolic acidosis is based on history/physical examination, biochemical test results (including blood glucose, kidney function tests, electrolytes, serum osmolality, toxin levels, etc.). A proposed approach to high AG metabolic acidosis is given in Fig. 6.4.

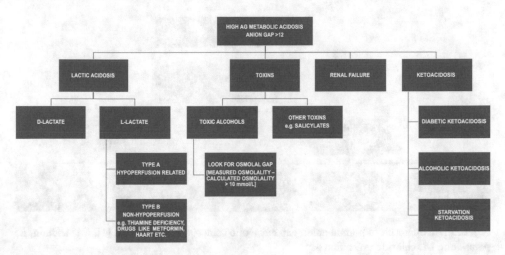

Fig. 6.4   Approach to high anion gap metabolic acidosis. Adapted from [1]. *HAART* highly active antiretroviral therapy, *AG* anion gap

Normal AG Metabolic Acidosis

- Further analysis of normal AG metabolic acidosis requires history/physical examination, serum and urinary electrolytes and urine pH. An approach to normal AG metabolic acidosis is shown in Fig. 6.5.

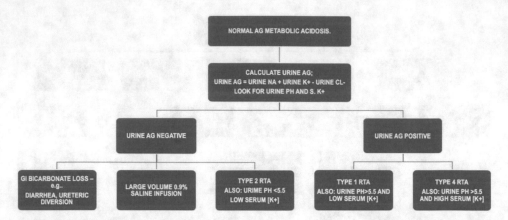

Fig. 6.5 An approach to normal anion gap metabolic acidosis. Adapted from [1]. *NA*+ sodium, *K*+ potassium, *Cl*− chloride, *AG* anion gap

Metabolic Alkalosis

- Metabolic alkalosis is either because of gain of alkali or excess renal retention of HCO_3^-. If the effective circulating volume is reduced, the renin–angiotensin–aldosterone system is activated and kidneys try to restore volume by re-absorption of filtered sodium, bicarbonate, and chloride. In these patients, spot urine chloride concentration is usually <25 mmol/L and the pH may be restored by the administration of 0.9% saline (chloride responsive).
- Metabolic alkalosis is also seen in conditions with mineralocorticoid excess (either true or functional) and in patients with K^+ deficiency. In these patients, excretion of sodium and chloride in urine is inappropriately high (urine chloride level >40 mmol/L) and pH is not restored by the administration of normal saline (chloride unresponsive).
- A suggested approach to metabolic alkalosis is shown in Fig. 6.6.

Step 4: Exploring the delta anion gap—look for the third disorder.

- The magnitude of increase in anion gap from upper limit of normal (12 mmol/L) (henceforth Δ AG) is closely related to the decrease in $[HCO_3^-]$ Δ AG. The relationship is 1:1 in case of ketoacidosis (i.e., $[HCO_3^-]$ value will decrease by Δ AG (the normal delta AG is zero)) but 1:0.6 in cases of lactic acidosis (i.e., $[HCO_3^-]$ value will decrease by 60% of Δ AG).
- This relationship can be explored further to calculate expected $[HCO_3^-]$ from Δ AG:
  - For ketoacidosis or any other high AG acidosis: expected $[HCO_3^-] = [24 - \Delta$ anion gap$] \pm 5$
  - For lactic acidosis: expected $[HCO_3^-] = [24 - (0.6 \times \Delta$ anion gap$)] \pm 5$
  - Actual $[HCO_3^-]$ < expected $[HCO_3^-]$ = additional normal AG metabolic acidosis
  - Actual $[HCO_3^-]$ > expected $[HCO_3^-]$ = additional metabolic alkalosis

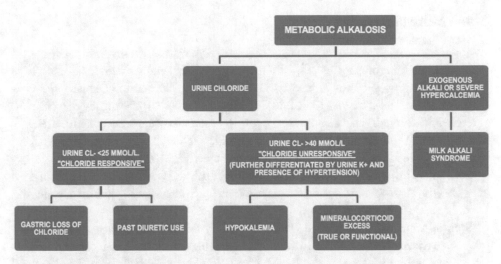

Fig. 6.6 An approach to metabolic alkalosis. Adapted from [1]. *Cl⁻* chloride

Case Vignette

Case 1: Looking into the case vignette (**1**) provided in the beginning of this chapter, we can interpret the acid-base disorders by following the steps mentioned.

Step 1: Here, two opposing disorders (low $PaCO_2$ and low HCO_3) are leading to the normalization of pH. The percentage of change of HCO_3 from the normal value (normal value 24 mmol/L) is marginally more than the percentage of change of $PaCO_2$ (normal value 40 mmHg). For the purpose of compensatory response calculation, we shall take "Metabolic Acidosis" as the primary disorder.

Step 2: Applying Winter's formula, expected $PaCO_2$ is 36.5 mmHg (range—34.5–38.5) [$1.5 \times 19 + 8 = 36.5$]. Since measured $PaCO_2$ < expected $PaCO_2$, there is an associated "Respiratory Alkalosis".

Step 3: Calculated AG is 34 [132 − (79 + 19)] classifying the condition as "High Anion Gap Metabolic Acidosis", possibly due to diabetic ketoacidosis (from the history and presence of ketonuria).

Step 4: On further analysis, Δ anion gap is 22 (34 − 12 = 22) and expected HCO_3 is (24 − 22) ± 5, i.e., 0–7 mmol/L. Actual HCO_3 is > expected HCO_3, confirming associated "Metabolic Alkalosis".

Final Diagnosis: High anion gap metabolic acidosis (possibly diabetic ketoacidosis) with metabolic alkalosis.

Some More Illustrative Cases

Case 2: Police brought a 22-year-old-man to the ED in an unconscious state. ABG: pH 7.27, $PaCO_2^-$ 26 mmHg, and HCO_3^- 11 mmol/L. The serum chemistry result showed Na^- 130 mmol/L, K^- 4 mmol/L, Cl^- 94 mmol/L, BUN 56 mg/dl, serum creatinine 2 mg/dl, and glucose 72 mg/dl. His measured serum osmolality is 320 mosmol/L. Serum lactate, ketones, and ethanol levels are all within normal range.

Step 1: With low pH and $[HCO_3^-]$, primary disorder is "Metabolic Acidosis".

Step 2: On calculating compensatory response, expected $PaCO_2$ is 24.5 mmHg (1.5 × 11 + 8 = 24.5 mmHg) which is close to the measured $PaCO_2$, ruling out additional respiratory disorder.

Step 3: Anion gap is 25 [130 − (94 + 11)] classifying the condition as "High Anion Gap Metabolic Acidosis". On further analysis, the calculated serum osmolality is 284 mosmol/L [2 × 130 + (72/18) + (56/2.8)] with an osmolal gap of 36 (320 − 284) raising high likelihood of toxic alcohol ingestion as the cause of high AG metabolic acidosis.

Step 4: Δ Anion gap is 13 (25 − 12). With this, expected $[HCO_3^-]$ is between 4 to 14 mmol/L. Actual $[HCO_3^-]$ is within this range, ruling out other metabolic abnormalities.

Final diagnosis: High anion gap metabolic acidosis possibly due to toxic alcohol ingestion.

Case 3: A 28-year-old-woman with a history of Sjogren's syndrome reports 3–4 episodes of watery diarrhea lasting for a day, 4-days before her visit to the Rheumatology clinic. ABG done in the clinic is revealed, pH 7.15, $PaCO_2$ 17 mmHg, and HCO_3^- 5 mmol/L. Serum chemistry results are Na^- 135 mmol/L, K 2.5 mmol/L and Cl^- 120 mmol/L/L.

Step 1: Low pH and $[HCO_3^-]$ suggests metabolic acidosis as the primary disorder.

Step 2: Expected $PaCO_2$ applying Winter's formula is 15.5 mmHg, that is closure to measured $PaCO_2$, ruling out additional respiratory disorder.

Step 3: An anion gap of 10 suggests normal AG metabolic acidosis.

Step 4: With normal AG, this step is not applicable in this case.

On further investigations (following approach provided in Fig. 6.5), to elucidate the underlying cause of normal AG acidosis: Urine K^- 31 mmol/L, urine Na 100 mmol/L, urine Cl^- 105 mmol/L and urine pH: 6. Calculated urine anion gap is +26 [(100 + 31) − 105]. Positive urine AG, urine pH >5.5 and low serum K^+ suggests Type 1 renal tubular acidosis as the underlying cause of normal AG acidosis.

Final diagnosis: Normal anion gap metabolic acidosis possibly due to Type 1 RTA.

Case 4: A 62-year-old woman was admitted with history of recurrent vomiting and was diagnosed as small bowel obstruction. She is on nasogastric suction. Arterial blood gases: pH 7.40, pCO$_2$ 40 mmHg, HCO$_3$ 25 mmol/L. Lab results showed Na 135 mEq/L, K 3.5 mEq/L, Cl 85 mEq/l, HCO$_3$ 25 mEq/l, blood glucose 90 mg/dl, blood urea nitrogen 110 mg/dl and serum creatinine 4.5 mg/dl.

Step 1 and 2: Normal pH, HCO$_3^-$ and PCO$_2$ makes compensatory response calculation is invalid.

Step 3: High anion gap of 25 mmol/L 135 − (85+25) is the only clue to underlying high anion gap metabolic acidosis.

Step 4: On further analysis, Δ anion gap is 13 (25 − 12) and expected [HCO$_3^-$] is between 6 and 16 mmol/L. Actual [HCO$_3^-$] is higher than this range, suggesting associated metabolic alkalosis.

Final diagnosis: High anion gap metabolic acidosis with metabolic alkalosis.

Case 5: A 65-year-old man collapsed in the general ward. He was admitted on the same day for acute exacerbation of COPD. The ward nurse noticed him to be apneic with an easily palpable carotid pulse. He was intubated by the rapid response team and was transferred to the ICU. ABG done while on bag ventilation and 15 L O$_2$/min: pH—7.10, PaO$_2$—147 mmHg, PaCO$_2$—135 mmHg and HCO$_3^-$ 36 mmol/L.

Step 1: Low pH with high PCO$_2$ suggests respiratory acidosis as the primary abnormality.

Step 2: For 95 mmHg increase in PaCO$_2$ above normal 40 mmHg, HCO$_3^-$ has changed by 12 mmol/L from normal; that is just 3 mmol/L for every 10 mmHg change in PaCO$_2$, suggesting some "Chronic respiratory acidosis".

Step 3 and 4: In the absence of any metabolic abnormality, these steps are not required.

Final diagnosis: Acute respiratory acidosis possibly related to respiratory arrest.

Conclusion

The biggest strength of the traditional approach is its simplicity, easy understanding, availability of variables used, wide acceptability and its ability to identify a vast majority of acid-base abnormalities in clinical medicine. But there are several limitations to this approach. Traditional approach describes PaCO$_2$ and [HCO$_3^-$] as independent determinants of respiratory and metabolic components, respectively. But the fact is [HCO$_3^-$] is not an independent variable and it varies with changing PaCO$_2$ as can be seen in the Henderson–Hasselbalch equation. Moreover, various formulae describing compensatory responses are empirical and based on animal experiments performed more than half a century ago.

Take Home Messages
- Traditional approach considers $PaCO_2$ and HCO_3^- concentration in plasma as independent variables to determine acid-base disorders. Any change in $PaCO_2$ or HCO_3^- beyond normal value produces respiratory or metabolic acid-base disorders.
- Change in $PaCO_2$ or HCO_3^- concentration leads to compensatory response through kidneys or lungs, respectively, in an effort to normalize pH.
- Various empirical formulae can quantify expected compensatory changes and provide an approach to interpret presence of any second base disorder.
- Traditional approach provides the concept of anion gap to further elucidate causes of metabolic acid-base disorders. The concept of anion gap is also useful in various other ways.
- The concept of delta anion gap provided in the traditional approach can be used to find out any third metabolic acid-base disorder.

Reference

1. Berend K, de Vries APJ, Gans ROB. Physiological approach to assessment of acid–base disturbances. N Engl J Med. 2014;371:1434–45. https://doi.org/10.1056/NEJMra1003327.

Acid Base Homeostasis: Stewart Approach at the Bedside

7

Supradip Ghosh

Contents

Introduction 156
Physicochemical Perspective 157
SID and Acid Base Balance 158
Total Nonvolatile Acid Anion (A_{tot}) and Acid Base Balance 158
Total CO_2 158
Stewart at Bedside: Fencl-Stewart Approach 159
Fencl-Stewart: Putting It All Together 159
Stewart at Bedside: Using Standard Base Excess 160
Effect of Different IV Fluids on Acid-Base Balance 161
Conclusion 164
Some More Illustrative Case 163
References 164

S. Ghosh (✉)
Department of Critical Care Medicine, Fortis - Escorts Hospital, Faridabad, Haryana, India

M. L. N. G. Malbrain et al. (eds.), *Rational Use of Intravenous Fluids in Critically Ill Patients*, https://doi.org/10.1007/978-3-031-42205-8_7

IFA Commentary (MLNGM)

The Stewart approach to acid-base balance is a fascinating method that is increasingly being used by the medical community and especially intensive care physicians. First presented by the late Peter Stewart around 1980, the approach completely clarifies any acid base disturbance [1]. One of the key concepts of the new Stewart approach is that bicarbonate, or HCO_3^-, does not play any role in acid-base balance as opposed to the traditional and still generally used approach. This is usually very counterintuitive for most clinicians as the commonly used Henderson Hasselbalch approach advocates otherwise. Interestingly, Stewart does not deny the value of the Henderson Hasselbalch equation. In fact, this equation is actually one of the six equations that Stewart proposes to describe the acid-base equilibrium (Table 7.1).

This implies that both approaches are mathematically compatible and that the Stewart approach may provide the overall and bigger picture. According to the Stewart approach, there are only three independent variables that determine the concentration of H^+ and thus pH in any fluid, including plasma (Fig. 7.1). These variables are first, the partial pressure of carbon dioxide (PCO_2), second, the total amount of not completely dissociated weak acids (Atot, mainly albumin) and finally, the so-called Strong Ion Difference (SID). The strong ion difference is the sum of all positively charged fully dissociated ions (mainly Na^+) minus the sum of all negatively charged fully dissociated ions (mainly Cl^-). If PCO_2 or Atot decrease, the patient will become more alkalotic. However, if the SID decreases the patient will become more acidotic. Thus, while HCO_3^- may follow the change in one of these independent variables, it can never cause a change in the pH by itself.

One of the most fascinating aspects of the Stewart approach is that it becomes very easy to see how fluid therapy may alter acid base status. Normal concentrations of plasma sodium and chloride are about 140 and 110 mEq/L, respectively, which results in a normal SID of 40 mEq/L. If we now infuse normal saline with a sodium and chloride content of 154 mEq/L and thus a SID of 0 mEq/L, it can easily be understood that plasma SID will decrease resulting in metabolic (hyperchloremic) acidosis.

Acidbase.org has been serving the critical care community for over a decade. The backbone of this online resource consists of Peter Stewart's original text "How to understand Acid-Base" which is freely available to everyone. In addition, Stewart's Textbook of Acid Base, which puts the theory in today's clinical context, is available for purchase from the website. However, many intensivists use acidbase.org on a daily basis for its educational content and in particular for its analysis module. A recent review provides an overview of the history of this website, a tutorial and descriptive statistics of over 10,000 queries submitted to the analysis module [2].

At first glance, the Stewart approach may appear difficult, especially because it involves a number of equations. However, in this chapter we will show you that the Stewart approach is actually very easy to use and understand at the bedside. We will focus on a number of difficult cases that will be solved at the end. This chapter will provide the reader the tools needed to apply the Stewart approach at the bedside. After completion you will be able to fully understand, quantify, and diagnose any acid base disturbance you may encounter in daily clinical practice.

Suggested Reading
1. Kellum JA, Elbers PWG. Stewart's textbook of acid-base. Amsterdam, 2009. AcidBase.org. Available online at www.acidbase.org.
2. Elbers PW, Van Regenmortel N, Gatz R. Over ten thousand cases and counting: acidbase.org is serving the critical care community. Anaesthesiol Intensive Ther. 2015;47(5):441–8. https://doi.org/10.5603/AIT.a2015.0060. Epub 2015 Oct 13. PMID: 26459229.

Table 7.1 The Stewart equations, all of which need to be satisfied simultaneously

1. Water dissociation equilibrium	$[H^+] \times [OH^-] = K'_W$
2. Weak acid dissociation equilibrium	$K_A \times [HA] = [H^+] \times [A^-]$
3. Conservation of mass for "A"	$A_{TOT} = [A^-] + [HA]$
4. Bicarbonate ion formation equilibrium	$[PCO_2] \times K_C = [H^+] \times [HCO_3^-]$
5. Carbonate ion formation equilibrium	$[K_3] \times [HCO_3^-] = [II^+] \times [CO_3^{2-}]$
6. Electrical neutrality equation	$SID + [H^+] - [HCO_3^-] - [A^-] - [CO_3^{2-}] - [OH^-] = 0$

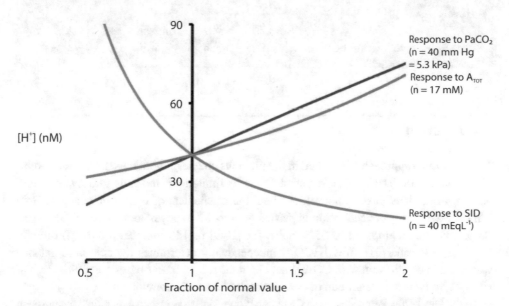

Fig. 7.1 The relative influence of the three independent parameters, SID, A_{TOT} and P_aCO_2 on H^+. pH 7.4 corresponds to $[H^+] = 40$ nM, whereas pH = 7 and pH =8 correspond to $[H^+]$ of 100 and 10 nM respectively. *SID* strong ion difference. Reprinted and adapted with permission from Elbers et al. under the Open Access CC BY Licence 4.0 [2]

Learning Objectives

After reading this chapter, you will have learned:

1. To understand independent variables determining acid base homeostasis.
2. To understand concepts of total carbon di-oxide, strong ion difference (SID) and total non-volatile acid anion (Atot), their individual components, and the effects of these variables on acid base physiology.
3. To learn about Fencl's simplified methods (and calculations) to understand Stewart at bedside.
4. To understand the unified concept of base excess and Stewart.
5. To understand the impact of large volume resuscitation on plasma acid base homeostasis in light of Stewart approach.

Case Vignette

Mr. M, a 46 year-old male with a history of alcoholic liver disease was admitted to the Intensive Care Unit in a hypotensive state following variceal bleeding. On examination, he had evidence of peripheral circulatory shock. Blood gases done on admission showed: pH—7.40, $PaCO_2$—39 mmHg, HCO_3—24 mEq/L, BE—0. Laboratory reports revealed: Na −125 mEq/L, K −5.2 mEq/L, Cl −98 mEq/L, Albumin −13 g/L, Ca −3.2 mEq/L, and Pi −0.9 mEq/L.

Questions

Q1. Do we expect any acid base disturbance in Mr. M? If the answer is yes, how do we elucidate it from the given clinical and biochemical information?

Introduction

The traditional approach (described in the previous chapter), though useful for interpretation of acid base issues in most patients, has its limitations and fails to answer certain pertinent questions. It does not tell us about the mechanism of metabolic changes. How can [H$^+$] with a tiny concentration in plasma (40 nmol/L at physiological pH of 7.4 and 38 °C temperature, compared to 55.3 mol/L for [H$_2$O] or 140 mmol/L for [Na$^+$]) directly manipulate plasma pH? How [HCO$_3^-$] independently determines the acid base balance when it is in equilibrium with CO$_2$? What about the role of buffer bases other than PaCO$_2$/HCO$_3^-$? What is the magnitude of changes in the metabolic component?

In the late 1970s, Peter Stewart, a Canadian biophysicist, described a quantitative approach to acid-base disorder. His approach was based on fundamental physicochemical properties of a solution that include principles of electroneutrality, law of conservation of mass, and dissociation equilibrium of all incompletely dissociated substances in a solution [1]. Although quite comprehensive, Stewart's original approach failed to gain popularity because it demands the user to solve complicated equations limiting its utility at the bedside. In last three decades, various researchers have proposed modifications of the original Stewart approach. These modifications have now made it possible to utilize Stewart at the bedside, without losing much of its precision. In this chapter, we shall discuss simple bedside approach to Stewart's physicochemical approach to acid-base and its usefulness in critically ill patients. See also Chap. 6 to learn more about the traditional approach to acid-base.

Physicochemical Perspective

As mentioned earlier, Stewart approach looks at acid-base balance from physicochemical perspective. According to Stewart, $[HCO_3^-]$ and pH in body fluids are dependent variables and are determined by three independent variables:

(a) Total CO_2 content (this incorporates $PaCO_2$, H_2CO_3, and HCO_3).
(b) Strong ion difference (SID).
(c) Concentration of weak nonvolatile acids (A_{tot}). Mostly determined by Albumin and Phosphate concentration.

Principle of electroneutrality states that concentration of all cations in plasma must be equal to the concentration of all anions to maintain the electrical equilibrium, as can be seen in the Gamblegram below (Fig. 7.2).

Strong ions are derived from substances that are almost completely dissociated in a solution. The strong ion difference (SID) is the sum of routinely measured strong plasma cations (Na^+, K^+, Ca^{2+}, Mg^{2+}) minus the sum of routinely measured strong plasma anions (mostly Cl^-) ("**Apparent SID**").

$$SID = \left(\left[Na^+ \right] + \left[K^+ \right] + \left[Ca^{++} \right] + \left[Mg^{++} \right] \right) - \left(\left[Cl^- \right] \right)$$

Fig. 7.2 Principle of electro-neutrality: concentrations of all cations same as concentrations of all anions. *Alb*- albuminate, *UA*- unmeasured anion, *Pi*- phosphate

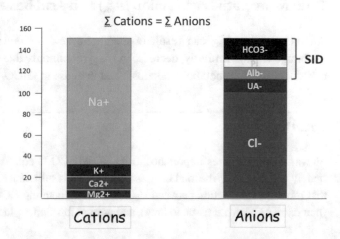

In physiological state, the gap between strong cations ($[Na^+]$, $[K^+]$, $[Ca^{++}]$, $[Mg^{++}]$) and strong anions($[Cl^-]$) or SID, is filled up mostly by $[HCO_3^-]$ and total amount of nonvolatile acids anions ($[A_{tot}]$ comprising mostly of $[Alb-]$ and to a lesser extent by $[Pi-]$) (as can be seen in Fig. 7.2). Thus, SID can also be calculated alternatively as the sum of $[HCO_3^-]$ and $[A_{tot}]$ (**"Effective SID"**).

$$SID \sim \left[HCO_3^-\right] + \left[A_{tot}\right]$$

Any change in electrical charge between strong cations or strong anions (SID) or change in nonvolatile acid anion concentration (A_{tot}) distorts the dissociation equilibrium of weakly dissociating substances in plasma (including water itself) altering the balance between $[H^+]$ and $[OH^-]$. Relative increase or decrease in $[H^+]$ (compared to $[OH^-]$) produces acidosis and alkalosis, respectively—Arrhenius definition of acid/base.

SID and Acid Base Balance

SID can decrease with any gain in unmeasured strong anions (e.g., beta hydroxybutyrate or lactate) without an equivalent increase in strong cations. Otherwise, a decrease in SID can simply be because of $[Cl^-]$ and $[Na^+]$ moving closer together. $[Na^+]$ and $[Cl^-]$ can move closer together either because of water excess (lowering $[Na^+]$) or an increase in $[Cl^-]$.

Decrease in SID in turn decreases the available space between strong cations and strong anions, resulting in a decrease in $[HCO_3^-]$ (see the Gamblegram above). Decrease in $[HCO_3^-]$ seen in metabolic acidosis is the effect (or marker) of metabolic acidosis rather than its cause.

On the other hand, an increase in SID results in metabolic alkalosis. SID can either increase as a result of an increase in $[Na^+]$ (reflecting water deficit) or because of a decrease in $[Cl^-]$. With more available space, $[HCO_3^-]$ increases with an increase in [SID].

Total Nonvolatile Acid Anion (A_{tot}) and Acid Base Balance

An increase in $[A_{tot}]$ can result in metabolic acidosis and decrease in $[HCO_3^-]$ (with unchanged SID). Similarly, decrease in $[A_{tot}]$ (commonly due to hypoalbuminemia in critically ill) results in metabolic alkalosis and increase in $[HCO_3^-]$.

Total CO$_2$

Stewart approach gives importance to $[H_2CO_3]/[HCO_3^-]$ equilibrium. But maintains that ultimately what counts is the total CO_2, as long as there is sufficient carbonic anhydrase (an enzyme that modifies the reaction between H_2O and CO_2 generating HCO_3^- and H^+), intact circulation (that carries CO_2 from tissue to lung), and normal functioning lungs (that regulate $PaCO_2$).

Stewart at Bedside: Fencl-Stewart Approach

Fencl and Leith proposed a simplified approach to Stewart's physicochemical concept by determining the plasma values of independent variables and getting direct insight into the mechanism of acid base abnormality [2]. Acid–base status of the plasma can be considered normal only when all independent variables are within normal range. In contrast, abnormality of any one of these independent variables leads to acid–base disturbances. Values for all independent variables can either be obtained directly or may be easily calculated from the arterial blood gas analyzer and routine biochemistry.

1. **Water excess/deficit**: Any deviation in $[Na^+]$ (**Normal value 140 ± 2 mEq/L**), low value signifying water deficit and high value water excess.
2. **$[Cl^-]$ excess or deficit:** Observed $[Cl^-]$ value needs correction for any dilution/ concentration of plasma. This can be done by following equation:
   (a) $[Cl^-]_{Corrected} = [Cl^-]_{Observed} \times ([Na^+]_{Normal}/[Na^+]_{Observed})$
   (b) Chloride excess/deficit = $[Cl^-]_{Normal} - [Cl^-]_{Corrected}$ (**Normal value—102 mEq/L**)
3. **Calculation of SID**: As can be seen from the Gamblegram above, the SID in plasma can be derived as the sum of $[HCO^+]$ plus the negative electric charges contributed by albumin [Alb-] and by inorganic phosphate [Pi-]. $[HCO_3^-]$ is available from arterial blood gas machine or routine biochemistry values. [Alb-] and [Pi-] (in mEq/L) can be calculated from the measured Albumin (in gm/L), [Pi] (mmol/L) and pH, as per equations proposed by Figge et al. [3] or more useful one by Fencl and colleagues [4].
   (a) [Alb-] in mEq/L = $(42 - [Alb-_{Measured}]) \times (0.148 \times pH - 0.818)$ **OR** [Alb-] = 0.25 × Alb (in g/L)
   (b) [Pi-] in mEq/L = $0.309 \times (pH - 0.46) \times (0.8 - [Phos_{Measured}])$ **OR** [Pi-] = 0.6 × Phosphate (in mg/dl)
   (c) SID = $[HCO_3^-] + [Alb-] + [Pi-]$ (**Normal Value—39 ± 1 mEq/L**)
4. **Unmeasured strong anions [UA-]:** [UA-] are strong anions other than Cl^- (included in the differential diagnosis of high Anion Gap metabolic acidosis e.g., lactate, keto-acids and other organic anions, sulfate). Value of [UA-] can be indirectly derived from the equation below:
   (a) Unmeasured Anion = $[Na^+] + [K^+] + [Ca^{2+}] + [Mg^{2+}] - [Cl^-] - [SID]$ (normal range—8 ± 2 mEq/L) (For routine purpose $[Mg^{2+}]$ may be replaced by 1.7.)

Fencl-Stewart: Putting It All Together

Following the discussion above, causes of acidosis (pH < 7.38) can be re-classified and are depicted in Fig. 7.3 [4].

Following schema can classify causes of alkalosis (pH > 7.42) following Fencl and Stewart approach (Fig. 7.4) [4].

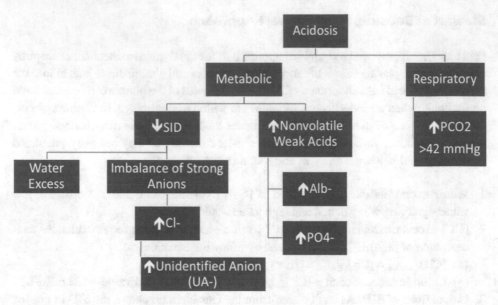

Fig. 7.3 Classification of acidosis

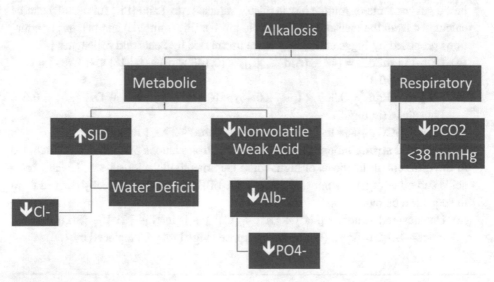

Fig. 7.4 Classification of alkalosis

Stewart at Bedside: Using Standard Base Excess

The concepts of base excess (BE) and standard base excess (SBE) were introduced by Siggaard-Anderson to provide a quantitative measure of the metabolic component of acid base disorders, independent of respiratory effect [5]. BE can be defined as the amount of acid (in equivalent) required to bring the blood pH back to 7.40 with $PaCO_2$ kept constant at 40 mmHg. To nullify the effect of hemoglobin on acid base balance, Siggaard-Anderson also introduced the concept of standard base excess (SBE) that assumes hemoglobin concentration of the whole extracellular compartment of 5 g/L. Both BE and SBE are parameters, easily available from routine printouts of all blood gas machine.

Since BE is the single variable that may be used to quantify the overall metabolic component of acid base status, it can be assumed that changes in Stewart independent variables (SID and A_{tot}) will impact the BE. Several authors have proposed simplified approaches to Stewart's concept of acid base by utilizing the concept of BE [6–8]. In all these simplified approaches base excess effects of SID and A_{tot} were determined to quantify unmeasured anion.

Story et al. calculated the effects of changes in free water or sodium concentration ("**Sodium Effect**"), chloride concentration ("**Chloride Effect**"), and albumin ("**Albumin Effect**") on base excess, by using formulae that can be easily used at the bedside [7]. They further combined Sodium effect and Chloride effect to give a simplified effect of SID (called Sodium-Chloride effect). Finally, they subtracted Sodium-Chloride effect and Albumin effect from SBE to quantify effect of Unidentified anion on SBE (called unmeasured ion effect).

- **Sodium effect (in mEq/L)** $= 0.3 \times [Na^+] - 140)$
- **Chloride effect (in mEq/L)** $= 102 - ([Cl^-] \times 140/[Na^+])$
- **Sodium-Chloride effect (in mEq/L)** = Sodium Effect + Chloride Effect
     OR
- **Sodium-Chloride effect (in mEq/L)** $= ([Na^+] + [Cl^-]) - 38$
- **Albumin effect (mEq/L)** $= 0.25 \times [42 - Albumin (g/L)]$
- **Unmeasured ion effect (mEq/L)** = SBE − (Sodium-Chloride effect + Albumin effect).

Effect of Different IV Fluids on Acid-Base Balance

Properties of intravenous fluids and consequences of large volume infusion of these fluids on plasma acid base balance can be explained by using Stewart's physicochemical approach. As crystalloid solutions do not contain Atot, rapid intravenous administration crystalloids will dilute plasma Atot, producing a trend towards metabolic alkalosis. The SID of all fluids including crystalloids also has its effect on plasma SID, potentially producing change in pH.

Infusion of large volumes of zero SID fluids (all saline solution with equivalent concentration of $[Na^+]$ and $[Cl^-]$ or Dextrose or Mannitol solutions without any strong ion) will reduce plasma SID by admixture and equilibration, forcing acid-base balance in the direction of a metabolic acidosis. Although this acidosis is commonly Hyperchloremic, it can also occur with low plasma $[Cl^-]$, depending on the fluid employed (as in cases of large volume Dextrose infusion resulting in water excess with low or normal $Cl^-_{Corrected}$).

Acidosis due to rapid infusion of large volume crystalloids can only be avoided by increasing crystalloid SID, which means replacing some [Cl^-] in the crystalloid with certain organic anions like lactate, acetate, gluconate, or maleate, that are rapidly metabolized in the body resulting in a large increase in SID. For example, Ringer's lactate contains L-Lactate at a concentration of 29 mEq/L. Unless there is severe impairment of hepatic function, L-Lactate is metabolized at 100 mEq/h, resulting in a calculated SID of 29 mEq/L. However, in normal body temperature, effective SID of RL is approximately 27 mEq/L because of incomplete dissociation.

In an in vitro experiment, Carlesso et al. had found that baseline [HCO_3^-] dictates the pH response to large volume rapid crystalloid infusion [8, 9]. If the [SID] of the crystalloid solution infused equals baseline [HCO_3^-], pH remains unchanged provided the $PaCO_2$ is constant. On the other hand, solutions with SID values higher or lower than plasma result in an increase or decrease in pH, respectively.

Case Vignette

Let us now look into the case vignette in the beginning of the chapter (**Case 1**) and try to understand acid base issues if any. With normal pH, $PaCO_2$, Base Excess and corrected Anion Gap (9.75) values, the patient apparently does not have any acid base disorder (following either Traditional or Siggaard-Anderson Approach). But that seems to be unusual considering the overall clinical status of the patient.

Following Fencl-Stewart approach as described above, following observations can be made.

- No respiratory abnormality ($PaCO_2$ 39 mmHg)
- Low [Na^+] (129 mEq/L) suggesting acidifying "Water Excess".
- High [$Cl_{corrected}$] (98 × (142/125) = 111 mEq/L) suggesting acidifying "Chloride Excess".
- Low [Albuminate-] (0.25 × 13 = 3.25 mEq/L) suggesting alkalinizing "Low [Alb-]".
- Normal Pi (0.9 mEq/L).
- High SID ([HCO_3^-] + [Alb-] + [Pi-]): 24 + 3.25 + 0.9 = 28.15 mEq/L) suggesting acidifying "Low SID".
- Normal unmeasured anion ([Na^+] + [K^+] + [Ca^{2+}] + [Mg^{2+}] − [Cl^-] − [SID] = 8.95 mEq/L).

Final Diagnosis: This patient has multiple acid base abnormalities including low SID "Metabolic Acidosis" (Water excess plus high corrected chloride) and hypoalbuminemic "Metabolic Alkalosis".

Some More Illustrative Case

Case 2: A 45 years old male, operated for Ileal perforation, developed multiple organ failure postoperatively. Arterial blood gas revealed, pH—7.33, PaCO$_2$—30 mmHg, HCO$_3$—15 mEq/L and BE—10. Serum biochemistry showed, Na −117mEq/L, K −3.9 mEq/L, Cl −92 mEq/L, Albumin −6 g/L, Ca −3 mEq/L, Pi −0.6 mEq/L.
Applying Fencl-Stewart approach:

- PaCO$_2$: 30 mmHg. Low value suggesting "Respiratory Alkalosis".
- [Na$^+$]: 117 mEq/L. Suggesting acidifying "Water Excess".
- [Cl$_{corrected}$]: 92 × (142/117) = 112 mEq/L. Suggesting acidifying "Chloride Excess"
- [Alb-]: 0.25 × 6 = 1.5 mEq/L. Alkalinizing "Low [Alb-]".
- [SID]: 15 + 1.5 + 0.6 = 17.1 mEq/L. Suggesting acidifying "Low SID".
- Normal Pi: 0.6 mEq/L
- Unmeasured Anion ([Na$^+$] + [K$^+$] + [Ca^{2+}] + [Mg^{2+}] − [Cl$^-$] − [SID]): 117 + 3.9 + 3 + 1.7 − 92 − 17.1 = 16.5 mEq/L. Acidifying "High [UA-]"

Final Diagnosis: This patient has "Metabolic Acidosis" due to a combination of "Low SID" (water excess and high corrected Chloride) and "High [UA-]" partially offset by "Metabolic Alkalosis" due to "Low [Alb-]" and "Respiratory Alkalosis".

Case 3: 72-years old female patient, a cardiac arrest survivor, was admitted to the ICU with hypoxic ischemic encephalopathy. Arterial blood gas revealed, pH—7.55, PaCO$_2$—29 mmHg, HCO$_3$—25.5 mEq/L, BE—+2. Biochemical analysis showed, Na −159 mEq/L, K −3.6 mEq/L, Cl −121 mEq/L, Albumin −9 g/L, Ca −4.2 mEq/L, Pi −0.5 mEq/L.
Applying Fencl-Stewart approach:

- PaCO$_2$: 29 mmHg. Suggesting presence of "Respiratory Alkalosis".
- [Na$^+$]: 159 mEq/L. Suggesting alkalinizing "Water deficit".
- [Cl$_{corrected}$]: 121 × (142/159) = 108 mEq/L. Suggesting acidifying "Chloride Excess"
- [Alb-]: 0.25 × 9 = 2.25 mEq/L. Presence of alkalinizing "Low [Alb-]".
- SID: 25.5 + 2.25 + 0.5 = 28.25 mEq/L. Suggesting acidifying "Low [SID]"
- Normal Pi: 0.6 mEq/L
- Unmeasured Anion ([Na$^+$] + [K$^+$] + [Ca^{2+}] + [Mg^{2+}] − [Cl$^-$] − [SID]): 159 + 3.6 + 4.2 + 1.7 − 121 − 28.25 = 19.25 mEq/L. High value suggesting presence of acidifying "High [UA-]".

Final Diagnosis: This patient has "Metabolic Alkalosis" due to "Water deficit" and "Low [Alb-]" along with "Metabolic Acidosis" due to "Chloride Excess" and "High [UA-]". She is also having evidence of "Respiratory Alkalosis".

Conclusion

Stewart's approach has the ability to identify and also quantify individual components of complex acid base abnormalities. Another unique ability of this approach is to identify hidden acid base disorder (not identified by traditional or base excess approach) as illustrated in the case vignette. By providing insight into the pathogenesis of complex metabolic acid base disorder, Stewart's approach can help the clinician in deciding probable ways to rectify the problem. Unmeasured anion, identified by modified Stewart's, is a powerful indicator of prognosis in critically ill patient. In a study on pediatric population, Balasubramanyan et al. found unmeasured anions to be more strongly associated with mortality compared to BE, anion gap, or lactate [5].

Take Home Messages
- Three variables independently determine acid base homeostasis in any fluid including plasma—total carbon di-oxide, strong ion difference (SID), and total nonvolatile acid anion (A_{tot}).
- These individual components can be easily quantified at the bedside by using modified Stewart approach provided by Fencl.
- Quantification of independent variables provides a direct insight into the mechanisms of acid base disturbances and any measure to be taken to correct them (if required).

References

1. Stewart PA. How to understand acid-base. A qualitative acid-base primer for biology and medicine. New York: Elsevier North Holland Inc.; 1981.
2. Fencl V, Leith DE. Stewart's quantitative acid–base chemistry: applications in biology and medicine. Respir Physiol. 1993;91:1–16.
3. Fencl V, Jabor A, Kazda A, Figge J. Diagnosis of metabolic acid–base disturbances in critically ill patients. Am J Respir Crit Care Med. 2000;162:2246–51.
4. Figge J, Mydosh T, Fencl V. Serum proteins and acid-base equilibria: a follow-up. J Lab Clin Med. 1992;120:713–9.
5. Andersen OS. The pH-log pCO_2 blood acid-base nomogram revised. Scand J Clin Lab Invest. 1962;14:598–604.

6. Balasubramanyan N, Havens P, Hoffman G. Unmeasured anions identified by the Fencl-Stewart method predict mortality better than base excess, anion gap, and lactate in patients in the pediatric intensive care unit. Crit Care Med. 1999;27:1577–81.
7. Story DA, Morimatsu H, Bellomo R. Strong ions, weak acids and base excess: a simplified Fencl-Stewart approach to clinical acid-base disorders. Br J Anaesth. 2004;92:54–60.
8. Magder S, Emami A. Practical approach to physical-chemical acid-base management. Stewart at the bedside. Ann Am Thorac Soc. 2015;12:111–7.
9. Carlesso E, Maiocchi G, Tallarini F, Polli F, Valenza F, Cadringher P, Gattinoni L. The rule regulating pH changes during crystalloid infusion. Intensive Care Med. 2011;37:461–8.

The 4-indications of Fluid Therapy: Resuscitation, Replacement, Maintenance and Nutrition Fluids, and Beyond

8

Manu L. N. G. Malbrain (ID), Michaël Mekeirele, Matthias Raes, Steven Hendrickx, Idris Ghijselings, Luca Malbrain, and Adrian Wong

Contents

Introduction 171
The Four Indications 172
  Resuscitation Fluids 172
  Maintenance Fluids 172
  Replacement Fluids 177
  Nutrition Fluids 177
The Four Questions 178
  When to Start IV Fluids? 178
  When to Stop IV Fluids? 179
  When to Start Fluid Removal? 179
  When to Stop Fluid Removal? 179

M. L. N. G. Malbrain (✉)
First Department of Anaesthesiology and Intensive Therapy, Medical University of Lublin, Lublin, Poland

M. Mekeirele · M. Raes · S. Hendrickx · I. Ghijselings
Intensive Care Department, University Hospital Brussels (UZB), Jette, Belgium

L. Malbrain
University School of Medicine, Katholieke Universiteit Leuven (KUL), Leuven, Belgium

A. Wong
Intensive Care and Anaesthesia, King's College Hospital NHS Foundation Trust, London, UK

© The Author(s) 2024
M. L. N. G. Malbrain et al. (eds.), *Rational Use of Intravenous Fluids in Critically Ill Patients*, https://doi.org/10.1007/978-3-031-42205-8_8

The Four (or Six) D's 180
    Diagnosis 180
    Drug 180
    Dose 181
    Duration 188
    De-escalation 188
    Discharge 189
The Four Hits 189
    First Hit: Initial Insult 189
    Second Hit: Ischemia-Reperfusion 189
    Third Hit: Global Increased Permeability Syndrome 189
    Fourth Hit: Hypoperfusion 190
The Four Phases (ROSE Concept) 191
    Resuscitation 192
    Optimization 193
    Stabilization 193
    Evacuation 193
The Other Fours 196
    The Four Compartments 196
    The Four Spaces 196
    The Four Losses 196
Conclusions 197
References 199

IFA Commentary (PN)

The administration of intravenous fluids is a crucial and one of the most frequent therapeutic options in critical care, but it is high time that clinicians begin to view fluids as drugs that require a systematic approach. To this end, a conceptual framework of the 7 D's has been proposed to provide a comprehensive understanding of fluid therapy and monitoring.

The 7 D's framework includes definitions of key terms, such as fluid status, preload, and fluid responsiveness. It also emphasizes the importance of accurate diagnosis, including hypo-, eu-, and hypervolemia, and monitoring organ and tissue perfusion. The framework also covers the drug aspect of fluid therapy, including the type of fluids, indications, contraindications, adverse effects, rate, objectives, and limits, followed by dose, duration, de-escalation, and discharge. Understanding these aspects is critical for selecting the appropriate fluids for patients and avoiding unnecessary complications.

The framework also addresses 4 critical questions, such as when to start and stop IV fluids, when to begin fluid evacuation, and when to stop fluid removal. The 4 indications for fluid administration are discussed: resuscitation, maintenance, replacement, and nutrition. It also outlines the four phases of fluid therapy, including resuscitation, optimization, stabilization, and evacuation (ROSE).

Furthermore, the framework explores the four hits and four compartments of fluid therapy. The four hits refer to the underlying conditions that may lead to fluid imbalances, including hypovolemia, redistribution, capillary leak, and interstitial edema. The four compartments refer to the various fluid compartments in the body and their unique characteristics, including intravascular, interstitial, intracellular, and transcellular fluids. Understanding these compartments is critical for selecting the appropriate fluids and monitoring their effectiveness.

Finally, the framework advocates for fluid stewardship, which refers to a coordinated series of interventions aimed at selecting the optimal fluid, dose, and duration of therapy to achieve the best clinical outcomes while minimizing adverse events and reducing costs. Fluid stewardship is critical in ensuring that patients receive the best possible care while minimizing the risks associated with fluid therapy.

In summary, the 7 D's framework provides a comprehensive approach to fluid therapy and monitoring, emphasizing the importance of accurate diagnosis, drug selection, and appropriate monitoring. By adopting this approach, clinicians can optimize patient outcomes, minimize adverse events, and reduce healthcare costs.

Learning Objectives
In this chapter we will discuss the different indications for intravenous (IV) fluid therapy in critically ill patients. After finishing this chapter, the reader will understand the differences between resuscitation, maintenance, replacement, and nutrition fluids. Each type of fluid has indications and contraindications and pros and cons, benefits, and adverse effects and the user must understand the different pitfalls that may affect the clinical outcome when one fluid is preferred over another. Resuscitation fluids should be given to save lives in patients with shock (trauma, sepsis, bleeding, burns, pancreatitis…). Maintenance fluids should be given to cover the daily needs of total body water, glucose, and electrolytes (mainly sodium and potassium). Replacement fluids should mimic the fluid that is lost (egammonium chloride or normal saline in case of gastrointestinal losses). And finally, nutrition fluids should cover the daily caloric needs with focus on proteins and/or nitrogen. In order to be able to administer the right dose of fluids, assessment of fluid status and hemodynamic function is mandatory, besides other monitoring techniques like indirect calorimetry or bioelectrical impedance analysis. Echocardiography should be seen as an additional tool or the modern stethoscope to assess cardiac function and to obtain a "volumetric" idea of preload in combination with cardiac function, afterload, and fluid responsiveness. Besides the four indications of fluid therapy, the reader will also understand other basic principles of fluid therapy like the four (or even six or seven) D's, the four questions, the four hits, and the four phases.

Case Vignette

Woman, 75 years old, bedridden, weighs 50 kg

Previous History: minimental state evaluation (MMSE) 19/30, arterial hypertension, type 2 diabetes mellitus, diverticulitis

Current problem: fever, increasing confusion, blood pressure 99/55 mmHg, pulse rate 119/min

Lab results: CRP 99 mg/dl, creatinine 2.1 mg/dl, urea 102 mg/dl, Na 145 mmol/L, K 3.5 mmol/L

Diagnosis: urosepsis. The patient appears dehydrated and has acute renal failure RIFLE I (injury), presumably prerenal. Now follow some questions. We ask the reader not to think too much or too long, but to choose the answer that first pops up in his/her mind.

Questions

Q1. You decide to administer a fluid bolus, how much do you give? 100—250—500—1000 ml?

Q2. How fast do you administer the fluid bolus? 10 to 15 min— 30 min—1 hour—2 hours?

Q3. What do you consider the most clinically relevant parameter to assess fluid responsiveness? Heart rate—mottled skin—capillary refill time—blood pressure—passive leg raise test—diuresis—respiratory rate?

Q4. What type of fluids did you administer during resuscitation phase? Normal saline (NaCl 0.9%)—Hypotonic saline (NaCl 0.45%)—Glucose 5%—Plasmalyte—Ringer's lactate—Ringer's acetate—Hartmann solution—Maintelyte—Volulyte—Gelatin—Albumin—Glucose 5% in NaCl 0.45%—Glucose 5% in NaCl 0.9%?

After fluid resuscitation (you gave twice 250 ml over 10 min), paracetamol (1 g IV in 100 ml bottle) and starting antibiotic therapy, the patient ameliorates, and on day 3, it is decided to transfer the patient to the normal ward. However, there are strong doubts about correct swallowing function, and the patient is kept nil per mouth until evaluation by ENT specialist.

Q5. What type of fluids did you administer as maintenance solution? Normal saline (NaCl 0.9%)—Hypotonic saline (NaCl 0.45%)—Glucose 5%—Plasmalyte—Ringer's lactate—Ringer's acetate—Hartmann solution—Maintelyte—Volulyte—Gelatin—Albumin—Glucose 5% in NaCl 0.45%—Glucose 5% in NaCl 0.9%?

Q6. How many ml of fluid do you administer to this patient on a daily basis? 500 ml—750 ml—1000 ml—1500 ml—2000 ml—2500 ml?

Q7. What is the daily need for sodium (mmol) in this patient? 15—25—50—75—100—150?

Q8. What is the daily need for potassium (mmol) in this patient? 15—25—50—75—100—150?

Q9. What is the daily need for glucose (g) in this patient? 15—25—50—75—100—150?

From the seventh day, the patient starts producing profound watery diarrhea (12 times a day) with nausea and vomiting (around 1500 ml of cumulative daily gastric aspirate volume). A lab result indicates a BE of 8.

Q10. What would be the best replacement fluid in addition to her daily maintenance solution? Normal saline (NaCl 0.9%)—Hypotonic saline (NaCl 0.45%)—Glucose 5%—Plasmalyte—Ringer's lactate—Ringer's acetate—Hartmann solution—Maintelyte—Volulyte—Gelatin—Albumin—Glucose 5% in NaCl 0.45%—Glucose 5% in NaCl 0.9%?

Introduction

In critically ill patients, the administration of intravenous (IV) fluids remains a major therapeutic challenge and one size does not fit all [1]. We are faced with many open questions regarding the type (crystalloids vs colloids), properties (balanced vs unbalanced), speed of administration, dose (intermittent bolus vs continuous), and timing (early vs late) of intravenous fluid administration [2, 3]. Figure 8.1 gives an overview of different IV fluids.

There are only four major indications for intravenous fluid administration: aside from resuscitation (in order to save lives), intravenous fluids have many other uses including maintenance (to cover the daily needs of total body water and electrolytes) and replacement (to replace the fluid that is lost) and for parenteral nutrition [4]. But there may even be more indications like fluids as carriers for medications (sedation, antibiotics,

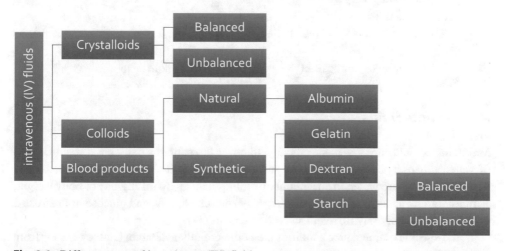

Fig. 8.1 Different types of intravenous (IV) fluids

analgesics…). In this chapter, we discuss not only the 4 major indications for fluid therapy in the critically ill, but also the different fluid management strategies including early adequate goal-directed fluid management (EAFM), late conservative fluid management (LCFM), and late goal-directed fluid removal (LGFR) [4]. In addition, and in analogy to antibiotics, we expand on the concept of the six (seven) D's of fluid therapy, namely (definitions), diagnosis, drug, dosing, duration, de-escalation, and documentation at discharge [5]. This chapter will elaborate further on the terms and definitions listed in Chap. 1.

The Four Indications

Resuscitation Fluids

Resuscitation fluids are given to correct an intravascular volume deficit in the case of absolute or relative hypovolemia [4]. In theory, the choice between colloids and crystalloids should take into account the revised Starling equation and the glycocalyx model of transvascular fluid exchange [4, 6]. When capillary pressure (or transendothelial pressure difference) is low, as in hypovolemia or sepsis and especially septic shock, or during hypotension (after induction and anesthesia), albumin or plasma substitutes have no advantage over crystalloid infusions, since they all remain intravascular. However, the glycocalyx layer is a fragile structure and is disrupted by surgical trauma-induced systemic inflammation or sepsis, but also by rapid infusion of fluids (especially saline). Under these circumstances, transcapillary flow (albumin leakage and risk of tissue edema) is increased; as is the risk to evolve to a state of global increased permeability syndrome (GIPS) [6]. Table 8.1 gives an overview of different resuscitation fluids.

> **Definitions and Key Messages**
> - Isotonic resuscitation fluids are administered to save lives.
> - A fluid bolus (or better a fluid challenge) should be small (4 ml/kg) and given fast (in 5–15 min).
> - Do not administer fluids until the patient is no longer fluid-responsive

Maintenance Fluids

Maintenance fluids are given, specifically, to cover the patient's daily basal requirements of water, glucose, and electrolytes. As such, they are intended to cover daily needs. The basic daily needs are water, in an amount of 1 ml/kg/h or 25–30 mL/kg/day of body weight, 1 mmol/kg/day potassium, 1–1.5 mmol/kg/day sodium per day, and glucose or dextrose 5 or 10% 1.4–1.6 g/kg/day (to avoid starvation ketosis) [7].

Some specific maintenance solutions are commercially available, but they are far from ideal. In Belgium, Glucion© 5% and Glucion© 10% are commercially available. During a

Table 8.1 Characteristics and composition of different resuscitation crystalloids

		Electrolytes												
		Cations (mEq/L)				Anions (mEq/L)								
	Nutrients														Osmolarity
	Gluc (g)	Na	K	Ca	Mg	Cl	P	Lactate	Acetate	Gluconate	Malate	SID	pH	(mOsm/L)
Unbalanced NaCl 0.9%	0	154	0	0	0	154	0	0	0	0	0	0	5.5	308
Glucose 5% + NaCl 0.9%	50	154	0	0	0	154	0	0	0	0	0	0	3.5–6.5	585
NaCl 3%	0	513	0	0	0	513	0	0	0	0	0	0	5.5	1026
GNaK	50	51	40	0	0	91	0	0	0	0	0	0	4.5	460
Balanced PlasmaLyte	0	140	5	0	3	98	0	0	27	23	0	50	7.4	295
Sterofundin ISO	0	145	4	5	2	127	0	0	24	0	5	29	5.1–5.9	309
Ionolyte	0	137	4	0	3	110	0	0	24	0	0	34	6.9–7.9	286
Hartmann	0	131	5	4	0	111	0	29	0	0	0	29	5–7	278

previous ISICEM (International Symposium on Intensive Care and Emergency Medicine) meeting in Brussels, the Baxter company launched a new ready from the shelve maintenance solution called Maintelyte©. There is a lot of debate whether isotonic or hypotonic maintenance solutions should be used. Data in children showed that hypotonic solutions carry the risk for hyponatremia and neurologic complications [8, 9]. However, studies in adults are scarce and indicate that administration of isotonic solutions will result in a more positive fluid balance as compared to hypotonic solutions [10]. This was confirmed in a recent pilot study (MIHMoSA) in healthy volunteers showing that isotonic solutions (glucose 5% in NaCl 0.9% + 40 mmolKCl/L) caused lower urine output (and thus more positive cumulative fluid balance at 48 h), characterized by decreased aldosterone concentrations indicating (unintentional) volume expansion, than hypotonic solutions (Glucion© 5%) [11]. The cumulative fluid balance at 48 h is shown in Fig. 8.2.

Despite their lower sodium and potassium content, hypotonic fluids were not associated with clinically significant hyponatremia or hypokalemia, as illustrated in Fig. 8.3 [11]. These results have been recently confirmed in 69 critically ill patients after major thoracic surgery (TOPMAST) using the same isotonic and hypotonic fluids as the MIHMoSA trial [12].

Figure 8.4 shows the TOPMAST study results with respect to cumulative fluid balance. The tonicity of the maintenance fluids was responsible for the clinical impact on perioperative fluid retention (4.5 L in isotonic vs 3.1 L in hypotonic group), independent of the administered volume (around 2.65 L in both groups). Isotonic maintenance fluids resulted in an estimated difference at 72 h of 1369 mL (95%CI 601–2137). An isotonic

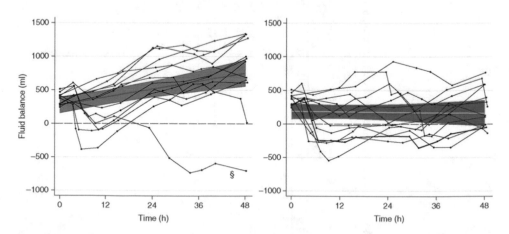

Fig. 8.2 Cumulative fluid balance over the course of each study period. Left panel shows the isotonic (glucose % + NaCl 0.9% + 40 mmol KCl/L) maintenance fluids (purple), while the right panel shows the effect of the hypotonic (Glucion© 5%, NaCl 0.32%) maintenance fluids (dark blue). Black lines are individual observations per subject. Colored lines are the marginal means estimated using the mixed effects model; the shaded areas represent 95% confidence intervals. Dashed lines are predicted values at 48 h (t_{48}). §Outlier with exaggerated natriuresis. The positive fluid balance at t_0 is attributable to oral fluid intake. Reproduced and adapted from Van Regenmortel et al. with permission according to the Open Access CC BY Licence 4.0 [11]

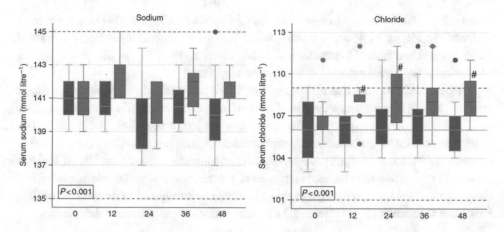

Fig. 8.3 Serum concentration of electrolytes, sodium (Na, left panel) and chloride (Cl, right panel), over the course of both study periods. In-graph *P*-values are indicated for the difference between the two fluids. Hypotonic fluids are indicated in blue and isotonic fluids in purple box plots. #Significantly different from t_0 on a fluid-specific level ($P < 0.05$). Black dashed lines represent the normal range of the electrolytes. Colored lines indicate the median value at t_0 for each fluid. Reproduced and adapted from Van Regenmortel et al. with permission according to the Open Access CC BY Licence 4.0 [11]

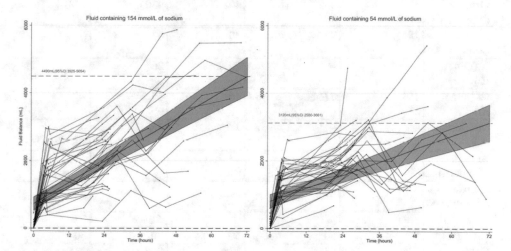

Fig. 8.4 TOPMAST study results. Cumulative fluid balance over the course of each study period. Black lines are individual observations of cumulative fluid balance over time per subject. Colored lines are the marginal means estimated using the mixed effects model; the shaded areas represent 95% confidence intervals. Fluid balance was estimated at 72 h (dashed line), as this is a typical duration for maintenance fluid therapy in the perioperative setting and the maximum duration of study treatment in the current study. The positive fluid balance at baseline is fluids that were administered immediately before surgery. Adapted from Van Regenmortel et al., with permission according to the Open Access CC BY Licence 4.0 [13]

maintenance fluid strategy was reported to cause hyperchloraemia (>109 mmol/L) in most patients (68.6% vs 11.8% $p < 0.001$), while hypotonic maintenance fluids decreased sodium levels and caused hyponatraemia (<135 mmol/L) in 11.8% vs 0% ($p = 0.04$), but no clinical effects were reported in adult surgical patients.

A recent study showed that maintenance and replacement fluids account for the largest amount (24.7%) of the average daily total fluid volume, exceeding by far resuscitation fluids (6.5%). Maintenance fluids are also the most important source of sodium and chloride [14]. Fluid creep caused by maintenance and replacement fluids represents on average one third of the daily fluid volume. In septic patients, non-resuscitation fluids have an even larger absolute impact on cumulative fluid balance compared to resuscitation fluids. Therefore, inadvertent daily loading of volume, sodium, and chloride should be considered when prescribing (isotonic) maintenance fluids [14]. Table 8.2 lists some common maintenance solutions.

Table 8.2 Characteristics and composition of different maintenance solutions

Fluids (1 l.)	Glucose 5% + 0.9% NaCl isotonic	Glucose 5% + 0.45% NaCl hypotonic	Maintelyte hypertonic[a]	Glucion 5% hypertonic	Glucose 5% hypotonic
Osm (mosm/L)	585	432	402	430	278
Na (mmol/L)	154	77	40	54	–
K (mmol /L)	–	–	20	26	–
Cl (mmol /L)	154	77	40	55	–
Mg (mmol /L)	–	–	1.5	2.6	–
Acetate (mmol /L)	–	–	23		–
Lactate (mmol/L)				25	
P (mmol/L)				6.2	
Glu (g/L)	50[a]	50[a]	50	50	50
Caloric value (KJ/L) (Kcal/L)	835 200	835 200	835 200	835 200	835 200
SID (mEq/L)	0	0	21.5	30	0
pH	4.5 ± 1.0	4.3	4.5–6.5	5–5.2	4.2

[a] It has to be noted that the new Maintelyte solution is slightly hypertonic (in vitro), but the mOsm includes the 5% glucose, which should not contribute to cellular tonicity in humans. Therefore, the rest of the content—Na, K, Cl, Mg, and acetate, are the components which can provide tonicity. Since glucose 5% exerts 278 mOsm/L, the balance of the mOsm/L is 124 mOsm/L

> **Definitions and Key Messages**
> - Maintenance fluids should always cover the daily needs.
> - The daily needs are 1 ml/kg/h or 20–25 ml/kg/day for water, 1–1.5 mmol/kg/day for sodium, 0.5–1 mmol/kg/day for potassium, 1–1.5 g/kg/day for glucose
> - Maintenance fluids are responsible for fluid creep, especially if they are isotonic.
> - It is not (only) the volume, that causes fluid overload, it's also the salt!

Replacement Fluids

Replacement fluids are administered to correct fluid deficits that cannot be compensated by oral intake. Such fluid deficits have a number of potential origins, like drains or stomata, vomiting, burns, diarrhea, vacuum dressings (like Abthera abdominal VAC, Acelity, USA), high output fistulas, fever or hyperthermia, open wounds, polyuria (salt wasting nephropathy, cerebral salt wasting, osmotic diuresis, or diabetes insipidus), during abdominal surgery, physical activity, and others [15].

Similar to maintenance fluids, data on replacement fluids are also scarce. Several recent guidelines advise matching the amount and composition of fluid and electrolytes as closely as possible to the fluid that is being or has been lost [16, 17]. An overview of the composition of the different body fluids can be found in the NICE guidelines [16]. Replacement fluids are usually isotonic balanced solutions. In patients with fluid deficit due to a loss of chloride-rich gastric fluid, high chloride solutions, like ammonium chloride (NH4Cl) or (ab)normal saline (0.9% NaCl), can be used as replacement fluid.

> **Definitions and Key Messages**
> - Replacement fluids should mimic the fluid that is lost
> - Gastrointestinal losses may be the only indication left for (ab)normal saline

Nutrition Fluids

Often overlooked, it is about time to consider parenteral nutrition as another source of intravenous fluids that may contribute to fluid overload or accumulation. On the other hand, enteral nutrition can also contribute to fluid overload in critical illness as the adaptive mechanisms to avoid water and sodium retention may not always function properly. Likewise, nutritional therapy in the critically ill should be seen as "medication" helping the healing process. As such, we might consider also the four D's of nutritional therapy in analogy to how we deal with antibiotics and fluids [3]: drug (type of feeding), dose (caloric and protein load), duration (when and how long), and de-escalation (stop enteral nutrition and/or parenteral nutrition when oral intake improves) [18]. It is noteworthy that in case of an open abdomen the patient is at risk for potentially significant fluid, electrolyte, and protein losses from the exposed viscera. In case of extensive fluid losses (open abdomen, abdominal drains, ascites paracentesis, or VAC dressings), there will be a substantial loss of nitrogen (on average 2g N/L fluid) [19].

> **Definitions and Key Messages**
> - Nutrition fluids should cover daily caloric needs
> - On average, 2g N are lost per L drainage fluid

The Four Questions

When to Start IV Fluids?

Early adequate fluid management (EAFM) is the initial hemodynamic resuscitation of patients with (septic) shock by administering fluids during the first 6 h after the initiation of therapy. Most studies looking at treatment of septic shock define achieving the early goal as giving 25–50 mL/kg (on average 30 mL/kg) of fluids given within the first 3 h [1]. However, the recent surviving sepsis campaign guidelines define EAFM as 30 mL/kg given in the first hour [20, 21]. However, it has been hypothesized that fluid resuscitation using such large volumes of fluid may lead to "iatrogenic salt water drowning" and that more conservative strategies for fluid resuscitation might be warranted [22]. As stated above, the best fluid is the one that has not been given unnecessarily to the patient. Most patients with a good cardiac function are on the steep slope of their Frank-Starling curve. It is a misconception that in critical illness fluid responsiveness always means that actual fluids need to be administered. There is no high-quality evidence to support the use of IV fluids to optimize the circulation, and especially there is no evidence for the use of higher volumes as recommended by international guidelines [20, 23]. In contrast, data from cohort studies, small trials, and systematic reviews in sepsis and large trials in other settings and patient groups suggest potential benefits from restriction of IV fluids in patients with septic shock [24–26]. Therefore, fluids should only be given when needed, i.e., when the patient is in shock (DO_2/VO_2 imbalance with lactate production) and fluid-responsive [27, 28]. In all other cases, it may be wise to withhold IV fluids [29, 30].

> **Definitions and Key Messages**
> - Early adequate fluid management (EAFM) is the initial hemodynamic resuscitation of patients with (septic) shock by administering adequate fluids during the first 6 h after the initiation of therapy.
> - Fluids should only be given when needed, i.e., when the patient is in shock (DO_2/VO_2 imbalance with lactate production) and fluid-responsive.

When to Stop IV Fluids?

Late Conservative Fluid Management (LCFM) describes a moderate fluid management strategy following the initial EAFM in order to avoid (or reverse) fluid overload. Recent studies showed that 2 consecutive days of negative fluid balance within the first week of the ICU stay is a strong and independent predictor of survival [31]. LCFM must be adapted according to the variable clinical course of septic shock during the first days of ICU treatment, e.g., patients with persistent systemic inflammation maintain transcapillary albumin leakage and do not reach the flow phase (see further) mounting up positive fluid balances. Once one has decided to administer IV fluids, one must immediately think of a fluid strategy stopping them. Fluids can be stopped when initial signs and symptoms of shock and hypovolemia have resolved. Usually this is based on normalization of macro-hemodynamic parameters like MAP, HR, CVP, GEDVI in combination with other clinical, biochemical, and/or imaging signs.

> **Definitions and Key Messages**
> - Late Conservative Fluid Management (LCFM) is defined as 2 consecutive days of negative fluid balance within the first week of the ICU stay.
> - After the initial Ebb phase, most patients enter the Flow phase spontaneously

When to Start Fluid Removal?

Because of the very nature of (septic) shock, fluids may accumulate in the body. Late Goal-Directed Fluid Removal (LGFR) describes that in some patients more aggressive and active fluid removal by means of diuretics or renal replacement therapy with net ultrafiltration is needed either or not in combination with hypertonic solutions to mobilize the excess interstitial edema [32]. This is referred to as de-resuscitation, a term that was coined for the first time in 2014 [28].

> **Definitions and Key Messages**
> - Late Goal-Directed Fluid Removal (LGFR) is defined as active fluid removal with diuretics or renal replacement therapy with net ultrafiltration and started within the first week of ICU stay also referred to as de-resuscitation

When to Stop Fluid Removal?

During de-resuscitation, it is important to assure adequate intravascular filling and to avoid hypovolemia and hypoperfusion as this may cause further harm. Hypertonic solutions can be used to "drive" fluids from the interstitium into the intravascular space. According to the revised Starling principle, this is usually obtained via lymphatic drainage.

> **Definitions and Key Messages**
> - The benefits of fluid removal should always outweigh the potential risks

The Four (or Six) D's

Diagnosis

Correct diagnosis of a state of shock, hypovolemia vs hypervolemia, and fluid responsiveness are all equally important. The American consensus definition states that shock is defined by a systolic blood pressure below 90 mmHg refractory to fluid administration. This definition is not useful at the bedside. The European definition states that shock is a situation of imbalance between oxygen delivery (DO_2) and oxygen consumption (VO_2) resulting in anaerobic metabolism and lactate production:

$$DO_2 = CO \times CaO_2 = HR \times SV \times (Hgb \times Sat \times 1.34 + pO_2 \times 0.0034)$$

Standardizing and driving adoption of hypovolemia screening and assessment tools, including hemodynamic monitoring, is the cornerstone in initial management of any shocked patient. Figure 8.5 lists some clinical signs, and the laboratory, imaging, hemodynamic, and organ function signs and effects related to hypovolemia are summarized in Fig. 8.6.

Drug

We should consider the different compounds: crystalloids vs. colloids, synthetic vs. blood derived, balanced vs. unbalanced, intravenous vs. oral; the osmolality, tonicity, pH, electrolyte composition (chloride, sodium, potassium, etc.) and levels of other metabolically active compounds (lactate, acetate, malate…). Clinical factors (underlying conditions, kidney or liver failure, presence of capillary leak, acid-base equilibrium, albumin levels, fluid balance…) must all be taken into account when choosing the type and amount of fluid for a given patient at a given time. Moreover, the type of fluid is different depending on the reason why they are administered.

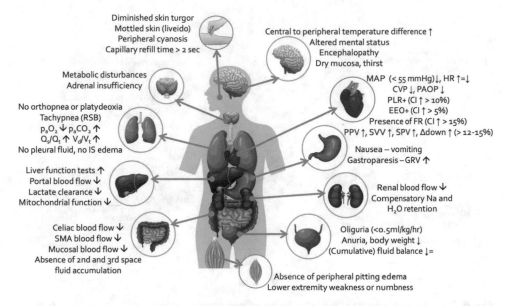

Fig. 8.5 Clinical signs and symptoms related to hypovolemia and hypoperfusion. *CVP* central venous pressure, *EEO* end-expiratory occlusion, *FR* fluid responsiveness, *GRV* gastric residual volume, *HR* heart rate, *MAP* mean arterial blood pressure, *Na* sodium, *PAOP* pulmonary artery occlusion pressure, *PLR* passive leg raising, *PPV* pulse pressure variation, *Qs/Qt* shunt fraction, *RSB* rapid shallow breathing, *SMA* superior mesenteric artery, *SPV* systolic pressure variation, *SVV* stroke volume variation, *Vt/Vd* dead space ventilation

Dose

As Paracelsus nicely stated: "All things are poison, and nothing is without poison; only the dose permits something not to be poisonous". Like other drugs, it is the dose of fluids that make them poisonous. As stated before, the risk of excessive fluid overload is well established.

Similar to other drugs, choosing the right dose implies that we take into account the pharmacokinetics and pharmacodynamics of intravenous fluids (Table 8.3).

Pharmacokinetics describes how the body affects a drug resulting in a particular plasma and effect site concentration [33]. Pharmacokinetics of intravenous fluids depends on distribution volume, osmolality, tonicity, oncoticity, and kidney function. Eventually, the half time depends on the type of fluid, but also on the patient's condition and the clinical context (Table 8.4). When administering one liter of fluid only, 10% of glucose solution, vs. 25% of an isotonic crystalloid solution, vs. 100% of a colloid solution will remain intravascularly after one hour, but as stated above the half-life is dependent on other conditions (like infection, inflammation, sedation, surgery, anesthesia, blood pressure,…) (Fig. 8.7) [34, 35].

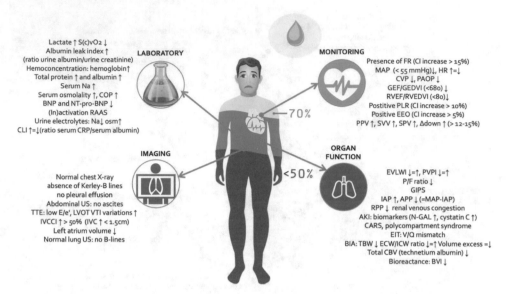

Fig. 8.6 Laboratory, imaging, hemodynamic and organ function signs and symptoms related to hypovolemia and hypoperfusion. Total body water accounts for 70% of body weight. Overt signs and symptoms of hypovolemia occur when circulating blood volume is reduced with more than 50%. *AKI* acute kidney injury, *APP* abdominal perfusion pressure, *BIA* bioelectrical impedance analysis, *BNP* brain natriuretic peptide, *BVI* blood volume index, *CARS* cardio-abdominal-renal syndrome, *CBV* circulating blood volume, *CI* cardiac index, *CLI* capillary leak index, *COP* colloid oncotic pressure, *CRP* C-reactive protein, *CVP* central venous pressure, *ECW* extracellular water, *EIT* electrical impedance tomography, *EEO* end-expiratory occlusion, *EVWLI* extravascular lung water index, *FR* fluid responsiveness, *GEDVI* global end-diastolic volume index, *GEF* global ejection fraction, *GIPS* global increased permeability syndrome, *HR* heart rate, *IAP* intra-abdominal pressure, *ICW* intracellular water, *IVC* inferior vena cava, *IVCCI* inferior vena cava collapsibility index, *LVOT* left ventricular outflow tract, *MAP* mean arterial blood pressure, *Na* sodium, *P/F ratio* pO_2 over FiO_2 ratio, *PAOP* pulmonary artery occlusion pressure, *PLR* passive leg raising, *PPV* pulse pressure variation, *PVPI* pulmonary vascular permeability index, *RAAS* renin angiotensin aldosterone system, *RPP* renal perfusion pressure, *RVEDVI* right ventricular end-diastolic volume index, *RVEF* right ventricular ejection fraction, *ScvO2* mixed central venous oxygen saturation, *SPV* systolic pressure variation, *SVV* stroke volume variation, *TBW* total body water, *TTE* transthoracic echocardiography, *US* ultrasound, *V/Q* ventilation/perfusion, *VTI* velocity time integral

Volume kinetics is an adaptation of pharmacokinetic theory that makes it possible to analyze and simulate the distribution and elimination of infusion fluids [35]. Applying this concept, it is possible, by simulation, to determine the infusion rate that is required to reach a predetermined plasma volume expansion. Volume kinetics may also allow the quantification of changes in the distribution and elimination of fluids (and calculation of the half-life) that result from stress, hypovolemia, anesthesia, and surgery [34].

Pharmacodynamics relates the drug concentrations to its specific effect. For fluids, the Frank-Starling relationship between cardiac output and cardiac preload is the equivalent of the dose effect curve for standard medications. Because of the shape of the Frank-Starling

Table 8.3 Analogy between the 4 D's of antibiotic and fluid therapy

Description	Terminology	Antibiotics	Fluids
Drug	Inappropriate therapy	More organ failure, longer ICU LOS, longer hospital LOS, longer MV	Hyperchloremic metabolic acidosis, more AKI, more RRT, increased mortality
	Appropriate therapy	Key factor in empiric AB selection is consideration of patient risk factors (e.g., prior AB, duration MV, corticosteroids, recent hospitalization, residence in nursing home)	Key factor in empiric fluid therapy is consideration of patient risk factors (e.g., fluid balance, fluid overload, capillary leak, kidney, and other organ function). Don't use glucose as resuscitation fluid
	Combination therapy	Possible benefits: e.g., broader spectrum, synergy, avoidance of emergency of resistance, less toxicity	Possible benefits: e.g., specific fluids for different indications (replacement vs maintenance vs resuscitation), less toxicity
	Class	Broad-spectrum or specific, Beta-lactam or glycopeptide, additional compounds as tazobactam. The choice has a real impact on efficacy and toxicity	Hypo- or hypertonic, high or low chloride and sodium level, lactate or bicarbonate buffer, glucose containing or not. This will impact directly acid-base equilibrium, cellular hydration, and electrolyte regulation
	Appropriate timing	Survival decreases with 7% per hour delay. Needs discipline and practical organization	In refractory shock, the longer the delay, the more microcirculatory hypoperfusion
Dosing	Pharmacokinetics	Depends on distribution volume, clearance (kidney and liver function), albumin level, tissue penetration	Depends on type of fluid: glucose 10%, crystalloids 25%, vs colloids 100% IV after 1 hour, distribution volume, osmolality, oncoticity, kidney function
	Pharmacodynamics	Reflected by the minimal inhibitory concentration. Reflected by "kill" characteristics, time (T>MIC) vs concentration (Cmax/MIC) dependent	Depends on type of fluid and desired location: IV (resuscitation), IS vs IC (cellular dehydration)
	Toxicity	Some AB are toxic to kidneys, advice on dose adjustment needed. However, not getting infection under control isn't helping the kidney either	Some fluids (HES) are toxic for the kidneys. However, not getting shock under control is not helping the kidney either

(continued)

Table 8.3 (continued)

Description	Terminology	Antibiotics	Fluids
Duration	Appropriate duration	No strong evidence, but trend towards shorter duration. Don't use AB to treat fever, CRP, or chest X-ray infiltrates but use AB to treat infections	No strong evidence, but trend towards shorter duration. Don't use fluids to treat low CVP, MAP, or UO, but use fluids to treat shock
	Treat to response	Stop AB when signs and symptoms of active infection resolve. Future role for biomarkers (PCT)	Fluids can be stopped when shock is resolved (normal lactate). Future role for biomarkers (NGAL, cystatin C, citrullin, L-FABP)
De-escalation	Monitoring	Take cultures first and have the guts to change a winning team	After stabilization with EAFM (normal PPV, normal CO, normal lactate), stop ongoing resuscitation and move to LCFM and LGFR (=deresuscitation)

Adapted from Malbrain et al. with permission [3]

AB antibiotic, *AKI* acute kidney injury, C_{max} maximal peak concentration, *CO* cardiac output, *CRP* C reactive protein, *CVP* central venous pressure, *EAFM* early adequate fluid management, *EGDT* early goal-directed therapy, *IC* intracellular, *ICU* intensive care unit, *IS* interstitial, *IV* intravascular, *LCFM* late conservative fluid management, *L-FABP* L-type fatty acid binding protein, *LGFR* late goal-directed fluid removal, *LOS* length of stay, *MAP* mean arterial pressure, *MIC* mean inhibitory concentration, *MV* mechanical ventilation, *NGAL* neutrophil gelatinase-associated lipocalin, *PCT* procalcitonin, *PPV* pulse pressure variation, *RRT* renal replacement therapy, *UO* urine output

Table 8.4 Overview of half-life (T1/2) of Ringer's, glucose, and colloid solutions as reported in different studies

Category	Study population	n	Fluid studied	$T_{1/2}$ (min)
Volunteers	Healthy adults	24	Glucose 2.5%	19
	Healthy adults	9	Glucose 5%	13
	Healthy adults	6	Ringer's acetate	22–46
	Healthy adults	8	Dextran 70	175
	Healthy adults	15	Plasma	197
	Healthy adults	15	Albumin 5%	110
	Healthy adults	20	HES 130/0.4	110
	Dehydrated adults	20	Ringer's acetate	76
	Healthy children	14	Ringer's lactate	30
Pregnancy	Normal	8	Ringer's acetate	71
	Preeclampsia	8	Ringer's acetate	12
	Before caesarian section	10	Ringer's acetate	175
Surgery	Before surgery	29	Ringer's acetate	23
	Before surgery		Ringer's lactate	169
	Thyroid	29	Ringer's acetate	327–345
	Laparoscopic cholecystectomy	12	Glucose 2.5%	492
	Laparoscopic cholecystectomy	12	Ringer's acetate	268
	Gynecological laparoscopy	20	Ringer's lactate	346
	Open abdominal	10	Ringer's lactate	172
	After hysterectomy	15	Glucose 2.5%	14
	After laparoscopy	20	Ringer's lactate	17

Adapted from Hahn [34]
HES hydroxyethyl starch

relationship, the response of cardiac output to the fluid-induced increase in cardiac preload is not constant [36]. The effective dose 50 (ED50), in pharmacology, is the dose or amount of drug that produces a therapeutic response or desired effect in 50% of the subjects receiving it, whereas lethal dose 50 (LD50) will result in death of 50% of recipients. Translated to IV fluids, this would be the dose of fluid that induces, respectively, a therapeutic response or death in 50% of the patients. The problem is that the therapeutic response varies from one patient to another (Fig. 8.8).

Fluid administration can be toxic (or even lethal) at a high enough dose, as demonstrated in 2007 when a California woman died of water intoxication (and hyponatremia) in a contest organized by a radio station (http://articles.latimes.com/2007/jan/14/local/me-water14). The difference between toxicity and efficacy is dependent upon the particular patient and the specific condition of that patient, although the amount of fluids administered by a physician should fall into the predetermined therapeutic window.

Unanswered questions remain: what is an effective dose of IV fluids? What is the exact desired therapeutic effect? What is the therapeutic window? In some patients, volume expansion increases the mean systemic filling pressure (the backward pressure of venous

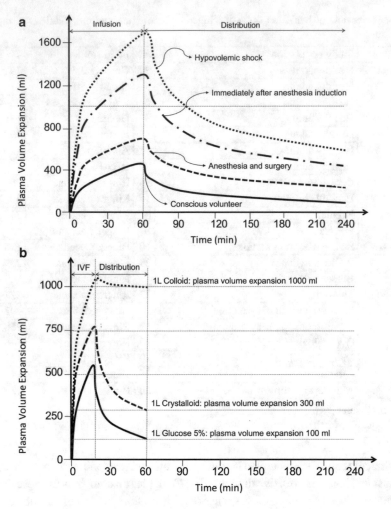

Fig. 8.7 Pharmacokinetics and pharmacodynamics fluids. Original artwork based on the work of Hahn R [34, 35]. (**a**) Volume kinetic simulation. Expansion of plasma volume (in ml) after intravenous infusion of 2 l of Ringer's acetate over 60 min in an adult patient (average weight 80 kg), depending on normal condition as conscious volunteer (solid line —), during anesthesia and surgery (dashed line - -), immediately after induction of anesthesia due to vasoplegia and hypotension with decrease in arterial pressure to 85% of baseline, (mixed line — ■) and after bleeding during hemorrhagic shock with mean arterial pressure below 50 mmHg (dotted line ••••), see text for explanation. (**b**) Volume kinetic simulation. Expansion of plasma volume (in ml) is 100, 300, and 1000 ml respectively after 60 min following intravenous infusion of 1 l of glucose 5% over 20 min in an adult patient (solid line —), vs. 1 l of crystalloid (dashed line - -), vs. 1 l of colloid (dotted line ••••), see text for explanation. (**c**) Volume kinetic simulation. Expansion of plasma volume (in ml) after intravenous infusion of 500 ml of hydroxyethyl starch 130/0.4 (Volulyte, solid line —) vs. 1 l of Ringer's acetate (dashed line - -) when administered in an adult patient (average weight 80 kg), over 30 min (RED) vs 60 min (BLACK), vs 180 min (BLUE). When administered rapidly and as long as infusion is ongoing, the volume expansion kinetics are similar between crystalloids and colloids, especially in case of shock, after induction and anesthesia and during surgery (see text for explanation)

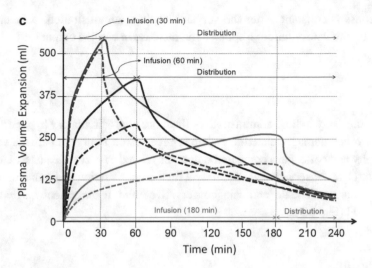

Fig. 8.7 (continued)

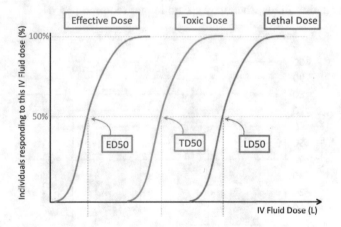

Fig. 8.8 Schematic representation of median IV Fluid doses. ED50: Median effective IV fluid dose: the dose of IV fluids required to achieve 50% of the desired response in 50% of the population. TD50: Median toxic IV fluid dose: the dose of IV fluids required to get 50% of the population reporting this specific toxic effect. LD50: Median lethal IV fluid dose: the dose of IV fluids required to achieve 50% mortality from toxicity

return), but it increases the right atrial pressure (the forward pressure of venous return) to the same extent, such that venous return and, hence, cardiac output does not increase [37]. Hence, venous congestion and backward failure may even play a more important and currently underestimated role [38]. The probability of the heart to "respond" to fluid by a significant increase in cardiac preload varies along the shock time course, and thus pharmacodynamics of fluids must be regularly evaluated. At the very early phase, fluid responsiveness is constant. After the very initial fluid administration, only one half of patients with circulatory failure respond to an increase in cardiac output [39].

Duration

The longer the delay in fluid administration, the more microcirculatory hypoperfusion and subsequent organ damage related to ischemia-reperfusion injury. In patients with sepsis [31], Murphy and colleagues compared outcomes related to early adequate vs. early conservative and late conservative vs. late liberal fluid administration and found that the combination of early adequate and late conservative fluid management carried the best prognosis [31] (Fig. 8.9).

De-escalation

As we will discuss below, the final step in fluid therapy is to consider withholding or withdrawing resuscitation fluids when they are no longer required [28, 41, 42].

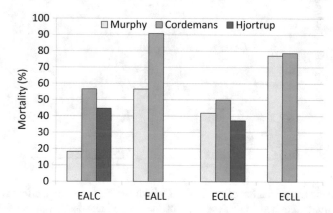

Fig. 8.9 Impact on outcome of appropriate timing of fluid administration. Bar graph showing outcome (mortality %) in different fluid management categories. Comparison of the data obtained from different studies: hospital mortality in 212 patients with septic shock and acute lung injury, adapted from Murphy et al. (black bars) [31], hospital mortality in 180 patients with sepsis, capillary leak and fluid overload, adapted and combined from 2 papers by Cordemans et al. (light grey bars) [32, 40], 90-day mortality in 151 adult patients with septic shock randomized to restrictive vs standard fluid therapy (CLASSIC trial), adapted from Hjortrup et al. (dark grey bars) [24]. See text for explanation. *EA* early adequate fluid management, defined as fluid intake >50 ml/kg/first 12–24 h of ICU stay, *EC* early conservative fluid management, defined as fluid intake <25 ml/kg/first 12–24 h of ICU stay, LC: late conservative fluid management, defined as 2 negative consecutive daily fluid balances within first week of ICU stay, *LL* late liberal fluid management, defined as the absence of 2 consecutive negative daily fluid balances within first week of ICU stay

Like for antibiotics (Table 8.3), the duration of fluid therapy must be as short as possible, and the volume must be tapered when shock is resolved. However, many clinicians use certain triggers to start, but are unaware of triggers to stop, fluid resuscitation, increasing the potential for fluid overload. As with duration of antibiotics, although there is no strong evidence, there is a trend towards shorter duration of intravenous fluids [24].

Discharge

Fluid therapy and prescription post-discharge from ICU or hospital must not be overlooked in order to assure adequate daily (oral) intake.

The Four Hits

First Hit: Initial Insult

After the initial insult (related to sepsis, burns, pancreatitis, trauma, haemorrhage...), the patient will enter the Ebb phase. This refers to the initial phase of septic shock when the patient shows hyperdynamic circulatory shock with decreased systemic vascular resistance due to vasodilation, increased capillary permeability, and severe absolute or relative intravascular hypovolemia. Fluids are mandatory and lifesaving in this phase. The patient in this stage needs EAFM [43].

Second Hit: Ischemia-Reperfusion

The second hit occurs within hours and refers to ischemia and reperfusion. Fluid accumulation reflects the severity of illness (and might be considered a "biomarker" for it). The greater the fluid requirement, the sicker the patient and the more likely organ failure (e.g., acute kidney injury) may occur.

Third Hit: Global Increased Permeability Syndrome

After the second hit, the patient can either further recover entering the "flow" phase with spontaneous evacuation of the excess fluids that have been administrated previously. Some patients will not transgress to the "flow" phase spontaneously and will remain in a "no flow" or persistent state of *global increased permeability syndrome* and ongoing fluid accumulation [44]. The global increased permeability syndrome can hence be defined as fluid overload in combination with new onset organ failure (Fig. 8.10). This is referred to as 'the third hit of shock' [32].

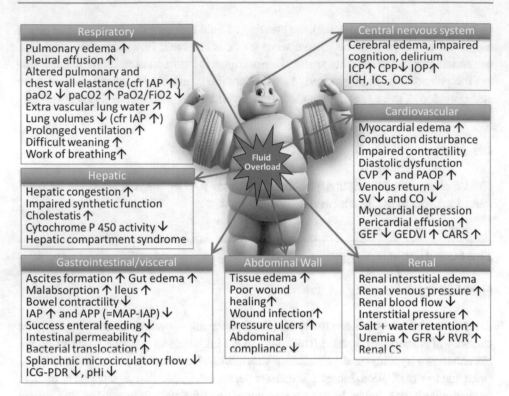

Respiratory
Pulmonary edema ↑
Pleural effusion ↑
Altered pulmonary and
chest wall elastance (cfr IAP ↑)
paO2 ↓ paCO2 ↑ PaO2/FiO2 ↓
Extra vascular lung water ↗
Lung volumes ↓ (cfr IAP ↑)
Prolonged ventilation ↑
Difficult weaning ↑
Work of breathing↑

Central nervous system
Cerebral edema, impaired
cognition, delirium
ICP↑ CPP↓ IOP↑
ICH, ICS, OCS

Cardiovascular
Myocardial edema ↑
Conduction disturbance
Impaired contractility
Diastolic dysfunction
CVP ↑ and PAOP ↑
Venous return ↓
SV ↓ and CO ↓
Myocardial depression
Pericardial effusion ↑
GEF ↓ GEDVI ↑ CARS ↑

Hepatic
Hepatic congestion ↑
Impaired synthetic function
Cholestatis ↑
Cytochrome P 450 activity ↓
Hepatic compartment syndrome

Fluid Overload

Gastrointestinal/visceral
Ascites formation ↑ Gut edema ↑
Malabsorption ↑ Ileus ↑
Bowel contractility ↓
IAP ↑ and APP (=MAP-IAP) ↓
Success enteral feeding ↓
Intestinal permeability ↑
Bacterial translocation ↑
Splanchnic microcirculatory flow ↓
ICG-PDR ↓, pHi ↓

Abdominal Wall
Tissue edema ↑
Poor wound
healing↑
Wound infection↑
Pressure ulcers ↑
Abdominal
compliance ↓

Renal
Renal interstitial edema
Renal venous pressure ↑
Renal blood flow ↓
Interstitial pressure ↑
Salt + water retention↑
Uremia ↑ GFR ↓ RVR ↑
Renal CS

Fig. 8.10 Potential adverse consequences of fluid overload on end-organ function. Adapted from Malbrain et al. with permission [4]. *APP* abdominal perfusion pressure, *IAP* intra-abdominal pressure, *IAH* intra-abdominal hypertension, *ACS* abdominal compartment syndrome, *CARS* cardio-abdominal-renal syndrome, *CO* cardiac output, *CPP* cerebral perfusion pressure, *CS* compartment syndrome, *CVP* central venous pressure, *GEDVI* global enddiastolic volume index, *GEF* global ejection fraction, *GFR* glomerular filtration rate, *ICG-PDR* indocyaninegreen plasma disappearance rate, *ICH* intracranial hypertension, *ICP* intracranial pressure, *ICS* intracranial compartment syndrome, *IOP* intraocular pressure, *MAP* mean arterial pressure, *OCS* ocular compartment syndrome, *PAOP* pulmonary artery occlusion pressure, *pHi* gastric tonometry, *RVR* renal vascular resistance, *SV* stroke volume

Fourth Hit: Hypoperfusion

Hypoperfusion is usually the result of hypovolemia. Hypovolemia is the term used to describe a patient with insufficient intravascular volume. It does not refer to total body fluid, but rather refers solely to the intravascular compartment. Total body fluid comprises approximately 60% of the body weight of men and 50% for women [45]. Blood volume can be estimated according to Gilcher's rule of fives at 70 mL/kg for men and 65 mL/kg for women [46]. Blood loss is frequently followed by recruitment of interstitial fluid from compartments distant to the central compartment. Vasoconstriction of the splanchnic mesenteric vasculature is one of the first physiologic responses [47]. Sodium and water retention results from activation of the renin-angiotensin-aldosterone system (RAAS) which replenishes the interstitial reserves and maintains transcapillary perfusion [48]. As a result, the body may lose up to 30% of blood volume before hypovolemia becomes clinically apparent [44]. Therefore, undiagnosed hypovolemia may be present long before clinical signs and symptoms occur. Hypovolemia can also occur in edematous patients, where total body water in increased, but intravascular volume is reduced (e.g., eclamptic patients). Finally, some patients are fluid-responsive, but not necessarily hypovolemic. Even the most basic of paradigms, such as the description of early sepsis and distributive shock being a hypovolemic state needing aggressive fluid resuscitation, have recently been called into question, [49] with data suggesting improved outcomes with less or even no administered intravenous fluid [24, 49]. Greater focus on the health and function of the microcirculation and the endothelial glycocalyx, potential new treatment paradigms calling for less fluids, and earlier vasopressor use have become the focus [3, 4, 49, 50]. These elements make accurate assessment of fluid status in the critically ill a challenging task.

The Four Phases (ROSE Concept)

Recently, a three (or even four) hit model of septic shock was suggested in which we can recognize four (or even five) distinct dynamic phases of fluid therapy [40]: Resuscitation, Optimization, Stabilization, and Evacuation (de-resuscitation) at the end (the acronym R.O.S.E.) (Table 8.3). On the other hand, too aggressive de-resuscitation may result in hypoperfusion again increasing end-organ damage. Logically, this acronym or mnemonic describes the different clinical phases of fluid therapy, occurring over the time course during which patients experience a different impact on end-organ function (Fig. 8.11). Similar principles were also suggested by others confirming the need for a multicenter prospective clinical trial with a biphasic fluid therapy approach, starting with initial early adequate goal-directed treatment followed by late conservative fluid management in those patients not transgressing spontaneously from the Ebb to the Flow phase [41, 42, 51–57]. The RADAR (Role of Active De-resuscitation After Resuscitation) trial may help to find such answers (http://www.hra.nhs.uk/news/research-summaries/radar-icu/). Clinicians should take into account the revised Starling equation and the glycocalyx model of transvascular fluid exchange [6]. When capillary pressure (or transendothelial pressure difference) is low, as in hypovolemia or sepsis, albumin or plasma substitutes have no advantage over crystalloid infusions, since they all remain intravascular. However, the glycocalyx layer is a fragile structure and is disrupted by surgical trauma-induced systemic inflammation or sepsis, but also by rapid infusion of fluids (especially saline). Under these circumstances, transcapillary flow (and risk of tissue edema) is increased; as is the risk to evolve to a state of global increased permeability syndrome (GIPS) [6].

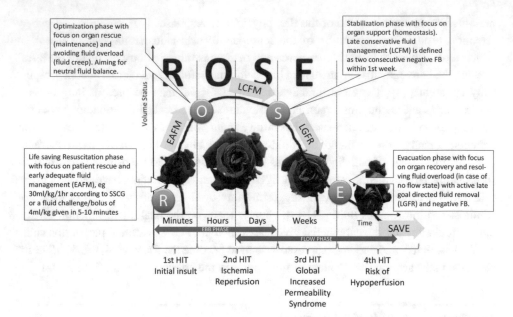

Fig. 8.11 Graph showing the four-hit model of shock with evolution of patients' cumulative fluid volume status over time during the five distinct phases of resuscitation: Resuscitation (R), Optimization (O), Stabilization (S), and Evacuation (E) (ROSE), followed by a possible risk of Hypoperfusion in case of too aggressive deresuscitation. On admission, patients are hypovolemic, followed by normovolemia after fluid resuscitation (EAFM, early adequate fluid management), and possible fluid overload, again followed by a phase going to normovolemia with late conservative fluid management (LCFM) and late goal-directed fluid removal (LGFR) or deresuscitation. In case of hypovolemia O_2 cannot get into the tissues because of convective problems, in case of hypervolemia O_2 cannot get into the tissue because of diffuse problems related to interstitial and pulmonary edema, gut edema (ileus and abdominal hypertension). Adapted according to the Open Access CC BY Licence 4.0 with permission from Malbrain et al. [4]

Resuscitation

After the **first hit** which can be sepsis (but also burns, pancreatitis, or trauma), the patient will enter the "ebb" phase of shock. This phase of severe circulatory shock, that can be life-threatening, occurs within minutes and is characterized by a low mean arterial pressure and microcirculatory impairment and can be accompanied with high cardiac output (hyperdynamic circulatory shock) or low cardiac output (e.g., septic shock with severe hypovolemia or septic shock with cardiomyopathy). Early adequate fluid management is not only useful but also lifesaving in this phase, but the goal should be individualized for every patient; also considering the patient's premorbid conditions [1, 58–60].

The lower autoregulatory threshold of the most vulnerable organs (kidney and brain) should be minimally reached [41]. In this phase, we try to find an answer to the first question: "When to start fluid therapy?", addressing the benefits of fluid resuscitation (restoration of organ perfusion).

Optimization

The **second hit** occurs within hours and refers to ischemia and reperfusion. Fluid accumulation reflects the severity of illness (and might be considered a "biomarker" for it) [55]. The greater the fluid requirement, the sicker the patient. In this phase, we try to find an answer to the second question: "When to stop fluid therapy?", avoiding potential risks of fluid administration (fluid overload).

Stabilization

After the Optimization phase follows the Stabilization phase (homeostasis) evolving over the next days. As previously described, the focus now is on organ support and this phase reflects the point at which a patient is in a stable steady state [28, 57]. Fluid therapy is now only used for ongoing maintenance and replacement fluids either in setting of normal fluid losses (i.e., renal, gastrointestinal, insensible), but this could also be fluid infusion (including rehydration) if the patient was experiencing ongoing losses because of unresolved pathologic conditions [28, 57]. However, this stage is distinguished from the prior two by the absence of shock (compensated or uncompensated) or the imminent threat of shock. Since persistence of a positive daily fluid balance over time is strongly associated with a higher mortality rate in septic patients [61], clinicians should also be aware of the hidden obligatory fluid intake, as it may contribute more than a liter each day [62].

Evacuation

After the second hit, the patient can either further recover entering the "flow" phase with spontaneous evacuation of the excess fluids that have been administrated previously, or, as is the case in many ICU patients, the patient remains in a "no flow" state followed by a **third hit** usually resulting from GIPS with ongoing fluid accumulation due to capillary leak [6, 63]. Further fluid administration at this stage becomes toxic. Peripheral and generalized edema is not only of cosmetic concern, as believed by some [64], but harmful to the patient as a whole as it results in organ dysfunction [28, 42]. In any case, the patient enters a phase of "de-resuscitation" (Table 8.5). This term was first suggested in 2012 [32] and finally coined in 2014 [28]. It specifically refers to *Late Goal-Directed Fluid Removal* and *Late Conservative Fluid Management*. Estimation of fluid overload measured by bioelectrical impedance (vector) analysis seems to predict mortality risk and is safe and easy to perform at the bedside [45, 65].

A vicious cycle may be established with further fluid loading. This will cause even more intestinal edema and visceral swelling leading to venous hypertension and deteriorating renal function (Fig. 8.12).

Table 8.5 The ROSE concept avoiding fluid overload (adapted from Malbrain et al. with permission [28])

	Resuscitation	Optimization	Stabilization	Evacuation
Hit sequence	First hit	Second hit	Second hit	Third hit
Time frame	Minutes	Hours	Days	Days to weeks
Underlying mechanism	Inflammatory insult	Ischemia and reperfusion	Ischemia and reperfusion	Global increased permeability syndrome
Clinical presentation	Severe shock	Unstable shock	Absence of shock or threat of shock	Recovery from shock, possible Global Increased Permeability Syndrome
Goal	Early adequate goal-directed fluid management	Focus on organ support and maintaining tissue perfusion	Late conservative fluid management	Late goal-directed fluid removal (de-resuscitation)
Fluid therapy	Early administration with fluid boluses, guided by indices of fluid responsiveness	Fluid boluses guided by fluid responsiveness indices and indices of the risk of fluid administration	Only for normal maintenance and replacement	Reversal of the positive fluid balance, either spontaneous or active
Fluid balance	Positive	Neutral	Neutral to negative	Negative
Primary result of treatment	Salvage or patient rescue	Organ rescue	Organ support (homeostasis)	Organ recovery
Main risk	Insufficient resuscitation	Insufficient resuscitation and fluid overload (e.g., pulmonary edema, intra-abdominal hypertension)	Fluid overload (e.g., pulmonary edema, intra-abdominal hypertension)	Excessive fluid removal, possibly inducing hypotension, hypoperfusion, and a "fourth hit"

At this stage, testing preload responsiveness may still be useful, since it is safe to remove fluid in patients who have no preload dependence [67]. The use of albumin seems to have positive effects on vessel wall integrity, facilitates achieving a negative fluid balance in hypoalbuminemia, and is less likely to cause nephrotoxicity [68]. In this phase, we try to find an answer to the third and fourth question: "When to start fluid removal?" and "When to stop fluid removal?" in order to find the balance between the benefits (reduction of second and third space fluid accumulation and tissue edema) and risk (hypoperfusion) of fluid removal and subsequent organ failure (Fig. 8.13).

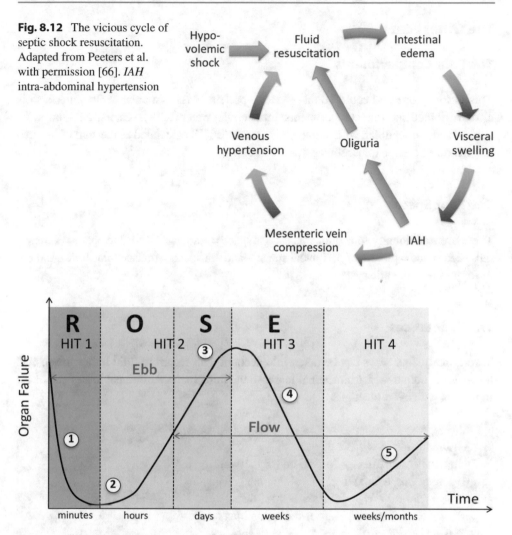

Fig. 8.12 The vicious cycle of septic shock resuscitation. Adapted from Peeters et al. with permission [66]. *IAH* intra-abdominal hypertension

Fig. 8.13 Graph illustrating the four-hit model of shock corresponding to the impact on end-organ function in relation to the fluid status. On admission patients are hypovolemic [1], followed by normovolemia [2] after fluid resuscitation, and fluid overload [3], again followed by a phase going to normovolemia with deresuscitation [4] and hypovolemia with risk of hypoperfusion [5]. In case of hypovolemia (phase 1 and 5), O_2 cannot get into the tissues because of convective problems, in case of hypervolemia (phase 3) O_2 cannot get into the tissue because of diffusion problems related to interstitial and pulmonary edema, gut edema (ileus and abdominal hypertension). See text for explanation

The Other Fours

The Four Compartments

This is tricky one and could be fat—water—protein—and minerals, while water also is also distributed into four compartments: intracellular water (ICW)—Interstitial—intravascular—and transcellular, with extracellular water (ECW) calculated as the sum of interstitial + intravascular + transcellular water content.

The Four Spaces

There are traditionally four fluid spaces: 1st space = intravascular—2nd space = interstitial—3rd space = pleural or peritoneal space—and 4th space = transcellular fluid. And not to forget the lymphatic system.

The Four Losses

Traditionally, four ways can be taken into account with regard to fluid losses: insensible loss—urine output—gastrointestinal losses—and third space. Additional losses can occur in trauma with overt bleeding.

Case Vignette

Below the correct answers are given for the case vignette.

Q1: You decide to administer a fluid bolus, how much do you give?

A1: 100–250 are correct. The lower dose would fit for a mini-fluid challenge as well.

Q2: How fast do you administer the fluid bolus?

A2: Bolus given in 10–15 min is the best answer.

Q3: What do you consider the most clinically relevant parameter to assess fluid responsiveness?

A3: The correct answer is passive leg raising test.

Q4: What type of fluids did you administer during resuscitation phase?

A4: The best fluid is a balanced isotonic solution like Plasmalyte–Ringer's lactate–Ringer's acetate–Hartmann solution.

Q5: What type of fluids did you administer as maintenance solution?

A5: The best fluid for maintenance (if at all needed) is a hypotonic balanced solution like Maintelyte–Glucion.

Q6: How many mls of fluid do you administer to this patient on a daily basis?

A6: In view of the body weight of 50 kg 20–25 mL/kg/day should be enough are thus around 1000 mL.

Q7: What is the daily need for sodium (mmol) in this patient?

A6: Sodium need is 1–1.5 mmol/kg/day or thus 50–75 mmol/day.

Q8: What is the daily need for potassium (mmol) in this patient?

A8: Potassium need is 1 mmol/kg/day or thus 50 mmol/day.

Q9: What is the daily need for glucose (grams) in this patient?

A9: Glucose need is 1–1.5 g/kg or thus 50–75 g/day.

Q10: What would be the best replacement fluid in addition to her daily maintenance solution?

A10: Normal saline (NaCl 0.9%) can be given in case of metabolic alkalosis as saline will induce hyperchloremic metabolic acidosis. This is the only indication left for "abnormal" saline, besides TBI.

Conclusions

There are only four major indications for fluid administration in the critically ill: resuscitation, maintenance, replacement, and nutrition (enteral or parenteral). In this chapter, a conceptual framework is presented looking at fluids as drugs by taking into account the four D's (drug selection, dose, duration, and de-escalation) and the four phases of fluid therapy within the ROSE concept (resuscitation, optimization, stabilization, evacuation). The four hits model is presented herein. This will provide answers to the four basic questions surrounding fluid therapy: (1) when to start IV fluids? (2) when to stop fluid administration? (3) when to start fluid removal, and finally (4) when to stop fluid removal? In analogy to the way we deal with antibiotics in critically ill patients, it is time for fluid stewardship.

Take Home Messages
- There are only 4 indications for fluid therapy: Resuscitation, maintenance, replacement, nutrition
- Resuscitation fluids should save lives
  - Fluid bolus should be small (4 ml/kg) and given fast (in 5–15 min)
  - Do not administer fluids until the patient is no longer fluid responsive
- Maintenance fluids should always cover the daily needs
  - The daily need for water is 1 ml/kg/h or 20–25 ml/kg/day
  - The daily need for sodium is 1–1.5 mmol/kg/day
  - The daily need for potassium is 0.5–1 mmol/kg/day
  - The daily need for glucose is 1–1.5 g/kg/day
  - Fluid creep is real: subtract unintended fluid administration (to dilute drugs in) from daily water need

- Maintenance fluids are responsible for fluid creep, especially if they are isotonic. It is not (only) the volume, that causes fluid overload, it's the salt!
- Replacement fluids should mimic the fluid that is lost
  - Gastrointestinal losses may be the only indication left for (ab)normal saline
- Nutrition fluids should cover the daily caloric needs
  - On average 2 g N are lost per L drainage fluid
- The best fluid is the one that has not been given unnecessarily
- The presence of fluid responsiveness does not mean that fluids need to be administered
- One must always try to find answers to the four basic questions
  - When to start fluids, or the benefits of fluid therapy
    Early adequate fluid management (EAFM) is the initial hemodynamic resuscitation of patients with (septic) shock by administering adequate fluids during the first 6 h after the initiation of therapy.
    Fluids should only be given when needed, i.e., when the patient is in shock (DO_2/VO_2 imbalance with lactate production) and fluid-responsive.
  - When to stop fluids, or the dangers of fluid therapy (fluid overload)
    Late Conservative Fluid Management (LCFM) is defined as 2 consecutive days of negative fluid balance within the first week of the ICU stay.
    After the initial Ebb phase, most patients enter the Flow phase spontaneously
  - When to start fluid removal, or the benefits of deresuscitation
    Late Goal-Directed Fluid Removal (LGFR) is defined as active fluid removal with diuretics or renal replacement therapy with net ultrafiltration, and started within the first week of ICU stay also referred to as de-resuscitation
  - When to stop fluid removal, or the dangers of deresuscitation (hypoperfusion)
    The benefits of fluid removal should always outweigh the potential risks
- Consider the 4-hit model during fluid therapy
  - 1st hit: initial insult
  - 2nd hit: following ischemia and reperfusion
  - 3rd hit: global increased permeability syndrome (GIPS) and fluid accumulation
  - 4th hit: hypoperfusion during deresuscitation
- Fluids are drugs, consider the 6 D's in analogy with antibiotic therapy
  - 1st D—Diagnosis: depending on underlying conditions, different types of fluids need to be administered
  - 2nd D—Drug: fluids are drug with indications and contraindications and possible adverse effects
  - 3rd D—Dose: the dose depends on the condition and indication
  - 4th D—Duration: stop IV fluids when they are no longer needed
  - 5th D—De-escalation: taper fluids when oral intake has resumed and remove excess fluids in case of fluid overload with diuretics or ultrafiltration
  - 6th D—Discharge: make sure the patient is able to cover his daily needs

- Fluid therapy is not static but dynamic, consider the four phases during critical illness (ROSE)
  - Resuscitation: early adequate goal-directed fluid therapy to rescue the patient and to save lives
  - Optimization: monitoring and support organ function
  - Stabilization: late conservative fluid management (2 consecutive negative daily fluid balances within first week of ICU stay)
  - Evacuation: late goal-directed fluid removal by means of diuretic therapy or ultrafiltration

Acknowledgments Parts of this chapter were published previously as open access under the creative commons Attribution 4.0 International Licence (CC BY 4.0) [4]. The European Commission announced it has adopted CC BY 4.0 and CC0 to share published documents, including photos, videos, reports, peer-reviewed studies, and data. The Commission joins other public institutions around the world that use standard, legally interoperable tools like Creative Commons licenses and public domain tools to share a wide range of content they produce. The decision to use CC aims to increase the legal interoperability and ease of reuse of authors' own materials.

References

1. Vandervelden S, Malbrain ML. Initial resuscitation from severe sepsis: one size does not fit all. Anaesthesiol Intensive Ther. 2015;47:44–55.
2. Malbrain ML, Van Regenmortel N, Owczuk R. The debate on fluid management and haemodynamic monitoring continues: between Scylla and Charybdis, or faith and evidence. Anaesthesiol Intensive Ther. 2014;46(5):313–8.
3. Malbrain ML, Van Regenmortel N, Owczuk R. It is time to consider the four D's of fluid management. Anaesthesiol Intensive Ther. 2015;47:1–5.
4. Malbrain MLNG, Van Regenmortel N, Saugel B, De Tavernier B, Van Gaal P-J, Joannes-Boyau O, et al. Principles of fluid management and stewardship in septic shock: it is time to consider the four D's and the four phases of fluid therapy. Ann Intensive Care. 2018;8(1):66.
5. Malbrain MLNG, Rice TW, Mythen M, Wuyts S. It is time for improved fluid stewardship. ICU Manage Pract. 2018;18(3):158–62.
6. Woodcock TE, Woodcock TM. Revised Starling equation and the glycocalyx model of transvascular fluid exchange: an improved paradigm for prescribing intravenous fluid therapy. Br J Anaesth. 2012;108(3):384–94.
7. Herrod PJ, Awad S, Redfern A, Morgan L, Lobo DN. Hypo- and hypernatraemia in surgical patients: is there room for improvement? World J Surg. 2010;34(3):495–9.
8. McNab S, Duke T, South M, Babl FE, Lee KJ, Arnup SJ, et al. 140 mmol/L of sodium versus 77 mmol/L of sodium in maintenance intravenous fluid therapy for children in hospital (PIMS): a randomised controlled double-blind trial. Lancet. 2015;385(9974):1190–7.
9. Moritz ML, Ayus JC. Maintenance intravenous fluids in acutely ill patients. N Engl J Med. 2015;373(14):1350–60.
10. Lobo DN, Stanga Z, Simpson JA, Anderson JA, Rowlands BJ, Allison SP. Dilution and redistribution effects of rapid 2-litre infusions of 0.9% (w/v) saline and 5% (w/v) dextrose on haematological parameters and serum biochemistry in normal subjects: a double-blind crossover study. Clin Sci. 2001;101(2):173–9.

11. Van Regenmortel N, De Weerdt T, Van Craenenbroeck AH, Roelant E, Verbrugghe W, Dams K, et al. Effect of isotonic versus hypotonic maintenance fluid therapy on urine output, fluid balance, and electrolyte homeostasis: a crossover study in fasting adult volunteers. Br J Anaesth. 2017;118(6):892–900.

12. Hendrickx S, Van Vlimmeren K, Baar I, Verbrugghe W, Dams K, Van Cromphaut S, et al. Introducing TOPMAST, the first double-blind randomized clinical trial specifically dedicated to perioperative maintenance fluid therapy in adults. Anaesthesiol Intensive Ther. 2017;49(5):366–72.

13. Van Regenmortel N, Hendrickx S, Roelant E, Baar I, Dams K, Van Vlimmeren K, et al. 154 compared to 54 mmol per liter of sodium in intravenous maintenance fluid therapy for adult patients undergoing major thoracic surgery (TOPMAST): a single-center randomized controlled double-blind trial. Intensive Care Med. 2019;45(10):1422–32.

14. Van Regenmortel N, Verbrugghe W, Roelant E, Van den Wyngaert T, Jorens PG. Maintenance fluid therapy and fluid creep impose more significant fluid, sodium, and chloride burdens than resuscitation fluids in critically ill patients: a retrospective study in a tertiary mixed ICU population. Intensive Care Med. 2018;44(4):409–17.

15. Van Regenmortel N, Jorens PG, Malbrain ML. Fluid management before, during and after elective surgery. Curr Opin Crit Care. 2014;20(4):390–5.

16. Padhi S, Bullock I, Li L, Stroud M, National Institute for H, Care Excellence Guideline Development G. Intravenous fluid therapy for adults in hospital: summary of NICE guidance. BMJ. 2013;347:f7073.

17. Soni N. British consensus guidelines on intravenous fluid therapy for adult surgical patients (GIFTASUP): cassandra's view. Anaesthesia. 2009;64(3):235–8.

18. De Waele E, Honore PM, Malbrain M. Does the use of indirect calorimetry change outcome in the ICU? Yes it does. Curr Opin Clin Nutr Metab Care. 2018;21(2):126–9.

19. Cheatham ML, Safcsak K, Brzezinski SJ, Lube MW. Nitrogen balance, protein loss, and the open abdomen. Crit Care Med. 2007;35(1):127–31.

20. Rhodes A, Evans LE, Alhazzani W, Levy MM, Antonelli M, Ferrer R, et al. Surviving sepsis campaign: international guidelines for management of sepsis and septic shock: 2016. Intensive Care Med. 2017;43(3):304–77.

21. Dellinger RP, Schorr CA, Levy MM. A users' guide to the 2016 surviving sepsis guidelines. Intensive Care Med. 2017;43(3):299–303.

22. Marik PE. Iatrogenic salt water drowning and the hazards of a high central venous pressure. Ann Intensive Care. 2014;4:21.

23. Machado FR, Levy MM, Rhodes A. Fixed minimum volume resuscitation: pro. Intensive Care Med. 2016;43:1678–80.

24. Hjortrup PB, Haase N, Bundgaard H, Thomsen SL, Winding R, Pettila V, et al. Restricting volumes of resuscitation fluid in adults with septic shock after initial management: the CLASSIC randomised, parallel-group, multicentre feasibility trial. Intensive Care Med. 2016;42(11):1695–705.

25. Perner A, Singer M. Fixed minimum fluid volume for resuscitation: Con. Intensive Care Med. 2016;43:1681–2.

26. Myles PS, Bellomo R, Corcoran T, Forbes A, Peyton P, Story D, et al. Restrictive versus liberal fluid therapy for major abdominal surgery. N Engl J Med. 2018;378(24):2263–74.

27. Marik PE, Malbrain M. The SEP-1 quality mandate may be harmful: how to drown a patient with 30 mL per kg fluid! Anaesthesiol Intensive Ther. 2017;49(5):323–8.

28. Malbrain ML, Marik PE, Witters I, Cordemans C, Kirkpatrick AW, Roberts DJ, et al. Fluid overload, de-resuscitation, and outcomes in critically ill or injured patients: a systematic review with suggestions for clinical practice. Anaesthesiol Intensive Ther. 2014;46(5):361–80.

29. Marik PE, Farkas JD, Spiegel R, Weingart S. POINT: should the surviving sepsis campaign guidelines be retired? Yes. Chest. 2019;155(1):12–4.

30. Spiegel R, Farkas JD, Rola P, Kenny JE, Olusanya S, Marik PE, et al. The 2018 surviving sepsis campaign's treatment bundle: when guidelines outpace the evidence supporting their use. Ann Emerg Med. 2019;73(4):356–8.
31. Murphy CV, Schramm GE, Doherty JA, Reichley RM, Gajic O, Afessa B, et al. The importance of fluid management in acute lung injury secondary to septic shock. Chest. 2009;136(1):102–9.
32. Cordemans C, De Laet I, Van Regenmortel N, Schoonheydt K, Dits H, Martin G, et al. Aiming for a negative fluid balance in patients with acute lung injury and increased intra-abdominal pressure: a pilot study looking at the effects of PAL-treatment. Ann Intensive Care. 2012;2(Suppl 1):S15.
33. Elbers PW, Girbes A, Malbrain ML, Bosman R. Right dose, right now: using big data to optimize antibiotic dosing in the critically ill. Anaesthesiol Intensive Ther. 2015;47(5):457–63.
34. Hahn RG, Lyons G. The half-life of infusion fluids: an educational review. Eur J Anaesthesiol. 2016;33(7):475–82.
35. Hahn RG. Volume kinetics for infusion fluids. Anesthesiology. 2010;113(2):470–81.
36. Monnet X, Marik P, Teboul JL. Prediction of fluid responsiveness: an update. Ann Intensive Care. 2017;6(1):111.
37. Guerin L, Teboul JL, Persichini R, Dres M, Richard C, Monnet X. Effects of passive leg raising and volume expansion on mean systemic pressure and venous return in shock in humans. Crit Care. 2015;19:411.
38. Verbrugge FH, Dupont M, Steels P, Grieten L, Malbrain M, Tang WH, et al. Abdominal contributions to cardiorenal dysfunction in congestive heart failure. J Am Coll Cardiol. 2013;62(6):485–95.
39. Bentzer P, Griesdale DE, Boyd J, MacLean K, Sirounis D, Ayas NT. Will this hemodynamically unstable patient respond to a bolus of intravenous fluids? JAMA. 2016;316(12):1298–309.
40. Cordemans C, De Laet I, Van Regenmortel N, Schoonheydt K, Dits H, Huber W, et al. Fluid management in critically ill patients: the role of extravascular lung water, abdominal hypertension, capillary leak and fluid balance. Ann Intensive Care. 2012;2(1):S1.
41. Benes J, Kirov M, Kuzkov V, Lainscak M, Molnar Z, Voga G, et al. Fluid therapy: double-edged sword during critical care? Biomed Res Int. 2015;2015:729075.
42. O'Connor ME, Prowle JR. Fluid overload. Crit Care Clin. 2015;31(4):803–21.
43. Cuthbertson DP. Observations on disturbance of metabolism produced by injury to the limbs. Quart J Med. 1932;25:233–46.
44. Duchesne JC, Kaplan LJ, Balogh ZJ, Malbrain ML. Role of permissive hypotension, hypertonic resuscitation and the global increased permeability syndrome in patients with severe hemorrhage: adjuncts to damage control resuscitation to prevent intra-abdominal hypertension. Anaesthesiol Intensive Ther. 2015;47(2):143–55.
45. Malbrain MLNG, Huygh J, Dabrowski W, De Waele J, Wauters J. The use of bio-electrical impedance analysis (BIA) to guide fluid management, resuscitation and deresuscitation in critically ill patients: a bench-to-bedside review. Anaesthesiol Intensive Ther. 2014;46(5):381–91.
46. Nadler SB, Hidalgo JH, Bloch T. Prediction of blood volume in normal human adults. Surgery. 1962;51(2):224–32.
47. Miller TE, Raghunathan K, Gan TJ. State-of-the-art fluid management in the operating room. Best Pract Res Clin Anaesthesiol. 2014;28(3):261–73.
48. Jacob G, Robertson D, Mosqueda-Garcia R, Ertl AC, Robertson RM, Biaggioni I. Hypovolemia in syncope and orthostatic intolerance role of the renin-angiotensin system. Am J Med. 1997;103(2):128–33.
49. Marik P, Bellomo R. A rational approach to fluid therapy in sepsis. Br J Anaesth. 2016;116(3):339–49.
50. Myburgh JA, Mythen MG. Resuscitation fluids. N Engl J Med. 2013;369(25):2462–3.
51. McDermid RC, Raghunathan K, Romanovsky A, Shaw AD, Bagshaw SM. Controversies in fluid therapy: type, dose and toxicity. World J Crit Care Med. 2014;3(1):24–33.
52. Rivers EP. Fluid-management strategies in acute lung injury-liberal, conservative, or both? N Engl J Med. 2006;354(24):2598–600.

53. Bellamy MC. Wet, dry or something else? Br J Anaesth. 2006;97(6):755–7.
54. Bagshaw SM, Bellomo R. The influence of volume management on outcome. Curr Opin Crit Care. 2007;13(5):541–8.
55. Bagshaw SM, Brophy PD, Cruz D, Ronco C. Fluid balance as a biomarker: impact of fluid overload on outcome in critically ill patients with acute kidney injury. Crit Care. 2008;12(4):169.
56. Vincent JL, De Backer D. Circulatory shock. N Engl J Med. 2013;369(18):1726–34.
57. Hoste EA, Maitland K, Brudney CS, Mehta R, Vincent JL, Yates D, et al. Four phases of intravenous fluid therapy: a conceptual model. Br J Anaesth. 2014;113(5):740–7.
58. Perel A, Saugel B, Teboul JL, Malbrain ML, Belda FJ, Fernandez-Mondejar E, et al. The effects of advanced monitoring on hemodynamic management in critically ill patients: a pre and post questionnaire study. J Clin Monit Comput. 2015;30(5):511–8.
59. Saugel B, Trepte CJ, Heckel K, Wagner JY, Reuter DA. Hemodynamic management of septic shock: is it time for "individualized goal-directed hemodynamic therapy" and for specifically targeting the microcirculation? Shock. 2015;43(6):522–9.
60. Saugel B, Malbrain ML, Perel A. Hemodynamic monitoring in the era of evidence-based medicine. Crit Care. 2016;20(1):401.
61. Acheampong A, Vincent JL. A positive fluid balance is an independent prognostic factor in patients with sepsis. Crit Care. 2015;19:251.
62. Bashir MU, Tawil A, Mani VR, Farooq U. Hidden obligatory fluid intake in critical care patients. J Intensive Care Med. 2016;32(3):223–7.
63. Malbrain ML, De Laet I. AIDS is coming to your ICU: be prepared for acute bowel injury and acute intestinal distress syndrome. Intensive Care Med. 2008;34(9):1565–9.
64. Pinsky MR. Hemodynamic evaluation and monitoring in the ICU. Chest. 2007;132(6):2020–9.
65. Samoni S, Vigo V, Resendiz LI, Villa G, De Rosa S, Nalesso F, et al. Impact of hyperhydration on the mortality risk in critically ill patients admitted in intensive care units: comparison between bioelectrical impedance vector analysis and cumulative fluid balance recording. Crit Care. 2016;20:95.
66. Peeters Y, Lebeer M, Wise R, Malbrain ML. An overview on fluid resuscitation and resuscitation endpoints in burns: past, present and future. Part 2 - avoiding complications by using the right endpoints with a new personalized protocolized approach. Anaesthesiol Intensive Ther. 2015;47:15–26.
67. Monnet X, Cipriani F, Camous L, Sentenac P, Dres M, Krastinova E, et al. The passive leg raising test to guide fluid removal in critically ill patients. Ann Intensive Care. 2016;6(1):46.
68. Vincent JL, De Backer D, Wiedermann CJ. Fluid management in sepsis: the potential beneficial effects of albumin. J Crit Care. 2016;35:161–7.

Part II

Available Intravenous Fluids

The Place of Crystalloids

9

Amandeep Singh and Aayush Chawla

Contents

Introduction 208
Fluid Physiology 208
Types of Crystalloids 210
Isotonic Crystalloids 212
Isotonic Saline or 0.9% Saline 213
Balanced Crystalloids 214
Clinical Evidence: 0.9% Saline Vs Balanced 215
    Observational Studies 215
    Randomized Controlled Studies 216
Hypotonic Crystalloids 218
Hypertonic Crystalloids 220
    Hypertonic Saline 220
    Sodium Bicarbonate Solution 221
Conclusion 223
References 224

> **IFA Commentary (MLNGM)**
>
> This chapter takes you back to the basics with an overview of basic definitions, terminology, and concepts. Crystalloids are solutions that contain electrolytes dissolved in water and other small water-soluble molecules, with or without dextrose or glucose. They are widely used as maintenance solutions, replacement solutions, or

A. Singh (✉)
Department of Critical Cate Medicine, Fortis Escorts Hospital, Faridabad, Haryana, India

A. Chawla
Amrita Hospital, Faridabad, India

© The Author(s) 2024
M. L. N. G. Malbrain et al. (eds.), *Rational Use of Intravenous Fluids in Critically Ill Patients*, https://doi.org/10.1007/978-3-031-42205-8_9

resuscitation fluids. Crystalloids are categorized by their tonicity relative to plasma and can be isotonic, hypotonic, or hypertonic. And they can be balanced (or buffered) with a strong ion difference (SID) close to plasma or unbalanced (like NaCl 0.9% with a SID of zero). The SID is important for the effect on the acid–base status after administration. There is more and more evidence that imprudent administration of crystalloids may lead to morbidity. There are two major concerns in administering crystalloids: First is the induction of hyperchloremic metabolic acidosis (HMA), a proven side effect of saline. Although animal studies showed HMA can lead to kidney dysfunction and it also seemed to induce morbidity in normal volunteers, there was little data on relevant clinical parameters. There is also rising evidence that saline can lead to a delay in micturition, although the exact mechanism is unclear. Second is the induction of fluid overload or accumulation. It is frequently shown that more crystalloids than colloids are needed to achieve clinical stability. Historically, colloid vs crystalloid studies showed conflicting data in this matter but in critically ill shocked patients the volume expansion effects of crystalloids and colloids may be similar based on their pharmacokinetic and dynamic properties. The induction of a positive sodium balance also accompanied with fluid accumulation is another explanation why saline may induce fluid accumulation. Even normal kidneys may take days if not weeks to get rid of the excess sodium. Other deleterious effects of saline are increased potassium levels, renal hypoperfusion, and increased need for vasopressors and renal replacement therapy. A recent systematic reviews and post-hoc analyses of the latest major fluid trials including almost 35,000 ICU patients have shown a 90% probability that balanced solutions reduce mortality by 1% (range −9 to +1%). Figure 9.1 shows the combined summary of findings.

Therefore, in patients with sepsis and septic shock, burns, or diabetic ketoacidosis, balanced or buffered crystalloids (not containing glucose) are a good first choice but not in patients with traumatic brain injury where saline is preferred. Gastrointestinal losses may be another indication for (ab)normal saline as it may help to correct hypochloremic metabolic alkalosis caused by losses. There is also growing body of evidence that maintenance solutions should be hypotonic crystalloids, although the pediatric community still favors isotonic solutions. Hypertonic crystalloids have been described for small volume resuscitation in specific patient populations (e.g., post cardiac arrest) but the sodium burden may outweigh the temporarily beneficial hemodynamic effects. In case of excessive losses, fluids should be substituted or replaced by those, mimicking the fluids that are lost (e.g., blood). Crystalloid solutions should be prescribed with the same care and caution as we do with medication, by giving the right dose of the right fluid at the right time. When using crystalloids, avoiding HMA by using balanced solutions seems to be important, although the critical dose for a switch from saline is not known. Fluid accumulation is to be avoided as it is proven to induce morbidity and mortality.

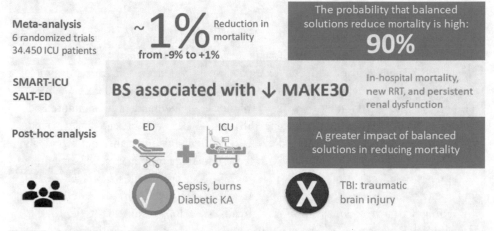

Fig. 9.1 Summary of findings of six randomized controlled trials showing the benefits of balanced solutions compared to saline. *BS* balanced solution, *KA* ketoacidosis, *MAKE* major adverse kidney event, *RRT* renal replacement therapy

Learning Objectives

After reading this chapter, you will understand that:

1. Half-life of intravenous fluids is dependent on the pharmacokinetics and pharmacodynamic properties of the specific fluid.
2. Nearly 75% of isotonic crystalloid fluids leaves intravascular space to interstitial after administration.
3. A 0.9% saline is not "normal" and can cause dilutional hyperchloremic metabolic acidosis, renal and splanchnic vasoconstriction, glycocalyx, and coagulation dysfunction, especially, when administered in large volumes.
4. The evidence on the benefit of balanced crystalloids over 0.9% saline is equivocal. Because of the physiological rationale of balanced salt solutions and the risk of harm associated with 0.9% saline, they are the resuscitation fluids of choice for most patients with sepsis, burns, or diabetic ketoacidosis.
5. Saline is preferred over balanced solutions in patients with traumatic brain injury and gastrointestinal losses.
6. Hypertonic saline may be used for small volume resuscitation or the treatment of raised intracranial pressure or severe symptomatic hyponatremia. However, frequent monitoring of serum sodium and osmolality is recommended with serum sodium not exceeding 12 mEq over 24 h and 18 mEq over 48 h.
7. Sodium bicarbonate administration may cause paradoxical acidosis with intracellular acidosis, and there is lack of evidence supporting the use of sodium bicarbonate for correction of metabolic acidosis on any patient-centered outcomes.

Case Vignette

Mr. B, an 82-year-old male, with past history of hypertension on hydrochlorothiazide, was admitted with history of acute central abdominal pain for the past few days, associated with vomiting. On examination, he was drowsy but obeying simple commands, his extremities were cool to touch with a heart rate of 108/min, he has a blood pressure of 70 mmHg systolic, respiratory rate 28/min, and temperature 36.9 °C. His abdomen was distended and diffusely tender with absent bowel sound. Arterial blood gas analysis showed evidence of high anion gap metabolic acidosis with lactate 5 mmol/L. Combined with the CT findings of a pneumoperitoneum, a diagnosis of bowel perforation with peritonitis and septic shock was made. He was planned for an emergency laparotomy after initial resuscitation. At laparotomy, he was found to have a duodenal perforation with bowel loop adhered to it. Perforation repair and peritoneal toileting was performed, and he was moved to the ICU.

Questions

Q1. What will be the most appropriate fluid for initial resuscitation of this patient?
Q2. Which fluid to be chosen for maintenance intravenous therapy now?

Introduction

Over the centuries, intravenous fluid therapy has become an integral part of therapeutic intervention in critically sick patients. Crystalloids and colloids have been the mainstay of intravenous fluid resuscitation. First successful use of a crystalloid solution was by Thomas Latta in 1832, who infused a solution of saline and sodium bicarbonate in cholera patients [1]. In 1876, Sidney Ringer developed a fluid comparable to blood plasma that enabled a frog's heart to continue beating in vitro [2]. In 1932, Alex Hartmann modified Ringer's solution by adding lactate as a buffer and used it to rehydrate children suffering from gastroenteritis [3].

Crystalloids are described as fluids containing electrolytes (e.g., sodium, potassium, chloride). They lack the large proteins and molecules found in colloids and plasma, and 0.9% saline has been the most commonly prescribed crystalloid over many years. But recently, balanced solutions are catching more attention. Despite the ubiquity of fluid therapy, this intervention remains a subject of an ongoing controversy. An "ideal fluid" remains elusive. More information on albumin use can be found in Chap. 10, while other colloid solutions like starches and gelatins are discussed in Chap. 11.

Fluid Physiology

All intravascular fluids tend to redistribute throughout the body. After administration, intravascular half-life of any given intravenous fluid varies depending on the pharmacokinetic and pharmacodynamic properties of the fluid. Some of the factors that determine the in vivo activity of intravenous fluids are its tonicity, oncotic pressure, acid–base properties, and integrity of the endothelial glycocalyx (see Chaps. 2 and 3). A fundamental rationale for intravascular fluid resuscitation is to sustain an effective circulating intravascular volume. Interestingly, around 75% of a crystalloid volume load ends up in the interstitium.

Total body water (TBW) is divided functionally into extracellular (ECW) and the intracellular water (ICW), confined to dedicated fluid spaces separated by the cell membrane. ECW is further divided into intravascular and interstitial fluid spaces (Table 9.1). Figure 9.2 illustrates fluid composition in a 70 kg male. These two compartments of ECW are separated by capillary membrane with pores. Intravascular volume depends on the net balance between plasma oncotic pressure and hydrostatic pressures. This relationship was mathematically expressed by Starling in his famous Starling equation [4]:

$$\text{Net driving pressure of intravascular fluid} = \left[(Pc - Pi) - (pc - pi) \right]$$

Pc hydrostatic pressure in the capillary, Pi hydrostatic pressure in the interstitium, pc oncotic pressure in the capillary, pi oncotic pressure in the interstitium.

Table 9.1 Fluid compartments and their composition

	ECW			ICW		
	Plasma	ISF	CSF	ICF_{ST}	ICF_{RBC}	TBW
% of body weight	4.7	20	0.3	31.5	3.5	60
Na^+ (mEq/L)	143	137	145	10	19	64
K^+ (mEq/L)	4	3	3	155	95	88
Ca^{2+} (mEq/L)	2	2	2	<0.1	<0.1	0.8
Mg^{2+} (mEq/L)	2	2	2	10	5	6
Cl^- (mEq/L)	107	111	125	10	52	54
Lac^- (mEq/L)	1	1	1.5	1	1	1
Other anions (mEq/L)	–	–	–	34	9	18
HCO_3^- (mEq/L)	25	31	24	11	15	19
Albumin (g/dL)	5	<1	<0.1	<0.1	<0.1	<1
A^- (mEq/L)	16	<1	1	118	42	66
SID (mEq/L)	42	31	24	130	57	85

Table summarizes the simplified composition of different body fluid compartments, schematically divided into extracellular (ECW) and intracellular (ICW) water. In addition, the theoretical average composition of total body water (TBW), resulting from the mixing of ICW and ECW, was calculated and reported in the table. Adapted with permission from Langer et al. according to the Open Access CC BY Licence 4.0 (Langer T, et al. Intravenous balanced solutions: from physiology to clinical evidence. Anaesthesiol Intensive Ther. 2015;47 Spec No: s78-88)

CSF cerebrospinal fluid, *ECW* extracellular water, *ICF*$_{RBC}$ red blood cells fluid, *ICF*$_{ST}$ "standard" intracellular fluid, *ICW* intracellular water, *ISF* interstitial fluid, *Na*$^+$ sodium concentration, *K*$^+$ potassium concentration, *Ca*$^{2+}$ ionized calcium concentration, *Mg*$^{2+}$ ionized magnesium concentration, *Cl*$^-$ chloride concentration, *Lac*$^-$ lactate concentration, *other anions* sum of the concentration of other anions, *HCO*$_3^-$ bicarbonate concentration, *A*$^-$ dissociated, electrically charged part of "noncarbonic buffers" (A$_{TOT}$), *SID* strong ion difference. All concentrations, except for albumin, are expressed in mEq/L

Fig. 9.2 Fluid distribution in a 70 kg man. The human body consists of 60% water. The total body water (TBW) is separated into intracellular water (ICW, 66%) and extracellular water (ECW, 33%). The ECW consists of the intravascular fluid (IVF, 25%) and extravascular fluid (EVF, 75%), mainly interstitial fluid

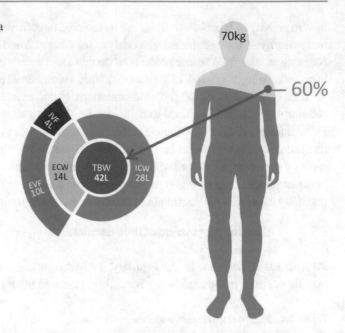

More recently, Starling's description of fluid dynamics has been challenged. With the discovery of endothelial glycocalyx, a lining inside the endothelium, it is now realized that movement of fluid is much more complex. Glycocalyx is negatively charged and contributes as a natural barrier of the vessel walls. Glycocalyx is fragile and is affected by various factors like ischemia, sepsis, hypoxia, and inflammation. Woodcock and colleagues proposed a revised Starling model that considers the composition of intravascular fluid, interstitial fluid, and physical characteristics of the transvascular barrier, i.e., endothelial glycocalyx [5]. This revised model shows that at low capillary hydrostatic pressures, transcapillary fluid losses for both crystalloids and colloids are similar [5]. Starling's model and its revised form are described in more detail in Chap. 2.

It is vital to understand the mechanism for acid–base disturbances in critically ill patients which is important for the appropriate prescription of intravenous fluid (traditional acid–base concepts are discussed in Chap. 6). Stewart's quantitative physical chemical approach enables us to understand the acid–base properties of intravenous fluids. Stewart's concept is described in Chap. 6.

Types of Crystalloids

Crystalloids have been classified on the basis of their tonicity (compared to that of plasma), their effects on acid–base balance, and their clinical use.

Tonicity Tonicity or "effective osmolality" is an important property of body fluids, as it determines movement of water between extracellular and intracellular compartments (see Chap. 2). Osmolality of a solution is defined as the amount of solute (in mmol/L) dissolved in the solvent (e.g., water) measured in kilogram (kg). Normal plasma tonicity is 270–290 mOsm/kg.

Another closely related term is **osmolarity**, defined as the amount of solute dissolved in a solution measured in liter (mOsm/L).

$$Osm_{serum} = 2 \times \left[Na^+ \text{ in mmol}/L \right] + \left[glucose \text{ in mg}/dL \right]/18 + \left[ureum \text{ in mg}/dL \right]/6$$

Isotonic Crystalloids Isotonic crystalloids have a tonicity close to plasma. When administered to a normally hydrated patient, isotonic crystalloids do not cause a significant shift of water between the blood vessels and the cells. Thus, there is no (or minimal) osmosis occurring. Commonly prescribed isotonic fluids are Ringer's lactate (Hartmann's), Ringer's acetate, Plasma-Lyte, or dextrose 5% in saline 0.9%.

Hypertonic Crystalloids Hypertonic crystalloids have a tonicity higher than plasma. Administration of a hypertonic crystalloids causes water to shift from the extravascular space into the intravascular space thereby increasing the intravascular volume. This osmotic shift occurs as the body attempts to dilute the higher concentration of electrolytes contained within the hypertonic fluid by moving water into the intravascular space. Hypertonic solutions may result in cellular dehydration. A commonly used hypertonic crystalloid is 3% saline. Other concentrations are 5%, 7.5%, and 23% saline.

Hypotonic Crystalloids Hypotonic crystalloids have a tonicity lower than plasma. Administration of a hypotonic crystalloid causes water to shift from the intravascular space to the extravascular space because of the higher concentration of electrolytes in the extravascular spaces. This shift of fluid eventually transmits into the tissue cells. Hypotonic solutions may result in cellular hydration. Commonly used hypotonic solutions are 5% dextrose, 10% dextrose, and dextrose in hypotonic saline (5% dextrose + 0.45% saline).

Unbalanced Crystalloids Unbalanced crystalloids have been described as intravenous crystalloid solutions having a high chloride concentration in comparison with plasma chloride levels (96–106 mEq/L). Examples of unbalanced crystalloids are 0.9% saline, 3% saline, etc.

Balanced Crystalloids Balanced (or buffered) crystalloids are defined as intravenous crystalloid solutions whose electrolyte composition is closer to that of plasma with a strong ion deficit (SID) around 24 mmol/L. They contain physiological or near physiological amounts of chloride. The commonest balanced fluids are Ringer's lactate, Ringer's acetate, Plasma-Lyte, and Sterofundin.

Isotonic Crystalloids

Crystalloids have been widely used in resuscitating patients with dehydration, trauma, burn, and other shock states including septic shock. They along with colloids have been the mainstay of resuscitation though the latter has fallen out of favor because of their deleterious effects on the human body (discussed in more detail in Chaps. 10 and 11). Major guidelines including surviving sepsis guidelines recommend isotonic crystalloid as the initial choice of fluid for resuscitation [6, 7]. Isotonic crystalloids are also routinely used as maintenance fluids especially in children. In this section, we shall discuss about isotonic crystalloids most widely used for resuscitation (Table 9.2).

Table 9.2 Characteristics of isotonic intravenous fluids and comparison to human plasma

	Plasma	Ringer's lactate	Ringer's acetate	D1% in balanced solution	D5% in 0.9% NaCl	Plasma -yte	NaCl 0.9%	Sterofundin ISO
Na$^+$ (mEq/L)	136–145	130	132	140	154	140	154	145
K$^+$ (mEq/L)	3.5–5	4	4	4	–	5	–	4
Ca^{2+} (mEq/L)	2.2–2.6	3	3	2	–	–	–	5
Mg^{2+} (mEq/L)	0.8–1	–	–	2	–	–	–	2
Cl$^-$ (mEq/L)	96–106	109	110	118	154	98	154	127
Lactate (mEq/L)	–	28	–	–	–	–	–	–
Acetate (mEq/L)	–	–	29	30	–	27	–	24
Phosphate (mEq/L)	–	–	–	–	–	–	–	–
Malate (mEq/L)	–	–	–	–	–	–	–	5
Gluconate (mEq/L)	–	–	–	–	–	23	–	–
Dextrose (mmol/L)	80–120	–	–	56	278	–	–	–
In vivo SID (mEq/L)	40	28	29	30	0	50	–	29
Osmolarity (mOsm/L)	270–290	274	278	296	308	296	308	312
Tonicity (mOsm/kg)	270–290	254	258	NA	286	NA	286	290

Intravenous fluids have been listed according to increasing tonicity

In-vivo strong ion deficit (SID) all organic molecules contained in balanced solutions are strong anions. The resulting calculated SID (in vitro SID) is equal to 0 mE/L. Once infused, the organic molecules are metabolized to CO_2 and water; the resulting in vivo SID corresponds to the number of organic anions metabolized. Tonicity (or effective osmolality) is the number of solutes to which cell membranes are impermeable. In this context, glucose, which rapidly crosses cell membranes, is not included in the calculation

Isotonic Saline or 0.9% Saline

Normal saline is a 0.9% preparation of sodium chloride, equivalent to 154 mmol/L of sodium (Na) and chloride (Cl). If sodium chloride completely dissociated in solution, the expected osmolality would be two times 154, or 308 mOsm/kg. Interestingly, in-vivo measured effective osmolality (tonicity) of 0.9% saline of 286 mOsmol/L makes it isotonic to plasma, because a small percentage remains non-ionized in water. As such, this fits nicely in the normal range of blood osmolality, of 275–290 mOsm/L.

The term "normal" is often misunderstood. Normal solution in physicochemistry is described as a solution where 1 mol, or 1 g weight equivalent, of the salt is dissolved in 1 kg of water. This is not the case with 0.9% saline, which derived its name from red-cell lysis studies performed in the 1880s which suggested that the concentration of salt in the blood is 0.9%; hence, it is "normal" ECF. However, this seems not correct, but is beyond the scope of this chapter.

The "isotonic," "0.9% saline," or normal saline was developed by Dr. Hartog Jacob Hamburger. It remains unknown how 0.9% saline became known as "normal." Despite being described as normal or physiological, 0.9% saline differs significantly from plasma including much higher chloride content, SID of 0, and absence of electrolytes except Na and Cl (Table 9.2).

A major issue associated with 0.9% saline is dilutional hyperchloremic metabolic acidosis, seen with infusion of large volumes of saline. Using the term "dilutional hyperchloremic metabolic acidosis" instead of hyperchloremic acidosis is more appropriate as it considers SID changes as well as variations in volume and chloride concentration.

Biological effects of 0.9% saline have been shown by numerous studies. In a study of patients awaiting intra-abdominal surgery, SID decreased from 40 to 31 mEq/l with a simultaneous increase in chloride from 105 to 115 mEq/l, following infusion of 6 l of 0.9% saline over 2 h [8].

Animal studies and some clinical data suggest hyperchloremic metabolic acidosis as a proinflammatory stimulus causing renal and splanchnic vasoconstriction and circulatory and coagulation dysfunction. Renal effects of dilutional hyperchloremic acidosis are most widely described. In a study in human volunteers, Chowdhury and colleagues demonstrated a decrease in renal blood flow and renal cortical perfusion following infusion of 0.9% saline compared to Plasma-Lyte [9]. However, these changes in renal blood flow and renal perfusion following 0.9% saline infusion were not associated with increased concentration of urinary neutrophil gelatinase-associated lipocalin (NGAL), an early marker of kidney injury. The decrease in renal blood flow is possibly related to high chloride content in the distal convoluted tubule following 0.9% saline and tubuloglomerular feedback. In a recent review, Lobo and Awad listed a number of adverse consequences of administering 0.9% saline (Table 9.3) [11]. However, some of these adverse effects may be manifested only at a very high dose and many of these effects are not seen in clinical studies.

The primary advantage of 0.9% saline, over balanced crystalloids, is cost, as it is significantly cheaper.

Table 9.3 Possible adverse consequences of large-volume saline administration

Metabolic	• Acid–base and pH alterations • Dilutional and hyperchloremic metabolic acidosis • Chloride overload • Sodium overload and accumulation • Increased potassium levels
Endothelium/fluid compartments	• Possible damage to endothelial glycocalyx • Increased interstitial fluid volume and edema formation • Capillary leak
Kidney	• Acute kidney injury • Increased need for renal replacement therapy • Renal edema and capsular stretch leading to intrarenal hypertension • Decreased renal blood flow and renal hypoperfusion • Decreased glomerular filtration rate leading to sodium retention • Fluid accumulation • Local renal compartment syndrome
Cardiovascular	• Increased vasopressor need • Hemodynamic instability
Gastrointestinal	• Gastrointestinal edema • Ileus • Possible anastomotic leak
Hematological	• Coagulopathy • Increased blood loss • Increased need for blood products

Adapted with permission from Lobo and Awad [10]

Balanced Crystalloids

Balanced (or buffered) solutions contain different organic anions (such as lactate, acetate, malate, pyruvate, and gluconate) to maintain the electrical neutrality. Metabolization of these organic anions increases the SID of these solutions in vivo. Hence, these solutions become hypotonic in vivo. Despite having an electrolyte content closer to plasma, balanced solutions are neither perfect nor physiological. The concentrations of these organic anions present in these solutions are much higher than those of plasma. For example, lactate content of Ringer's lactate is >25 times than that of plasma. These organic anions have variable effects in vivo. Compared to lactate, acetate has less effect on oxygen consumption and carbon dioxide elimination, and it is also metabolized by extrahepatic tissues. But high levels of acetate may lead to hypotension and myocardial toxicity. Gluconate is metabolized more slowly than lactate. Interestingly, plasma gluconate elevations following Plasma-Lyte infusion can cause false-positive tests for galactomannan (a marker used for early detection of systemic mycoses especially aspergillosis). Effects of organic anion (or buffering substances) are discussed in greater detail in Chap. 24. The SID of balanced crystalloids is different (29 mEq/l for Ringer's lactate compared to 50 mEq/l for Plasma-Lyte) producing variable effect on acid–base balance (discussed in Chaps. 6 and 7).

Traditionally, it is believed that balanced crystalloids are contraindicated in the presence of hyperkalemia or in patients at a higher risk of hyperkalemia (e.g., chronic kidney disease) because of their K^+ content. However, multiple studies have failed to confirm this concept. In a randomized controlled trial (RCT), O'Malley and colleagues compared the effects of 0.9% saline vs Ringer's lactate for intraoperative intravenous fluid therapy in kidney transplant patients [10]. The study was prematurely terminated after enrolling 51 patients as a significantly higher number of patients in saline group developed hyperkalemia (defined as serum K^+ >6 mmol/L) requiring anti-hyperkalemic measures. There are two possible explanations of balanced fluid not producing hyperkalemia. First, K^+ content of balanced crystalloids gets rapidly diluted in the large extracellular fluid compartment. Second, contrary to 0.9% saline, balanced crystalloids do not produce dilutional hyperchloremic metabolic acidosis and mobilize K^+ from intracellular compartment.

Another possible issue is related to co-administration of balanced crystalloids with blood transfusion, because of the theoretical concern about calcium salt being present in certain balanced fluids (e.g., Ringer's lactate or Sterofundin) and possible precipitation of citrate and clot formation. Again, this has not been proven in clinical studies [12]. Plasma-Lyte is approved by the U.S. FDA as suitable for use with blood products.

Buffering substances in the balanced solutions (lactate, acetate, maleate, and gluconate) are metabolized primarily in the liver, and compromised liver function may affect the metabolism of these substances. The metabolism of lactate is affected most, compared to acetate (as acetate is metabolized in other organs too). In a rat model of hemorrhagic shock, Egin and colleagues tested Ringer's lactate, Ringer's acetate, Plasma-Lyte, and 0.9% saline in the presence or absence of a 70% partial liver resection [13]. The authors concluded that 0.9% saline is the most inappropriate fluid for resuscitation during shock in the presence of hepatic failure. Buffering capacity of lactate is overwhelmed by hepatic failure, whereas acetate metabolism remains uncompromised. Gluconate is excreted largely unchanged in urine, not being affected by hepatic dysfunction and not having much buffering effects. Differential effects of different buffers are discussed further in Chap. 23.

Clinical Evidence: 0.9% Saline Vs Balanced

Observational Studies

In a before-and-after single center study, Yunos and colleagues tested the effect of restricting chloride-rich fluid on renal outcome and mortality. They collected baseline data for 6 months when the ICU was predominantly using chloride-rich fluids (0.9% saline, succinylated gelatin, and 5% albumin) followed by a phaseout period of 6 months before switching to chloride-restricted fluid strategy (Plasma-Lyte, hyperoncotic albumin) [14].

Rise in creatinine, incidence of new-onset acute kidney injury (AKI) with RIFLE I and F class, and need for renal replacement therapy (RRT) were significantly reduced during the chloride restriction period. However, there was no difference in mortality or hospital/ICU length of stay between two periods. In a subsequent study, Yunos and colleagues extended the chloride restriction strategy for another 6 months and also collected retrospective data for chloride liberal period for additional 6 months [15]. The chloride-restricted strategy continued to be associated with decreased incidence of AKI and need for RRT. But interestingly, the incidence of AKI in the extended chloride-restricted period was higher compared to the original observation period! Both of Yunos' studies were criticized for following reasons—open-label design, change in the bundle of care, not a single intervention, and possible Hawthorne effect. In a large retrospective observational study, Raghunathan and colleagues evaluated the effect of 0.9% saline vs some balanced crystalloids as resuscitation fluid in the first 2 days [16]. The balanced crystalloids group had lower mortality, and mortality was further reduced in patients receiving higher percentage of balanced crystalloids.

Randomized Controlled Studies

In the SPLIT study, a double-blind, double-crossover, cluster RCT conducted in four ICUs, patients requiring intravenous crystalloids were randomized to receive either 0.9% saline or Plasma-Lyte [17]. The incidence of AKI at 90 days, the primary outcome of the study, was not different between two groups. There was no difference in 90-day mortality, need for RRT, or other secondary outcomes between the groups. However, the study was criticized because of following reasons: First, indications for crystalloid use (resuscitation, maintenance, or replacement) were not specified. Second, mostly postoperative patients were enrolled. Third patients enrolled were not so sick (median APACHE II score ~14, 4% patients with sepsis or 2.5% with traumatic brain injury). Fourth, chloride levels were not measured. Finally, median volume of fluid received was only 2000 ml [17].

The SALT-ED study was a single-center, unblinded, multiple-crossover trial comparing balanced crystalloids (Ringer's lactate or Plasma-Lyte) vs 0.9% saline among adults treated with intravenous fluid in the emergency department (ED) and were admitted to the hospital outside the ICU [18]. A total of 13,347 patients were enrolled, with a median crystalloid volume administered in ED of ~1000 ml. There was no difference in the number of hospital free days, the primary outcome of the study, between two groups. However, the incidence of major adverse kidney events (a combination of death, persistent AKI at day 30, or new need of RRT, MAKE30), a secondary outcome, was significantly lower in the balanced crystalloids group (4.7% vs 5.6%, $P = 0.01$). It was primarily driven by the lower incidence of AKI (defined as doubling of creatinine), not mortality nor the need of RRT [18].

In the SMART study, more than 15,000 patients admitted in five ICUs of a university hospital were randomized to receive either 0.9% saline or balanced crystalloids (Ringer's lactate or Plasma-Lyte) as intravenous fluid [19]. The primary outcome, MAKE30, was significantly lower in the balanced crystalloid group (14.3% vs 15.4%, $p = 0.04$). There was also a trend towards higher 30-day mortality in the 0.9% saline group. However, the individual components of MAKE30, mortality before discharge or at day 30, need for new RRT, and persistent kidney dysfunction at 30 days were not different between two groups. There were important limitations of both (SMART and SALT-ED) studies: First, both were single-center, nonblinded studies requiring external validation of the data. Second, patient populations were not so sick with low overall mortality. Third, balanced crystalloids with different compositions (Ringer's lactate and Plasma-Lyte) were clubbed together. Fourth, overall fluid volume received were low (median volume received in SMART ~1000 ml; median volume ED admission to wards in SALT-ED ~1000 ml). Finally, composite outcome of MAKE30 with giving similar weightage to death, RRT, and persistent renal dysfunction to decide MAKE30 may not be a true patient centered outcome [19].

Afterwards, the BASICS trial randomized 11,052 patients from 75 Brazil ICUs. They performed a factorial 2×2 randomization in 1:1:1:1 ratio to each fluid (balanced solution: Plasma-Lyte and 0.9% sodium chloride) and each rate of administration (333 ml/h and 999 ml/h). The conclusions were that the use of a balanced crystalloid compared to 0.9% sodium chloride did not reduce 90-day mortality [20] nor did the use of slower infusion rates, when a fluid bolus is required compared to a faster rate of infusion [21]. A post-hoc analysis showed that there is a high probability that balanced solution use in the ICU reduces 90-day mortality in patients who exclusively received balanced fl-uids before trial enrollment [22]. Another post-hoc analysis showed that among patients with sepsis, the effect of balanced crystalloids vs 0.9% saline on mortality was greater for those whom fluid choice was controlled starting in the ED compared with starting in the ICU [23].

Finally, another recent RCT (the PLUS study) compared Plasma-Lyte 148 to 0.9% saline, involving 5,037 patients from 53 ICUs of Australia and New Zealand. No increased risk of the 90 days mortality was observed with 0.9% saline (22% vs 21.8%, $p = 0.9$) compared to Plasma-Lyte 148. There was also no significant increased incidence of AKI (mean maximal risk in creatinine of 0.41 ± 1.02 mg/dl vs 0.41 ± 1.06 mg/dl) or need of RRT (12.9% vs 12.7%) with the use of 0.9% saline compared to Plasma-Lyte 148. The study was prematurely terminated due to disruptions from the COVID-19 pandemic. However, the futility cutoff was achieved before the termination and it was unlikely that results would have been different, if the trial continued. There were a large number of protocol deviations, with the use of nonstudy fluids in both groups. Finally, fluids used outside ICUs were not controlled and recorded [24].

Subsequently, researchers from these RCTs performed a metanalysis including13 RCTs and 35,884 patients. From the six RCTs with a low risk of bias (34,450 patients), including the PLUS study, the use of balanced crystalloids compared to 0.9% saline in critically ill patients was found to produce 9% relative reduction in mortality to 1% relative increase in mortality. There was high probability of 90% of reduction of mortality with the balanced crystalloids. In patients with sepsis, the effect was further pronounced with a range of 14% relative reduction of mortality to 1% increase [25].

To conclude, the negative effects of dilutional hyperchloremic acidosis on patient-centered outcome have not yet been documented unequivocally. But from a physiological standpoint and from limited evidence available so far, balanced fluids are superior over saline especially when administered in larger volumes during resuscitation. The use of 0.9% saline may still have a limited role in resuscitating patients with possible raised intracranial pressure, in replacing gastric fluid loss, as drug diluent (when dextrose 5% is contraindicated), or when no other isotonic crystalloid is available for resuscitation.

Hypotonic Crystalloids

Hypotonic fluids have tonicity lower than plasma and the osmolality varies, depending on its constituents. The addition of dextrose to hypotonic fluids helps to create isosmotic environment to prevent intravascular hemolysis with their administration. However, with the intracellular movement or metabolism of dextrose, the fluid becomes hypotonic. They are freely redistributed to the interstitium and intracellular compartment based on total body water composition, i.e., nearly two-third of the infused volume will move into the intracellular space.

Hypotonic crystalloid solutions are mainly used as maintenance fluids. Other use includes the treatment of hypernatremia with solute-free water deficits and drug diluents. The maintenance fluids are required to replace sensible (e.g., urine, feces, sweat) and insensible (e.g., cutaneous or respiratory evaporative losses, fever) losses, in those who are unable to replace them enterally. The best maintenance fluid is the one that has not been administered. One should only start maintenance solutions if the patient is not able to cover his/her daily fluid needs (25 ml/kg/day) orally or enterally.

Solute-free water is lost with insensible losses, and therefore more water than solutes are needed for maintaining fluid balance. The sodium concentration in these fluids is between 40 and 77 mEq/L and can contain other additional anions and cations to replaces the daily losses (Table 9.4). Table 9.4 gives an overview of the different hypotonic solutions. The main indication is to deliver free water in case of cellular dehydration. Recent evidence from the MIHMOSA and TOPMAST trials show that hypotonic balanced maintenance solutions are preferred over isotonic ones since they will lead to a less positive fluid and sodium balance.

Table 9.4 Composition of different crystalloids

	Plasma	Dextrose 5%	NaCl 0.3%	NaCl 0.45%	D 5% in NaCl 0.45%	Glucion 5%	Isolyte M	Isolyte P	Isolyte G	D 5% in Plasma-Lyte 56	Water
Na^+ (mEq/L)	136–145	–	51	77	77	54	40	25	65	40	<1
K^+ (mEq/L)	3.5–5	–	–	–	–	26	35	20	17	13	<0.1
Ca^{2+} (mEq/L)	2.2–2.6	–	–	–	–	–	–	–	–	–	2.5
Mg^{2+} (mEq/L)	0.8–1	–	–	–	–	5	–	3	–	1.5	2.5
Cl^- (mEq/L)	96–106	–	51	77	77	55	38	22	150	40	<0.1
Phosphate (mEq/L)	–	–	–	–	–	6	15	3	–	–	–
Lactate (mEq/L)	–	–	–	–	–	25	–	–	–	–	–
Acetate (mmol/L)	–	–	–	–	–	–	20	23	–	16	–
Dextrose (g/L)	50	50	–	–	50	50	50	50	50	50	
Dextrose (mmol/L)	80–120	278	–	–	278	278	278	278	278	278	–
In vivo SID (mEq/L)	40	–	–	–	–	30	37	36	NA	14.5	–
Osmolarity (mOsm/L)	270–290	0	102	154	154	170	80	50	130	80	10

Hypertonic Crystalloids

Hypertonic Saline

Hypertonic saline refers to any saline having concentration greater than 0.9% saline. These hypertonic crystalloids are available in varying concentrations ranging from 2% to 23% saline, but the commonly prescribed is 3% saline. Hypertonic saline 3% is indicated in critically ill for small-volume resuscitation, in patients with severe hyponatremia presenting with seizures or altered sensorium, and in patients of serve traumatic brain injury (having features of raised intracranial hypertension). Hypertonic saline exerts an osmotic effect by drawing fluid out of edematous tissues, as it has a higher concentration of sodium compared to interstitium.

Hypertonic saline acts on various body systems in different ways: Firstly, it affects hemodynamics by raising mean arterial pressure, raising cardiac output and stroke volume; it also increases left ventricular end-diastolic volume and reduces pulmonary vascular resistance. Secondly, it increases the total plasma volume and plasma vasopressin concentrations due to increased plasma osmolality. Thirdly, neurologic effects are related to increases in plasma osmolarity, and higher sodium concentration causes blood to be hypertonic compared to cerebral tissue (which has low sodium concentration). This difference leads to an osmotic gradient promoting the flow of excess water to move out of cerebral tissue. Trials showed an ICP improvement for approximately 72 h when sodium levels were increased by 10–15 mEq/l with hypertonic saline therapy [26]. Hypertonic saline increases capillary vessel inner diameter and plasma volume counteracting vasospasm and hypoperfusion by increased cerebral blood flow. These fluids have immune modulation and neurochemical properties too.

Hypertonic saline can be administered as bolus or continuous infusion in traumatic brain injury. The target serum osmolarity is less than 320 mOsmol/L. When treating patients of increased intracranial pressure with continuous 3% saline infusion, the optimal therapy is monitored by sodium levels and targeted between 145 and 155 mEq/l [27]. Hypertonic saline can be used as bolus in emergency situations, in concentrations ranging from 1.7% to 30% saline, and most often as bolus doses of 250 ml. The serum sodium level should be measured within 6 h of administration of bolus doses given. Readministration of hypertonic saline should not occur until the serum sodium concentration is <155 mEq/l. In head injury, when used in infusion, the rate of infusion has varied from 30 to 150 ml/h in light of the sodium levels.

For correction of severe hyponatremia, hypertonic saline is used in form of infusion guided by the sodium deficit calculated as total body water × wt (kg) × (desired sodium − actual sodium). The rate of sodium correction should be 6–12 mEq/L (0.5 mEq/h) in the first 24 h and 18 mEq per L or less in 48 h. A bolus of 100–150 mL of hypertonic 3% saline can be given to correct severe symptomatic hyponatremia until sodium levels reach 120 mEq/L. Limited evidence-supported resuscitation with 3% saline can reduce the total volume infused, less postoperative complications, and short ICU stay [28]. However, a recent a monocentric RCT failed to found any significant reduction in volume infused with the resuscitation using 7.3% saline vs 0.9% sodium chloride in postoperative cardiac surgery patients. Besides, a transient but considerable electrolytes and acid–base disturbance was noted in the hypertonic saline group [29].

The most serious potential complication of hypertonic saline administration is central pontine myelinolysis, characterized by a rapid and irreversible demyelination of the pons. Acute renal insufficiency has been seen in patients with traumatic brain injury receiving hypertonic saline, and this can be minimized by maintaining euvolemic state in such patients.

In comparison to mannitol, hypertonic saline causes less "rebound" ICP and lower nephrotoxicity, has no obligatory osmotic diuresis, and can be easily monitored by serial sodium levels.

Sodium Bicarbonate Solution

Bicarbonate is the leading source of CO_2 transport in the plasma. However, the regulation of bicarbonate is mainly through the kidneys via secretion and absorption. Sodium bicarbonate ($NaHCO_3$) is the most frequently used buffer to prevent or treat the metabolic acidosis and treat severe hyperkalemia. $NaHCO_3$ is available in various forms: oral tablets, IV injections, and IV infusions. Injectable sodium bicarbonate is mainly available in two concentrations: 7.5% (44.6 mEq $NaHCO_3$) and 8.5% (50 mEq $NaHCO_3$). Injectable $NaHCO_3$ has high osmolality and can cause thrombophlebitis with prolonged peripheral venous administration. However, bicarbonate administration can stimulate release of pro-inflammatory cytokines, superoxide radical production, apoptosis, and paradoxical intracellular acidosis due to production of CO_2.

Indications of $NaHCO_3$

- Hyperkalemia (>6 mEq/l) and arrhythmias, especially in the setting of resuscitation
- Alkalization in salicylate intoxication
  - Alkalization is essential (urinary pH 7.5–8.0, arterial <7.6).
  - Higher renal excretion, less fat soluble and less penetration by blood–brain barrier (BBB)
  - No standard dose: 1–2 mEq/kg bolus + maintenance infusion
- Alkalinization in rhabdomyolysis [30]
- Alkalinization of urine (pH> 6.5) prevents myoglobin casts formation and helps in AKI prevention. No RCTs compared $NaHCO_3$ infusion to "classic" IV hydration. The criteria of rhabdomyolysis for $NaHCO_3$ administration is a creatinine kinase (CK) increase to 5 times the upper limit of normal value. Start $NaHCO_3$ from CK >10,000.
- Sodium-channel blocker toxicity (e.g., tricyclic antidepressants)
  - Mainly based on animal experiments and case reports

- Bolus 8.4% $NaHCO_3$ 1–2 mEq/kg on electrocardiogram abnormalities, malignant ventricular arrhythmias, or hemodynamic instability followed by maintenance infusion
- During CVVH or intermittent hemodialysis for metabolic correction to a base excess of 0 to −5 (with or without substitution fluid or as a separate SPP)
- Prevention of contrast-induced nephropathy (CIN) [31]
    - The use of NaHCO3 may reduce the risk of CIN (serum creatinine may increase by 0.5 mEq/l or increase by 25%), but no effect on the need of new dialysis or mortality.
    - Moderate heterogeneity, varying study patients, setting, and type of contrast agent.
    - More effect with emergency scans. More effect in studies published before 2008. The bolus is better than continuous infusion and in combination with N-acetylcysteine (NAC).
    - A meta-analysis of 125 studies favored $NaHCO_3$ infusion over 0.9% saline along with N-acetylcysteine, vitamin C, statins, and adenosine antagonists for prevention of CIN after coronary angiography [32].
- Another meta-analysis including 21,450 patients from 107 studies reported saline and N-acetylcysteine are the most effective treatment options that can reduce short-term mortality. However, none of the drugs could reduce the requirement of RRT or adverse cardiovascular events [33]. However, a recent RCT found no benefit of $NaHCO_3$ infusion over saline in reduction of CIN, mortality, or need of RRT, after coronary angiography [34]. Metabolic acidosis with normal anion gap, correcting base excess to 0-5 (e.g., pronounced gastrointestinal loss, renal tubular acidosis) [35].
    - Dose = 0.3 × weight × −BE
- $NaHCO_3$ in the management of metabolic acidosis with high anion gap has been a matter of debate since long (BE of <−10 [aim is to achieve homeostasis of the internal environment as soon as possible]) [36, 37].
- The multicenter open-label (BICAR-ICU) RCT evaluated the use of $NaHCO_3$ infusion (vs no infusion) in critically ill patients with metabolic acidosis (pH ≤7.20) to target a pH >7.3. Sepsis and AKI were present in 61% and 47% of patients, respectively. Patients were sick with 83% on invasive mechanical ventilation and 80% on vasopressors. There was no benefit with $NaHCO_3$ in the primary outcome, composite of mortality from any cause at day 28, and one or more organ failure at day 7. However, in subgroup of patients with AKI, the $NaHCO_3$ infusion produced significant difference in composite outcome and individual components of mortality and organ failure [38].

Recent Surviving Sepsis Campaign guidelines suggested against using sodium bicarbonate therapy for the purpose of improving hemodynamics or reducing vasopressor requirements in patients with septic shock and hypoperfusion-induced lactic acidemia [39]. (Low quality of evidence). The following are side effects of $NaHCO_3$:

- Sodium overload (166.6 mmol/L)
- fluid overload
- Hypokalemia
- Hyperosmolality: cellular dehydration

- Hypocalcemia
- Metabolic alkalosis: vasoconstriction
- Extravasation
- Very careful use in elderly patients
- Possible pCO_2 increase due to CO_2 accumulation

Case Vignette

Q1. What will be the most appropriate fluid for initial resuscitation of this patient?

Recent studies have shown that balanced crystalloids are the best first choice in this setting. In case of profound shock and liver failure, exogenous lactate (from Ringer's lactate) may accumulate. Hence, serum lactate values may lose their ability to discriminate between ongoing lactate production (DO_2/VO_2 mismatch) and diminished lactate clearance. Therefore, balanced crystalloids not containing lactate may be preferred (e.g., Plasma-Lyte).

Q2. Which fluid to choose for maintenance intravenous therapy now?

The best maintenance fluid is the one that has not been administered. One should only start maintenance solutions if the patient is not able to cover his/her daily fluid needs (25 ml/kg/day) orally or enterally. Recent studies showed that over 30% of the total fluid amount administered comes from fluids given to deliver antibiotics, pain killers, or other drugs. This is called fluid creep and should be reduced to a minimum. Fluid creep is defined as the sum of the volumes of electrolytes, the small volumes to keep venous lines open (saline or glucose 5%) and the total volume used as a vehicle for medication.

Conclusion

Crystalloids are the most common used fluids for critically ill patients. Despite an ongoing debate, balanced crystalloids are the preferred resuscitation fluid in most patients, except those with traumatic brain injury. Crystalloids should be prescribed like any other ICU medication, and selecting the right fluid, indication, dose, and duration is crucial for optimal outcomes.

Take Home Messages

- Crystalloids like other medications should be used in the right patient, right indication, right dose, and for right duration.
- Balanced crystalloids are resuscitation fluids of choice in patients with sepsis and septic shock, burns, or diabetic ketoacidosis.
- 0.9% sodium chloride is not normal nor physiological and its administration may cause harm in critically ill patients.

- Hypertonic saline is mainly used for the treatment of raised intracranial pressure and symptomatic hyponatremia.
- Maintenance solutions should be only considered if the patient is not able to cover his/her daily fluid needs orally or enterally.
- Evidence does not support the use sodium bicarbonate therapy in patients with septic shock and hypoperfusion-induced lactic acidemia to support hemodynamics.

References

1. Latta TA. Malignant cholera. Documents communicated by the Central Board of Health, London, relative to the treatment of cholera by the copious injection of aqueous and saline fluids into the veins. Lancet. 1832;18:274–80.
2. Ringer S. Regarding the action of the hydrate of soda, hydrate of ammonia, and the hydrate of potash on the ventricle of the frog's heart. J Physiol. 1880;3:195–202.
3. Hartmann AF, Senn MJ. Studies in the metabolism of sodium R-lactate. I. Response of normal human subjects to the intravenous injection of sodium R-lactate. J Clin Invest. 1932;11:327–35.
4. Starling EH. On the absorption of fluids from the connective tissue spaces. J Physiol. 1896;19:312–26.
5. Woodcock TE, Woodcock TM. Revised Starling equation and the glycocalyx model of transvascular fluid exchange: an improved paradigm for prescribing intravenous fluid therapy. Br J Anaesth. 2012;108:384–94.
6. NICE. Intravenous fluid therapy in adults in hospital. London: National Institute for Health and Care Excellence; 2013. https://www.nice.org.uk/guidance/cg174.
7. Rhodes A, Evans LE, Alhazzani W, Levy MM, Antonelli M, Ferrer R, et al. Surviving sepsis campaign: international guidelines for management of sepsis and septic shock: 2016. Intensive Care Med. 2017;43:304–77.
8. Rehm M, Finsterer U. Treating intraoperative hyperchloremic acidosis with sodium bicarbonate or tris-hydroxymethyl aminomethane: a randomized prospective study. Anesth Analg. 2003;96:1201–8.
9. Chowdhury AH, Cox EF, Francis ST, Lobo DN. A randomized, controlled, double-blind crossover study on the effects of 2-L infusions of 0.9% saline and plasmalyte-148 on renal blood flow velocity and renal cortical tissue perfusion in healthy volunteers. Ann Surg. 2012;256:18–24.
10. O'Malley CM, Frumento RJ, Hardy MA, Benvenisty AI, Brentjens TE, Mercer JS, Bennett-Guerrero E. A randomized, double-blind comparison of lactated Ringer's solution and 0.9% NaCl during renal transplantation. Anesth Analg. 2005;100:1518–24.
11. Lobo DN, Awad S. Should chloride-rich crystalloids remain the mainstay of fluid resuscitation to prevent 'pre-renal' acute kidney injury? Con. Kidney Int. 2014;86:1096–105.
12. Cull DL, Lally KP, Murphy KD. Compatibility of packed erythrocytes and Ringer's lactate solution. Surg Gynecol Obstet. 1991;173:9–12.
13. Ergin B, Kapucu A, Guerci P, Ince C. The role of bicarbonate precursors in balanced fluids during haemorrhagic shock with and without compromised liver function. Br J Anaesth. 2016;117:521–8.
14. Yunos NM, Bellomo R, Hegarty C, Story D, Ho L, Bailey M. Association between a chloride-liberal versus chloride-restrictive intravenous fluid administration strategy and kidney injury in critically ill adults. J Am Med Assoc. 2012;308:1566–72.

15. Yunos NM, Bellomo R, Glassford N, Sutcliffe H, Lam Q, Bailey M. Chloride-liberal vs. chloride-restrictive intravenous fluid administration and acute kidney injury: an extended analysis. Intensive Care Med. 2015;41:257–64.
16. Raghunathan K, Shaw A, Nathanson B, Stürmer T, Brookhart A, Stefan MS, Setoguchi S, Beadles C, Lindenauer PK. Association between the choice of IV crystalloid and in-hospital mortality among critically ill adults with sepsis. Crit Care Med. 2014;42:1585–91.
17. Young P, Bailey M, Beasley R, et al. Effect of a buffered crystalloid solution vs saline on acute kidney injury among patients in the intensive care unit. The SPLIT randomized clinical trial. JAMA. 2015;314:1701–10.
18. Self WH, Semler MW, Wanderer JP, Wang L, Byrne DW, Collins SP, et al. Balanced crystalloids versus saline in noncritically ill adults. N Engl J Med. 2018;378(9):819–28.
19. Semler MW, Self WH, Wanderer JP, Ehrenfeld JM, Wang L, Byrne DW, et al. Balanced crystalloids versus saline in critically ill adults. N Engl J Med. 2018;378:829–39.
20. Zampieri FG, Machado FR, Biondi RS, Freitas FGR, Veiga VC, Figueiredo RC, et al. Effect of intravenous fluid treatment with a balanced solution vs 0.9% saline solution on mortality in critically ill patients: the BaSICS randomized clinical trial. JAMA. 2021;326(9):1–12.
21. Zampieri FG, Machado FR, Biondi RS, Freitas FGR, Veiga VC, Figueiredo RC, et al. Effect of slower vs faster intravenous fluid bolus rates on mortality in critically ill patients: the BaSICS randomized clinical trial. JAMA. 2021;326(9):830–8.
22. Zampieri FG, Machado FR, Biondi RS, Freitas FGR, Veiga VC, Figueiredo RC, et al. Association between type of fluid received prior to enrollment, type of admission, and effect of balanced crystalloid in critically ill adults: a secondary exploratory analysis of the BaSICS clinical trial. Am J Respir Crit Care Med. 2022;205:1419–28.
23. Jackson KE, Wang L, Casey JD, Bernard GR, Self WH, Rice TW, et al. Effect of early balanced crystalloids before ICU admission on sepsis outcomes. Chest. 2021;159(2):585–95.
24. Finfer S, Micallef S, Hammond N, Navarra L, Bellomo R, Billot L, Delaney A, et al. Balanced multielectrolyte solution versus saline in critically ill adults. N Engl J Med. 2022;386(9):815–26.
25. Hammond NE, Zampieri FG, Di Tanna GL, Garside T, Adigbli D, Cavalcanti AB, et al. Balanced crystalloids versus saline in critically ill adults – a systematic review with meta-analysis. NEJM Evid. 2022;1(2):10. https://doi.org/10.1056/EVIDoa2100010.
26. Khanna S, Davis D, Peterson B, Fisher B, Tung H, O'Quigley J, et al. Use of hypertonic saline in the treatment of severe refractory posttraumatic intracranial hypertension in pediatric traumatic brain injury. Crit Care Med. 2000;28(4):1144–51.
27. Qureshi AI, Suarez JI, Bhardwaj A, Mirski M, Schnitzer MS, Hanley DF, et al. Use of hypertonic (3%) saline/acetate infusion in the treatment of cerebral edema: Effect on intracranial pressure and lateral displacement of the brain. Crit Care Med. 1998;26(3):440–6.
28. Pfortmueller CA, Schefold JC. Hypertonic saline in critical illness - a systematic review. J Crit Care. 2017;42:168–77.
29. Pfortmueller CA, Kindler M, Schenk N, Messmer AS, Hess B, Jakob L, et al. Hypertonic saline for fluid resuscitation in ICU patients post-cardiac surgery (HERACLES): a double-blind randomized controlled clinical trial. Intensive Care Med. 2020;46(9):1683–95.
30. Chavez LO, Leon M, Einav S, Varon J. Beyond muscle destruction: a systematic review of rhabdomyolysis for clinical practice. Crit Care. 2016;20(1):135. https://doi.org/10.1186/s13054-016-1314-5.
31. Silver SA, Shah PM, Chertow GM, Harel S, Wald R, Harel Z. Risk prediction models for contrast induced nephropathy: systematic review. BMJ. 2015;351:h4395. https://doi.org/10.1136/bmj.h4395.
32. Ali-Hasan-Al-Saegh S, Mirhosseini SJ, Ghodratipour Z, Sarrafan-Chaharsoughi Z, Rahimizadeh E, Karimi-Bondarabadi AA, et al. Strategies preventing contrast-induced nephropathy after

coronary angiography: a comprehensive meta-analysis and systematic review of 125 random-ized controlled trials. Angiology. 2017;68(5):389–413.

33. Ma WQ, Zhao Y, Wang Y, Han XQ, Zhu Y, Liu NF. Comparative efficacy of pharmacological interventions for contrast-induced nephropathy prevention after coronary angiography: a net-work meta-analysis from randomized trials. Int Urol Nephrol. 2018;50(6):1085–95.

34. Weisbord SD, Gallagher M, Jneid H, Garcia S, Cass A, Thwin SS, et al. Outcomes after angiog-raphy with sodium bicarbonate and acetylcysteine. N Engl J Med. 2018;378(7):603–14.

35. Adeva-Andany MM, Fernandez-Fernandez C, Mourino-Bayolo D, Castro-Quintela E, Dominguez-Montero A. Sodium bicarbonate therapy in patients with metabolic acidosis. Sci World J. 2014;2014:627673. https://doi.org/10.1155/2014/627673, indexed in Pubmed: 25405229.

36. Velissaris D, Karamouzos V, Pierrakos C, Koniari I, Apostolopoulou C, Karanikolas M. Use of sodium bicarbonate in cardiac arrest: current guidelines and literature review. J Clin Med Res. 2016;8(4):277–83.

37. Kitabchi AE, Umpierrez GE, Murphy MB, Barrett EJ, Kreisberg RA, Malone JI, et al. Hyperglycemic crises in diabetes. Diabetes Care. 2004;27(1):94–102.

38. Jaber S, Paugam C, Futier E, Lefrant JY, Lasocki S, Lescot T, et al. Sodium bicarbonate therapy for patients with severe metabolic acidaemia in the intensive care unit (BICAR-ICU): a multi-centre, open-label, randomised controlled, phase 3 trial. Lancet. 2018;392(10141):31–40.

39. Evans L, Rhodes A, Alhazzani W, Antonelli M, Coopersmith CM, French C, et al. Surviving sepsis campaign: international guidelines for management of sepsis and septic shock 2021. Intensive Care Med. 2021;47(11):1181–247.

The Case for Albumin as Volume Expander and beyond

10

Prashant Nasa, Rajesh Kumar, Deven Juneja, and Supradip Gosh

Contents

Introduction 230
Albumin in Health 231
Albumin in Critical Illness 232
Evidence on Albumin as a Plasma Expander 232
Timing of Albumin Administration during Resuscitation 234
Comparison of Different Strengths of Albumin 234
Albumin beyond Resuscitation 235
   Patients with Liver Disease 235
   Treatment of Hypoalbuminemia with Peripheral Oedema 235
   Deresuscitation 236
   Other Indications 236
Caution with the Use of Albumin 236
Conclusion 238
References 239

P. Nasa (✉)
Department of Critical Care Medicine, NMC Specialty Hospital, Dubai, UAE

Internal Medicine, College of Medicine and Health Sciences, Al Ain, UAE
e-mail: dr.prashantnasa@hotmail.com

R. Kumar
Department of Critical Care Medicine, NMC Specialty Hospital, Dubai, UAE

D. Juneja
Institute of Critical Care Medicine, Max Super Specialty Hospital, Saket, New Delhi, India

S. Gosh
Department of Critical Care Medicine, Fortis Escorts Hospital, Faridabad, Haryana, India

© The Author(s) 2024
M. L. N. G. Malbrain et al. (eds.), *Rational Use of Intravenous Fluids in Critically Ill Patients*, https://doi.org/10.1007/978-3-031-42205-8_10

IFA Commentary (MLNGM)

The plasma oncotic pressure, which is primarily determined by endogenous albumin, is a critical factor in maintaining fluid balance and microvascular fluid dynamics. In addition to its contribution to oncotic pressure, albumin plays a crucial role in endothelial glycocalyx layer function, which affects fluid dynamics in the microvasculature. While some studies have suggested that albumin may be useful for fluid resuscitation in patients with sepsis and septic shock, the evidence supporting this approach is largely based on post-hoc analysis, rather than predefined studies. Furthermore, the use of albumin is associated with a significantly higher cost compared to crystalloids, and its efficacy remains controversial due to a lack of sound clinical evidence. Ongoing randomised trials, such as the ALBumin Italian Outcome Septic Shock-BALANCED Trial (ALBIOSS-BALANCED) and the albumin replacement therapy in septic shock (ARISS), may provide more definitive answers to these issues.

While the role of albumin in sepsis remains a matter of debate, it has a well-established role in the management of patients with decompensated cirrhosis and complications such as hepatorenal syndrome, spontaneous bacterial peritonitis, and large volume paracentesis. In these patients, albumin infusion is a critical component of treatment and has been shown to improve outcomes. Additionally, albumin has been used in other clinical scenarios such as cardiac surgery, burns, and trauma, where it may help to maintain oncotic pressure and prevent fluid shifts. However, further studies are needed to determine the optimal dosing and duration of albumin therapy in these contexts. Despite some controversies, albumin remains an important therapeutic option in critical care, and ongoing research is likely to refine our understanding of its role in fluid management.

A recent paper addresses 10 myths about albumin therapy (Fig. 10.1).

Myth #1. Albumin leaks from the intravascular space into the interstitial compartment and contributes to oedema.

No, it does not.

Myth #2. Albumin is less effective for intravascular volume expansion than artificial colloids.

No, it is more effective.

Myth #3. Albumin administration prevents acute kidney injury.

Yes, in specific settings.

Myth #4. Albumin improves survival in sepsis.

Maybe, but it is still uncertain.

Myth #5. Albumin improves the effects of diuretics.

Yes, but only temporarily.

Myth #6. Albumin administration improves fluid removal during KRT.

Yes, it does.

Myth #7. Albumin decreases mortality in liver cirrhosis.

Yes, but only in specific subgroups.

Myth #8. Albumin increases mortality in traumatic brain injury (TBI).

Maybe, but we are not sure.

Myth #9. Albumin substitution to correct hypoalbuminemia from all causes reduces mortality.

No, it does not.

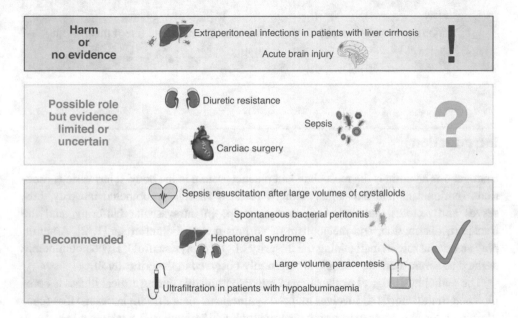

Fig. 10.1 Albumin therapy in critical care. (Adapted from Joannidis M. et al. [1])

Learning Objectives

In this chapter, we will learn the physiology of albumin and the relation of hypoalbuminemia to clinically meaningful outcomes. We will review the evidence on plasma expansion with exogenous albumin in different indications.

Case Vignette

A 46-year-old female, 76 kg, with a history of inflammatory bowel disease, presented with pain in the abdomen for three days. On examination, she was anxious, with cold extremities, dry oral mucosa, heart rate of 132/min, and blood pressure (BP) of 78/46 mmHg. She was resuscitated with crystalloids (0.9% sodium chloride and Plasma-Lyte™). Despite, fluid resuscitation with 4.5 L crystalloids, norepinephrine 0.4 µg/kg/min, and vasopressin 0.04 units/min, she stayed hypotensive (MAP 60 mmHg); arterial blood gas showed metabolic acidosis with lactates 4.6. Passive leg raising test using pulse pressure variation confirmed fluid responsiveness.

Questions

Q1: Which intravenous fluids will you use for further resuscitation of this patient?
Q2: What will be the end points of resuscitation?

Introduction

Endogenous albumin is the most abundant plasma protein in the body. It has various functions (antioxidant and anti-inflammatory), restores vascular endothelial integrity, preserves and restores endothelial glycocalyx, helps in intravascular buffering, and the transport, distribution, and metabolism of various protein-bound drugs [1, 2]. Albumin plays a crucial role in maintaining the integrity of glycocalyx scaffold. Hypoalbuminemia defined as serum albumin <35 g/L is commonly observed in the critically ill.

The pathophysiological explanation of hypoalbuminemia during critical illness is complex and multifactorial. It involves reduced synthesis or malnutrition, increased loss (capillary leak, renal loss, protein-losing enteropathy), and/or increased catabolism [3].

Various observational studies explored the association between hypoalbuminemia and outcomes. In a meta-analysis of 90 cohort studies and five controlled trials, including 291,968 patients, hypoalbuminemia was an independent predictor of worse outcomes. Each 10 g/L drop in serum albumin was associated with a higher risk of mortality (137%), morbidity (89%), ICU or hospital length of stay (28% and 71%, respectively), and increased resource utilisation (66%). Exogenous albumin administration reduced the incidence of complications when targeting serum albumin concentrations of more than 30 g/L. However, the authors recommended prospective well-designed trials to verify the therapeutic effect of exogenous albumin in patients with hypoalbuminemia [4]. Intravenous (IV) exogenous albumin is often used in the intensive care unit (ICU) for various indications, from resuscitation to deresuscitation [5]. However, the evidence on the use of exogenous albumin as a plasma expander is conflicting. In this chapter, we will review the pharmacokinetics of albumin and the use of exogenous albumin for plasma expansion and other indications.

More information on crystalloid solutions can be found in Chap. 9, while other colloid solutions like starches and gelatins are discussed in Chap. 11.

Albumin in Health

The human albumin accounts for 50–60% of plasma protein with a median half-life of 18–19 days. Albumin contributes to 70–80% of intravascular colloid oncotic pressure. Albumin is a negatively charged molecule constituted by 585 amino acids in a single polypeptide chain with a molecular weight of 66.5 KDa. Disulphide bridges provide structural resilience to the albumin; denaturation only occurs at highly abnormal conditions (extreme of temperature, pH, or chemical environment).

Serum albumin concentration depends on factors like rate of synthesis, degradation, and distribution in body compartments. The albumin pool measures about 3.5–5.0 g/kg/body weight, nearly 40% intravascular. The distribution half-time of endogenous albumin is 15 hours. Intravascular albumin leaks into the extravascular space at a rate of 5% per hour, known as transcapillary escape rate (TER). However, most of the leaked albumin is absorbed via the lymphatic systems and enters back in the blood. Small amount of albumin is lost in the gastrointestinal tract (1 g/day) and minimally through normal kidneys (10–20 mg/day).

In a normal state, around 9–14 g of albumin is synthesised daily by the liver and released in portal circulation. The liver has a limited capacity to increase the synthesis (by 2–2.7 times) and primarily depends on nutritional intake. Fasting decreases synthesis and insulin in combination with corticosteroids increase synthesis. However, corticosteroid plays a complex role in albumin metabolism as it increases its catabolism too.

Nearly 5% of albumin is degraded daily, with a turnover of around 9–14 g/day. The degradation occurs in most organs of the body, muscle, and skin (40–60%), liver (15%), kidneys, gastrointestinal tract, and others (10% each) .

Albumin plays a crucial role in microvascular fluid dynamics [6]. Greater understanding of the glycocalyx and its impact on fluid dynamics has challenged the "Starling equation" of protein-based transcapillary fluid exchange. The intravascular functional barrier is constituted by endothelial glycocalyx (made up of peptidoglycans, syndecan and glypican, glycoproteins, and plasma constituents, including albumin). The glycocalyx gets damaged during inflammation, sepsis, and trauma.

In healthy volunteers, 20% IV albumin administration causes significant plasma expansion via recruitment of interstitium. The plasma volume expansion peaks at 20 mins post-infusion and lasts beyond 5 h [7]. The low-concentration (4 to 5%) albumin can cause plasma expansion by approximately 80% of the administered volume and high-concentration albumin by approximately 210% (20% albumin) to 260% (25% albumin) [8]. Theoretically, this may translate to one-fourth of 20% albumin compared to balanced crystalloids required for resuscitation.

Albumin in Critical Illness

The critical illness alters the metabolism and distribution of endogenous albumin. During the early phase of illness, there is decreased synthesis and increased degradation, with altered distribution between body compartments. Inflammation, sepsis, and trauma decrease the rate of transcription of albumin mRNA. This may be due to a higher TER because of inflammatory damage to the endothelial barrier function and glycocalyx [1]. In septic shock, TER may increase by 300%, which saturates the absorption capacity of the lymphatic system. The pharmacokinetics of exogenous albumin is also altered in critically ill patients. The ratio of 4% albumin to 0.9% NaCl in the saline versus albumin fluid evaluation (SAFE) study to achieve hemodynamic targets was 1:1.4 [9]. This may be due to a higher TER because of inflammatory damage to the endothelial barrier function and glycocalyx [1].

Evidence on Albumin as a Plasma Expander

The role of albumin for plasma expansion during resuscitation is a matter of investigation for decades. Physiological rationale of albumin as plasma expansion is supported by higher blood pressure, both early and later resuscitation points, higher filling pressures, and lower cumulative fluid balance with albumin [9–11].

In a 1998 Cochrane meta-analysis involving 30 randomised controlled trials (RCTs), albumin administration was linked to an increased risk of mortality in critically ill patients [12]. The pooled risk of death with albumin administration was 1.02 (95% CI 0.95 to 1.16). In patients with hypovolemia, the pooled risk was 1.02 (95% CI 0.92 to 1.13). It influenced the practice around the world, especially in the United Kingdom. Since then, various large RCTs have evaluated the role of albumin for fluid resuscitation in the SAFE study, Early Albumin Resuscitation during Septic Shock (EARSS), or albumin replacement (ALBIOS) study in patients with sepsis [8, 13, 14].

The SAFE trial from 16 centres in Australia and New Zealand involving 6997 patients compared 4% albumin vs 0.9% sodium chloride (NaCl) as a resuscitation fluid in a heterogenous population of intensive care unit (ICU). No significant difference was found in day-28 mortality, duration of mechanical ventilation, need for renal replacement therapy, and length of ICU stay. A trend towards increased mortality was found with 4% albumin in the subgroup of patients with trauma (relative risk [RR] 1.36 [95% CI 0.99–1.86]; p = 0.06) [8]. Despite a mega RCT of 7000 patients, the study design had few issues. The study recruited a heterogenous population with mild to moderate severity of illness and recieved only a modest amount of fluid for replacement.

In a *post-hoc* analysis of the SAFE trial, statistically significant lower mortality was found with 4% albumin resuscitation in patients with severe sepsis (adjusted odds ratio 0.71 (95% CI 0.52–0.97]) [15]. Hence, the SAFE study demonstrated the safety aspect of administering exogenous albumin for fluid resuscitation and a trend towards benefit in patients with sepsis.

The multi-centre, open-label RCT (the EARSS study) from France, presented only in LIVES 2011, Berlin, Germany, comparing 20% albumin (8 hourly for 3 days) vs 0.9% NaCl, did not find any significant mortality difference between the two groups (24.1% vs 26.3%). However, the vasopressor requirement was significantly lower in the albumin group [14].

The ALBIOS trial, involving 1818 patients, compared crystalloids vs crystalloids and 20% albumin to correct hypoalbuminemia (targeting a serum albumin >30 gm/L or more) in the first 28 days of patients with sepsis and septic shock. The study design was different from the SAFE study and EARSS as end point of the study was the correction of albumin. There was no significant difference in day-28 and day-90 mortality [13]. The *post-hoc* analysis in patients with septic shock showed a significant 6.3% absolute reduction in mortality (43.6% vs 49.9%; RR: 0.87; 95% CI: 0.77–0.99) and quicker resolution of shock in the albumin group (3 vs 4 days, $p = 0.007$). The albumin group also had a lower cumulative negative fluid balance (347 ml vs 1220 ml, $p = 0.004$) [15].

Subsequently, the meta-analysis, including these trials, showed mixed results.

The meta-analysis of 16 RCTs by Patel et al. yielded no difference in outcome with albumin vs control fluid. However, most of the trials (13 out of 16) included were small, with fewer than 60 patients [16]. In another meta-analysis of five RCTs, comparing albumin with crystalloid, a trend to lower day-90 mortality was reported in patients with severe sepsis (0.88; 95% CI: 0.76–1.01; $P = 0.08$) who received albumin, which was significantly lower in patients with septic shock (OR 0.81; 95% CI: 0.67– 0.97; $P = 0.03$) [17]. An exploratory meta-analysis by Wiedermann et al., including three large RCTs, found a significant reduction in mortality with albumin use. However, this was not a formal meta-analysis and may need further analysis [18].

Recently, the albumin role has been investigated in a specific population of patients with sepsis. A single-centre, double-blind RCT, the Lactated Ringer Versus Albumin in Early Sepsis Therapy (RASP) study, investigated the effects of 4% albumin and Ringer's lactate compared to Ringer's lactate alone in 360 cancer patients with sepsis. No significant difference in day-28 (26% vs 22%) and day-90 (53% vs 46%) mortality was found between the groups and any other secondary outcomes [19].

In cirrhotic patients with sepsis, two single-centre RCTs investigated the role of albumin vs 0.9% NaCl (FRISC study) or Plasma-Lyte (ALPS study). The FRISC study reported significantly higher reversal of sepsis-induced hypotension, reduction of heart rate, lactate clearance, and lower day-7 mortality (38.3% vs 43.5%, p = 0.03), with 5% albumin resuscitation [20]. The ALPS study also reported a significantly higher proportion of patients attaining improvement in haemodynamics (mean arterial pressure of 65 mm hg or higher at 3 h) with 20% albumin compared to Plasma-Lyte (62% vs 22%). The albumin group also had higher lactate clearance. However, there was no difference in day-28 survival between the two groups [21].

An open-label pilot study evaluated the role of 100 ml of 20% albumin bolus (up to two treatments) in postoperative cardiac surgery patients with a crystalloid fluid bolus. The albumin group was associated with less median fluid balance at 24 h (1100 vs 1970, $p = 0.001$), shorter time to cessation of vasopressors (17 vs 28 h, $p = 0.002$), and decreased overall vasopressors requirement in the first 24 h (19 vs 47 µg/kg/24 h, $p = 0.025$) [22]. Despite no significant effect on coagulation function and lower volume required for resuscitation than 0.9% NaCl, albumin did not have any advantage over crystalloids in reducing mortality in patients with haemorrhagic shock [23]. The CRISTAL trial also failed to show any survival difference with colloids, including albumin [24].

Timing of Albumin Administration during Resuscitation

In a recent meta-analysis, including 55 RCTs and 27,036 patients, comparing crystalloids vs colloids for fluid resuscitation in ICU, crystalloid was found to be less efficient than colloids, including albumin, in achieving haemodynamic stabilisation end points [9]. The Surviving Sepsis Campaign 2021 guidelines suggested using albumin for fluid resuscitation in patients who received large volumes of crystalloid [25]. However, the optimal time to switch from crystalloids to albumin is still being determined. The SAFE and ALBIOS studies administered albumin within 28 days of randomisation and the RASP study within 6 h of randomisation [8, 13, 18]. No RCT has evaluated the optimal timing of albumin administration during fluid resuscitation. Recently, an expert group from the Chinese Society of Critical Care Medicine gave consensus recommendations on the timing of albumin administration in patients with septic shock. They recommended albumin administration in fluid-responsive patients along with haemodynamically unstablity even after resuscitation with crystalloids. The haemodynamic instability was defined as (1) failure to maintain a MAP ≥65 mmHg, despite receiving at least 30 mL/kg crystalloids and norepinephrine at a dose of ≥0.4 µg/kg/min, (2) frequent fluctuations in blood pressure, and (3) signs of apparent capillary leakage [2].

Comparison of Different Strengths of Albumin

Different concentration of albumin was used in studies, low (4% or 5%) and high concentrations (20% or 25%). Low-concentration albumin was used in the SAFE, FRISC and RASP trials [9120,21], and high-concentration was used in the ALBIOS and ALPS trials [12, 21]. Evidence supports adverse outcomes in patients with a positive cumulative fluid balance after the first week of ICU admission. A proposition of "small-volume resuscitation" using hyperoncotic albumin to reduce the total amount of fluid administered sparked interest in the ICU community. This utilises the oncotic properties of albumin to draw fluid from the interstitium and maximise the proportion of fluid staying in the intravascular compartment. A multi-centre RCT from Australia and the United Kingdom (the SWIPE study) compared 20% albumin vs 5% albumin for fluid resuscitation. The cumulative fluid balance was lower in the 20% albumin group at 48h (median difference: −576 ml; 95% CI: −1033 to −119; $p = 0.01$). There was no significant difference in secondary outcomes like duration of mechanical ventilation, the need for renal replacement therapy, or proportions of patients discharged from ICU [26]. However, no adverse events were reported with hyperoncotic albumin, and authors recommended further exploration of "small-volume resuscitation" in larger RCTs.

A recent meta-analysis of 26,351 patients in 58 clinical trials indicated no significant difference in the fatality rate or amount of resuscitation fluid between patients with sepsis who were administered low- and high-concentration albumin solutions [27]. Both concentrations of albumin can be used for volume expansion. In a recent survey by the International Fluid Academy, including 1045 participants, 54% agreed to use 20% albumin and 49% agreed to use 5% albumin for sepsis [28].

Albumin beyond Resuscitation

Patients with Liver Disease

Critically ill patients with cirrhosis are often admitted to ICU with complications like variceal bleeding, hepatic encephalopathy, and hepatorenal syndrome (HRS). Hypoalbuminemia is a poor prognostic marker in patients with cirrhosis. However, routine replacement of albumin in patients with decompensated cirrhosis failed to show any survival benefit [29].

Replacement of albumin (the ANSWER study) after large-volume paracentesis (LVP) was found to have lower mortality (HR 0.62; 95% CI: 0.35–0.64) and risk of refractory ascites (HR 0.43; 95% CI: 0.29–0.62) [30]. However, subsequent meta-analysis found conflicting results on the survival benefit of albumin replacement [31, 32].

Combined treatment with albumin with terlipressin is effective for the treatment of acute kidney injury associated with HRS and superior to albumin alone or in combination with other vasoconstrictors like midodrine and octreotide [33]. For patients with spontaneous bacterial peritonitis, albumin replacement with antibiotics can reduce mortality and the risk of AKI [34]. In a recent RCT, terlipressin alone or in combination with albumin was found to be an alternative therapeutic option in high- risk SBP [35].

Treatment of Hypoalbuminemia with Peripheral Oedema

In single-centre RCT, 20% albumin replacement to correct hypoalbuminemia (<31 g/dL) was associated with a greater improvement of organ failure compared to placebo [36]. Subsequent meta-analysis demonstrated that exogenous albumin administration in patients with hypoalbuminemia to achieve a serum albumin level > 30 g/L might be associated with lesser morbidity [4]. However, the multicentre ALBOIS study failed to show any survival benefit with albumin replacement to correct hypoalbuminemia [14].

Deresuscitation

Furosemide is commonly used in ICU for the treatment of fluid accumulation or peripheral oedema. However, hypoalbuminemia reduces the diuretic effect of the furosemide [37]. Combination of albumin and furosemide is synergistic in patients with hypoalbuminemia who need fluid removal. Two small trials have tested this combination for deresuscitation in patients with acute respiratory distress syndrome (ARDS). The retrospective case–control study, evaluated PAL (combination of PEEP, 20% albumin, and furosemide) treatment in patients with ARDS, and found a combination of albumin and furosemide was associated with improved clinical outcomes and lower net negative fluid balance, extravascular lung water, and intrabdominal pressure [38]. See Chap. 25.

In a small RCT of 40 patients, the intervention (albumin) group received a loading dose of 100 mL 25% albumin, followed by the initiation of a furosemide infusion. It was followed by 100 ml 25% albumin IV, repeated every 8 h for 3 days. The control group received 100 mL 0.9% saline every 8 h along with an infusion of furosemide. The albumin group had a significantly higher net negative fluid balance (−5480 mL vs −1490 mL) at the end of the study and greater improvement in their oxygenation index [39].

Other Indications

Albumin is also considered for fluid resuscitation in a patient with burns and extracorporeal membrane oxygenation. Albumin has the theoretical advantage of reducing the net positive cumulative balance, replacing plasma protein lost because of increased capillary permeability. However, the evidence on albumin for the resuscitation of patients with burns is conflicting.

Caution with the Use of Albumin

1. High Sodium chloride load
     Chloride-rich fluids administration has been linked to adverse outcomes in critically ill patients. Few commercial low-concentration albumin (4–5% albumin) solutions contain high sodium chloride. On the other hand, 20% albumin as a chloride-limited strategy was associated with a significantly lower incidence of hyperchloremia, despite no benefits in reducing adverse renal outcomes [40].
2. Traumatic Brain Injury

The *post-hoc* analysis of the SAFE trial (the SAFE-TBI study) involving 460 patients with TBI found higher mortality with 4% albumin compared to 0.9% NaCl. Furthermore, in patients with intracranial pressure (ICP) monitoring, significantly higher ICP and more interventions were required in the albumin group. There was a higher proportion of deaths in the albumin group when the ICP monitoring was discontinued within the first week (34.4% vs 17.4%, p = 0.006) [41]. However, higher mortality could result from hypotonic 4% albumin used in the SAFE study [42]. Hence, these findings need verification in well-planned RCTs, and at present it is pragmatic to avoid albumin in traumatic brain injury.

3. Leakage of albumin and contributes to edema

Systemic inflammation associated with sepsis, trauma, and surgery can affect the endothelial barrier function and glycocalyx. This may cause the extravascular leak of albumin through higher TER. However, albumin does not stay in the interstitium and re-enters the intravascular compartment through absorption into the lymphatic system. Leakage from pulmonary vessels and resulting pulmonary oedema depend on the transcapillary difference between oncotic and interstitial pressures. Exogenous albumin infusion can restore the oncotic pressure gradient because of hypoalbuminemia associated with sepsis [1].

4. Adverse reactions related to blood products

Albumin is produced from pooled human plasma, and the same vigilance is required as other blood products, though pasteurisation during production reduces the risk of microbial transmission [43].

5. Cost-benefit

The cost of albumin is nearly 40–80 times that of a crystalloid. In a cost–benefit analysis based on the *post-hoc* analysis of the ALBIOS study in patients with sepsis, the number needed to treat is 16. The additional cost per life saved was $14,384 in 2017 [44].

Case Vignette

Q1: Which intravenous fluids will you use for further resuscitation of this patient?

A1: The patient is haemodynamically unstable and received 4.5 L of crystalloids for fluid resuscitation, and 20% albumin can be considered for further resuscitation if the patient continues to be haemodynamically unstable (MAP <65 mmHg) and fluid responsive.

Q2: What will be the end points of resuscitation?

A2: The end points of resuscitation can be haemodynamic end points (MAP ≥65 mmHg) or fluid tolerance. Despite fluid-responsive state, if there is evidence of global increased permeability syndrome, vasopressors should be considered early to avoid fluid accumulation.

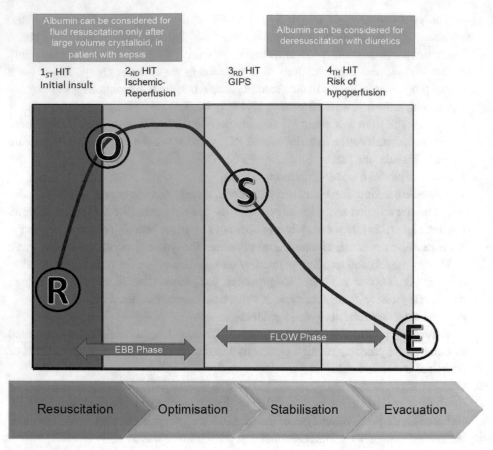

Fig. 10.2 Different roles for albumin use in all phases of fluid management in ICU (resuscitation, stabilisation, optimisation, and deresuscitation)

Conclusion

Albumin is the most promising plasma expander among colloids. The evidence supports the safety of albumin as a plasma expander in patients with septic shock and post-operative cardiac surgery. Albumin has different roles in all phases of fluid management in ICU (resuscitation, stabilisation, optimisation, and deresuscitation) (Fig. 10.2). Appropriate patient selection with cost–benefit analysis may justify its use. Despite reducing the administered volume of IV fluids, the evidence on mortality outcomes is inconclusive. In the era of precision-based medicine, exogenous albumin can be considered for plasma expansion in fluid-responsive patients who have received a considerable amount of crystalloids and/or hypoalbuminemia.

Take-Home Messages
- Both high- and low-concentration albumin solutions can be used for resuscitation if the patient continues to require fluid, despite receiving a considerable volume of crystalloids.
- Albumin is a safe and effective plasma expander in patients with sepsis and septic shock.
- Albumin resuscitation should be avoided in patients with traumatic brain injury.
- Albumin is a blood product and is costlier than crystalloid. Like any other blood product, judicious and vigilant use of albumin is recommended.
- There is no evidence to support that exogenous albumin administration contributes to oedema formation in patients with sepsis.

References

1. Joannidis M, Wiedermann CJ, Ostermann M. Ten myths about albumin. Intensive Care Med. 2022;48(5):602–5.
2. Yu YT, Liu J, Hu B, Wang RL, Yang XH, Shang XL, et al. Expert consensus on the use of human serum albumin in critically ill patients. Chin Med J. 2021;134(14):1639–54.
3. Franch-Arcas G. The meaning of hypoalbuminaemia in clinical practice. Clin Nutr Edinb Scotl. 2001;20:265–9.
4. Vincent JL, Dubois MJ, Navickis RJ, Wilkes MM. Hypoalbuminemia in acute illness: is there a rationale for intervention? A meta-analysis of cohort studies and controlled trials. Ann Surg. 2003;237(3):319–34.
5. Malbrain MLNG, Langer T, Annane D, Gattinoni L, Elbers P, Hahn RG, et al. Intravenous fluid therapy in the perioperative and critical care setting: executive summary of the international fluid academy (IFA). Ann Intensive Care. 2020;10(1):64.
6. Caironi P. POINT: should intravenous albumin be used for volume resuscitation in severe sepsis/ septic shock? Yes. Chest. 2016;149(6):1365–7.
7. Zdolsek M, Hahn RG, Zdolsek JH. Recruitment of extravascular fluid by hyperoncotic albumin. Acta Anaesthesiol Scand. 2018;62(9):1255–60.
8. Jacob M, Chappell D, Conzen P, Wilkes MM, Becker BF, Rehm M. Small-volume resuscitation with hyperoncotic albumin: a systematic review of randomized clinical trials. Crit Care. 2008;12(2):R34.
9. Finfer S, Bellomo R, Boyce N, French J, Myburgh J, Norton R. SAFE study investigators: a comparison of albumin and saline for fluid resuscitation in the intensive care unit. N Engl J Med. 2004;350(22):2247–56.
10. Martin GS, Bassett P. Crystalloids vs. colloids for fluid resuscitation in the intensive care unit: a systematic review and meta-analysis. J Crit Care. 2019;50:144–54.
11. Tseng CH, Chen TT, Wu MY, Chan MC, Shih MC, Tu YK. Resuscitation fluid types in sepsis, surgical, and trauma patients: a systematic review and sequential network meta-analyses. Crit Care. 2020;24(1):693.
12. Cochrane Injuries Group Albumin Reviewers. Human albumin administration in critically ill patients: systematic review of randomised controlled trials. BMJ. 1998;317(7153):235–40.

13. Charpentier J, Mira JP. EARSS study group: efficacy and tolerance of hyperoncotic albumin administration in septic shock patients: the EARSS study. Intensive Care Med. 2011;37(Suppl 1):S115–S0438.
14. Caironi P, Tognoni G, Masson S, Fumagalli R, Pesenti A, Romero M, et al. Albumin replacement in patients with severe sepsis or septic shock. N Engl J Med. 2014;370:1412–21.
15. SAFE Study Investigators, Finfer S, Mc Evoy S, Bellomo R, Mc Arthur C, Myburgh J, Norton R. Impact of albumin compared to saline on organ function and mortality of patients with severe sepsis. Intensive Care Med. 2011;37(1):86–96.
16. Patel A, Laffan MA, Waheed U, Brett SJ. Randomised trials of human albumin for adults with sepsis: systematic review and meta-analysis with trial sequential analysis of all-cause mortality. BMJ. 2014;349:g4561.
17. Xu JY, Chen QH, Xie JF, Pan C, Liu SQ, Huang LW, et al. Comparison of the effects of albumin and crystalloid on mortality in adult patients with severe sepsis and septic shock: a meta-analysis of randomized clinical trials. Crit Care. 2014;18(6):702.
18. Wiedermann CJ, Joannidis M. Albumin replacement in severe sepsis or septic shock. N Engl J Med. 2014;371:83.
19. Park CHL, de Almeida JP, de Oliveira GQ, Rizk SI, Fukushima JT, Nakamura RE, et al. Lactated Ringer's versus 4% albumin on lactated ringer's in early sepsis therapy in cancer patients: a pilot single-center randomized trial. Crit Care Med. 2019;47:e798–805.
20. Philips CA, Maiwall R, Sharma MK, Jindal A, Choudhury AK, Kumar G, et al. Comparison of 5% human albumin and normal saline for fluid resuscitation in sepsis induced hypotension among patients with cirrhosis (FRISC study): a randomized controlled trial. Hepatol Int. 2021;15(4):983–94.
21. Maiwall R, Kumar A, Pasupuleti SSR, Hidam AK, Tevethia H, Kumar G, et al. A randomized-controlled trial comparing 20% albumin to plasmalyte in patients with cirrhosis and sepsis-induced hypotension [ALPS trial]. J Hepatol. 2022;77(3):670–82.
22. Wigmore GJ, Anstey JR, St John A, Greaney J, Morales-Codina M, Presneill JJ, et al. 20% human albumin solution fluid bolus administration therapy in patients after cardiac surgery (the HAS FLAIR study). J Cardiothorac Vasc Anesth. 2019;33(11):2920–7.
23. Roberts I, Blackhall K, Alderson P, Bunn F, Schierhout G. Human albumin solution for resuscitation and volume expansion in critically ill patients. Cochrane Database Syst Rev. 2011;11:CD001208.
24. Annane D, Siami S, Jaber S, Martin C, Elatrous S, Declère AD, et al. Effects of fluid resuscitation with colloids vs crystalloids on mortality in critically ill patients presenting with hypovolemic shock: the CRISTAL randomized trial. JAMA. 2013;310:1809–17.
25. Evans L, Rhodes A, Alhazzani W, Antonelli M, Coopersmith CM, French C, et al. Surviving sepsis campaign: international guidelines for Management of Sepsis and Septic Shock 2021. Crit Care Med. 2021;49(11):e1063–143.
26. Mårtensson J, Bihari S, Bannard-Smith J, Glassford NJ, Lloyd-Donald P, Cioccari L, et al. Small volume resuscitation with 20% albumin in intensive care: physiological effects : the SWIPE randomised clinical trial. Intensive Care Med. 2018;44(11):1797–806.
27. McIlroy D, Murphy D, Kasza J, Bhatia D, Wutzlhofer L, Marasco S. Effects of restricting perioperative use of intravenous chloride on kidney injury in patients undergoing cardiac surgery: the LICRA pragmatic controlled clinical trial. Intensive Care Med. 2017;43(6):795–806.
28. Nasa P, Wise R, Elbers PWG, Wong A, Dabrowski W, Regenmortel NV, et al. Intravenous fluid therapy in perioperative and critical care setting-knowledge test and practice: an international cross-sectional survey. J Crit Care. 2022;71:154122.
29. China L, Freemantle N, Forrest E, Kallis Y, Ryder SD, Wright G, et al. A randomized trial of albumin infusions in hospitalized patients with cirrhosis. N Engl J Med. 2021;384:808–17.

30. Caraceni P, Riggio O, Angeli P, Alessandria C, Neri S, Foschi FG, et al. Long-term albumin administration in decompensated cirrhosis (ANSWER): an open-label randomised trial. Lancet. 2018;391:2417–29.
31. Kütting F, Schubert J, Franklin J, Bowe A, Hoffmann V, Demir M, et al. Insufficient evidence of benefit regarding mortality due to albumin substitution in HCC-free cirrhotic patients undergoing large volume paracentesis. J Gastroenterol Hepatol. 2017;32:327–38.
32. Benmassaoud A, Freeman SC, Roccarina D, Plaz Torres MC, Sutton AJ, Cooper NJ, et al. Treatment for ascites in adults with decompensated liver cirrhosis: a network meta-analysis. Cochrane Database Syst Rev. 2020;1:CD013123.
33. Best LM, Freeman SC, Sutton AJ, Cooper NJ, Tng EL, Csenar M, et al. Treatment for hepatorenal syndrome in people with decompensated liver cirrhosis: a network meta-analysis. Cochrane Database Syst Rev. 2019;9:CD013103.
34. Salerno F, Navickis RJ, Wilkes MM. Albumin infusion improves outcomes of patients with spontaneous bacterial peritonitis: a meta-analysis of randomized trials. Clin Gastroenterol Hepatol. 2013;11(2):123–30.e1.
35. Salman TA, Edrees AM, El-Said HH, El-Abd OL, El-Azab GI. Effect of different therapeutic modalities on systemic, renal, and hepatic hemodynamics and short-term outcomes in cirrhotic patients with spontaneous bacterial peritonitis. Eur J Gastroenterol Hepatol. 2016;28(7):777–85.
36. Dubois MJ, Orellana-Jimenez C, Melot C, De Backer D, Berre J, Leeman M, et al. Albumin administration improves organ function in critically ill hypoalbuminemic patients: a prospective, randomized, controlled, pilot study. Crit Care Med. 2006;34(10):2536–40.
37. Oh SW, Han SY. Loop diuretics in clinical practice. Electrolyte Blood Press. 2015;13:17–21.
38. Cordemans C, De Laet I, Van Regenmortel N, Schoonheydt K, Dits H, Martin G, et al. Aiming for a negative fluid balance in patients with acute lung injury and increased intra-abdominal pressure: a pilot study looking at the effects of PAL-treatment. Ann Intensive Care. 2012;2(Suppl 1):S15.
39. Martin GS, Moss M, Wheeler AP, Mealer M, Morris JA, Bernard GR. A randomized, controlled trial of furosemide with or without albumin in hypoproteinemic patients with acute lung injury. Crit Care Med. 2005;33(8):1681–7.
40. SAFE Study Investigators, Australian and New Zealand Intensive Care Society clinical trials group, Australian red cross blood service, George Institute for International Health, Myburgh J, Cooper DJ, et al. Saline or albumin for fluid resuscitation in patients with traumatic brain injury. N Engl J Med. 2007;357:874–84.
41. Cooper DJ, Myburgh J, Heritier S, Finfer S, Bellomo R, Billot L, et al. Albumin resuscitation for traumatic brain injury: is intracranial hypertension the cause of increased mortality? J Neurotrauma. 2013;30(7):512–8.
42. Melia D, Post B. Human albumin solutions in intensive care: a review. J Intensive Care Soc. 2021;22(3):248–54.
43. Coz Yataco AO, Flannery AH, Simpson SQ. Counterpoint: should intravenous albumin be used for volume resuscitation in severe sepsis/septic shock? No. Chest. 2016;149(6):1368–70.
44. Joint Formulary Committee. British national formulary. 79th ed. London: BMJ Group and Pharmaceutical Press; 2020.

The Place for Starches and Other Colloids

11

Ripenmeet Salhotra, Adrian Wong, and Manu L. N. G. Malbrain

Contents

Introduction 245
Hydroxyethyl Starch 246
   Pharmacology 246
Is Hydroxyethyl Starch Beneficial? 248
Evidence in Critically Ill Patients 248
Perioperative Use of HES 253
Controversies and Restrictions on HES 254
Gelatins 254
Dextrans 255
Conclusion 256
References 256

R. Salhotra (✉)
Department of Anaesthesiology and Critical Care, Amrita Hospital, Faridabad, India

A. Wong
Intensive Care Unit, King's College Hospital, London, UK

Manu L. N. G. Malbrain
First Department of Anaesthesiology and Intensive Therapy, Medical University of Lublin, Lublin, Poland

International Fluid Academy, Lovenjoel, Belgium

Medical Data Management, Medaman, Geel, Belgium

© The Author(s) 2024
M. L. N. G. Malbrain et al. (eds.), *Rational Use of Intravenous Fluids in Critically Ill Patients*, https://doi.org/10.1007/978-3-031-42205-8_11

IFA Commentary (MLNGM)

This chapter provides a review of the different types of colloids mainly hydroxyethyl starch (HES) solutions and the differences between balanced and unbalanced starches. It tackles many questions like the never-ending crystalloid vs. colloid debate: Where are we now? Is there merely a difference in cosmetics or also in outcome? What are the strengths and flaws of the different big fluid trials and meta-analyses? Are there specific situations or patient groups where colloids behave differently and may have an advantage? This chapter will basically focus on the results of five major trials comparing the use of crystalloids versus colloids in critically ill patients: The 6S and VISEP study, the CRYSTMAS trial, the CRISTAL study, and the CHEST trial.

At the time of the First International Fluid Academy Day in November 2011, the evidence base for the use of colloids versus crystalloids in critically ill patients was rather weak. Except for the SAFE and VISEP studies, no randomized intervention studies were available. Crucially, neither of these addressed the use of the more recent lower molecular weight starch derivatives (HES 130) or the use of 'balanced' solutions. Subgroup analysis and meta-analysis indicated equipoise for most subgroups, with the exception of trauma patients where harm could be expected with the use of colloids on one side and sepsis, cardiopulmonary bypass, and malaria patients on the other side where the use of albumin might be advantageous. In the '6S study' and the 'CHEST trial', the colloid was one of the HES 130 solutions, and, while failing to find benefit of these solutions in critically ill patients, both trials indeed confirmed earlier suspicions of renal damage associated with them. The EMA's safety committee, PRAC, suspended in 2013 the use of HES solutions in critically ill, septic, and burn patients or those with kidney injury. HES solutions could only be used in the perioperative setting, e.g., haemorrhagic shock.

However, many questions and controversies remained: Is molecular weight the only parameter that counts or do we need to take into account the charge? Are smaller starches safer and is the origin of the starch (maize vs. potatoes) important? Does the buffer solution in balanced solutions (lactate, acetate, malate, etc.) matter? Do we have to fear for the kidneys and the coagulation with the latest perioperative indications for starches? Should we bother about anaphylactic reactions or prior disease when using gelatins? What to use in haemorrhagic shock: colloids or crystalloids or just blood products? However, the final curtain may fall over HES as EMA's safety committee, PRAC, has recommended in February 2022 that the marketing authorizations for HES solutions for infusion should be suspended across the European Union. This was based on new results of an ongoing safety analysis which showed that HES solutions for infusion are still being used outside the recommendations included in the product information. The committee concluded that the further restrictions introduced in 2018 have not sufficiently ensured that the medicines are used safely and that HES solutions continue to be used in certain groups of patients in whom serious harm has been demonstrated.

Learning Objectives

After reading this chapter, you will understand that:

1. Various types of colloids can be used in critically ill and perioperative patients.
2. Structures, properties, benefits, and harms of synthetic colloids are listed.
3. Evidence for use of synthetic colloids is reviewed.
4. Starches should no longer be used in critically ill patients with sepsis, burns, and kidney injury.

Case Vignette

A 74-year-old male with a past history of poorly controlled diabetes mellitus with diabetic nephropathy and coronary artery disease with severe left ventricular systolic dysfunction (global ejection fraction ~25%) was admitted to the coronary care unit with acute left ventricular failure. He was managed with medical therapy and required invasive ventilation support for the initial 2 days. On the fourth day of hospital stay, he developed fever and shortness of breath. On examination, he was a little confused with a heart rate 112/min, blood pressure 84/56 mmHg, respiratory rate 24/min, and SpO2 of 96% on 4 litres of O2. Chest X-ray showed new infiltrate in the left lower zone. Arterial blood gas revealed pH 7.36, PO2 64 mmHg, PaCO2 32.8 mmHg, HCO3 19.2 mmol/L, and lactate 4.6 mmol/L.

One of your colleagues suggested giving a bolus of 6% hydroxyethyl starch (140/0.4) for rapid correction of hypotension. He argued that the bolus of synthetic colloid will reduce the overall fluid requirement for this patient with septic shock and underlying cardiac dysfunction.

Questions

Q. What is the evidence in favour of or against the use of synthetic colloids in critically ill patients?

Introduction

Colloids, like crystalloids, are types of intravenous fluids used for resuscitation in critically ill, perioperative, or trauma patients. Colloids consist of large molecules which at least theoretically stay in the intravascular space for a longer duration before leaking into the interstitium. Colloids can be natural (e.g. human albumin, fresh frozen plasma) or synthetic (e.g. starches, gelatins, or dextran). Synthetic colloids were popular resuscitation fluids until a few years ago. However, they have lost their popularity because of increasing uncertainty about their benefit, high cost, and numerous adverse effects. In this chapter, we shall discuss various aspects of synthetic colloids including their role in current practice (Fig. 11.1). More information on crystalloid solutions can be found in Chap. 9, while albumin use is discussed in Chap. 10.

Fig. 11.1 Overview of colloids

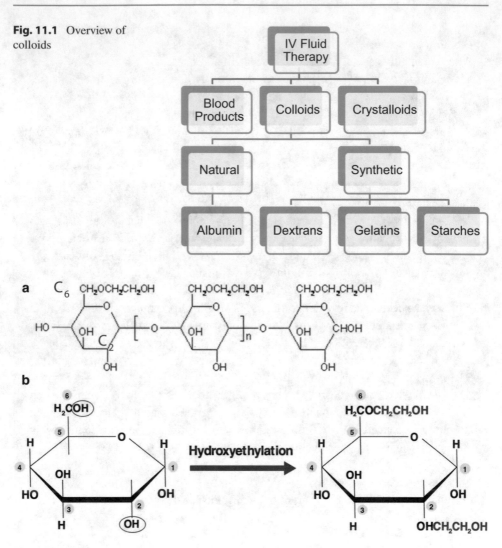

Fig. 11.2 (**a**) Schematic drawing of starch molecule. (**b**) Hydroxyethylation of starch molecule

Hydroxyethyl Starch Pharmacology

HES solutions are hydroxyethylated polysaccharides (carbohydrates) prepared from maize or potato (Fig. 11.2). The process of hydroxyethylation makes them relatively stable against degradation by alpha-amylase in serum and also increases their solubility. Typical commercially available HES product is characterized by three numbers: concentration of HES in solution (e.g. 6%), mean molecular weight (MW) (e.g. 200 kDa), and molecular substitution (MS) (e.g. 0.4) (Fig. 11.3). For example, a product labelled 6% HES 200/0.4

Fig. 11.3 Typical commercially available HES product is characterized by three numbers: concentration of HES in solution (e.g. 6%), mean molecular weight (MW) (e.g. 130 kDa), and molecular substitution (MS) (e.g. 0.42)

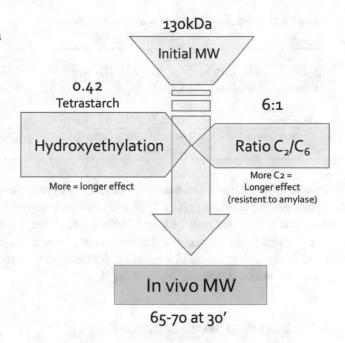

contains a 6% solution of HES of mean MW 200 kDa and a molecular substitution of 0.4. These properties influence the therapeutic profile as well as the adverse effects of a particular HES solution.

HES solutions are a polydisperse system consisting of particles of different molecular mass. The MW of a particular product denotes the average of these diversely sized particles. Osmotic effectiveness depends on the number of particles and not size and hence MW has little impact on the volume expanding effect of the solution. The concentration of HES in a solution determines the oncotic property of a particular HES solution. Commonly available concentrations are 6% and 10% which make them iso-oncotic and hyperoncotic, respectively. MS describes the degree of hydroxyethyl substitution per glucose unit. The higher the substitution, the more resistant it is to degradation by alpha-amylase and hence the longer the plasma retention time. Another chemical property is the C2/C6 ratio which is generally omitted from the product name (Fig. 11.3). It is the ratio of hydroxyethyl substitution at C2 and C6 carbon atoms of glucose subunit [1]. Greater hydroxyethylation at C2 inhibits degradation and hence a higher ratio leads to longer plasma retention. However, longer persistence in plasma may not necessarily mean a better volume effect. Newer or third-generation HES solutions have lower MS and MW resulting in more rapid metabolism and clearance and fewer adverse effects without loss of efficacy. Finally, the carrier solution can influence the adverse effects of some HES solutions. Different combinations of these three parameters account for a wide variety of commercially available products as depicted in Table 11.1.

In total, 30 to 40% of HES is eliminated renally and the remaining may be stored in tissues. Being a polydisperse solution, the smallest particles (< 60–70 kDa) are quickly

Table 11.1 Available HES solutions and composition

Parameter.	Types available	Effect
Concentration	6%,10%	Iso-oncotic, hyperoncotic
Molecular weight (MW)	130, 200, 450, 600, 670	Not significant
Molecular substitution (MS)	0.4, 0.5, 0.6, 0.7	Plasma retention time, adverse effects
C2/C6 ratio	4.5:1, 5:1, 9:1, 6:1, 3:1	
Carrier solution	Normal saline, balanced solutions	Adverse effects, acid–base status

excreted. Larger molecules are first broken down by alpha-amylase into smaller fragments before getting excreted renally. HES molecules are also phagocytosed by the reticuloendothelial system and may be found in the liver, spleen, kidneys, and bone marrow even after several years. Its deposition in cutaneous nerves is the cause of pruritus that may be debilitating and quite often long-lasting. Similarly, deposition in renal tubular cells is the cause of osmotic nephrosis like lesions [2].

Is Hydroxyethyl Starch Beneficial?

In the past, it was thought that colloids are 3–4 times more effective than crystalloids for restoring intravascular volume. This assumption was based on Starling's equation which states that maintenance of intravascular volume depends on the balance between plasma oncotic pressures and hydrostatic pressure. More recently, Starling's principle has been challenged after the discovery of the subendothelial glycocalyx layer and a revised Starling's equation has been proposed (described in greater detail in Chap. 2) [3]. In the 6S trial, the ratio of crystalloid to colloid to achieve the similar hemodynamic goal was 1.06 [4]. In the CHEST trial, the similar ratio was 1.17 [5]. Overall, resuscitation with HES requires somewhat less volume of fluid compared to crystalloid. But the benefit of this lesser volume requirement on patient outcomes remains less clear. In contrast, the association of HES with several adverse effects like renal injury, bleeding, pruritus, and allergic reactions is well established. In the following sections, we shall discuss available evidence from clinical trials on HES.

Evidence in Critically Ill Patients

Three large multicentre investigator-initiated randomized controlled trials (RCTs) demonstrated increased renal failure associated with starches in critically ill and septic patients [4, 5, 6]. In the VISEP trial,10% HES (200/0.5) in normal saline as the carrier solution was compared with lactated Ringer's solution for resuscitation of patients with severe sepsis

[6]. The trial was terminated after enrolling 600 patients as there was a trend towards increased 90-day mortality in the HES group. As expected, the total fluid required was less in HES group. There was a trend towards increased 28-day mortality (primary outcome) in the HES group, but it did not reach statistical significance. Higher cumulative doses of HES was clearly associated with an increase in 90-day mortality. Other secondary outcome measures like the incidence of acute kidney injury (AKI), the need for renal replacement therapy (RRT), and the need for red blood cell transfusion were significantly higher in the HES group. The trial was criticized for its two-by-two factorial (patients were simultaneously randomized for tight vs. conventional glucose control arm) and open-label design, use of more harmful pentastarch, and use of 0.9% saline as the carrier which may itself cause renal injury.

In the 6S trial, 798 patients with severe sepsis were randomized to receive either 6% HES (130/0.42) in Ringer's acetate or Ringer's acetate as resuscitation fluid [4]. The primary outcome, a composite of death or dependence on RRT at 90 days, was significantly higher in the HES group. Compared to Ringer's acetate, patients in the HES group also had significantly higher mortality at 90 days (51% vs. 43%). A significantly higher percentage of patients in the HES group required RRT during study period (22% vs. 16%). RRT-free and hospital-free days at 90 days were significantly lower in the HES group. However, 28-day mortality and the incidence of severe bleeding or allergic reactions were not different between the two groups. In the pre-specified subgroup analysis, the deleterious effects of HES were significant only in patients with septic shock at enrolment.

The CHEST trial, the largest of the HES trials, randomized 7000 patients admitted to ICU requiring fluid resuscitation (unlike only severe sepsis patients included by the previous trials) to receive either 6% HES (130/0.4) in 0.9% saline or 0.9% saline [5]. Primary outcome, i.e. mortality at 90 days, was not different between the HES group and the saline group (18% vs. 17%). However, more patients in the HES group had worsened renal outcome (higher RIFLE-R and RIFLE-I class but similar RIFLE-F class) and required RRT (7% vs. 5.8%). Interestingly, the incidence of new cardiovascular failure during study period was lower in the HES group. Patients in the HES group also received less study or non-study fluid, and the positive net fluid balance was significantly lower in the HES group compared to saline (921 ml vs. 982 ml).

Some experts argue that the aforementioned trials lacked a rational protocol for fluid therapy. Indication for fluid therapy included static parameters like central venous pressure (CVP) and none of these trials used dynamic parameters for fluid responsiveness (described in more detail in Chap. 5). Randomization happened late after ICU admission, possibly in the 'stabilization' phase of fluid therapy, missing the early 'resuscitation' phase (see ROSE concept described in Chap. 25). This is illustrated in Fig. 11.4. This is supported by the fact that mean CVP was 12 mmHg in VISEP and about 9 mmHg in the CHEST trial at baseline. About 40% of patients in both groups of the 6S trial had already received between 500 ml and 700 ml synthetic colloids prior to randomization, and in the VISEP trial patients had received a median of 2 litres of crystalloids and 850 ml of colloids

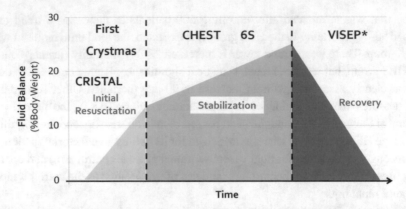

Fig. 11.4 Timeline vs. fluid balance expressed as a percentage of body weight. In the VISEP study, colloids were still administered late in the course of the disease

in 12 hours preceding randomization. Besides, resuscitation fluids could be administered from 21 to 90 days after randomization [4, 5, 6]. Thus, these trials might have ended up administering HES to 'non-hypovolemic' patients who should not have received fluids in the first place.

In the multicentre CRISTAL trial, 2857 patients of hypovolemic shock were randomized to receive either colloid (HES and gelatins, dextrans, or 4% or 20% of albumin) or crystalloid (isotonic or hypertonic saline or Ringer's lactate solution) for all fluid interventions other than fluid maintenance throughout the ICU stay [7]. The primary outcome (28-day mortality) was not different between the two groups. However, 90-day mortality and the use of RRT were significantly lower and mechanical ventilation–/vasopressor-free days at day 28 were significantly higher in the colloid group. The biggest strength of the trial was that it included patients in the very early phase of disease process. HES was given only on days zero to two of ICU admission and the median cumulative dose of HES was only 1500 ml, much less than in trials just described. However, the trial had its own flaws that cannot be ignored. Clinicians were free to use the colloid of their choice including HES, albumin, or gelatins, the trial was open-label, the recruitment period lasted unusually long (nine years), and like other trials subjects received substantial amounts of colloids before randomization.

To conclude evidence does exist for harm from the use of HES in critically ill and septic patients. Additional research is needed to establish or refute the role of 'early and limited' use of HES in 'initial' resuscitation of critically ill patients. Till that time, it is reasonable to avoid the use of HES for resuscitation of critically ill patients (especially patients with sepsis).

The importance for attention to detail is exemplified by the fact that commentaries in scientific journals and lectures at scientific meetings dealing with the major fluid trials often cite information only contained in the appendices of the original publications. Given the frequent emotional nature of the debate on this subject, this phenomenon might ironically be termed 'appendicitis' [8]. The appendices are indeed necessary for accurate interpretation of data. The population, intervention, comparator, and outcome (PICO) method was applied on the two highly cited 6S and CHEST trials on fluid therapy in critically ill patients. The analysis shows that, going over all PICO criteria, the main text of both publications provide insufficient information (Table 11.2).

Table 11.2 Analysis of the 6S and CHEST trials using the population, intervention, comparator, and outcome (PICO) method

Patients	6S	CHEST
N	804	7000
Setting	ICU, Scandinavia	ICU, Australia and New Zealand
Inclusion criteria	Patients requiring fluid resuscitation in the ICU fulfilling the criteria of severe sepsis during the preceding 24 hours. Severe sepsis (100%). Definition of severe sepsis: Sepsis (focus of infection and at least two SIRS criteria) and at least one organ failure. Excluded were patients with intracranial haemorrhage or renal replacement therapy	Patients requiring fluid resuscitation over and above that required for maintenance. Hypovolaemia in medical and surgical ICU patients; sepsis in 29.2% and 28.4% of patients, respectively. Excluded were patients after cardiac surgery or with intracranial haemorrhage
Age and sex	66–67 years; 60–61% male	63 years; 60% male
Illness severity at baseline	Median SAPS II score 50 and 51, respectively; mechanical ventilation in 60 and 61% of patients, respectively; acute kidney injury in 36 and 35% of patients, respectively	Apache II score 17; mechanical ventilation in 64.1 and 64.9% of patients, respectively; no patients with impending or current renal failure
Vital signs at baseline	'Shock' (mean arterial pressure < 70 mmHg, need for inopressors, or serum lactate > 4 mmol/L < 1 h before randomization), in 84% of patients. CVP 10 mmHg; ScvO2 75 and 73%, respectively; serum lactate 2.0 and 2.1 mmol/L, respectively; arterial hypertension in 39% of patients	Heart rate 89 bpm; mean arterial pressure 74 mmHg; CVP 9.5 and 8.9 mmHg, respectively; serum lactate 2.1 and 2.0 mmol/L, respectively
Non-trial fluids before randomization	Median amounts of 3500 and 3000 mL in 96 and 97% of patients, respectively	Not specifically reported; included in 'day 0' = day of randomization. Excluded were patients having had received >1000 mL HES before screening
Blood products before randomization	Median amounts of 838 and 600 mL in 23 and 22% of patients, respectively	Not specifically reported; included in 'day 0' = day of randomization

(continued)

Table 11.2 (continued)

Patients	6S	CHEST
Synthetic colloids before randomization	Median amounts of 700 and 500 mL in 42% of patients, respectively	HES in 15% of patients
Time from admission to randomization	Medians of 3.7 and 4.0 h, respectively	Mean 10.9 ± 156.5 and 11.4 ± 165.4 h, respectively
Intervention	6S	CHEST
Fluid	6% HES with molecular weight of 130 kDa, and substitution ratio of 0.42. Na + 140 m Mol/L, K+ 4 mmol/L, ca++ 2.5 mmol/L, mg++ 1.0 mmol/L, cl- 118 mmol/L, malate 5 mmol/L, acetate 24.0 mmol/L	6% HES with molecular weight 130 kDa, and substitution ratio of 0.42. Na + 154 mmol/L, cl- 154 mmol/L
Indication	Hypovolaemia as perceived by clinical judgment	Hypovolaemia as perceived by clinical judgment +1 physiological criterion (i.e. heart rate > 90 bpm, systolic or mean arterial pressure < 100 or < 75 mmHg, respectively, CVP < 10 mmHg, PAOP < 12 mm hg, respiratory pressure variation > 5 mmHg, capillary refill time > 1 s, urine output 0.5) ml/kg)
Maximum dose and duration	33/ml/kg/d IBW, 90 days	50 ml/kg BW/d, 90 days
Comparator	6S	CHEST
Fluid	Na+ 145 mmol/L, K+ 4 mmol/L, Ca2+ 2.5 mmol/L, Mg2+ 1.0 mmol/L, cl- 127 mmol/L, malate 5 mmol/L, acetate 24 mmol/L	Na + 154 mmol/L, cl- 154 mmol/L
Outcomes	6S	CHEST
Primary outcome	Composite death or dependence on dialysis 90 days after randomization	All-cause mortality 90 days after randomization
Modified intension-to-treat analysis primary outcome	Dead at 90 days: HES vs. comparator, RR 1.17 (1.01–1.36), $p = 0.03$. Survival time censored at 90 days: $p = 0.07$	Death at 90 days: HES vs. comparator, RR 1.06 (0.96–1.18), $p = 0.26$. Survival time censored at 90 days: $p = 0.27$
Per-protocol analyses primary outcome	Death at 90 days: Per-protocol analysis 1: HES vs. comparator, RR 1.14 (0.97–1.34), $p = 0.12$. Per-protocol analysis 2: HES vs. comparator, RR 1.16 (0.97–1.37), $p = 0.07$	Death at 90 days if sepsis at randomization: RR 1.07 (0.92–1.25), $p = 0.38$. Death at 90 days, adjusted: RR 1.05 (0.95–1.16), $p = 0.33$
Secondary outcome	Renal replacement therapy	Renal replacement therapy

Table 11.2 (continued)

Patients	6S	CHEST
Modified intension-to-treat analysis secondary outcome	HES vs. comparator: RR 1.35 (1.01–1.80), $p = 0.04$	HES vs. comparator: RR 1.21 (1.00–1.45), $p = 0.04$. Adjusted: RR 1.20 (1.00–1.44), $p = 0.05$
Trial fluid	Day 1: Median amount of 1500 mL Days 1–3: Median amount of 4000 mL	Day 1: Mean amount of approx. 480 and 570 mL, respectively. Days 0–3: 2104 and 2464 mL, respectively
ICU fluid balance	Median amounts 5452 and 4616 mL, respectively	Days 0–3: Mean amounts of approx. 3120 and 3340, respectively
Circulatory variables at 24 h after randomization	CVP 11 and 10 mmHg, respectively; ScvO2 75 and 73%, respectively; serum lactate 2.0 mmol/L	Heart rate 87 bpm; mean arterial pressure 81 mmHg; CVP approx. 10.5 and 11.5, respectively; serum lactate approx. 1.5 mmol/L

Bold text indicates information that is only available in the appendix or in the legend of figures. Adapted with permission from Priebe et al. According to the Open Access CC BY Licence 4.0 [8].

Perioperative Use of HES

The settings of trauma and surgery are different from that of septic shock as they are not associated with the disruption of capillary glycocalyx to as great an extent as sepsis, burn, or pancreatitis with probably less leaky capillaries. This may offer an advantage to colloids like HES, perhaps producing a similar haemodynamic effect (compared to crystalloid) with lesser volume. In fact, most perioperative studies examining the goal-directed therapy (GDT) approach to fluid therapy used colloids – specifically HES. The GDT approach involves the use of invasive haemodynamic monitoring and giving fluids to reach a predetermined goal, for example, a stroke volume variation (SVV) of less than 10%. HES was compared to crystalloids in a recent trial of the GDT approach to fluid management in elective abdominal surgery [9]. Total intraoperative fluid and net fluid balance were significantly lower in the HES group. The HES group also had significantly lower postoperative morbidity score and lower incidence of postoperative complications. Authors attributed the beneficial effect of HES to the decrease in total intraoperative fluid administered. No renal adverse effects were noted even on long-term (up to 1 year) follow-up of the patients [10]. However, two other smaller RCTs on abdominal surgery patients didn't find any benefit or harm associated with use of HES [11, 12]. In addition, several meta-analyses failed to suggest any difference in outcome either benefit or associated harm (including nephrotoxicity) [13, 14] .

To conclude, there is no evidence to suggest harm associated with the use of hydroxyethyl starch in perioperative settings. However, in the absence of definite benefit and substantial cost involved, the use of HES cannot be strongly recommended even in this setting.

Controversies and Restrictions on HES

Between the year 2008 and 2012, several large multicentre randomized controlled trials indicated that HES increased the risk of renal failure requiring renal replacement therapy and death in critically ill patients in general and septic patients in particular [4, 5, 6]. By 2012, investigations were initiated by the U.S. Food and Drug Administration (U.S. FDA) and European Medicines Agency (EMA) pertaining to the safety of HES. In October 2013, EMA concluded that HES should no longer be used in patients with sepsis or burn injury or in critically ill patients; however, it can be prescribed to patients with hypovolaemia due to acute blood loss if treatment with crystalloids was inadequate. HES could still be used in surgical and trauma patients. The EMA also stated that no more than 30 ml/kg of HES should be administered and kidney function of patients receiving HES should be monitored. The U.S. FDA also issued a black box warning regarding the use of HES in November 2013. It prohibited the use of HES in critically ill patients and patients with sepsis, severe liver disease, and pre-existing coagulopathy.

Based on the studies conducted by the agencies suggesting widespread non-compliance to restrictions imposed on the use of HES including its use in prohibited (critically ill, sepsis) settings, EMA initiated a proposal in 2017 to ban HES completely. However, several experts argued against the complete ban on HES. They felt that the complete ban is potentially hazardous as this would lead to unmet medical needs with scarce and costly alternatives (i.e. albumin) [15]. Afterwards, the proposal to completely withdraw HES was withheld by the European Commission and HES continued to be available with restrictions and warnings imposed since 2013. However, the final curtain may fall over HES as EMA's safety committee, PRAC, has recommended in February 2022 that the marketing authorizations for HES solutions for infusion should be suspended across the European Union. This was based on new results of an ongoing safety analysis which showed that HES solutions for infusion are still being used outside the recommendations included in the product information. The committee concluded that the further restrictions introduced in 2018 have not sufficiently ensured that the medicines are used safely and that HES solutions continue to be used in certain groups of patients in whom serious harm has been demonstrated.

Gelatins

Gelatins are polypeptides derived from bovine collagen. Gelatin particles are smaller than other synthetic colloids (average MW 35000 Da) and therefore have a shorter clinical effect. Commonly available gelatin products are urea cross-linked (e.g. Haemaccel, originally marketed by Hoechst AG) and succinylated or modified fluid gelatins (e.g. Gelofusine, B. Braun Medical). The capacity of gelatin for plasma expansion, expressed by a mean crystalloid to colloid ratio of 1.4, is also not different from other colloids.

In a recent meta-analysis, including both randomized and non-randomized animal and human trials, comparing gelatin with crystalloids and albumin found that gelatin is associated with an increase in the risk of anaphylaxis (more than threefold), AKI, need for RRT, and need for blood transfusion [16]. There was also a trend towards increased mortality in the gelatin group though not statistically significant. However, a recent Cochrane systematic review failed to substantiate these findings [17]. Results of an ongoing trial on gelatin are awaited [18].

Gelatins are not approved for use by the U.S. FDA since 1978 due to its association with deranged coagulation parameters and prolonged bleeding time. Concerns over adverse effects, doubtful benefits, and short clinical effects lead several guidelines (including Surviving Sepsis Campaign) to recommend crystalloids over gelatins for fluid resuscitation.

Dextrans

Dextrans are a mixture of glucose polymers of various sizes. They are derived from the bacteria named *Leuconostoc mesenteroides* and have an average MWs of 40 kDa and 70 kDa. The formulations commonly available are 10% dextran-40 and 6% dextran-70. Following intravenous administration, dextran is almost exclusively eliminated by the kidneys except for a small fraction eliminated via the gastrointestinal tract. The length of time that dextran stays in the intravascular compartment is dependent on particle size. Approximately 60% to 70% of dextran-40 is cleared within 5 h. Dextran-70 has a duration of action of 6–8 h [19].

Dextrans are used to improve blood rheologic properties and for decreasing blood viscosity and indirectly to improve microcirculatory flow after vascular surgery. There is little evidence to support dextran as a resuscitation fluid. Moreover, dextrans cause more anaphylactic reactions than gelatins or starches and their use is also associated with renal failure and impaired coagulation.

Case Vignette

The patient in the case vignette is in septic shock (due to hospital-acquired pneumonia), and fluid resuscitation is indicated in view of hypotension and poor perfusion. Though giving a bolus of HES may lead to faster resolution with lesser volume, it now becomes clear that this leads to worse outcomes as strong evidence exists that the use of HES in sepsis may lead to kidney injury and increased mortality. Both the EMA and U.S. FDA forbid the use of HES in this setting. The case is more or less similar for other synthetic colloids. Balanced crystalloids remain the fluid of choice in septic shock, and if the need to use a colloid is inevitable albumin remains an option, especially at a later stage.

Conclusion

On May 24, 2022, the European Commission issued a legal decision confirming the suspension of the marketing authorizations of HES solutions for infusion. If necessary for public health reasons, individual EU member states may delay the suspension for no longer than 18 months and keep HES solutions on the market, subject to agreed risk minimization measures. Outside of the EU, as of now, the use of HES and other synthetic colloids should be restricted to resuscitation in perioperative setting or maybe in trauma settings in limited volumes (30 ml/kg) and with extreme caution.

Take-Home Messages
- The natural colloid albumin and several synthetic colloids are at the disposal of the acute care physician.
- Though marginally lesser volume of colloids produces similar hemodynamic effect, it has not resulted in any outcome benefit in clinical trials.
- The synthetic colloid HES is associated with renal failure and increased use of renal replacement therapy in critically ill and septic patients and its use remains restricted by several regulatory authorities across the world.
- HES solutions cannot be used in patients with sepsis, burns, and (acute) kidney injury and have recently been suspended in the ICU.
- Use of synthetic colloids in perioperative patients is unsafe as strong evidence showing their superiority over crystalloids is lacking.
- When given (outside the ICU) in the peri- and postoperative phase, the dose should be limited to 30 ml/kg.

References

1. Jung F, Koscielny J, Mrowietz C, Förster H, Schimetta W, Kiesewetter H, Wenzel E. The effect of molecular structure of hydroxyethyl starch on the elimination kinetics and fluidity of blood in human volunteers. Arzneimittelforschung. 1993;43:99–105.
2. Dickenmann M, Oettl T, Mihatsch MJ. Osmotic nephrosis: acute kidney injury with accumulation of proximal tubular lysosomes due to administration of exogenous solutes. Am J Kidney Dis. 2008;51(3):491–503.
3. Levick JR, Michel CC. Microvascular fluid exchange and the revised starling principle. Cardiovasc Res. 2010;87(2):198–210.
4. Perner A, Haase N, Guttormsen AB, Tenhunen J, Klemenzson G, Aneman A, et al. Hydroxyethyl starch 130/0.42 versus Ringer's acetate in severe sepsis. N Engl J Med. 2012;367:124–34.
5. Myburgh JA, Finfer S, Bellomo R, Billot L, Cass A, Gattas D, et al. Hydroxyethyl starch or saline for fluid resuscitation in intensive care. N Engl J Med. 2012;367:1901–11.
6. Brunkhorst FM, Engel C, Bloos F, Meier-Hellmann A, Ragaller M, Weiler N, et al. Intensive insulin therapy and pentastarch resuscitation in severe sepsis. N Engl J Med. 2008;358:125–39.

7. Annane D, Siami S, Jaber S, Martin C, Elatrous S, Declère AD, et al. Effects of fl uid resuscitation with colloids vs crystalloids on mortality in critically ill patients presenting with hypovolemic shock: the CRISTAL randomized trial. JAMA. 2013;310(17):1809–17.
8. Priebe HJ, Malbrain ML, Elbers P. The great fluid debate: methodology, physiology and appendicitis. Anaesthesiol Intensive Ther. 2015;47(5):437–40.
9. Joosten A, Delaporte A, Ickx B, Touihri K, Stany I, Barvais L, et al. Crystalloid versus colloid for intraoperative goal-directed fluid therapy using a closed-loop system: a randomized, double-blinded, controlled trial in major abdominal surgery. Anesthesiology. 2018;128(1):55–66.
10. Joosten A, Delaporte A, Mortier J, Ickx B, Van Obbergh L, Vincent JL, et al. Long-term impact of crystalloid versus colloid solutions on renal function and disability-free survival after major abdominal surgery. Anesthesiology. 2019;130(2):227–36.
11. Yates DR, Davies SJ, Milner HE, Wilson RJ. Crystalloid or colloid for goal-directed fluid therapy in colorectal surgery. Br J Anaesth. 2014;112:281–9.
12. Feldheiser A, Pavlova V, Bonomo T, Jones A, Fotopoulou C, Sehouli J, Wernecke KD, Spies C. Balanced crystalloid compared with balanced colloid solution using a goal-directed haemodynamic algorithm. Br J Anaesth. 2013;110:231–40.
13. Raiman M, Mitchell CG, Biccard BM, Rodseth RN. Comparison of hydroxyethyl starch colloids with crystalloids for surgical patients: a systematic review and meta-analysis. Eur J Anaesthesiol. 2016;33(1):42–8.
14. Gillies MA, Habicher M, Jhanji S, Sander M, Mythen M, Hamilton M, Pearse RM. Incidence of postoperative death and acute kidney injury associated with i.v. 6% hydroxyethyl starch use: systematic review and meta-analysis. Br J Anaesth. 2014;112(1):25–34.
15. Annane D, Fuchs-Buder T, Zoellner C, Kaukonen M, Scheeren TWL. EMA recommendation to suspend HES is hazardous. Lancet. 2018;391:736–8.
16. Moeller C, Fleischmann C, Thomas-Rueddel D, Vlasakov V, Rochwerg B, Theurer P, et al. How safe is gelatin? A systematic review and meta-analysis of gelatin-containing plasma expanders vs crystalloids and albumin. J Crit Care. 2016;35:75–83.
17. Lewis SR, Pritchard MW, Evans DJ, Butler AR, Alderson P, Smith AF, Roberts I. Colloids versus crystalloids for fluid resuscitation in critically ill people. Cochrane Database Syst Rev. 2018;8:CD000567.
18. Marx G. Gelatin in ICU and sepsis (GENIUS). Available online at https://clinicaltrials.gov/ct2/show/NCT02715466
19. Svensén C, Hahn RG. Volume kinetics of ringer solution, dextran 70 and hypertonic saline in male volunteers. Anesthesiology. 1997;87:204–12.

How to Use Blood and Blood Products

12

Kapil Dev Soni and Rahul Chaurasia

Contents

Introduction 261
Anemia and Red Cell Administration 262
Age of RBC and Transfusion Outcomes 265
Thrombocytopenia and Platelet Transfusion 266
Coagulopathy and Plasma Transfusion 267
Adverse Transfusion Reactions in Critical Care 269
Alternatives to Transfusion 270
Conclusion 271
References 272

> **IFA Commentary (MLNGM)**
> Blood transfusions are an integral part of treatment in the critical care setting. Like any other medical interventions, transfusions are also associated with serious adverse reactions which may affect patient outcomes. Evidence from various RCTs show that adhering to a restrictive RBC transfusion strategy is more beneficial than liberal transfusion strategies. The age of the transfused RBCs shows minimal to no effect on patient outcomes. Similarly, plasma and platelet components are also

K. D. Soni (✉)
Critical and Intensive Care, JPN Apex Trauma Center, All India Institute of Medical Sciences, New Delhi, India

R. Chaurasia
Department of Transfusion Medicine, All India Institute of Medical Sciences, New Delhi, India

© The Author(s) 2024
M. L. N. G. Malbrain et al. (eds.), *Rational Use of Intravenous Fluids in Critically Ill Patients*, https://doi.org/10.1007/978-3-031-42205-8_12

recommended by experts and guidelines for therapeutic purposes or prophylactically prior to any intervention or prevention of life-threatening bleeding. Point-of-care tests such as thromboelastography (TEG) or rotational thromboelastometry (ROTEM) are useful aids in guiding transfusion therapy. Use of transfusion alternatives such as erythropoietin and tranexamic acid reduce the overall need for blood transfusions and hence the associated adverse effect.

In hemorrhagic shock, the macrocirculation, microcirculation, and tissue perfusion are impaired due to massive blood loss. Infusion strategy aims at restoring the volume of the intravascular space and, thereby, facilitating oxygen transport. The clinical questions include indication and differential indication of crystalloid and colloid fluids, clinical targets, and dosing. Intravenous fluids are required in order to restore microcirculation and to prevent organ dysfunction and death in massive bleeding. Deliberate hypotension is recommended in uncontrolled hemorrhage. In uncontrolled hemorrhage in general, pre-warmed fluids should be administered in order to prevent hypothermia-dependent coagulation disturbance. In hemorrhagic shock with lactate acidosis, additional hyperchloremic acidosis due to saline-based infusions should be avoided by the use of chlorine-balanced solutions.

Various crystalloid and colloid solutions are available. In a theoretical pathophysiology-driven approach, crystalloids are indicated to replace extravascular deficits and colloids are indicated for intravascular volume replacement. The use of crystalloids only cannot fulfill a pathophysiology-driven fluid strategy because of high volume loss into the interstitial compartment. Historically, in countries with predominant crystalloid resuscitation, coagulation management was based on a 1:1:1 ratio concept of red blood cell concentrates vs. fresh frozen plasma (FFP) vs. platelet concentrates. Ratio-based transfusion regimens deliver relevant amounts of volume (three components together about 600 ml). The volume expanding capacity of the 8.5% protein solution in FFP, however, is unknown. Albumin is used in some countries as an endogenous colloidal solution in massive bleeding but both FFP and albumin also have their disadvantages, risks, and costs.

Coagulation factor concentrate-based coagulation management delivers procoagulant activity in small carrier solutions (50 ml), and synthetic colloids with a context-sensitive volume expanding effect of around 100% are often used in this setting. Synthetic colloids, however, may aggravate bleeding by inducing intravascular dilutional coagulopathy. Accordingly, maximum doses need to be considered. In acute bleeding, the endothelial barrier is suggested to be intact.

Fluid strategy in hemorrhagic shock is heterogeneous (from liberal to restrictive) throughout countries and continents. Studies comparing traditional regimens are warranted. In a pathophysiology-based concept, balanced crystalloids plus colloids are given individualized according to metabolic (and preload) parameters with monitoring for (dilutional) coagulopathy and active avoidance of overdosing and hypervolemia.

Learning Objectives

The learning objectives of this chapter are:

1. To list the indications for red blood cell (RBC) transfusions in various subgroups of critically ill patients.
2. To assess the effect of the age of RBC on patient outcomes.
3. To review the indications for platelet transfusion in critically ill patients.
4. To explain the role of plasma transfusion in coagulopathic, critically ill patients.
5. To list the frequently encountered and serious transfusion reactions in ICU.
6. To discuss alternatives to blood transfusions.

Case Vignette

Mr. G, a 34-year-old male, presented to the emergency department with a road traffic injury. On arrival, he was conscious but agitated with heart rate of 150 beats per min, respiratory rate of 30 breaths per minute, and blood pressure of 80/50 mmHg. He was immediately put on oxygen. Two large-bore IV lines were placed and a liter of crystalloid solution was started. Massive transfusion protocol was initiated. Further examination revealed pelvic fracture and hemoperitoneum. He underwent exploratory laparotomy, which revealed splenic laceration and retroperitoneal hematoma. Splenectomy was performed with approximately 3 liters of blood loss. The patient was transferred to ICU with vasopressor support and ongoing packed red blood cell (PRBC) transfusion.

Questions

Q1. What are the indications for blood and its components in ICU?
Q2. Does the age of RBCs matter?
Q3. What is the management of coagulopathy in critical illness?
Q4. What are the adverse effects of blood transfusion?

Introduction

Blood transfusions are administered in over half of all patients admitted to ICU. The decision to transfuse blood and blood components in the ICU setting is often determined by present need and the underlying comorbidities in the patient. However, it is now more evident that adverse consequences of blood transfusions are common in ICU. Thus, it is necessary to balance the risks and the benefits, before the decision is made. Evidence-based practice in the ICU can provide valuable guidance in these situations. In this chapter, we discuss the available evidence for blood transfusion in various subgroups of critically ill patients. We will also address other common issues pertaining to the transfusion of blood and blood components that can affect the outcomes in these patients.

Anemia and Red Cell Administration

It is estimated that approximately 25% of patients admitted to the ICU are anemic at the time of presentation, whereas nearly 40% of patients become anemic (Hb <9 g/dl) during the course of their ICU stay [1, 2]. Anemia in critical illness results from factors such as blood loss, hemodilution, and decreased production and/or increased destruction of red blood cells (RBC). In these patients, RBC transfusion is most commonly performed for immediate correction of anemia with the aim to improve oxygen-carrying capacity and thus tissue oxygenation. However, RBCs are also transfused to promote hemostasis through its rheological effect. This effects allows the RBCs to preferentially move towards the center of blood vessel, causing margination of platelets and plasma, ensuring improved hemostasis [3].

Traditionally, the trigger for RBC transfusion is Hb <10 g/dL or hematocrit level < 30%, known as the 10/30 rule. Although RBC transfusions can often be lifesaving in the critically ill, there is an increasing body of evidence that it is associated with increased risk of infection, hospital stay, acute lung injury, multiple-organ failure, and mortality in a dose-dependent manner. In 1998, a national survey among critical care physicians in Canada demonstrated significant variations in transfusion thresholds, highlighting the need for randomized controlled trials to determine the optimal transfusion strategy in critically ill patients [4]. This was followed by the TRICC trial, where Hebert and colleagues compared transfusion with trigger Hb of 10 to 12 g/dl (liberal strategy) with a more restrictive strategy for transfusion at a trigger Hb of 7 to 9 g/dl in critically ill patients [5]. The authors observed that while the outcome, measured as 30-day mortality, was similar in both groups (18.7 percent vs. 23.3%, $p = 0.11$), the restrictive transfusion strategy was associated with a significant decrease in the number of patients being transfused as well as the total number of units transfused during the study period. The results from TRICC favored restrictive transfusion strategies and elucidated potential harm with the liberal transfusion strategy. But its generalizability to various subgroups of critically ill patients remains controversial. Until further evidence becomes available, we believe we can safely set a transfusion threshold of 7 g/dl in a stable patient without comorbidities and 10 g/dl for bleeding patients and those with active myocardial ischemia. The results of the RCTs looking at different subgroups of critically ill patients are summarized in Table 12.1.

Table 12.1 Randomized trials comparing liberal versus restrictive transfusion strategies in different subgroups of critically ill patients

Study	Clinical settings	No of patients	Groups (trigger)	Outcome
Transfusion requirements in septic shock (TRISS) [6]	ICU patients with septic shock	998	High, Hb ≤9 g/dl Vs. low, Hb ≤7 g/dl	• No significant difference in mortality rates at 90 days. • Significant decrease in number of patients transfused and total number of units transfused.
Villanueva et al. [7]	Patients with acute upper gastrointestinal bleeding	921	Liberal Hb ≤9 g/dl Vs. restrictive Hb ≤7 g/dl	• Significant decrease in mortality at 45 days in the restrictive strategy. • Significant decrease in number of patients transfused and total number of units transfused.
Transfusion in Gastrointestinal Bleeding (TRIGGER) trial [8]	Patients with acute upper Gastrointestinal bleeding	936	Liberal; Hb <10.0 g/dl Vs. restrictive; Hb <8.0 g/dl	• No significant difference in bleeding, thromboembolic or ischemic events, infections, and 28-day mortality. • Significant decrease in number of patients transfused.
Liberal or restrictive transfusion in high-risk patients after hip surgery (FOCUS) [9]	Patients aged ≥50 years after hip fracture surgery with History or risk factors for cardiovascular disease	2016	Liberal, Hb <10.0 g/dl, Vs. restrictive, Hb <8.0 g/dl	• No significant difference in terms of 30-day mortality or inability to walk independently on 60-day follow-up. • Significant decrease in number of patients transfused.

(continued)

Table 12.1 (continued)

Study	Clinical settings	No of patients	Groups (trigger)	Outcome
Transfusion Requirements In frail elderly (TRIFE) [10]	Patients ≥65 years of age post hip fracture surgery	284	Liberal, Hb <11.3 g/dl, Vs. restrictive, Hb <9.7 g/dl	• No significant difference in repeated measures of daily living activities or mortality at 90 days. • Significant reduction in median number of units transfused per patient. • Higher 30-day mortality in restrictive group as per protocol.
Transfusion Requirements After cardiac Surgery (TRACS) [11]	Patients undergoing cardiac surgery	502	Liberal, maintain HCT ≥30% vs. restrictive, maintain HCT ≥24%	• No significant reduction in all-cause mortality at 30 days and severe morbidity. • Significant decrease in number of patients transfused. • Number of units transfused was an independent risk factor for clinical complications/mortality at 30 days.
Transfusion Indication Threshold Reduction (TITRe2) [12]	Patients (≥16 years) undergoing cardiac surgery	2007	Liberal, Hb ≤9 g/dl, Vs. restrictive, Hb ≤7.5 g/dl	• No significant difference in development of serious infection, ischemic event, myocardial infarction, infarction of the gut, or acute kidney injury at three months. • Significant decrease in number of patients transfused.

Table 12.1 (continued)

Study	Clinical settings	No of patients	Groups (trigger)	Outcome
Transfusion Requirements In surgical Oncology Patients [13]	Adult cancer patients undergoing major abdominal surgery	198	Liberal, Hb ≤9 g/dl, Vs. restrictive, Hb ≤7.0 g/dl	• A liberal transfusion strategy had significantly lower rate of all cause death/severe complications at 30-day follow-up • Significant decrease in number of patients transfused with restrictive strategy
Bergamin et al. [14]	Adult cancer patients with septic shock	300	Liberal, Hb ≤9 g/dl, Vs. restrictive, Hb ≤7.0 g/dl	• Though statistically nonsignificant, a trend towards an increased mortality rate in the liberal group was observed. • Significant decrease in number of patients transfused and total number of units transfused.

Age of RBC and Transfusion Outcomes

RBCs are currently stored up to 42 days after collection as per the regulatory authority, depending upon the type of anticoagulant and additive solution used during the preparation process. During storage, RBCs undergo structural, biochemical, and metabolic changes, known as the "storage lesion." As a result of prolonged storage, RBCs may become ineffective and accumulation of bioactive substances can also lead to unwanted biological effects. Blood transfusion services usually issue the oldest compatible RBC units available as a part of FIFO policy (first in, first out) to minimize waste of blood components; this usual practice can lead to harm in critically ill patients. Though various observational studies and systematic reviews have reported adverse outcomes associated with stored/old blood, recent RCTs have refuted the claim. As shown in Table 12.2, to date, four RCTs have evaluated the fresh vs. old RBCs or standard issue RBCs and have not shown a difference in mortality or other outcomes based on RBC age. Therefore, we believe RBC age does not have clinically relevant effects on patient condition.

Table 12.2 Randomized trials comparing fresh versus old RBC transfusion in critically ill

Study	Clinical settings	No of patients	Groups	Outcome
ABLE (age of blood evaluation) [15]	Critically ill Multicenter	2510	<8 days vs. oldest	• No difference in 90-day all-cause mortality.
INFORM (informing fresh vs. old red cell management) [16]	All hospitalized patients Multicenter	24,736	Short vs. longest	• No difference in-hospital mortality.
RECESS (red cell storage duration study) [17]	Cardiac surgery Multicenter	1098	≤10 days vs. ≥21 days	• No difference in change in MODS from preoperative baseline through postoperative day 7, hospital discharge, or death, whichever occurred first.
TRANSFUSE (standard issue transfusion vs. fresher red blood cell use in intensive care) [18]	ICU patients Multicenter	4994	Fresh vs. standard	• 90-day mortality • Trial underway

Thrombocytopenia and Platelet Transfusion

Thrombocytopenia is a frequent complication encountered during critical illness, with a reported prevalence between 8.3% and 67.6% at the time of admission and up to 44.1% in patients with normal platelet counts during admission [19]. Thrombocytopenia in critically ill patients results from hemodilution, increased platelet consumption, decreased production, increased sequestration, and destruction. In addition, platelet dysfunction due to the underlying disease itself and due to medications can further add to the increased risk of bleeding in these patients. Platelet transfusions are required to treat thrombocytopenia-related bleeding and as a prophylactic measure for patients at risk of bleeding or with impaired platelet function.

In the ICU setting, 10% to 30% of patients will receive platelet transfusions, the majority of which are used as a prophylactic measure to prevent bleeding [20]. While platelet transfusions are an established trigger in thrombocytopenic patients with bleeding, prophylactic platelet transfusion in ICU setting are highly debated due to lack of evidence. Recommendations for platelet transfusion thresholds are largely based on expert opinion.

As critically ill patients are prone to bleeding and frequently undergo invasive procedures (surgery, catheters), the need for platelet transfusion should be balanced against the risks of transfusions. It is important to assess the risk of bleeding, cause and pattern of thrombocytopenia, and presence of comorbidities before making the decision to transfuse.

Table 12.3 Clinical indications for platelet transfusion

Indication for transfusion	Threshold
Therapeutic	
• Acute hemorrhage	• 50×10^9/l.
• Acute hemorrhage (part of massive transfusion).	• 100×10^9/l.
• Intracranial hemorrhage with involvement of eyes/lungs/spinal cord.	• 100×10^9/l.
Prophylactic	
• Non-bleeding stable patient.	• 10×10^9/l.
• Non-bleeding patient with additional risk factors for bleeding.	• 20×10^9/l.
• Minimal invasive procedure.	• $20\text{-}30 \times 10^9$/l.
• Invasive procedure with increased risk of bleeding.	• 50×10^9/l.

While hemorrhage in the presence of thrombocytopenia is an established trigger for therapeutic platelet transfusion, there is no predefined level of platelet count to be maintained in such patients. Based on expert opinion, several guidelines recommend a threshold of 50×10^9/ml in acutely bleeding patients. In fact, in severely injured trauma patients with massive hemorrhage, early platelet transfusion with target platelet count of 100×10^9/ml is recommended to prevent the coagulopathy of trauma. The degree of thrombocytopenia alone is not a prominent contributor to the hemorrhage and its consequences. Prophylactic platelet transfusions in the ICU setting are often required when there is a need for surgical or radiological intervention or if the patient is at increased risk of bleeding due to presence of additional risk factors such as fever, infection, concomitant diffuse intravascular coagulopathy (DIC), severe hepatic or renal dysfunction, and use of anti-platelet medications. Based on consensus, prophylactic platelet transfusion in non-bleeding patients are recommended at a threshold level of 10×10^9/l in the absence of additional risk factors for hemorrhage and $20\text{--}30\times10^9$/l for those with additional risk factors. Higher thresholds of 50×10^9/l for platelet transfusions are recommended if there is a possibility of platelet dysfunction, even if the patient is not thrombocytopenic. Similarly, for patients with neurological complications such as intracranial bleeding, a higher threshold of 100×10^9/l has been suggested. A summary of the recommended threshold for platelet transfusions is shown in Table 12.3. Though the threshold for platelet transfusion in ICU patients undergoing invasive procedures has been defined, the evidence base to guide the same is poor.

Coagulopathy and Plasma Transfusion

Coagulopathy is another condition frequently encountered in the ICU, occurring in up to two-third of critically ill patients [21]. Presence of coagulopathy in critical illness can increase the risk of developing hemorrhagic complications fivefold compared to patients with a normal coagulation status [22]. To assess bleeding risk and the effectiveness of plasma transfusion, prothrombin time (PT) or international normalized ratio (INR) is most widely used [23, 24]. However, as the coagulation status of a patient is the net result of a balance between procoagulant and antifibrinolytic activity, these tests poorly represent in-vivo hemostatic potential.

FFP and cryoprecipitate transfusions are used in the treatment and prevention of hemorrhage. Approximately 13% of ICU patients will receive a plasma transfusion during their admission, 70% of which are used prophylactically prior to an invasive procedure or to correct abnormal coagulation tests [24, 25]. Despite the lack of evidence to support the use of prophylactic plasma transfusion for correction of laboratory anomalies and during low-risk procedures such as central venous catheter insertion, percutaneous tracheostomy, thoracentesis, and lumbar puncture, prophylactic FFP transfusion is still a common practice in the ICU. Table 12.4 summarizes the indications for FFP and cryoprecipitate transfusions. There is increasing concern that adverse reactions associated with such transfusions will affect the risk vs. benefit balance of prophylactic FFP transfusion.

Given the poor ability of conventional coagulation tests to predict bleeding, viscoelastic methods have gained importance in the monitoring of coagulation status, especially in bleeding patients. These tests offer numerous advantages over the conventional coagulation tests and are able to better guide transfusion in critically ill patients. These tests, e.g., thromboelastography (TEG) or rotational thromboelastometry (ROTEM), provide an overall picture of hemostasis, including coagulation and fibrinolytic pathways (Fig. 12.1). Additionally, they can be performed at the point of care giving more accurate information about the patient's dynamic coagulation status with faster turnaround times. While the use of TEG has been shown to reduce bleeding-related morbidity and mortality in cardiac surgery and trauma patients, more clinical research is required to validate its utility in the critically ill patient population.

Table 12.4 indications for FFP and cryoprecipitate transfusion

FFP	Not indicated for • Volume replacement. • Prophylaxis for patients with abnormal coagulation tests in the absence of bleeding. • Immediate reversal of warfarin. Indicated for • Single factor deficiencies such as factor V deficiency and combined deficiency of factor V and factor VIII. • Other rare coagulation disorders in emergencies where a more specific replacement therapy is unavailable or diagnosis is uncertain. • Multifactor deficiencies associated with severe bleeding: Massive transfusion, DIC, liver disease, reversal of warfarin. • Replacement fluids during therapeutic plasma exchange.
Cryoprecipitate	Indicated only when specific factor concentrates are unavailable for • Hypofibrinogenemia/dysfibrinogenemia. • Factor VIII deficiency. • Factor XIII deficiency. • vWF (von Willebrand factor) deficiency.

Fig. 12.1 Specific TEG parameters represent the three phases of the cell-based model of hemostasis: initiation, amplification, and propagation

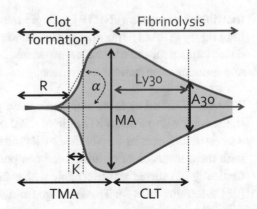

- R value = reaction time (s), time of latency from start of test to initial fibrin formation (amplitude of 2 mm), initiation phase, dependent on clotting factors (normal 4–8 min). Corresponding terminology for ROTEM is clotting time (CT).
- K = kinetics (s), time taken to achieve a certain level of clot strength (amplitude of 20 mm), amplification phase, dependent on fibrinogen (normal 1–4 min). Corresponding terminology for ROTEM is clot formation time (CFT).
- alpha (α) = angle (slope of line between R and K), measures the speed at which fibrin build up and cross-linking takes place, hence assesses the rate of clot formation, "thrombin burst" or propagation phase, dependent on fibrinogen (normal α-angle: 47–74°).
- TMA = time to maximum amplitude(s).
- MA = maximum amplitude (mm), represents the ultimate strength of the fibrin clot; i.e., overall stability of the clot, dependent on platelets (80%) and fibrin (20%) interacting via GPIIb/IIIa (normal 55–73 mm). Corresponding terminology for ROTEM is maximum clot firmness (MCF).
- A30 or LY30 = amplitude at 30 mins, percentage decrease in amplitude at 30 mins post-MA, fibrinolysis phase (normal 0–8%). Corresponding terminology for ROTEM is clot lysis (CL).
- CLT = clot lysis time (s).

Approximate normal values (kaolin-activated TEG, values differ if native blood used, and between types of assay).

Adverse Transfusion Reactions in Critical Care

Transfusion of blood and blood components is often lifesaving but can be associated with adverse effects including metabolic complications (e.g., hypothermia, acidosis), transfusion-transmitted infections (e.g., HIV, HCV, HBV), transfusion-associated circulatory overload (TACO), hemolytic transfusion reactions (HTR), febrile nonhemolytic transfusion reactions (FNHTR), allergic transfusion reactions, transfusion-related acute lung injury (TRALI), transfusion-associated graft versus host disease (TA-GVHD), nosocomial infection, and transfusion-associated immunomodulation (TRIM). TRALI, TACO, and nosocomial infections are frequently encountered in the ICU setting.

TRALI Defined as acute non-cardiogenic pulmonary edema developing within 6 h of transfusion with a PaO2:FiO2 ratio of <300 mmHg in room air and bilateral infiltrates on a chest radiograph in the absence of left atrial hypertension. It occurs more commonly with the transfusion of cellular blood components rather than plasma-based components. Critically ill patients are susceptible with estimated incidence up to 8% in this population [26]. Mortality rates for TRALI range from 9 to 15% but can be as high as 40% in critically ill patients [27].

TACO Defined as acute respiratory distress with pulmonary edema, tachycardia, increased blood pressure, and evidence of a positive fluid balance after a blood transfusion. Although all blood components have been implicated as potential causes of TACO, recent studies have identified FFP transfusion as a frequent cause [28]. The exact incidence of TACO is unknown but is common in critically ill patients. TACO accounted for 44% of the transfusion-related deaths reported to the UK Haemovigilance during 2010 to 2017 [29].

Nosocomial infections and transfusion The risk of infection following RBC transfusion is related to the amount of transfused blood and RBC storage duration. An increased risk of nosocomial infection following blood transfusion in critically ill patient populations has been demonstrated in a number of studies [30, 31]. Similarly, platelet and plasma transfusions have also been associated with postoperative infection in cardiac surgery and critically ill patients recovering from sepsis. As RBCs are often administered together with plasma and platelets, it is difficult to ascertain the exact component as the causative factor.

Alternatives to Transfusion

As previously discussed, anemia in critical illness is primarily due to functional iron deficiency (presence of chronic illness) and blunted erythropoietin response. The use of alternative strategies can reduce the incidence and severity of anemia and need for RBC transfusion and may reduce morbidity and mortality. Intravenous (IV) iron was studied as an alternative treatment for anemia in critically ill patients. However, the IRONMAN study failed to demonstrate a decrease in RBC transfusion requirements, although patients who received intravenous iron had significantly higher hemoglobin concentration at hospital discharge [32]. The use of IV iron preparation does have increased theoretical risks of infections and adverse reactions.

The use of erythropoietin in critically ill patients has also been evaluated in several RCTs. Significant decrease in RBC usage was observed in earlier studies but subsequent trials failed to demonstrate a consistent effect, suggesting that the benefits of using erythropoietin became negligible once the restrictive transfusion trigger of 7.0 g/dl became the standard [33]. No differences in other patient outcomes were noted.

Tranexamic acid, an antifibrinolytic agent, has been shown in the CRASH-2 study to reduce the need for blood transfusion in the trauma setting without an increase in thromboembolic events [34]. Its use is also recommended in postpartum hemorrhage, high-risk surgery, and other non-trauma settings [35, 36]. However, utility of tranexamic in the highly variable population of critically ill patients needs further evaluation.

Case Vignette
The patient in the vignette was given component therapy transfusion based on thromboelastography. Components were titrated to the results until the bleeding was effectively controlled. Thereafter, transfusion was stopped. As a consequence of the treatment, the patient developed TRALI which was managed successfully. The indications for blood and its components in ICU are either active bleeding or prophylactic. The age of RBCs does not matter. The management of coagulopathy in critical illness should be individualized. The potential adverse effects of blood transfusion include infection, TRALI, TACO, hemolysis, graft versus host disease, and immune modulation.

Conclusion

Blood and blood products constitute major lifesaving therapy especially in critically ill patients who are actively bleeding or at risk of major bleeding. The threshold for initiation of transfusion should be based on individual factors. However, the evidence supports restrictive use in the majority of cases. The risk–benefit ratio of adverse events should be considered when making the decision to transfuse. The use of newer viscoelastic tests provides dynamic assessment and can help in rationalizing the decision for component therapy.

Take-Home Messages
- RBC transfusion is required to improve oxygen-carrying capacity and also promote hemostasis.
- Restrictive RBC transfusion strategy in critically ill patients is more beneficial in reducing the volume of transfusion requirement and improved patient outcomes.
- RBC age does not have clinically significant effects on patient outcomes.

- Platelet transfusion is indicated to treat thrombocytopenic bleeding.
- Prophylactic platelet transfusion in critically ill should be administered after risk assessment for bleeding, cause and pattern of thrombocytopenia, and presence of underlying comorbidities.
- FFP and cryoprecipitate transfusions are used in the treatment and prevention of coagulopathy in critically ill patients.
- Use of point-of-care tests such as thromboelastography (TEG) or rotational thromboelastometry (ROTEM) have gained importance in the monitoring of coagulation status and can be used to guide to blood transfusion.
- TRALI, TACO, and nosocomial infections are frequently encountered transfusion reactions in the ICU setting.
- Transfusion alternatives such as IV iron, erythropoietin, and tranexamic acid should be considered whenever feasible.

References

1. Vincent JL, Baron J-F, Reinhart K, Gattinoni L, Thijs L, Webb A, et al. Anemia and blood transfusion in critically ill patients. JAMA. 2002;288(12):1499–507.
2. Corwin HL. Anemia and blood transfusion in the critically ill patient: role of erythropoietin. Crit Care. 2004;8(Suppl 2):S42–4.
3. Litvinov RI, Weisel JW. Role of red blood cells in haemostasis and thrombosis. ISBT Sci Ser. 2017;12(1):176–83.
4. Hebert PC, Wells G, Martin C, Tweeddale M, Marshall J, Blajchman M, et al. A Canadian survey of transfusion practices in critically ill patients. Transfusion requirements in critical care investigators and the Canadian critical care trials group. Crit Care Med. 1998 Mar;26(3):482–7.
5. Hebert PC, Tinmouth A, Corwin H. Anemia and red cell transfusion in critically ill patients. Crit Care Med. 2003 Dec;31(12 Suppl):S672–7.
6. Holst LB, Haase N, Wetterslev J, Wernerman J, Guttormsen AB, Karlsson S, et al. Lower versus higher hemoglobin threshold for transfusion in septic shock. N Engl J Med. 2014;371(15):1381–91.
7. Villanueva C, Colomo A, Bosch A, Concepcion M, Hernandez-Gea V, Aracil C, et al. Transfusion strategies for acute upper gastrointestinal bleeding. N Engl J Med. 2013;368(1):11–21.
8. Jairath V, Kahan BC, Gray A, Dore CJ, Mora A, James MW, et al. Restrictive versus liberal blood transfusion for acute upper gastrointestinal bleeding (TRIGGER): a pragmatic, open-label, cluster randomised feasibility trial. Lancet (London, England). 2015;386(9989):137–44.
9. Carson JL, Terrin ML, Noveck H, Sanders DW, Chaitman BR, Rhoads GG, et al. Liberal or restrictive transfusion in high-risk patients after hip surgery. N Engl J Med. 2011;365(26):2453–62.
10. Gregersen M, Borris LC, Damsgaard EM. Postoperative blood transfusion strategy in frail, anemic elderly patients with hip fracture: the TRIFE randomized controlled trial. Acta Orthop. 2015 Jun;86(3):363–72.
11. Hajjar LA, Vincent J-L, Galas FRBG, Nakamura RE, Silva CMP, Santos MH, et al. Transfusion requirements after cardiac surgery: the TRACS randomized controlled trial. JAMA. 2010;304(14):1559–67.

12. Murphy GJ, Pike K, Rogers CA, Wordsworth S, Stokes EA, Angelini GD, et al. Liberal or restrictive transfusion after cardiac surgery. N Engl J Med. 2015;372(11):997–1008.
13. de Almeida JP, Vincent JL, Galas FR, de Almeida EP, Fukushima JT, Osawa EA, et al. Transfusion requirements in surgical oncology patients: a prospective, randomized controlled trial. Anesthesiology. 2015 Jan;122(1):29–38.
14. Bergamin FS, Almeida JP, Landoni G, Galas F, Fukushima JT, Fominskiy E, et al. Liberal versus restrictive transfusion strategy in critically ill oncologic patients: the transfusion requirements in critically ill oncologic patients randomized controlled trial. Crit Care Med. 2017 May;45(5):766–73.
15. Cooper DJ, McQuilten ZK, Nichol A, Ady B, Aubron C, Bailey M, et al. Age of red cells for transfusion and outcomes in critically ill adults. N Engl J Med. 2017;377(19):1858–67.
16. Heddle NM, Cook RJ, Arnold DM, Liu Y, Barty R, Crowther MA, et al. Effect of short-term vs. long-term blood storage on mortality after transfusion. N Engl J Med. 2016;375(20):1937–45.
17. Steiner ME, Ness PM, Assmann SF, Triulzi DJ, Sloan SR, Delaney M, et al. Effects of red-cell storage duration on patients undergoing cardiac surgery. N Engl J Med. 2015;372(15):1419–29.
18. Kaukonen KM, Bailey M, Ady B, Aubron C, French C, Gantner D, et al. A randomised controlled trial of standard transfusion versus fresher red blood cell use in intensive care (TRANSFUSE): protocol and statistical analysis plan. Crit Care Resusc. 2014 Dec;16(4):255–61.
19. Hui P, Cook DJ, Lim W, Fraser GA, Arnold DM. The frequency and clinical significance of thrombocytopenia complicating critical illness: a systematic review. Chest. 2011;139(2):271–8.
20. McIntyre L, Tinmouth AT, Fergusson DA. Blood component transfusion in critically ill patients. Curr Opin Crit Care. 2013;19(4):326–33.
21. Chakraverty R, Davidson S, Peggs K, Stross P, Garrard C, Littlewood TJ. The incidence and cause of coagulopathies in an intensive care population. Br J Haematol. 1996;93(2):460–3.
22. Levi M, Hunt BJ. A critical appraisal of point-of-care coagulation testing in critically ill patients. J Thromb Haemost. 2015;13(11):1960–7.
23. Dara SI, Rana R, Afessa B, Moore SB, Gajic O. Fresh frozen plasma transfusion in critically ill medical patients with coagulopathy. Crit Care Med. 2005;33(11):2667–71.
24. Stanworth SJ, Walsh TS, Prescott RJ, Lee RJ, Watson DM, Wyncoll D. A national study of plasma use in critical care: clinical indications, dose and effect on prothrombin time. Crit Care. 2011;15(2):R108.
25. Stanworth SJ, Grant-Casey J, Lowe D, Laffan M, New H, Murphy MF, et al. The use of fresh-frozen plasma in England: high levels of inappropriate use in adults and children. Transfusion. 2011;51(1):62–70.
26. Gajic O, Rana R, Winters JL, Yilmaz M, Mendez JL, Rickman OB, et al. Transfusion-related acute lung injury in the critically ill: prospective nested case-control study. Am J Respir Crit Care Med. 2007;176(9):886–91.
27. Benson AB, Moss M, Silliman CC. Transfusion-related acute lung injury (TRALI): a clinical review with emphasis on the critically ill. Br J Haematol. 2009 Nov;147(4):431–43.
28. Roubinian NH, Hendrickson JE, Triulzi DJ, Gottschall JL, Michalkiewicz M, Chowdhury D, et al. Contemporary risk factors and outcomes of transfusion-associated circulatory overload*. Crit Care Med. 2018;46(4):577–85.
29. Annual Shot Report 2017.
30. Lelubre C, Vincent JL. Relationship between red cell storage duration and outcomes in adults receiving red cell transfusions: a systematic review. Crit Care. 2013;17(2):R66.
31. Lacroix J, Hebert PC, Fergusson DA, Tinmouth A, Cook DJ, Marshall JC, et al. Age of transfused blood in critically ill adults. N Engl J Med. 2015;372(15):1410–8.

32. Litton E, Baker S, Erber WN, Farmer S, Ferrier J, French C, et al. Intravenous iron or placebo for anaemia in intensive care: the IRONMAN multicentre randomized blinded trial : a randomized trial of IV iron in critical illness. Intensive Care Med. 2016;42(11):1715–22.

33. Corwin HL, Gettinger A, Fabian TC, May A, Pearl RG, Heard S, et al. Efficacy and safety of epoetin alfa in critically ill patients. N Engl J Med. 2007;357(10):965–76.

34. Shakur H, Roberts I, Bautista R, Caballero J, Coats T, Dewan Y, et al. Effects of tranexamic acid on death, vascular occlusive events, and blood transfusion in trauma patients with significant haemorrhage (CRASH-2): a randomised, placebo-controlled trial. Lancet (London, England). 2010;376(9734):23–32.

35. Simmons J, Sikorski RA, Pittet J-F. Tranexamic acid: from trauma to routine perioperative use. Curr Opin Anaesthesiol. 2015;28(2):191.

36. Effect of early tranexamic acid administration on mortality. Hysterectomy, and other morbidities in women with post-partum haemorrhage (WOMAN): an international, randomised, double-blind, placebo-controlled trial. Lancet (London, England). 2017;389(10084):2105–16.

Nutrition Delivery in Critically Ill Patients

13

Ranajit Chatterjee and Ashutosh Kumar Garg

Contents

Introduction	281
Goals of Nutrition in the ICU	282
Nutrition Assessment	282
Assessment of Energy Needs	283
Initiate Early EN	283
Dosing of EN	284
Monitoring Tolerance and Adequacy of EN	285
Selection of Appropriate Enteral Formulation	285
When to Use PN	285
When Indicated, Maximize Efficacy of PN	286
Special Situations	286
Pulmonary Failure	286
Renal Failure	286
Hepatic Failure	287
Acute Pancreatitis	287
Trauma	287
Burns	288
Sepsis	288
Postoperative Major Surgery	288
Obese Patients	288
Fluid Therapy and Nutrition	289
Conclusion	290
References	292

R. Chatterjee (✉)
Intensive Care Unit and Accident and Emergency Swami Dayanand Hospital, New Delhi, India

A. K. Garg
Kailash Deepak Hospital, Karkardooma, New Delhi, India

© The Author(s) 2024
M. L. N. G. Malbrain et al. (eds.), *Rational Use of Intravenous Fluids in Critically Ill Patients*, https://doi.org/10.1007/978-3-031-42205-8_13

IFA Commentary (MLNGM)

Often overlooked, nutritional fluids with total enteral (TEN) and parenteral nutrition (TPN) form a major part (33%) of fluid volume administration in critically ill patients. This chapter will help to define a reasonable strategy to optimize nutrition in the critical care setting. Some key variables to consider in obtaining nutritional adequacy in combination with the evidence related to optimal amount of calories will be listed. Nutritional deficits will eventually lead to adverse outcomes, and prolonged critical illness will eventually lead to a state of malnutrition. Important clinical level 1 studies and meta-analyses have been published in the past that assist the practicing intensivists in choosing a nutritional support plan for his patients [1–9]. A nutritional screening process should always precede the provision of artificial nutrition. Scores such as the nutritional risk score or the NUTRIC score are imperfect options. The caloric target should be individualized, even though we do not really know if or how many exogenous macronutrients can prevent or correct a nutritional deficit in most of our patients. Indirect calorimetry has never been shown to improve outcome in level one RCTs. The methodology is neither applicable in most ICUs nor in many patients. Therefore, formulas for calculating caloric target are still the recommended albeit flawed tool. There is good evidence for preferring enteral nutrition (EN) over parenteral nutrition (PN), and there are sufficient scientific arguments to advocate early EN within 24–48 h of admission. The gastric residual volume is the most frequently used parameter for monitoring tolerance to EN. As compared to the past, threshold values for intolerance can definitely be relaxed to values of 300 ml and above. Controversy about the risks or benefits of hypocaloric versus normocaloric (feeding to target) feeding has been ongoing for decades. In 2011, the EPaNIC trial showed that during the first week of ICU stay a substantial caloric deficit is not detrimental for outcome and thereby questioned the intrinsic value of PN in this time frame. Strong evidence has emerged from three level 1 trials that at least for the first week of ICU stay there is no benefit from a normocaloric feeding strategy. A hypocaloric regime might even be advantageous for outcome. Indeed, withholding PN and not reaching the currently recommended caloric targets seemed to be of benefit for the vast majority of critically ill patients during the first 7 days. Relevant studies addressing hypocaloric versus normocaloric feeding included the following. In a large, randomized trial (the EDEN trial, $n = 1000$) conducted in critically ill patients with acute lung injury, Rice et al. compared "trickle enteral feeding" to "full enteral feeding" [9]. Trickle feeding resulted in a large cumulative energy debt (after 6 days, a mean of 1300 kcal/d versus 400 kcal/d). However, morbidity and mortality were not different. Follow-up after 1 year also showed no difference for physical function, survival, or multiple secondary outcomes. A second smaller ($n = 305$) randomized trial assessed whether delivery of 100% of the energy target from day four to eight in ICU with EN plus PN as opposed to only EN could optimize clinical outcome [4]. This controversial study concluded that optimizing individual energy delivery with the aid of indirect calorimetry could reduce nosocomial infections. A third randomized trial addressed early PN versus standard care in 1372 critically ill patients with relative contraindications to early EN [3]. In the standard care group, 29.2% of patients commenced with EN, 27.3% with PN, and 40.8% remained unfed for variable periods of time. There was no significant difference between groups for either the primary end point (death by study day 60) or for ICU or LOS. Time on mechanical ventilation was significantly reduced by 0.47 days with early PN. Finally, subanalysis of the EPaNIC trial showed that a) tolerating a substantial macronutrient deficit early during critical illness did not affect muscle wasting but allowed for faster recovery from weakness and b) that caloric dose had a negative inverse relation with infectious morbidity [2, 5]. Other relevant observations from RCTs of the past 2 years with potential impact for clinical practice include the following: early provision of glutamine or antioxidants did not improve clinical outcomes, and not monitoring gastric residual volume did not increase the rate of VAP [6, 8].

The quality of clinical research aimed at optimizing nutritional strategies in the critically ill has improved significantly in recent years and is filling important knowledge gaps. Strong evidence from several RCTs supports the conclusion that tolerating a substantial caloric deficit in the first 5–7 days of ICU stay will influence mortality or length of stay. However, best evidence indicates that hypercaloric or even normocaloric feeding during this time frame will worsen morbidity.

Therefore, it is time for nutrition stewardship with the 7 D's. Nutrition stewardship is defined, in analogy with fluid stewardship, as a series of coordinated interventions, introduced to select the optimal type of nutrition, dose, and duration of therapy that results in the best clinical outcome, prevention of adverse events, and cost reduction [10]. This can be accomplished by adhering to the 7 D's (definitions, diagnosis, drug, dose, duration, de-escalation, discharge) [10–11]. The first D stands for definitions: correct and uniform definitions should be used when prescribing nutritional therapy. The second D is diagnosis: correct diagnosis should be made, as correct nutritional therapy starts with an adequate assessment of the patient's nutritional status and metabolic evaluation via indirect calorimetry in combination with other monitoring tools, such as BIA and nitrogen balance. Third D is drug: critical care physicians should consider nutrition as drugs that have indications and contraindications, and potential adverse effects, and pay particular attention to the different compounds and their specificities (calories, nitrogen, protein, glucose, lipids, and micronutrients) (Fig. 13.1). For each type of nutrition, there are distinct indications and specific side effects.

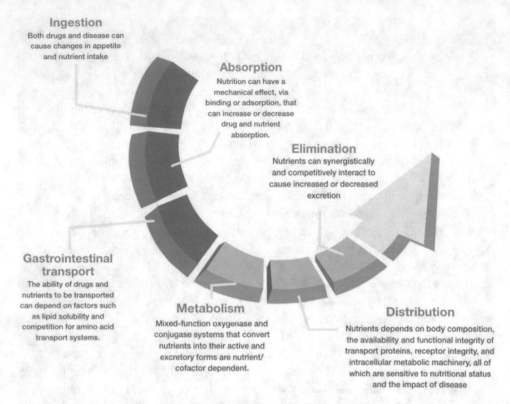

Fig. 13.1 Potential mechanism of nutrients–drugs interaction. Adpated from Pisani D. et al. with permission according to the Open Access CC BY License 4.0 [12]

The fourth D is dose: "sola dosis facit venenum" or "the dose makes the poison." As discussed earlier, there are various important considerations for nutritional prescription, as calorie and protein dosing are correlated with mortality, and pharmacokinetics and dynamics need to be taken into account, as well as volume kinetics, since nutrition may also contribute to fluid accumulation [10, 11]. The fifth D is duration: the duration of total or supplemental artificial nutritional therapy is equally important, and parenteral nutrition must be tapered when shock is resolved and the gastrointestinal tract is normally functioning [13]. The sixth D is de-escalation: the final step in artificial EN or PN nutrition therapy is to consider withholding or withdrawing when they are no longer required. Finally, the seventh D is discharge: correct (dis)continuation or tapering of artificial nutritional therapy and (when needed and indicated) prescription post-discharge from ICU, or hospital, is part of the nutritional care plan and should meet quality standards (Fig. 13.2) [11].

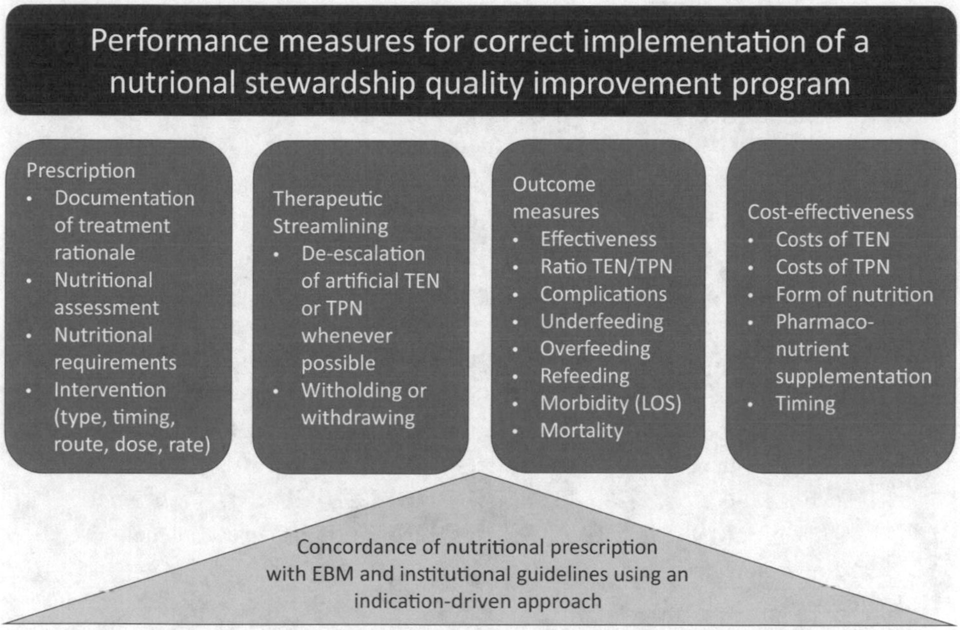

Performance measures for correct implementation of a nutrional stewardship quality improvement program

Prescription
- Documentation of treatment rationale
- Nutritional assessment
- Nutritional requirements
- Intervention (type, timing, route, dose, rate)

Therapeutic Streamlining
- De-escalation of artificial TEN or TPN whenever possible
- Witholding or withdrawing

Outcome measures
- Effectiveness
- Ratio TEN/TPN
- Complications
- Underfeeding
- Overfeeding
- Refeeding
- Morbidity (LOS)
- Mortality

Cost-effectiveness
- Costs of TEN
- Costs of TPN
- Form of nutrition
- Pharmaco-nutrient supplementation
- Timing

Concordance of nutritional prescription with EBM and institutional guidelines using an indication-driven approach

Fig. 13.2 Performance measures for nutritional stewardship program. EBM: cvidence-based medicine; ICU: intensive care unit; LOS: length of stay; TEN: total enteral nutrition; TPN: total parenteral nutrition. Adpated from Pisani D. et al. with permission according to the Open Access CC BY License 4.0 [12]

Suggested Reading
1. Casaer MP, Mesotten D, Hermans G, et al. Early versus late parenteral nutrition in critically ill adults. NEJM 2011;365(6):506–517.
2. Casaer MP, Wilmer A, Hermans G, Wouters PJ, Mesotten D, Van den Berghe G. Role of disease and macronutrient dose in the randomized controlled EPaNIC trial: a post hoc analysis. Am J Respir Crit Care Med 2013;187:247–255.
3. Doig GS. Early parenteral nutrition in critically il patients with short-term relative contraindications to early enteral nutrition. JAMA 2013;309:2130–2138.
4. Heidegger CP, Berger MM, Graf S, et al. Optimisation of energy provision with supplemental parenteral nutrition in critically ill patients: a randomised controlled clinical trial. Lancet 2013;381:385–393.
5. Hermans G. Effect of tolerating macronutrient deficit on the development of intensive-care unit acquired weakness: a subanalysis of the EPaNIC trial. Lancet Resp Med 2013;1(8):621–629.
6. Heyland D. A randomized trial of glutamine and oxidants in critically ill patients. NEJM 2013;368:1489–1497.

7. Needha DM et al. One year outcomes in patients with acute lung injury randomised to initial trophic or full enteral feeding. BMJ 2013;346:f1532.
8. Reignier J. Effect of not monitoring residual gastric volume on risk of VAP in adults receiving mechanical ventilation and early enteral feeding. JAMA 2013;309:249–256.
9. Rice TW, Wheeler AP, Thompson BT, et al. National Heart, Lung, and Blood Institute acute respiratory distress syndrome (ARDS) clinical trials network. Initial trophic vs full enteral feeding in patients with acute lung injury: the EDEN randomized trial. JAMA 2012;307(8):795–803.
10. Malbrain MLNG, Van Regenmortel N, Saugel B, De Tavernier B, Van Gaal PJ, Joannes-Boyau O, Teboul JL, Rice TW, Mythen M, Monnet X. Principles of fluid management and stewardship in septic shock: it is time to consider the four D's and the four phases of fluid therapy. Ann Intensive Care 2018 May 22;8(1):66. Doi: 10.1186/s13613-018-0402-x. PMID: 29789983; PMCID: PMC5964054.
11. De Waele E, Malbrain MLNG, Spapen H. Nutrition in sepsis: a bench-to-bedside review. Nutrients 2020;12:395. Doi: 10.3390/nu12020395.
12. Pisani D, Navalesi P, De Rosa S. Do we need a 6D's framework of nutritional stewardship in critical care? J Anesth Analg Crit Care 2021;1(5). Doi: 10.1186/s44158-021-00009-4.
13. Blaser AR, Starkopf J, Alhazzani W, Berger MM, Casaer MP, Deane AM, Fruhwald S, Hiesmayr M, Ichai C, Jakob SM. Early enteral nutrition in critically ill patients: ESICM clinical practice guidelines. Intens Care Med 2017, 43, 380–398. [Google Scholar] [CrossRef].

Learning Objectives

The learning objectives of this chapter are:

1. To understand "medical nutrition therapy" and goals of nutrition in intensive care unit (ICU).
2. To explain nutrition assessment in critically ill patients admitted to ICU.
3. To learn assessment of energy expenditure in critically ill patients.
4. To learn how to start enteral nutrition (EN) in critically ill patients.
5. To explain the dosing, monitoring of tolerance, and adequacy of EN.
6. To help the clinician with selection of appropriate EN.
7. To learn the indications of parenteral nutrition (PN).
8. To assist in diet formulation in special medical conditions like pulmonary failure, renal failure, hepatic failure, acute pancreatitis, trauma, sepsis, burns, postoperative case of major surgery, and obese patients.
9. To understand the impact of nutrition on fluid therapy and accumulation.
10. To introduce nutrition stewardship.

Case Vignette

A 57-year-old man was admitted to ER with history of 3 days of increasing shortness of breath, sputum production, and fever. He had a past medical history of diabetes, hypertension, and alcoholism. He did not consume alcohol since the last 3 days. He had around 8–10 kg weight loss over the past 2 months due to poor oral intake. Past surgical and family histories were not significant. On examination, the patient appeared anxious and diaphoretic. There was no jugular venous distension. Bitemporal wasting was present. There were cold and clammy skin and extremities. There were ronchi and bronchial breath sounds over the right axillae. The remainder of the clinical examination was unremarkable. Vital signs were as follows: heart rate 110/min, blood pressure 90/40 mmHg, respiratory rate 26/min, temperature 38.9 °C, and Spo2 84% on room air. The body mass index (BMI) was 19.9. Laboratory values are as follows: white blood cell count 19500 per microliter, serum potassium 2.8 mmol/L, phosphate 1.4 mg/dL, magnesium 1.1 mg/dL, bicarbonate 18 mmol/L, serum creatinine 2.8 mg/dL, and lactic acid 6 mmol/L. Serum albumin level was 1.8 g/dL. Arterial blood gas shows pH of 7.32, partial pressure carbon dioxide of 40 mmHg, partial pressure oxygen of 76 mmHg, and oxygen saturation of 90% on 10 liters oxygen. Chest radiograph shows right middle lobe opacity. Clinical diagnosis was sepsis with acute hypoxemic respiratory failure secondary to community acquired pneumonia.

Questions

Q1. What is the role of nutrition in a critically ill patient in the ICU?

Q2. How will you assess nutritional risk in this patient?

Q3. What will be the nutritional management strategy for this patient?

Introduction

Critical illness is a state of catabolic stress in which the patient shows a systemic inflammatory response along with complications of increased risk for infections, multiple-organ dysfunction, prolonged hospitalization, and disproportionate mortality. Traditionally, nutrition support in critically ill patients was regarded as adjunctive care designed to provide exogenous fuels to preserve lean body mass and support the patient during the stress response. Recently, this strategy has changed to medical nutrition therapy, in which feeding is thought to help attenuate the metabolic response to stress, prevent oxidative cellular injury, and favorably modulate immune responses. Delivering early nutrition therapy, primarily by the enteral route, is seen as a proactive therapeutic strategy that may maintain gut integrity, reduce disease severity, diminish complications, decrease length of stay (LOS) in the ICU, and favorably impact patient outcomes. In recently published guidelines, the term "medical nutrition therapy" has replaced "artificial nutrition." This term encompasses oral nutritional supplements, enteral nutrition (EN), and parenteral nutrition (PN) [1, 2]. Nutrition is one indication for fluid therapy, intravenous fluids to cover the other indications: resuscitation, replacement and maintenance are discussed elsewhere. More information on crystalloid solutions can be found in Chap. 9, albumin is discussed in Chap. 10, and other colloid solutions like starches and gelatins are discussed in Chap. 11.

Goals of Nutrition in the ICU

1. To preserve the lean body mass.
2. To maintain the immune function.
3. To avoid metabolic complications.

Nutrition Assessment

General clinical assessment should be performed to assess nutrition status in every critically ill patient admitted to the ICU [2]. This should include a detailed history of percentage weight loss (if any) in the last 6 months, appetite, nausea, food intake or decrease in physical performance before ICU admission, and physical examination focusing on body composition, muscle mass, and strength, where possible [3]. Weight loss of 20–30% suggests moderate protein calorie malnutrition, while 30% or greater indicates severe protein calorie malnutrition. Weight loss of 10% or greater over a short span of time is also clinically important. [4] The general appearance of a patient with emphasis on the temporalis and upper extremity wasting of skeletal muscle mass provides a quick, inexpensive, and clinically useful measure of nutritional status.

Formal assessment of nutrition status is performed using a nutrition scoring system, several of which exist. Examples include (1) subjective global assessment (SGA), (2) malnutrition universal screening tool (MUST), (3) nutritional risk screening (NRS), (4) mini nutritional assessment (MNA), and (5) NUTRIC score.

Although many of these scoring systems have not been validated in critically ill patients, the American Society for Parenteral and Enteral Nutrition (ASPEN) guidelines have recommended determination of nutrition risk by NRS score or NUTRIC score on all patients admitted to the ICU. As per the European Society for Clinical Nutrition and Metabolism (ESPEN) guidelines, NRS 2002 and MUST scores are easy and quick in calculation and have the strongest predictive value for mortality. Among the assessment tools available, SGA is inexpensive, quick, and can be conducted at the bedside. It is a reliable tool for determining outcomes in critically ill patients. High nutrition risk scores identify those patients most likely to benefit from early EN therapy. To complete the nutrition assessment, the history of comorbid conditions, function of the gastrointestinal (GI) tract, and aspiration risk must be evaluated.

Traditional nutrition indicators or surrogate markers are not validated in critical care. For example, traditional serum protein markers (albumin, prealbumin, transferrin, retinol binding protein, total lymphocyte count) are a reflection of the acute-phase response (increases in vascular permeability and reprioritization of hepatic protein synthesis) and hence do not accurately depict nutrition status in the ICU setting. Similarly, anthropometrics (body mass index, triceps skin fold thickness, mid-arm circumference area) are not reliable in assessment of nutrition status or adequacy of nutrition therapy. Individual levels of calcitonin, C-reactive protein, interleukin-1, tumor necrosis factor, interleukin-6, and citrulline are still under investigation as to their utility and should not be used as surrogate markers.

Ultrasound is emerging as a tool to expediently measure muscle mass and determines changes in muscle tissue at the bedside in the ICU, given its ease of use and availability. A computed tomography (CT) scan provides a precise quantification of skeletal muscle and adipose tissue depots; however, this would be unfeasible given the prohibitive cost and radiation exposure unless a scan is coincidently being performed for other clinical indication.

Assessment of Energy Needs

In critically ill patients on mechanical ventilation, energy expenditure (EE) can be most accurately determined by indirect calorimetry. However, in the absence of indirect calorimetry, a simple weight-based eq. (25–30 kcal/kg/d) would be adequate in determining energy requirements [5].

Initiate Early EN

Medical nutrition therapy should be considered for all patients admitted to the ICU for more than 48 h [6]. Enteral feeding preserves gut integrity and barrier and immune function. Oral diet is preferred over EN or PN in critically ill patients who are able to eat. If oral intake is not possible, early EN (within 48 h) should be initiated. Presence of bowel sounds is not a prerequisite for initiation of EN. Where there are contraindications to oral feeding and EN, early PN should be implemented within 3–7 days in severely malnourished patients. EN/PN feed should be gradually increased to the calorie target to avoid overfeeding. Gastric access should be used as the standard approach for EN. Post-pyloric feeding is a suitable alternative in patients with gastric feeding intolerance not resolved with prokinetic agents (intravenous erythromycin/metoclopramide). For patients at high risk for aspiration, post-pyloric, mainly jejunal, feeding should be considered. Continuous rather than bolus EN may have an advantage and is a must in post-pyloric feeding.

Early EN is preferred especially in the following conditions:

1. Patients receiving neuromuscular blocking agents, in prone position, and on ECMO.
2. Patients with traumatic brain injury (TBI), stroke (ischemic or hemorrhagic), and spinal cord injury.
3. Patients with severe acute pancreatitis, GI surgery, and open abdomen.
4. Patients after abdominal aortic surgery.
5. Patients with abdominal trauma when the continuity of the GI tract is confirmed/restored.
6. Regardless of the presence of bowel sounds unless bowel ischemia or obstruction is suspected in patients with diarrhea.

In following conditions, early EN should be delayed:

1. If shock is uncontrolled and hemodynamic and tissue perfusion goals are not reached, low dose EN can be started as soon as shock is recovered with fluids and vasopressors/inotropes while remaining vigilant for signs of bowel ischemia.
2. In case of uncontrolled life-threatening hypoxemia, hypercapnia, or acidosis. However, EN can be started in patients with stable hypoxemia and compensated or permissive hypercapnia and acidosis.
3. In the presence of active upper GI bleeding, EN can be started when the bleeding has stopped and no signs of re-bleeding are observed.
4. Patients with overt bowel ischemia.
5. Patients with high-output intestinal fistula if reliable feeding access distal to the fistula is not achievable.
6. Patients with abdominal compartment syndrome.
7. If gastric aspirate volume is above 500 ml/6 h.

Dosing of EN

If predictive equations are used to estimate the energy need, hypocaloric nutrition (below 70% estimated needs) is preferred over isocaloric nutrition in the early phase of acute illness. After day three, caloric delivery can be increased to 80–100% of measured EE. During critical illness, protein requirement is expected to be 1.2–2.0 g/kg actual body weight per day and is likely to be higher in burns or multitrauma patient [7]. The amount of carbohydrates administered to ICU patients should not exceed 5 mg/kg/min [8].

Low-dose EN should be administered in the following situations:

1. Patients receiving therapeutic hypothermia with an increased dose after rewarming.
2. Patients with intra-abdominal hypertension without abdominal compartment syndrome: temporary reduction or discontinuation of EN should be considered if intra-abdominal pressure values increase during EN.

3. Patients with acute liver failure when acute, immediately life-threatening metabolic derangements are controlled with or without liver support strategies, independent of grade of encephalopathy.

Monitoring Tolerance and Adequacy of EN

Patients should be monitored daily for tolerance of EN. Ordering a feeding status of nil per os (NPO) for diagnostic tests or procedures should be minimized to limit propagation of ileus and to prevent inadequate nutrient delivery. Gastric residual volume should not be used as part of routine care to monitor ICU patients receiving EN. A volume-based feeding protocol or a top-down multistrategy protocol should be considered.

In all intubated ICU patients receiving EN, the head of the bed should be elevated 30–45° and use of chlorhexidine mouthwash twice a day should be considered.

EN should not be automatically interrupted for diarrhea but rather that feeding should be continued while evaluating the etiology of diarrhea in an ICU patient to determine appropriate management.

Where there are contraindications to oral feeding and EN, early and progressive PN should be implemented within 3–7 days in severely malnourished patients.

Selection of Appropriate Enteral Formulation

A standard isotonic polymeric formula should be used for the initiation of EN in the ICU setting. Avoid the routine use of all specialty formulas in critically ill patients in a medial ICU and disease-specific formulas in the surgical ICU.

Immune-modulating enteral formulations (arginine with other agents, including eicosapentaenoic acid [EPA], docosahexaenoic acid [DHA], glutamine, and nucleic acid) should not be used routinely in the medical ICU. Except for burns and trauma patients, supplemental enteral glutamine(0.2–0.3 g/kg/d) should not be added to an EN regimen routinely in critically ill patients.

In unstable and complex ICU patients, particularly in those with hepatic and renal failure, parenteral glutamine should not be administered [9]. High doses of omega-3-enriched enteral formulas should not be given on a routine basis. The same holds true for other supplements like selenium, arginine, or vitamin C.

When to Use PN

ASPEN guidelines recommend that use of supplemental PN should be considered after 7–10 days if unable to meet >60% of energy and protein requirements by the enteral route alone in patients with both low and high nutrition risk. Initiating supplemental PN prior to this 7- to 10-day period in critically ill patients on some EN does not improve outcomes and may be detrimental to the patient. In the patient at low nutrition risk (e.g., NRS 2002 ≤3 or NUTRIC score ≤5), exclusive PN should be withheld over the first 7 days following ICU admission if unable to maintain volitional intake and if early EN is not feasible.

In the patient determined to be at high nutrition risk (e.g., NRS 2002 ≥ 5 or NUTRIC score ≥5) or severely malnourished, when EN is not feasible, ASPEN guidelines recommend initiating exclusive PN as soon as possible following ICU admission.

ESPEN guidelines recommends PN in patients who do not tolerate full-dose EN during the first week in the ICU. PN should not be started until all strategies to maximize EN tolerance have been attempted.

When Indicated, Maximize Efficacy of PN

ASPEN guidelines recommend that hypocaloric PN dosing (≤20 kcal/ kg/d or 80% of estimated energy needs) with adequate protein (≥1.2 g protein/kg/d) should be considered in appropriate patients (high risk or severely malnourished) requiring PN, initially over the first week of hospitalization in the ICU.

The target blood glucose range is 140–180 mg/dL for the general ICU population. As tolerance to EN improves, the amount of PN energy should be reduced and finally discontinued when the patient is receiving >60% of target energy requirements from EN.

Special Situations

Pulmonary Failure

ASPEN guidelines recommend that high-fat/low-carbohydrate formulations designed to manipulate the respiratory quotient and reduce CO_2 production should not be used in ICU patients with acute respiratory failure. Fluid-restricted energy-dense EN formulations should be considered for patients with acute respiratory failure (especially in the presence of volume overload). Serum phosphate level should be monitored closely when appropriate and phosphate replacement when needed.

Renal Failure

ASPEN guidelines recommend that ICU patients with acute kidney injury (AKI) should be placed on a standard enteral formulation (protein 1.2–2 g/kg actual body weight per day and energy 25–30 kcal/kg/day). Patients on renal replacement experience a loss of protein along with vitamins and micronutrients which can affect the patient adversely. Protein calorie malnutrition is an independent predictor of mortality in AKI patients. Energy consumption is not increased and is only 130% of REE. The loss (selenium, zinc, fat, lactate, glucose) is termed as "depletion syndrome."

A higher energy prescription do not induce a more positive nitrogen balance and is associated with a higher incidence of hyperglycemia and hypertriglyceridemia and a more positive fluid balance.

Energy provision should be composed of 3–5 (maximum 7) g per kilogram body weight carbohydrates and 0.8–1.0 g per kilogram body weight fat (KDIGO 2012) [10].

Administer 0.8–1.0 g/kg/d of protein in noncatabolic AKI patients without need for dialysis (KDIGO 2012) [10].

Administer 1.0–1.5 g/kg/d of protein in patients with AKI on RRT (KDIGO 2012, 2D) [12] up to a maximum of 1.7 g/kg/d in patients on CRRT and in hypercatabolic patients (KDIGO 2012) [10].

Hepatic Failure

ASPEN guidelines recommend that standard enteral formulations should be used in ICU patients with acute and chronic liver disease. Dry weight should be used instead of actual weight in predictive equations to determine energy and protein in patients with cirrhosis and hepatic failure, due to complications of ascites, intravascular volume depletion, edema, and hypoalbuminemia. There is no evidence of benefit of branched-chain amino acid (BCAA) formulations in patients with encephalopathy.

Acute Pancreatitis

Patients with moderate to severe acute pancreatitis should have a naso-/oroenteric tube placed and EN started at a trophic rate and advanced to goal as fluid volume resuscitation is completed (within 24–48 h of admission). EN should be provided to patients with severe acute pancreatitis by either the gastric or jejunal route, as there is no difference in tolerance or clinical outcomes between these two levels of infusion.

Trauma

Similar to other critically ill patients, early enteral feeding with a high-protein polymeric diet should be initiated in the immediate post-trauma period (within 24–48 hours of injury) once the patient is hemodynamically stable. Either arginine-containing immune-modulating formulations or EPA/DHA supplement with standard enteral formula are appropriate in patients with traumatic brain injury.

Table 13.1 Nutritional recommendations in sepsis

Nutrient	Recommended dose
Caloric needs	Determined by indirect calorimetry
Protein	0.8–1.3 g/kg/day
Lipids	0.7–1.5 g/kg/day
Glucose	1–1.5 g/kg/day
Glutamine	<0.35 g/kg/day IV or <0.5 g/kg/day enterally in TPN fed patients
Fluid	1 mL/kg/h

TPN Total Parenteral Nutrition

Burns

EN should be provided to burn patients whose GI tracts are functional and for whom voli-tional intake is inadequate to meet estimated energy needs. PN should be reserved for those burns patients for whom EN is not feasible or not tolerated. Patients with burn injury should receive protein in the range of 1.5–2 g/kg/d.

Sepsis

Critically ill patients should receive EN therapy within 24–48 h of the diagnosis of severe sepsis/septic shock as soon as resuscitation is complete and the patient is hemodynami-cally stable. Trophic feeding (defined as 10–20 kcal/h or up to 500 kcal/d) should be pro-vided for the initial phase of sepsis, advancing as tolerated after 24–48 h to >80% of target energy goal over the first week with a target protein delivery of 1.2–2 g /kg/d (Table 13.1).

Postoperative Major Surgery

EN should be provided when feasible in the postoperative period within 24 h of surgery, as it results in better outcomes than use of PN. Routine use of an immune-modulating formula (containing both arginine and fish oils) in the SICU for the postoperative patient who requires EN therapy. In a patient who has undergone major upper GI surgery and EN is not feasible, PN should be initiated early (only if the duration of therapy is anticipated to be ≥7 days).

Obese Patients

An iso-caloric high-protein diet can be administered with energy intake guided by indirect calorimetry if available. If indirect calorimetry is unavailable, energy intake can be based on "adjusted body weight" calculated as ideal body weight + 1/3 actual body weight.

Protein delivery should be guided by urinary nitrogen losses or lean body mass determination (using CT or other tools). If urinary nitrogen losses or lean body mass determinations are not available, protein intake can be 1.3 g/kg "adjusted body weight"/day.

Fluid Therapy and Nutrition

It has to be understood that nutrition and fluid therapy go hand in hand and nutrition therapy may be a major cause of fluid creep. The intensivist has to be vigilant while calculating the amount of fluid to be given to the patient when there is ongoing parenteral/enteral nutrition. He should be mindful that he is injecting a hyperosmolar fluid in the form of parenteral nutrition to the critically ill which has its own complications (electrolyte disturbances, hyperglycemia). The following points regarding "volume" and "electrolytes" should be noted:

1. TPN should not be used to completely replenish the fluid requirement of the patient. The intensivist must provide a *"maintenance fluid"* in addition to TPN.
2. As large amounts of fluid are being prescribed, it is crucial to assess the "need for fluid restriction," to "avoid volume overload," particularly in patients with congestive heart failure and renal failure.
3. There should be judicious use of ultrasound and dynamic parameters to assess fluid responsiveness while using fluid therapy along with nutrition; fluid overloading must be avoided.
4. Regular (12 hourly) electrolyte checks are necessary in patients on EN and PN. A standard TPN has 30–80 meq/L of sodium, 30–40 meq/L of potassium, 4–12 meq/L of magnesium, and 10–15 mmol/L of phosphate. So potassium, magnesium, and phosphate replacement should be considered with the initiation of parenteral therapy.

Case Vignette
Questions and Answers
Q1. What is the role of nutrition in a critically ill patient in the ICU?
A1. The earlier case scenario is very common in the ICU. Triggers such as trauma, infections, respiratory failure, and burns activate the metabolic response to stress which culminates in uncontrolled catabolism and resistance to anabolic signals, leading to proteolysis. Uncontrolled catabolism leads to a cumulative calorie deficit. Combination of proteolysis, stress-mediated anabolic resistance, immobilization, and muscle disuse accelerates loss of muscle mass. Loss of lean body mass has been associated with muscle weakness, poor wound healing, mechanical ventilator dependency, increased risk for nosocomial infection, increased hospital length of stay, and increased morbidity and mortality. Exogenous nutrient delivery via enteral or parenteral routes can provide sufficient calories, micronutrients, and antioxidants for energy substrate repletion and maintenance of daily caloric balance.

Q2. How will you assess nutritional risk in this patient?

A2. Patient is a 57-year-old man with a past medical history of diabetes, hypertension, and alcoholism admitted for respiratory failure and sepsis secondary to community-acquired pneumonia. The patient's history of poor oral intake and weight loss suggests pre-hospitalization malnutrition. Age, comorbidities, and severity of current illness leading to critical illness place this patient at high nutritional risk (NUTRIC score ≥ 5), suggesting he may have poor outcomes due to a lack of nutrition or insufficient nutrition. The patient also has major risk factors for refeeding syndrome.

Q3. What will be the nutritional management strategy for this patient?

A3. High nutritional risk suggests the patient will benefit from early nutrition. However, the patient's preexisting malnutrition (history of poor oral intake and weight loss) and significant electrolyte depletions put the patient at risk for refeeding syndrome, which may limit early aggressive nutrition. The patient has no reported contraindications for EN, which include hemodynamic instability requiring escalating vasopressor support, vomiting, ileus, active gastrointestinal bleed, and bowel ischemia. So EN is recommended using a standard (isocaloric) formula with a goal calorie prescription of 25 kcal/kg/day and at least 1.2 g/kg/day protein. EN would be started through a nasogastric tube at an initial rate of 10–20 mL/h and titrated to goal slowly while monitoring for refeeding syndrome. Serum phosphate, potassium, and magnesium should be checked frequently for repletion. Since the protein goal will not be achieved using a trophic EN rate, additional enterally delivered supplemental protein can be added. If the patient does not tolerate EN, early exclusive PN has been demonstrated to be safe and efficacious for calorie provision.

Conclusion

Nutrition stewardship is defined, in analogy with fluid stewardship, as a series of coordinated interventions, introduced to select the optimal type of nutrition, dose, and duration of therapy that results in the best clinical outcome, prevention of adverse events, and cost reduction. This can be accomplished by adhering to the 6 D's (diagnosis, drug, dose, duration, de-escalation, discharge).

Diagnosis Correct nutrition therapy starts with an adequate assessment of the patient's nutritional status (including body weight and body mass index, laboratory analysis with kidney function and electrolytes, urine analysis, etc.) and metabolic evaluation via indirect calorimetry in combination with other monitoring tools, such as body composition assessed with bio-electrical impedance analysis and nitrogen balance.

Drug Critical care physicians should consider nutrition as any other drug administered to our patients with distinct indications and contraindications and potential adverse and side effects. Particular attention should be paid to the different compounds and their specifications (calories, nitrogen, protein, glucose, lipids, and micronutrients).

Dose "Sola dosis facit venenum" or "only the dose makes the poison." There are various important considerations while prescribing a nutritional formula, not only calories and protein dosing as they are correlated with mortality, but also pharmacokinetics and pharmacodynamics need to be taken into account, as well as volume kinetics, since nutrition may also contribute to fluid accumulation.

Duration The duration of total or supplemental artificial nutritional therapy is equally important.

De-escalation The final step in artificial EN or PN nutrition therapy is to consider tapering, withholding, or withdrawing when they are no longer required, e.g., when shock is resolved and the gastrointestinal tract is normally functioning.

Discharge Correct (dis)continuation or tapering of artificial nutritional therapy and (when needed and indicated) prescription post-discharge from ICU, or hospital, is part of the nutritional care plan and should meet quality standards.

> **Take-Home Messages**
> - All the critically ill patients should undergo nutrition assessment, on admission by well-qualified and trained nutritionists using SGA/NRS/NUTRIC/MUST score as per local ICU protocol.
> - Observation of signs of malnutrition (e.g., cachexia, edema, muscle atrophy, BMI <20 kg/m²) is critical.
> - Enteral nutrition should be started early, preferably within the first 24–48 h.
> - The nasogastric route should be the first choice of enteral feeding.
> - Continuous formula feeding with pumps or gravity bags can be preferably done via fine bore (8F–12F) tubes.
> - Feeding should be tailored as per the patient's requirement and level of tolerance.
> - Calories should be in range of 25–30 Kcal/kg body weight/ day for most critically ill patients.
> - Protein requirement for most critically ill patients is in the range of 1.2–2.0 g/kg body weight/day.
> - Scientific formula feeding should be preferred over blended feeding to minimize contamination.
> - In case the nutrition requirement is not met adequately with EN even after 7 days of ICU admission, then usage of parenteral nutrition (PN) may be considered.
> - Give sufficient insulin for glycemic control using established protocols.

- Calorie deficits must be avoided because it is harder to catch up.
- It is time for nutrition stewardship taking into account the 4 D's: drug, dose, duration, de-escalation.

References

1. Singer P, Berger MM, Van den Berghe G, Biolo G, Calder P, Forbes A, et al. ESPEN guidelines on parenteral nutrition: intensive care. Clin Nutr. 2009;33:246e51.
2. Singer P, Blaser AR, Berger MM, Alhazzani W, Calder PC, et al. ESPEN guideline on clinical nutrition in the intensive care unit: intensive care. Clin Nutr. 2018;38:48. https://doi.org/10.1016/j.clnu.2018.08.037.
3. Singer P, Weinberger H, Tadmor B. Which nutrition regimen for the comorbid complex intensive care unit patient? World Rev Nutr Diet. 2013;105:169e74.
4. Sheean PM, Peterson SJ, Chen Y, Liu D, Lateef O, Braunschweig CA. Utilizing multiple methods to classify malnutrition among elderly patients admitted to the medical and surgical intensive care units (ICU). Clin Nutr. 2013;32:752e7.
5. Taylor BE, McClave SA, Martindale RG, Warren MM, Johnson DR, Braunschweig C, et al. Guidelines for the provision and assessment of nutrition support therapy in the adult critically ill patient: society of critical care medicine (SCCM) and American society for parenteral and enteral nutrition (A.S.P.E.N.). Crit Care Med. 2016;44:390e438.
6. Reintam Blaser A, Starkopf J, Alhazzani W, Berger MM, Casaer MP, Deane AM, et al. Early enteral nutrition in critically ill patients: ESCIM clinical practice guidelines. Intensive Care Med. 2017;43:380e98.
7. Zusman O, Theilla M, Cohen J, Kagan I, Bendavid I, Singer P. Resting energy expenditure, calorie and protein consumption in critically ill patients: a retrospective cohort study. Crit Care. 2016;20:367.
8. Burke JF, Wolfe RR, Mullany CJ, Mathews DE, Bier DM. Glucose requirements following burn injury. Parameters of optimal glucose infusion and possible hepatic and respiratory abnormalities following excessive glucose intake. Ann Surg. 1979;190:274e85.
9. Heyland DK, Elke G, Cook D, Berger MM, Wischmeyer PE, Albert M, et al. Glutamine and antioxidants in the critically ill patient: a post hoc analysis of a large-scale randomized trial. J Parenter Enter Nutr. 2015;39:401e9.
10. KDIGO 2012;Vol 2, Issue 1.

Part III

Fluid Therapy in Special Conditions

Fluid Management in Septic Shock

14

Supradip Ghosh and Garima Arora

Contents

Introduction.. 300
Septic Shock: Pathophysiology.. 300
Septic Shock: Diagnosis... 301
Septic Shock: Management... 302
Resuscitation... 303
Which Fluid?... 303
Dose of Fluid... 306
Interaction with Vasopressors.. 306
Septic Shock: Monitoring... 307
Limiting Cumulative Fluid Balance... 308
Conclusion.. 309
References.. 310

IFA Commentary (MLNGM)

Sepsis is a life-threatening organ dysfunction caused by a maladaptive and dysregulated host response to an infection in the bloodstream. That infection can be a virus (e.g., COVID), a bacteria, or a fungus. Without prompt recognition and adequate intervention, this can lead to septic shock, in which several organs usually fail simultaneously, resulting in death. It is therefore crucial to be alert from the first subtle clinical signs and symptoms. According to the World Health Organization, about 50

S. Ghosh (✉)
Department of Critical Care Medicine, Fortis-Escorts Hospital, Faridabad, Haryana, India

G. Arora
Department of Critical Care Medicine, Werribee Mercy Hospital, Werribee, VIC, Australia

© The Author(s) 2024
295
M. L. N. G. Malbrain et al. (eds.), *Rational Use of Intravenous Fluids in Critically Ill Patients*, https://doi.org/10.1007/978-3-031-42205-8_14

million people suffer from sepsis each year, resulting in 11 million deaths. Sepsis is responsible for as much as 20% of all deaths worldwide. This means that every 2.8 s someone dies from sepsis. However, as we speak, sepsis is poorly dealt with in many countries and education and training of healthcare workers can be substantially improved.

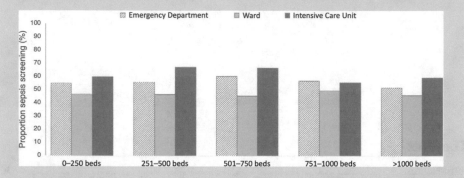

Proportion (in %) of departments (emergency room, general ward, or intensive care unit) with a standardized protocol or screening tool in place specifically for the (early) recognition or detection of sepsis. Adapted from the International Fluid Academy presentation by Scheer C. "Preliminary results of a global survey on sepsis acute care awareness with Christian Scheer" under the Open Access CC BY License 4.0 (video recording minute 11:10 https://whova.com/portal/ifad_202211/videos/3cTO2czN4YTM/).

Often, basic information and data are lacking regarding how many patients have had sepsis, where they were admitted, what the cause was, what treatment or organ support they received (mechanical ventilation, renal replacement therapy, etc.), and whether they died or not. Sepsis nevertheless has a huge impact on our society and the cost of healthcare. In addition, the physical and psychological complaints of sepsis survivors can drag on for a long time with an incremental cost and impact on work reintegration. Just to name a few, think of the post-intensive care syndrome and the recent emergence of long COVID.

Different quality improvement initiatives have been started via the Global and European Sepsis Alliance and the Surviving Sepsis Campaign. The introduction of sepsis stewardship is advocated in analogy with fluid and antimicrobial stewardship. Stewardship is a combination of coordinated actions whereby the right diagnosis is made and the correct treatment, medication, antibiotics, or fluids are administered to the right patient at the right time, in order to prevent complications and adverse effects, improve outcomes, and reduce costs. There are several early clinical signs that can point to sepsis and that can be used in early warning scores. Hospital staff, general practitioners, and even citizens should be trained to recognize them early.

Depending on those scores, we can establish general and specific guidelines (for hospitals and primary care) on how best to intervene. Early recognition and prompt treatment of sepsis are essential to prevent permanent damage and save lives. The World Health Organization therefore passed a resolution in 2017 to urge governments to develop a national sepsis plan with guidelines for early diagnosis, treatment, and aftercare. Several European countries, including Germany, the Netherlands, and the United Kingdom, have already undertaken appropriate action by including measurable quality indicators on sepsis in healthcare. The guidelines of the European Society of Intensive Care Medicine include the guiding principle with five main points for immediate resuscitation and treatment in patients with sepsis and septic shock:

1. Protocol-driven early recognition of sepsis and septic shock, with specific attention in case of immune depression or neutropenia. Measuring the amount of lactate in the blood (as a parameter for diagnosing sepsis and septic shock).
2. Taking blood cultures (preferably at least two sets) before administering antibiotics to determine the source of bloodstream infections and sepsis.
3. Immediately starting an IV for adequate fluid resuscitation up to 30 ml/kg.
4. Early administration of vasoactive medication in patients with persistent septic shock despite fluid resuscitation.
5. Administration of antibiotics based on local antibiotic guidelines.

Specifically for patients admitted to the emergency department with sepsis or septic shock, rapid administration of antibiotics (within 1 h in case of shock or within 3 h in other cases) is recommended as one of the important quality indicators, with the aim of treatment as short as possible.

Septic shock is a subset of sepsis in which underlying circulatory, cellular, and metabolic abnormalities are profound enough to substantially increase mortality [1]. In order to address the circulatory dysfunction, early aggressive fluid therapy has been one of the cornerstones in the treatment of septic shock using an early goal-directed therapy [2]. The revised Surviving Sepsis Campaign guidelines advocate the start of 30 ml/kg of IV fluid within the first hour [3]. However, adequate fluid management in sepsis requires a thoughtful approach. While early aggressive fluid therapy is generally required in the very early phases of patients with profound shock, one should also be aware of the risks of overzealous administration of large volumes of intravenous fluids as the body of evidence has grown that positive daily and cumulative fluid balances during ICU stay increase morbidity and mortality [4]. Furthermore, studies have shown that the type of IV fluid given during resuscitation also has an impact on the patients' outcome [5–7].

This chapter will discuss the pathophysiologic mechanisms of sepsis and the different diagnostic tools to assess volemic status, perfusion, and fluid responsiveness. It also emphasizes the importance of looking at fluids as drugs. A new framework is suggested, with the acronym EROS looking at early recognition, resuscitation, optimization, and source control. However, sepsis should be also seen within the overarching framework that can be divided in four distinct phases, each requiring a different fluid strategy: resuscitation, optimization, stabilization, and evacuation. Phase-by-phase guidance using this ROSE conceptual model is proposed. This led to two important concepts. The first concept being the fact that fluids should be considered as drugs. They come with indications, contraindications, and potential adverse effects. Similar to antibiotic stewardship, a more thoughtful administration of fluids is necessary, hence giving birth to the concept fluid stewardship. This addresses the importance of choosing the right fluid, applying the right dose, using it for the correct duration, and thinking timely about de-escalation. This concept is named the four D's of fluid therapy referring to drug, dose, duration, and de-escalation [8].

Even more important, the second concept states that adequate fluid therapy during sepsis requires a different strategy depending on the phase of illness. The first phase is one of a more aggressive resuscitation to rescue the patient's life; second, we need to optimize organ perfusion by more diligently titrating fluids. In a third phase, we aim at stabilizing the fluid balance to a neutral daily fluid balance, and in the final phase we try to evacuate the potentially accumulated fluids. Hence, the ROSE acronym has been proposed as a mnemonic for this conceptual model [8, 9].

- Fluids in sepsis are drugs and should be treated accordingly with indications, contraindications, and adverse effects.
- One should consider the four D's of fluid therapy: drug, dose, duration, de-escalation.
- We need to consider the four dynamic phases of fluid therapy in sepsis applying the ROSE conceptual model: resuscitation, optimization, stabilization, evacuation.

Suggested Reading

1. Singer M, Deutschman CS, Seymour CW, Shankar-Hari M, Annane D, Bauer M, et al. The third international consensus definitions for sepsis and septic shock (Sepsis-3). JAMA 2016;315(8):801–10.
2. Rivers E, Nguyen B, Havstad S, Ressler J, Muzzin A, Knoblich B, et al. Early goal-directed therapy in the treatment of severe sepsis and septic shock. N Engl J Med 2001;345(19):1368–77.
3. Levy MM, Evans LE, Rhodes A. The surviving sepsis campaign bundle: 2018 update. Intensive Care Med 2018;44(6):925–8.

4. Vincent JL, Sakr Y, Sprung CL, Ranieri VM, Reinhart K, Gerlach H, et al. Sepsis in European intensive care units: results of the SOAP study. Crit Care Med 2006;34(2):344–53.
5. Perner A, Haase N, Guttormsen AB, Tenhunen J, Klemenzson G, Åneman A, et al. Hydroxyethyl starch 130/0.42 versus Ringer's acetate in severe sepsis. N Engl J Med 2012;367(2):124–34.
6. Brunkhorst FM, Engel C, Bloos F, Meier-Hellmann A, Ragaller M, Weiler N, et al. Intensive insulin therapy and pentastarch resuscitation in severe sepsis. N Engl J Med 2008;358(2):125–39.
7. Myburgh JA, Finfer S, Bellomo R, Billot L, Cass A, Gattas D, et al. Hydroxyethyl starch or saline for fluid resuscitation in intensive care. N Engl J Med 2012;367(20):1901–11.
8. Malbrain MLNG, Van Regenmortel N, Saugel B, De Tavernier B, Van Gaal PJ, Joannes-Boyau O, et al. Principles of fluid management and stewardship in septic shock: it is time to consider the four D's and the four phases of fluid therapy. Ann Intensive Care 2018;8(1):66.
9. Mekeirele M, Vanhonacker D, Malbrain MLNG. Fluid Management in Sepsis. In: Prabhakar H, S Tandon, M., Kapoor, I., Mahajan, C. (eds) Transfusion practice in clinical neurosciences. Springer, Singapore. 2022. https://doi.org/10.1007/978-981-19-0954-2_20.

Learning Objectives

The learning objectives of this chapter are:

1. To learn the basic pathophysiology and hemodynamic changes observed in septic shock.
2. To get an insight about the steps towards diagnosis of septic shock.
3. To learn about timing, choice, and dosing of resuscitation fluids in septic shock.
4. To learn about the interaction between fluids and vasopressors and timing of initiation of vasopressors in septic shock.
5. To understand goals of resuscitation in septic shock.

Case Vignette

Mr. X, a 64-year-old male, was brought to ED with complaints of burning micturition and pain in the groin for the past two days. He is a known hypertensive and has history of coronary artery disease with poor LV function (LVEF ~ 45%). On examination, he is drowsy but easily arousable with HR of 110/min, blood pressure of 70/40 mmHg, RR of 20/min, and SpO2 of 96% on room air. His extremities are cold and clammy. The ED physician decides to infuse him with 500 ml of Ringer's lactate solution. Even after fluid bolus, he continues to be dull, with HR of 104/min, BP of 88/48 mmHg, and SpO2 of 95%. Blood gas analysis shows metabolic acidosis with lactate value of 4 mmol/ liter. The ED physician calls you to assess the patient and discuss further resuscitation plan.

Questions
Q1: How do you plan to resuscitate this gentleman now?

Introduction

Sepsis and septic shock remain a common and potentially lethal entity among the critically ill adult patients requiring prompt recognition and management [1]. The new Sepsis-3 definition has defined sepsis as a life-threatening organ dysfunction due to dysregulated host response to infection [2]. Septic shock is defined as persisting hypotension requiring vasopressors to maintain a mean arterial pressure more than 65 mmHg or a lactate of more than 2 mmol/l despite adequate fluid resuscitation [2]. Key principles in the management of septic shock are early recognition, administration of adequate antimicrobial(s), source control, organ support, and early aggressive resuscitation. As recommended by international guidelines, resuscitation starts with rapid intravenous fluid bolus, followed by further fluid administration guided by physiological parameters [3]. However, an inevitable consequence of aggressive fluid resuscitation is fluid overload and its complications, especially when the resuscitation is not monitored carefully. In this chapter, we shall be discussing on key aspects of fluid resuscitation in septic shock, potential ways to limit fluid overload including timely initiation of vasopressors, and goals of septic shock resuscitation. This chapter will focus on adult patients, and more information on fluid therapy in children can be found in Chap. 20. The next chapters will discuss fluids in specific populations: heart failure (Chap. 15), trauma (Chap. 16), neurocritical care (Chap. 17), perioperative setting (Chap. 18), burns (Chap. 19), liver failure (Chap. 21), abdominal hypertension (Chap. 22), and COVID-19 (Chap. 26).

Septic Shock: Pathophysiology

The fundamental features of septic shock include vasodilation, relative and true hypovolemia, increased permeability, and myocardial dysfunction. Vasodilatation in septic shock is due to underlying inflammatory state compounded by decreased responsiveness to natural catecholamines and relative deficiency of vasopressin [4, 5]. Profound vasodilation leads to decreased stress volume and lower mean systemic filling pressure, in turn leading to a decrease in venous return, cardiac output, and arterial pressure. In some patients, true hypovolemia may worsen the scenario, e.g., patients with abdominal sepsis and GI losses.

Increased capillary permeability is a hallmark feature in nearly all patients of sepsis. In response to infection, there is activation of neutrophils, release of a large number of inflammatory mediators, reactive oxygen species, and activation of coagulation pathways [6]. All these lead to endothelial dysfunction and an increase in vascular permeability [7]. Aggressive fluid resuscitation may compound this vascular permeability further by producing an increase in capillary transmural hydrostatic pressure worsening interstitial edema and organ dysfunction [8]. This explains why patients with sepsis and high fluid balances have worse outcomes [9].

An increasingly recognized entity that contributes to the pathophysiology of septic shock is septic cardiomyopathy, a condition characterized by transient decrease in left ventricular contractility with normal filling pressure. Incidence of septic cardiomyopathy widely varies in the literature from 10% to as high as 70% and reflects lack of standardized definition as well as variations in the patient population studies. [10] Right ventricular dysfunction can complicate septic shock further. It is characterized by poor right ventricular contractility with reduction in tricuspid annular plane systolic excursion (TAPSE) and dilatation of right ventricle observed in echocardiography. Using a definition of RV fractional area change (FAC) <35% or TAPSE <1.6 cm, a recent study has reported incidence of right ventricular dysfunction in septic shock as 48%.[11] Reduction in cardiac output resulting from left and right ventricular dysfunction worsens tissue perfusion further. Tachycardia observed in septic shock patients may sometimes be inappropriate and results in poor diastolic filling and loss of ventriculo-aortic coupling. [12].

Apart from endothelial dysfunction and capillary leak, septic shock is also characterized by lack of homogeneity in the distribution of blood flow at the level of microcirculation with both poorly perfused and adequately perfused areas in close vicinity to each other. [13] These alterations at the microvascular level have profound impact in the pathophysiology of septic shock, worsening organ dysfunction further and unfavorable outcomes. In the early stages of septic shock, improvement in systemic hemodynamics (macrocirculation) leads to improvement in microcirculation ("hemodynamic coherence"). However, in the late stages, this coherence between macro- and microcirculation is lost, leading to refractory shock. [14].

Septic Shock: Diagnosis

Early recognition of shock state is of utmost importance to improve hemodynamics and restore tissue perfusion [3]. Detailed history and clinical examination are essential first step towards diagnosing septic shock and identifying the source of infection. Look for history of altered sensorium, decreased urine output, and signs of poor peripheral perfusion such as cold extremities, increased capillary refill time, or mottling. Low blood pressure and a need for vasopressor to maintain MAP of at least 65 mmHg is a must to define septic shock as per current definition [2]. However, hypotension may not be there at the time of presentation in some patients especially in previously hypertensive patients on irregular or no medication in some patients because of compensatory response. In fact, high lactate values without hypotension in patients with septic shock (the so-called "cryptic shock") have similar bad prognosis as overt shock with hypotension. [15] Invasive blood pressure monitoring not only helps in accurate BP monitoring but also gives important information by giving variables for fluid responsiveness such as pulse pressure variation and systolic pressure variation or can be used for cardiac output monitoring.

Current definition of septic shock mandates measurement of lactate. High lactate may be an indicator for global tissue hypoperfusion, especially when correlated with other clinical hypoperfusion parameters. Serial measurement of lactate is also of value in following resuscitation process and is recommended by guideline. [3, 16] However, lactate may not be elevated in every patient of septic shock; but this lack of lactate elevation is associated with better prognosis. [15] One should also remember that lactate may be elevated in several other conditions apart from tissue hypoperfusion (type B lactic acidosis), e.g., hepatic dysfunction, mitochondrial dysfunction, thiamine deficiency, and medications (metformin, antiretroviral drugs). Elevated lactate may also be related to hyperglycemia and increased production of pyruvate, stress-related adrenergic hyperactivity, and increased glycolysis. Other markers of global hypoperfusion states used for monitoring resuscitation are mixed venous (or central venous) oxygen saturation (SvO2 or ScvO2) or venoarterial carbon dioxide pressure difference (Pv-aCO2). SvO2>65% or ScvO2>70% has been suggested by sepsis guideline as end point of resuscitation [3].

Point-of-care ultrasound can now be considered as an extension of clinical examination in critically ill patients. A focused ultrasonographic examination in appropriate clinical context is extremely useful in identifying mechanism of circulatory shock at the bedside and to determine appropriate mean to rectify it. [17] Apart from identifying type of shock, detailed ultrasonographic examination is helpful in recognizing possible source of infection in patients with septic shock, for example, consolidation pattern in lung ultrasound for pneumonia or fluid collection in body cavities, localized abscess in liver, or hydronephrosis of kidney. In appropriate patient, respirophasic variation in inferior caval diameter can help in taking a decision about further fluid resuscitation.

In some patients, more advanced hemodynamic monitoring may become necessary. Despite its limitations, pulmonary artery (PA) catheter is still considered as the gold standard for advanced hemodynamic monitoring. But with the availability of advanced noninvasive or minimally invasive diagnostic tests and potential concern about the safety of PA catheter, it is now gradually falling out of favor [18, 19].

Septic Shock: Management

The four pillars of septic shock management are (1) **E**arly recognition of shock state and identification of source of infection, (2) **R**esuscitation and rapid establishment of tissue reperfusion, (3) Providing support to failing **O**rgans, and (4) **S**ource control including early adequate antibiotics and drainage/debridement of infectious focus (if feasible). The pneumonic "EROS" may be useful as a checklist at the bedside (Fig. 14.1).

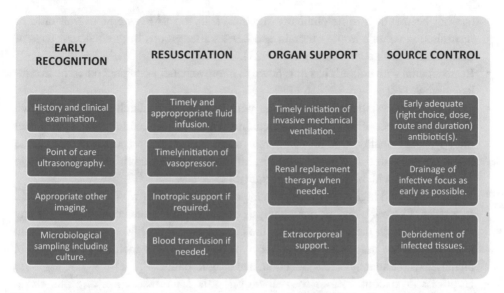

EARLY RECOGNITION	RESUSCITATION	ORGAN SUPPORT	SOURCE CONTROL
History and clinical examination.	Timely and appropropriate fluid infusion.	Timely initiation of invasive mechanical ventilation.	Early adequate (right choice, dose, route and duration) antibiotic(s).
Point of care ultrasonography.	Timely initiation of vasopressor.	Renal replacement therapy when needed.	Drainage of infective focus as early as possible.
Appropriate other imaging.	Inotropic support if required.		
Microbiological sampling including culture.	Blood transfusion if needed.	Extracorporeal support.	Debridement of infected tissues.

Fig. 14.1 EROS principle: summarizing principles of managing septic shock (Adapted from Ghosh S. with permission [20])

Resuscitation

The goal of resuscitation is to rapidly establish tissue reperfusion. This can be achieved by increasing delivery of oxygen and/or by maintaining oxygen content of blood and/or by increasing mean arterial pressure (upstream pressure for organ perfusion). Different tools are available to achieve these goals: fluid infusion, vasopressors, inotropic support, and blood transfusion, if required. In this chapter, we shall be focusing on fluid resuscitation in septic shock, its potential interaction with vasopressors, and appropriate indications to initiate inotropic support.

Despite several caveats associated with it, intravenous fluid infusion remains the first-line resuscitation option in septic shock resuscitation. Physiological principles behind fluid resuscitation are described elsewhere in this book. Briefly, intravenous fluid infusion can potentially increase cardiac output by increasing circulatory stressed volume and may also increase mean arterial pressure provided ventriculo-aortic coupling is maintained.

Which Fluid?

Colloids Versus Crystalloids Current evidence does not support colloids as the resuscitation fluid of choice in septic shock.

- Theoretical advantage of colloids remaining in the intravascular compartment for a longer period of time and thus potentially limiting overall resuscitation fluid volume has not been shown to be clinically significant. In the SAFE study, overall ratio of resuscitation volume in 4% albumin and 0.9% saline groups in the first four days of resuscitation was approximately 1:1.4. [21].

- Resuscitation with colloids has not shown to improve patient-centered outcome in clinical studies. [22].
- Compared to crystalloids, resuscitation with hydroxyethyl starch (HES) has shown increasing number of adverse events including renal failure, need for renal replacement therapy, coagulopathy, need for blood transfusion, and allergic reactions. [23–25] In the 6S study, compared to Ringer's acetate, infusion with hetastarch in Ringer's acetate was associated with higher 90-day mortality. [25].
- There are limited high-quality data available for resuscitation with gelatin or dextran. In a recent Cochrane review, meta-analysis of all available evidence does not find any advantage of both these colloids over the control group. [26] Moreover, both gelatin and dextrans are associated with number of adverse effects including renal failure, anaphylaxis (or anaphylactoid) reaction, and coagulopathy.
- Hypo- or iso-oncotic (4% or 5%) albumin is safe for resuscitation of septic shock patients and may possibly have some beneficial effect. [21, 27] However, cost–benefit ratio must be considered while prescribing 4% or 5% albumin for volume resuscitation in septic shock. Albumin should not be used for resuscitation of a patient with underlying traumatic brain injury or any evidence of raised intracranial pressure. [28].
- In a small study, hyperoncotic (20 or 25%) albumin infusion was found to be beneficial in limiting resuscitation volume compared to hypo- or iso-oncotic albumin. [29] However, this finding needs to be validated in a larger multicenter study, before recommending it for wider use.
- However, effects of albumin infusion in septic shock may not only be limited to improvement of hypoperfusion state. In the multicenter Italian ALBIOS trial, supplemental 20% albumin infusion in addition to crystalloid infusion was associated with mortality benefit in subgroup of patients with septic shock. [30].

Crystalloids: Saline or Balanced Over the years, 0.9% saline has been the most commonly administered crystalloid. But in recent years, its safety has been questioned because of its high chloride load and potential for renal hypoperfusion through tubuloglomerular feedback mechanism. Moreover, with a strong ion difference of 0, large volume 0.9% saline infusion may lead to hyperchloremic metabolic acidosis. Based on the current evidence, the Surviving Sepsis Campaign guidelines recommend balanced crystalloids as the first-line resuscitation fluid in septic shock [3].

- In a study on human volunteers, 0.9% saline has shown to reduce renal perfusion. [31].
- Restricting use of chloride-liberal fluids have shown to improve renal outcome in before and after studies. [32, 33].

- In a large observational study, increasing utilization of balanced salt solutions during septic shock resuscitation was shown to be associated with better survival outcome. [34].
- In the single-center SMART randomized control study, resuscitation with balanced crystalloids (mostly Ringer's lactate) had shown to lower composite outcome of death, renal dysfunction, and new requirement of RRT at 30 days (major advanced kidney event at 30 days or MAKE30) compared to 0.9% saline. [35].
- In the SALT-ED study, compared to 0.9% saline, resuscitation with balanced salt solutions was shown to reduce hospital length of stay in adult patients who needed fluid infusion in the ED and were admitted in the wards. [34] Balanced fluid group also had lower incidence of MAKE30. [36].
- In four more randomized control studies, balanced salt solutions were not associated with worse clinical outcome compared to 0.9% saline. [37–40].
- However, 0.9% saline is still useful in certain clinical scenarios like resuscitating patients with raised intracranial pressure, hypovolemic hyponatremia, hypovolemia with metabolic alkalosis, or in resource-limited settings.

Which Balanced Fluid? Currently, there is no high-quality clinical evidence comparing different balanced salt solutions. Choosing the right balanced fluid is largely based on physiological data and cost.

- Balanced salt solutions vary significantly in their composition including electrolyte content, buffer base, and strong ion difference. Lactate present in Ringer's lactate is largely metabolized in the liver and the metabolism may get overwhelmed, at least theoretically, in patients with severe hepatic dysfunction. In contrast, acetate present in Plasma-Lyte, Ringer's acetate, and Sterofundin is metabolized in almost all tissues.
- With higher SID, Plasma-Lyte can potentially correct metabolic acidosis faster. [41] However, clinical benefit of this earlier resolution of metabolic acidosis needs to be further evaluated in larger human studies.
- However, cost and availability of a particular balance fluid solution also should be considered before deciding the choice of fluid.

To Summarize Current evidence supports use of balanced salt solution as the preferred resuscitation fluid in most clinical circumstances.

- Synthetic colloids (HES, gelatins, and dextrans) should be avoided in septic shock resuscitation because of potential safety concern.
- Albumin can be given safely in patients requiring large volumes of fluid, thus decreasing cumulative fluid balance. However, high cost of albumin needs to be balanced with this small benefit.

Dose of Fluid

As discussed earlier, the rationale for fluid resuscitation is to possibly increase mean systemic filling pressure in massively vasodilated patients and also to cater for volume already lost or to replace ongoing losses. But volume infusion must be balanced against the possible increase in interstitial edema resulting from the capillary leak. Studies have shown a strong association between over-resuscitation and positive fluid balance with worse patient-centric outcomes. [42, 43] To maintain a balance between benefit and harm associated with fluid infusion, patients should be assessed frequently and every effort should be made to limit overall cumulative fluid volume without compromising tissue perfusion.

- SSC Guidelines recommend liberal fluid resuscitation with at least 30 ml/kg of crystalloids in the first 3 h of resuscitation in a septic shock patient [3]. However, the recommendation is not based on sound clinical evidence and has been widely criticized. [44].
- Instead of going ahead with empirical weight-based fluid resuscitation, fluid dosing should be individualized, based on clinical and hemodynamic parameters and evidence of no apparent harm associated with it. We suggest small frequent fluid boluses, with frequent monitoring of clinical response to the bolus, as proposed in the original description of intravenous fluid therapy. [45] Minimal fluid bolus to be given for substantive improvement in hemodynamic parameter is at least 4 ml/kg body weight. [46].
- After initial bolus, all subsequent fluid boluses should be administered only after assessment of fluid responsiveness parameters. [47].
- When fluid responsiveness parameters are not available or not applicable, it is advisable to perform a standard fluid challenge or mini-fluid challenge to guide further fluid therapy. [48, 49] Further fluid bolus should be administered only if the patient is fluid responsive or fluid challenge (or mini-fluid challenge) is positive. Fluid challenge should not be repeated if the initial response is negative or equivocal. [50].
- Underlying clinical status and possible harm associated with fluid infusion also should be considered before administering further fluid boluses. One should be extra cautious in patients at a higher risk of harm from fluid, for example, patients with profound baseline hypoxia or raised intra-abdominal pressure.

Interaction with Vasopressors

Prolonged hypotension is associated with increased mortality in septic shock and early initiation of vasopressors has shown to improve outcome, but not before infusion of some fluid. [51–53] Infusion of norepinephrine can potentially increase cardiac output by its positive effect on stressed volume through venoconstrictor effect. [54] Early initiation of norepinephrine infusion has also shown to reverse shock state earlier. [55] But these potential beneficial effects of early vasopressor initiation must be balanced against potentially adverse effects.

- Norepinephrine infusion may actually decrease cardiac output by increasing resistance to venous return, particularly in the presence of hypovolemia (both relative and absolute). [56].
- Vasopressors can potentially increase organ ischemia by vasospasm. In the multicenter SEPSISPAM study, incidences of acute myocardial infarction, mesenteric ischemia, and digital ischemia were 1.8%, 2.3%, and 2.6%, respectively, in the "high MAP" target group. [57].
- All vasopressors are associated with risk of potentially life-threatening cardiac arrhythmias. In the SOAP II study, overall incidences of arrhythmias were 24.1% in "dopamine arm" and 12.4% in "norepinephrine arm." [58].
- Other metabolic disturbances like hyperlactatemia are also known with certain vasopressor infusion. In the multicenter CAT study, 12.9% patients included in the "epinephrine group" withdrew because of transient but significant metabolic side effects especially hyperlactatemia. [59].

When to Initiate Vasopressor Infusion?   The Surviving Sepsis Guidelines suggest initiation of vasopressor infusion after adequate volume resuscitation [3]. However, at the bedside, timing of vasopressor initiation should be individualized. We suggest the following guidelines based on available evidence:

- In patients with diastolic blood pressure of <50 mmHg, vasopressor infusion should be started along with fluid boluses. DBP is the upstream pressure for coronary perfusion. Rise in cardiac enzymes was observed in pregnant ladies with persistent DBP <50 mmHg following postpartum hemorrhage. [60].
- Vasopressors also should be initiated simultaneously with fluid infusion, in patients with profound vasodilatation as suggested by diastolic shock index >2.3. [61] Diastolic shock index is defined as the ratio between heart rate and diastolic blood pressure.
- Otherwise, it is reasonable to start vasopressor infusion after initial 1–2 liters of crystalloid infusion. In the REFRESH study, a strategy of initiating norepinephrine infusion after one liter of fluid had shown to reduce cumulative fluid balance. [62] In an observational study, dose of vasopressor in the first six hours after septic shock onset was shown to be associated with increased mortality, and this effect was mitigated if vasopressors were initiated only after two liters of fluids. [53] However, further fluid administration should not be limited after starting norepinephrine infusion.

Septic Shock: Monitoring

Throughout the process of resuscitation, patients should be monitored for improvement of physiological parameters including heart rate, mean arterial pressure, increase in urine output, improvement of peripheral perfusion parameters (especially capillary refill time), gradual normalization of central venous (or mixed venous) oxygen saturation, and gradual improvement in lactate. Monitoring should also be done for harmful consequences of resuscitation including evidence of fluid overload (fall in oxygen saturation, B-profile in lung ultrasound, extravascular lung water, rising intra-abdominal pressure), or adverse effects of vasopressors (myocardial, mesenteric, digital ischemia, or arrhythmias).

- In the landmark early goal-directed therapy (EGDT) study, Rivers and colleagues applied protocolized resuscitation aiming to achieve certain hemodynamic and other parameters like central venous pressure, mean arterial pressure, oxygen saturation, and hemoglobin with an ultimate goal of ScvO2 > 65%, very early in septic shock resuscitation at ED. [63] This early protocolized resuscitation achieved remarkable mortality benefit compared to usual care. However, three recent studies conducted across several continents could not confirm the benefits of EGDT strategy targeting ScvO2 > 70%. [64–66].
- Serial measurement of lactate has shown to improve clinical outcome. [16] Guideline has suggested lactate measurement for initial diagnosis of sepsis, for following progress of resuscitation, and as an end point of resuscitation [3]. However, in a randomized study of septic shock resuscitation in emergency department, a strategy aiming to normalize lactate clearance did not show any outcome benefit compared to a strategy of normalizing ScvO2. [67].
- Capillary refill time is an easily available bedside clinical parameter with no additional cost involved to monitor. It is shown to have the fastest recovery kinetics among all available physiological parameters, and its normalization is shown to be associated with better regional perfusion and better prognosis. [14] In the ANDROMEDA-SHOCK trial, patients with septic shock were randomized to either be resuscitated based on capillary refill time (CRT) monitoring every 30 minutes or to 2-hourly lactate measurement. Compared to lactate group, CRT group received lower volume of fluid and also had less organ dysfunction. [68] In a subsequent Bayesian analysis of the ANDROMEDA-SHOCK data, mortality rate was better in the CRT group. [69].
- To summarize, a holistic approach should be followed while monitoring a patient with septic shock and multiple parameters should be considered to decide specific treatment measure during resuscitation process and to take a final call for the end point of resuscitation.

Limiting Cumulative Fluid Balance

The relationship between fluid volume and mortality follows a "U"-shaped curve with both too little and too much fluid increasing death. Every effort should be made to limit fluid infusion without compromising perfusion of organs.

Protocolized "restrictive fluid" strategy has yielded mixed result so far with CLASSIC pilot study showing beneficial effect and larger study showing no beneficial effect. [70, 71].

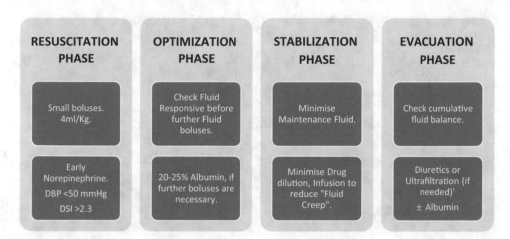

Fig. 14.2 Suggested approach to limit cumulative fluid balance in different stages of resuscitation. (Adapted from Ghosh S. with permsission [20])

A more prudent approach perhaps is to apply restrictive strategies in every stage of resuscitation [8]. We suggest the following approach in limiting cumulative fluid balance in different stages of shock (Fig. 14.2).

Case Vignette
Mr. X is likely a case of urosepsis with septic shock. He has already received 1 L of fluids. Despite that, he continues to be hypotensive with high lactates. Vasopressors should be initiated early along with appropriate antibiotics after obtaining cultures. He has a low ejection fraction. Hence, further fluid should be in the form of small boluses with frequent assessment for fluid responsiveness.

Conclusion

Balanced isotonic crystalloids are generally the fluid of choice in sepsis resuscitation, while there might be a place for human albumin in patients with septic shock and an albumin level below 30 g/l. Hypotonic crystalloids are the maintenance fluids of choice when enteral or parenteral feeding is insufficient. There is strong evidence against using HES or NaCl 0.9% in sepsis. There is no convincing evidence to support the use of Gelatins or Dextran. Early use of vasopressors can increase the stressed volume hence limiting the need for ongoing fluid resuscitation.

Take-Home Messages
- Fluid resuscitation remains the vital part of management of septic shock patients.
- Resuscitation should be initiated early with balanced crystalloids with frequent assessment of clinical parameters followed by variables to measure fluid responsiveness.
- Care must be taken to frequently assess for end point of hemodynamic resuscitation, thus avoiding increase in cumulative fluid balance and overload.
- Early introduction of vasopressors may improve clinical outcome.
- The goal is to achieve early and adequate resuscitation to prevent end-organ damage followed by measures to evacuate fluid and minimize cumulative balance once the shock has settled.

References

1. Rudd KE, Johnson SC, Agesa KM, Shackelford KA, Tsoi D, Kievlan DR, et al. Global, regional, and national sepsis incidence and mortality, 1990-2017: analysis for the global burden of disease study. Lancet. 2020;395:200–11.
2. Seymour CW, Liu VX, Iwashyna TJ, Brunkhorst FM, Rea TD, Scherag A, et al. Assessment of clinical criteria for sepsis: for the third international consensus definitions for sepsis and septic shock (Sepsis-3). JAMA. 2016;315:762–74.
3. Evans L, Rhodes A, Alhazzani W, Antonelli M, Coopersmith CM, French C, et al. Surviving sepsis campaign: international guidelines for management of sepsis and septic shock 2021. Intensive Care Med. 2021;47:1181–247.
4. Benedict CR, Rose JA. Arterial norepinephrine changes in patients with septic shock. Circ Shock. 1992;38:165–72.
5. Cumming AD, Dredger AA, McDonald JW, Lindsay RM, Solez K, Linton AL. Vasoactive hormones in the renal response to systemic sepsis. Am J Kidney Dis. 1988;11:23–32.
6. Angus DC, van der Poll T. Severe sepsis and septic shock. N Engl J Med. 2013;369:2063.
7. Khakpour S, Wilhelmsen K, Hellman J. Vascular endothelial cell toll-like receptor pathways in sepsis. Innate Immun. 2015;21(8):827–46.
8. Malbrain MLNG, Van Regenmortel N, Saugel B, De Tavernier B, Van Gaal P-J, Joannes-Boyau O, et al. Principles of fluid management and stewardship in septic shock: it is time to consider the four D's and the four phases of fluid therapy. Ann Intensive Care [Internet]. 2018;8(1)
9. Silversides JA, Fitzgerald E, Manickavasagam US, Lapinsky SE, Nisenbaum R, Hemmings N, et al. Deresuscitation of patients with iatrogenic fluid overload is associated with reduced mortality in critical illness. Crit Care Med. 2018;46:1600–7.
10. Beesley SJ, Weber G, Sarge T, Nikravan S, Grissom CK, Lanspa MJ, Shahul S, Brown SM. Septic cardiomyopathy. Crit Care Med. 2018;46:625–34.
11. Lanspa MJ, Cirulis MM, Wiley BM, Olsen TD, Wilson EL, Beesley SJ, Brown SM, Hirshberg EL, Grissom CK. Right ventricular dysfunction in early sepsis and septic shock. Chest. 2021;159:1055–63.
12. Morelli A, Ertmer C, Westphal M, Rehberg S, Kampmeier T, Ligges S, et al. Effect of heart rate control with esmolol on hemodynamic and clinical outcomes in patients with septic shock: a randomized clinical trial. JAMA. 2013;310:1683–91.

13. De Backer D, Ricottilli F, Ospina-Tascón GA. Septic shock: a microcirculation disease. Curr Opin Anaesthesiol. 2021;34:85–91.

14. Hernández G, Teboul J-L. Is the macrocirculation really dissociated from the microcirculation in septic shock? Intensive Care Med. 2016;42:1621–4.

15. Hernandez G, Bruhn A, Castro R, Regueira T. The holistic view on perfusion monitoring in septic shock. Curr Opin Crit Care. 2012;18:280–6.

16. Jansen TC, van Bommel J, Schoonderbeek FJ, Sleeswijk Visser SJ, van der Klooster JM, Lima AP, Willemsen SP, Bakker J, LACTATE study group. Early lactate-guided therapy in intensive care unit patients: a multicenter, open-label, randomized controlled trial. Am J Respir Crit Care Med. 2010;182:752–61.

17. Lichtenstein D. Fluid administration limited by lung sonography: the place of lung ultrasound in assessment of acute circulatory failure (the FALLS-protocol). Expert Rev Respir Med. 2012;6:155–62.

18. Connors AF Jr, Speroff T, Dawson NV, Thomas C, Harrell FE Jr, Wagner D, et al. The effectiveness of right heart catheterization in the initial care of critically ill patients. JAMA. 1996;276:889–97.

19. Richard C, Warszawski J, Anguel N, Deye N, Combes A, Barnaud D, et al. Early use of the pulmonary artery catheter and outcomes in patients with shock and acute respiratory distress syndrome: a randomized controlled Trial. JAMA. 2003;290:2713–20.

20. Ghosh S. Fluid resuscitation in septic shock. In: Handbook of intravenous fluids. Singapore: Springer; 2022. https://doi.org/10.1007/978-981-19-0500-1_11.

21. Finfer S, Bellomo R, Boyce N, French J, Myburgh J, Norton R, et al. A comparison of albumin and saline for fluid resuscitation in the intensive care unit. N Engl J Med. 2004;350(22):2247–56.

22. Annane D, Siami S, Jaber S, Martin C, Elatrous S, Declère AD, et al. Effects of fluid resuscitation with colloids vs crystalloids on mortality in critically ill patients presenting with hypovolemic shock: the CRISTAL randomized trial. JAMA. 2013;310:1809–17.

23. Brunkhorst FM, Engel C, Bloos F, Meier-Hellmann A, Ragaller M, Weiler N, et al. Intensive insulin therapy and pentastarch resuscitation in severe sepsis. N Engl J Med. 2008;358(2):125–39.

24. Myburgh JA, Finfer S, Bellomo R, Billot L, Cass A, Gattas D, et al. Hydroxyethyl starch or saline for fluid resuscitation in intensive care. N Engl J Med. 2012;367(20):1901–11.

25. Perner A, Haase N, Guttormsen AB, Tenhunen J, Klemenzson G, Åneman A, et al. Hydroxyethyl starch 130/0.42 versus Ringer's acetate in severe sepsis. N Engl J Med. 2012;367(2):124–34.

26. Lewis SR, Pritchard MW, Evans DJW, Butler AR, Alderson P, Smith AF, Roberts I. Colloids versus crystalloids for fluid resuscitation in critically ill people. Cochrane Database Systematic Rev. 2018;8:CD000567.

27. Finfer S, McEvoy S, Bellomo R, McArthur C, Myburgh J, Norton R. Impact of albumin compared to saline on organ function and mortality of patients with severe sepsis. Intensive Care Med. 2011;37:86–96.

28. Myburgh J, Cooper DJ, Finfer S, Bellomo R, Norton R, Bishop N, Kai Lo S, Vallance S. Saline or albumin for fluid resuscitation in patients with traumatic brain injury. N Engl J Med. 2007;357:874–84.

29. Mårtensson J, Bihari S, Bannard-Smith J, Glassford NJ, Lloyd-Donald P, Cioccari L, et al. Small volume resuscitation with 20% albumin in intensive care: physiological effects: the SWIPE randomised clinical trial. Intensive Care Med. 2018;44:1797–806.

30. Caironi P, Tognoni G, Masson S, Fumagalli R, Pesenti A, Romero M, et al. Albumin replacement in patients with severe sepsis or septic shock. N Engl J Med. 2014;370:1412–21.

31. Chowdhury AH, Cox EF, Francis ST, Lobo DN. A randomized, controlled, double-blind cross-over study on the effects of 2-L infusions of 0.9% saline and plasma-lyte® 148 on renal blood flow velocity and renal cortical tissue perfusion in healthy volunteers. Ann Surg. 2012;256:18–24.

32. Yunos NM, Bellomo R, Hegarty C, Story D, Ho L, Bailey M. Association between a chloride-liberal vs chloride-restrictive intravenous fluid administration strategy and kidney injury in critically ill adults. JAMA. 2012;308:1566–72.

33. Yunos NM, Bellomo R, Glassford N, Sutcliffe H, Lam Q, Bailey M. Chloride-liberal vs. chloride-restrictive intravenous fluid administration and acute kidney injury: an extended analysis. Intensive Care Med. 2015;41:257–64.

34. Raghunathan K, Shaw A, Nathanson B, Stürmer T, Brookhart A, Stefan MS, Setoguchi S, Beadles C, Lindenauer PK. Association between the choice of IV crystalloid and in-hospital mortality among critically ill adults with sepsis. Crit Care Med. 2014;42:1585–91.

35. Semler MW, Self WH, Wanderer JP, Ehrenfeld JM, Wang L, Byrne DW, et al. Balanced crystalloids versus saline in critically ill adults. N Engl J Med. 2018;378:829–39.

36. Self WH, Semler MW, Wanderer JP, Wang L, Byrne DW, Collins SP, et al. Balanced crystalloids versus saline in noncritically ill adults. N Engl J Med. 2018;378:819–28.

37. Young P, Bailey M, Beasley R, Henderson S, Mackle D, McArthur C, et al. Effect of a buffered crystalloid solution vs saline on acute kidney injury among patients in the intensive care unit: the SPLIT randomized clinical trial. JAMA. 2015;314:1701–10.

38. Semler MW, Wanderer JP, Ehrenfeld JM, Stollings JL, Self WH, Siew ED, et al. Balanced crystalloids versus saline in the intensive care unit. The SALT randomized trial. Am J Respir Crit Care Med. 2017;195:1362–72.

39. Zampieri FG, Machado FR, Biondi RS, Freitas FGR, Veiga VC, Figueiredo RC, et al. Effect of intravenous fluid treatment with a balanced solution vs 0.9% Saline Solution on mortality in critically ill patients: the Basics randomized clinical trial. JAMA. 2021;326(29):818.

40. Finfer S, Micallef S, Hammond N, Navarra L, Bellomo R, Billot L, et al. Balanced multielectrolyte solution versus saline in critically ill adults. N Engl J Med. 2022;386:815–26.

41. Rauserova-Lexmaulova L, Prokesova B, Blozonova A, Vanova-Uhrikova I, Rehakova K, Fusek M. Effects of the administration of different buffered balanced crystalloid solutions on acid–base and electrolyte status in dogs with gastric dilation–volvulus syndrome: a randomized clinical trial. Top Companion Anim Med. 2022;46:100613. https://doi.org/10.1016/j.ajem.2016.10.007.

42. Wiedemann HP, Wheeler AP, Bernard GR, Thompson BT, Hayden D, deBoisblanc B, et al. Comparison of two fluid-management strategies in acute lung injury. N Engl J Med. 2006;354:2564–75.

43. Boyd JH, Forbes J, Nakada TA, Walley KR, Russell JA. Fluid resuscitation in septic shock: a positive fluid balance and elevated central venous pressure are associated with increased mortality. Crit Care Med. 2011;39:259–65.

44. Prowle JR, Kirwan CJ, Bellomo R. Fluid management for the prevention and attenuation of acute kidney injury. Nat Rev Nephrol. 2014;10(1):37–47.

45. Latta T. Saline venous injection in cases of malignant cholera, performed while in the vapour-bath. Lancet. 1832;19(480):208–9.

46. Aya HD, Rhodes A, Chis Ster I, Fletcher N, Grounds RM, Cecconi M. Hemodynamic effect of different doses of fluids for a fluid challenge: a quasi-randomized controlled study. Crit Care Med. 2017;45:e161–8.

47. Monnet X, Marik PE, Teboul JL. Prediction of fluid responsiveness: an update. Ann Intensive Care. 2016;6(1):111.

48. Vincent JL, Weil MH. Fluid challenge revisited. Crit Care Med. 2006;34:1333–7.

49. Muller L, Toumi M, Bousquet PJ, Riu-Poulenc B, Louart G, Candela D, et al. AzuRéa group. An increase in aortic blood flow after an infusion of 100 ml colloid over 1 minute can predict fluid responsiveness: the mini-fluid challenge study. Anesthesiology. 2011;115:541–7.

50. Cecconi M, Hofer C, Teboul JL, Pettila V, Wilkman E, Molnar Z, et al. Fluid challenges in intensive care: the FENICE study: a global inception cohort study. Intensive Care Med. 2015;41:1529–37.

51. Bai X, Yu W, Ji W, Lin Z, Tan S, Duan K, Dong Y, Xu L, Li N. Early versus delayed administration of norepinephrine in patients with septic shock. Crit Care. 2014;18:532.

52. Waechter J, Kumar A, Lapinsky SE, Marshall J, Dodek P, Arabi Y, et al. Interaction between fluids and vasoactive agents on mortality in septic shock: a multicenter, observational study. Crit Care Med. 2014;42:2158–68.

53. Roberts RJ, Miano TA, Hammond DA, Patel GP, Chen JT, Phillips KM, et al. Evaluation of vasopressor exposure and mortality in patients with septic shock. Crit Care Med. 2020;48:1445–53.

54. Persichini R, Silva S, Teboul JL, Jozwiak M, Chemla D, Richard C, Monnet X. Effects of norepinephrine on mean systemic pressure and venous return in human septic shock. Crit Care Med. 2012;40:3146–53.

55. Permpikul C, Tongyoo S, Viarasilpa T, Trainarongsakul T, Chakorn T. Udompanturak S. Early Use of Norepinephrine in Septic Shock Resuscitation (CENSER). A randomized trial. Am J Respir Crit Care Med. 2019;199:1097–105.

56. Guyton AC, Coleman TG, Granger HJ. Circulation: overall regulation. Annu Rev Physiol. 1972;34:13–46.

57. Asfar P, Meziani F, Hamel JF, Grelon F, Megarbane B, Anguel N, et al. High versus low blood-pressure target in patients with septic shock. N Engl J Med. 2014;370:1583–93.

58. De Backer D, Biston P, Devriendt J, Madl C, Chochrad D, Aldecoa C, et al. Comparison of dopamine and norepinephrine in the treatment of shock. N Engl J Med. 2010;362:779–89.

59. Myburgh JA, Higgins A, Jovanovska A, Lipman J, Ramakrishnan N, Santamaria J, CAT Study investigators. A comparison of epinephrine and norepinephrine in critically ill patients. Intensive Care Med. 2008;34:2226–34.

60. Karpati PCJ, Rossignol M, Pirot M, Cholley B, Vicaut E, Henry P, et al. High incidence of myocardial ischemia during postpartum hemorrhage. Anesthesiology. 2004;100:30–6.

61. Ospina-Tascón GA, Teboul JL, Hernandez G, Alvarez I, Sánchez-Ortiz AI, Calderón-Tapia LE, et al. Diastolic shock index and clinical outcomes in patients with septic shock. Ann Intensive Care. 2020;10:41.

62. Macdonald SPJ, Keijzers G, Taylor DM, Kinnear F, Arendts G, Fatovich DM, et al. Restricted fluid resuscitation in suspected sepsis associated hypotension (REFRESH): a pilot randomised controlled trial. Intensive Care Med. 2018;44:2070–8.

63. Rivers E, Nguyen B, Havstad S, Ressler J, Muzzin A, Knoblich B, Peterson E, Tomlanovich M, Early Goal-Directed Therapy Collaborative Group. Early goal-directed therapy in the treatment of severe sepsis and septic shock. N Engl J Med. 2001;345:1368–77.

64. Yealy DM, Kellum JA, Huang DT, Barnato AE, Weissfeld LA, Pike F, et al. A randomized trial of protocol-based care for early septic shock. N Engl J Med. 2014;370:1683–93.

65. Peake SL, Delaney A, Bailey M, Bellomo R, Cameron PA, Cooper DJ, et al. Goal-directed resuscitation for patients with early septic shock. N Engl J Med. 2014;371:1496–506.

66. Mouncey PR, Osborn TM, Power GS, Harrison DA, Sadique MZ, Grieve RD, et al. Trial of early, goal-directed resuscitation for septic shock. N Engl J Med. 2015;372:1301–11.

67. Jones AE, Shapiro NI, Trzeciak S, Arnold RC, Claremont HA, Kline JA. Lactate clearance vs central venous oxygen saturation as goals of early sepsis therapy: a randomized clinical trial. JAMA. 2010;303:739–46.

68. Hernández G, Ospina-Tascón GA, Damiani LP, Estenssoro E, Dubin A, Hurtado J, et al. Effect of a resuscitation strategy targeting peripheral perfusion status vs serum lactate levels on 28-day mortality among patients with septic shock: the ANDROMEDA-SHOCK randomized clinical trial. JAMA. 2019;321:654–64.
69. Zampieri FG, Damiani LP, Bakker J, Ospina-Tascón GA, Castro R, Cavalcanti AB, Hernandez G. Effects of a resuscitation strategy targeting peripheral perfusion status versus serum lactate levels among patients with septic shock. A Bayesian reanalysis of the ANDROMEDA-SHOCK trial. Am J Respir Crit Care Med. 2020;201:423–9.
70. Hjortrup PB, Haase N, Bundgaard H, Thomsen SL, Winding R, Pettilä V, et al. Restricting volumes of resuscitation fluid in adults with septic shock after initial management: the CLASSIC randomised, parallel-group, multicentre feasibility trial. Intensive Care Med. 2016;42:1695–705.
71. Meyhoff TS, Hjortrup PB, Wetterslev J, Sivapalan P, Laake JH, Cronhjort M, et al. Restriction of intravenous fluid in ICU patients with septic shock. N Engl J Med. 2022;386:2459–70.

Fluid Management in Cardiogenic Shock

15

Shrikanth Srinivasan and Riddhi Kundu

Contents

Introduction 316
Fluid Management of Left-Ventricular Failure 317
How Should Fluid Responsiveness Be Assessed and Fluid Therapy Titrated
   in these Patients? 318
Fluid Management in Right-Ventricular Failure 321
How to Assess Fluid Responsiveness and Titrate Fluids in RV Failure? 324
Conclusion 327
References 327

IFA Commentary (MLNG)

Cardiogenic shock is a life-threatening medical condition where the heart fails to pump enough blood to meet the metabolic demands of tissues. Managing fluids in patients with cardiogenic shock can be challenging, as even small volumes of intravenous fluids can lead to worsening symptoms. Classification of subtypes of cardiogenic shock can aid in determining the underlying pathophysiology and initial management approach. There is a critical need for research on appropriate fluid management strategies in patients with cardiogenic shock. While pulmonary artery catheterization remains the gold-standard monitoring tool, noninvasive or minimally invasive

---

S. Srinivasan (✉)
Critical Care Medicine Manipal Hospitals, New Delhi, India

R. Kundu
Critical Care Medicine, Ruby Hall Clinic, Pune, India

© The Author(s) 2024
M. L. N. G. Malbrain et al. (eds.), *Rational Use of Intravenous Fluids in Critically Ill Patients*, https://doi.org/10.1007/978-3-031-42205-8_15

hemodynamic tools such as focused echocardiography, PICCO, or other continuous cardiac output monitors can guide fluid management in patients with left-ventricular failure. For patients with right-ventricular failure, optimizing preload is essential to maintain forward flow, and fluid administration can be guided by echocardiography, dynamic changes in central venous pressure (CVP), passive leg raising, or a pulmonary artery catheter. Fluid administration should be guided by hemodynamic monitoring and targeted to end points of improvement in tissue oxygen delivery.

Learning Objectives
1. To introduce cardiogenic shock and subtypes.
2. To overview and understand the spectrum of clinical presentation.
3. To learn about assessment of fluid responsiveness and fluid management in left- and right-ventricular failures.

Case Vignette
Mr. H, aged 72, is brought to the emergency room with sudden-onset chest pain, excessive sweating, nausea, and dyspnea. He has a history of type II diabetes mellitus on diet control, has arterial hypertension on medications which he takes irregularly, and is a chronic smoker (20 pack-years). He is agitated upon arrival and unable to give any history. Vital signs upon arrival are as follows: heart rate (HR) 145/min, blood pressure (BP) 80/50 mmHg, respiratory rate (RR) 35–40/min, SpO$_2$ 62% on room air. He has cold clammy skin and cyanosed extremities. Bilateral diffuse crackles and gallop rhythm are present on auscultation,

Questions
Q1. How do you resuscitate this patient?
Q2. Is there a role for fluid boluses during the resuscitation process?

Introduction

Cardiogenic shock is frequently encountered by physicians in the intensive care unit (ICU). It manifests as a state of end-organ ischemia secondary to a decreased cardiac output. The established criteria for the diagnosis of cardiogenic shock are as follows [1]:

- Sustained hypotension: systolic blood pressure < 90 mmHg for 30 min or requirement of vasopressors to achieve a blood pressure ≥ 90 mmHg.
- Reduced cardiac index (<2.2 L/min/m^2).

– Pulmonary congestion or elevated left-ventricular filling pressures with a pulmonary capillary wedge pressure (PCWP) or pulmonary artery occlusion pressure (PAOP) >15 mmHg or right-ventricular end-diastolic pressure (RVEDP) >10 mmHg.
– Signs of impaired organ perfusion manifesting as.

  altered mental status, cold, clammy skin, and prolonged capillary refill time (>2 s),
  oliguria (<0.5 mL/kg/h),
  increased serum lactate (or decreased mixed venous or central venous oxygen saturation).

These signs of impaired perfusion are present despite adequate intravascular volume and persist even after attempting to correct hypovolemia, arrhythmia, hypoxia, and acidosis.

Cardiogenic shock is a life-threatening clinical entity that occurs as a progression of dysfunction in the right or left side of the heart. Right- and left-sided heart failure are distinct clinical entities though there may be considerable overlap in signs and symptoms with disease progression.

– Left-ventricular (LV) failure is more likely to present with symptoms of pulmonary congestion in the form of hypoxemia, orthopnea, paroxysmal nocturnal dyspnea, pink frothy sputum production, cough, and wheezing.
– Right-ventricular (RV) failure on the other hand presents with symptoms of systemic venous congestion, an elevated jugular venous pulse, congestive hepatomegaly, extremity edema, and anasarca.

Since both chambers (right and left) share a common interventricular septum (interventricular independence) and are in series, both forms of heart failure will ultimately manifest in the form of decreased end-organ perfusion resulting in oliguria, hypotension, exercise intolerance, fatigue, and cold clammy extremities leading to life-threatening cardiogenic shock. This chapter will focus on adult patients, and more information on fluid therapy in children can be found in Chap. 20. Some other chapters will discuss fluids in specific populations: sepsis (Chap. 14), trauma (Chap. 16), neurocritical care (Chap. 17), perioperative setting (Chap. 18), burns (Chap. 19), liver failure (Chap. 21), abdominal hypertension (Chap. 22), and COVID-19 (Chap. 26).

Fluid Management of Left-Ventricular Failure

Cardiogenic shock may arise de novo, manifesting as acute heart failure, or it may arise on a background of chronic heart failure. Conventionally, most patients with chronic heart failure are believed to be fluid overloaded with little scope for further fluid resuscitation. They belong to Forrester subgroup IV (Fig. 15.1), have a low cardiac index, high systemic vascular resistance and would benefit from vasopressor and inotropic support. Some of these patients, especially those presenting with acute-on-chronic cardiac failure, may be volume overloaded and conversely may be better treated with diuresis. This situation is common in the ICU.

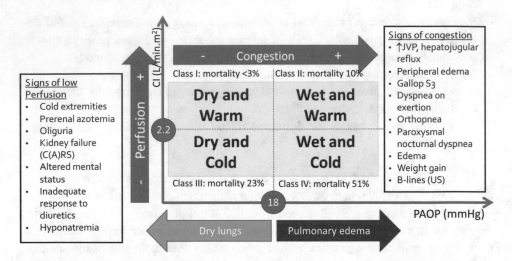

Fig. 15.1 Spectrum of hemodynamic presentation in cardiogenic shock according to Forrester (adapted from Forrester JS, Diamond G, Chatterjee K, Swan HJ. Medical therapy of acute myocardial infarction by application of hemodynamic subsets. N Engl J Med. 1976;295(24):1356–1362). *C(A)RS* cardio (abdominal) renal syndrome, *CI* cardiac index, *JVP* jugular vein pressure, *PAOP* pulmonary artery occlusion pressure, *US* ultrasound

The achievement of an adequate circulating volume is a vital part of the management for most patients with chronic heart failure (Fig. 15.1). Many of these patients will be volume deficient and will therefore respond to a fluid challenge.

It is a common misconception that the pulmonary edema in all acute de novo heart failure is the result of excessive blood volume. This is not generally the case; in fact, many such patients respond favorably to fluid challenge [2]. The elevation of venous pressure observed in these patients is the result of reduced forward flow, causing an increased "back pressure" and congestion in the venous circulation. The role of loop diuretics in the management of acute heart failure seems to contradict this. In fact, the beneficial effect of furosemide is often the result of its vasodilator effect rather than diuresis. It is not uncommon to see large doses of diuretics given to patients with acute pulmonary edema irrespective of their volume status; this can lead to hypovolemia and subsequent hypotension and deterioration of kidney function.

How Should Fluid Responsiveness Be Assessed and Fluid Therapy Titrated in these Patients?

Literature on fluid management of patients with cardiogenic shock is scarce. The pulmonary artery catheter remains the gold standard in providing reliable continuous and reproducible measures of filling pressures of both the right and left heart and monitoring the response of cardiac output to volume therapy. Traditional markers such as central venous or pulmonary artery wedge pressure continues to be used widely but are relatively poor markers of predicting fluid responsiveness [3]. Empiric fluid boluses of 250 mL (4 mL/kg) over 10–15 min of isotonic saline have been advocated previously as long as there is no evidence of pulmonary congestion on physical examination, chest X-ray, or lung ultrasound (B-lines). However, such indiscriminate fluid challenges in patients with impaired ventricular function carry the risk of precipitating pulmonary edema. Use of fluid challenges in left-ventricular failure has to be titrated carefully perhaps guided by dynamic markers of fluid responsiveness. Continuous monitoring of cardiac output is strongly advocated in these patients using transpulmonary thermodilution in combination with pulse wave contour analysis along with measurement of central venous or mixed venous oxygen saturation [4].

In a retrospective study by Adler and colleagues, in patients with cardiogenic shock following cardiac arrest, the PICCO (Pulsion Medical Systems, Munich, Germany) was used as a modality of monitoring fluid therapy guided by additional functional hemodynamic variables (Fig. 15.2) such as PPV (pulse pressure variation), SVV (stroke volume variation), and volumetric indices such as EVLW (extravascular lung water) and GEDV (global end-diastolic volume). The targets for SVV/PPV were set at <10% and a GEDV of 700–800 mL/m^{-2}, while the risk of pulmonary edema was minimized by keeping EVLW

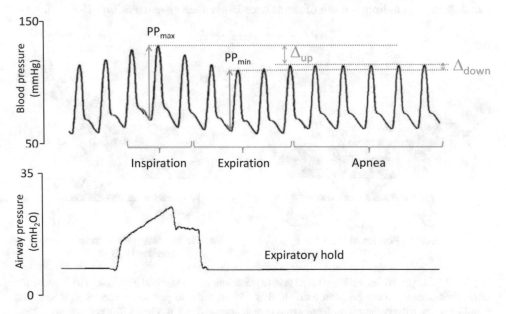

Fig. 15.2 Example of fluid unresponsiveness. Increased pulse (PPV) and systolic pressure variations (SPV) in a patient with IAP of 16 mmHg and cardiorenal syndrome. The PPV can be calculated as [(PPmax – PPmin)/PPmean] × 100 (%). After an apnea test it becomes clear that the increased SPV and PPV seen on the monitor is mainly related to a Δup phenomenon as only a smaller portion is caused by Δdown. This means that the increased PPV and SPV are not necessarily correlated to fluid responsiveness and higher thresholds are probably needed.

<10 mL/kg. This led to a greater use of fluids (5449 ± 449 mL vs. 4375 ± 1285 mL, $p = 0.007$) in the first 24 h following arrest and a lower incidence of AKI compared to conventional treatment (4.3% vs. 28.6%, $p = 0.03$) suggesting the potential role of more liberal fluid administration guided by advanced hemodynamic variables in patients post cardiac arrest with compromised cardiac function [5].

Passive leg raising (PLR) is a reversible fluid challenge that predicts whether cardiac output will increase with volume expansion. By transferring a volume of around 300 mL of venous blood from the lower body toward the right heart, PLR mimics an endogenous fluid challenge (Fig. 15.3). However, no fluids are actually infused, and the hemodynamic effects are rapidly reversible. The ability of PLR to correctly predict fluid responsiveness in patients with compromised cardiac function was explored in study by Xiang and colleagues [6]. The authors found that the ability of PLR to correctly predict fluid responsiveness was dependent on the systolic function of the heart with sensitivity, specificity, and AUC all higher in the near-normal systolic function group than in the group with impaired systolic function.

With the widespread use of bedside echocardiography, cardiac function can be reliably assessed at the bedside and repeated echocardiographic assessment is probably the way forward in titrating fluid therapy in these group of patients. The FALLS protocol (fluid administration limited by lung sonography) emphasizes the use of lung sonography as a valuable adjunct to limit the use of fluids once B-lines are visualized (Fig. 15.4) [7].

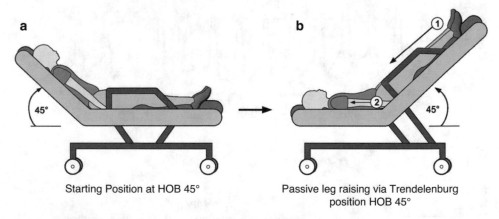

Fig. 15.3 The passive leg raising (PLR) test. (**a**). Starting position with HOB at 45. (**b**). Passive leg raising via Trendelenburg position with HOB at 45°. In order to perform a correct PLR test, one should not touch the patient in order to avoid sympathetic activation. The PLR is performed by turning the bed from the starting position with head of bed elevation at 30–45° (Panel A) to the Trendelenburg position (Panel B). The PLR test results in an autotransfusion effect via the increased venous return from the legs and the splanchnic mesenteric pool. Monitoring of cardiac output volume is required as a positive PLR test is defined by an increase in SV of at least 10% (adapted with permission from [8])

Fig. 15.4 The FALLS protocol. A decision tree facilitating the understanding of the FALLS protocol. According to the Weil classification, cardiac and lung ultrasound sequentially rule out obstructive, cardiogenic (from left heart), hypovolemic, and finally distributive shock, i.e., septic shock in current practice. Adapted from (33). FALL protocol, fluid administration limited by lung sonography; BLUE protocol, bedside lung ultrasound in emergency; *RV* right ventricle, *PneumoTx* pneumothorax. Adapted with permission from [9]

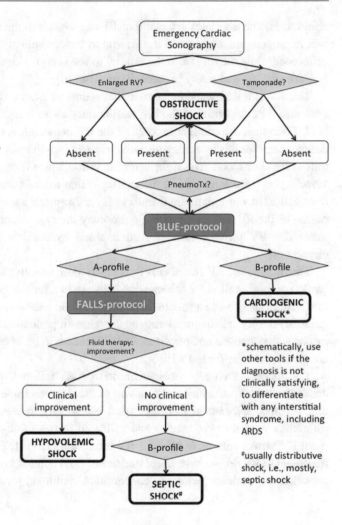

Fluid Management in Right-Ventricular Failure

Failure of the right heart is characterized by inadequate right-ventricular forward flow eventually leading to a decreased left-ventricular preload. The failing right ventricle generates back-pressure changes manifested by systemic venous congestion, pulsatile liver, and lower extremity edema. The goals of therapy in RV failure encompasses the basic principles of maintaining an optimal RV preload, decreasing RV afterload, and augmenting RV contractility through the use of inotropes and mechanical circulatory support as indicated.

The use of fluids in RV failure to augment RV stroke volume requires an in-depth understanding of RV physiology. The RV pumps its blood against a low-pressure pulmonary circuit in contrast to the LV which pumps blood against a high-pressure systemic circulation. The arterioles act as the resistance vessels in the systemic circulation leading to a large pressure drop across the arterial to venous side of the circulation. The pressure difference while moving from the arterial to the venous side in the pulmonary circulation is markedly less and rarely exceeds 10 mmHg [10].

The RV is a thin-walled chamber that seems to wrap around the more muscular left ventricle. The thickness of the RV wall is only about one-third that of the left ventricle [11]. Therefore, the contractile force of the RV is much less compared to the LV. The RV compensates for this by achieving a much larger end-diastolic volume and surface area per unit volume of blood. The right ventricle musculature is arranged in a superficial transverse layer and a longitudinal muscle layer that extends from apex to base. Sequential contraction of the longitudinal muscle layer from the apex to base dilates the outflow region of the RV and the proximal pulmonary artery to accommodate the RV stroke volume. The RV forward flow is further aided by the low pressure in the pulmonary circulation.

The thin-walled RV chamber is thus much more sensitive to acute changes in afterload, while the thick-walled LV tolerates an increase in afterload better than the RV. The LV is much more sensitive to an acute increase in preload because of its thick muscular walls. In contrast, the RV seems to tolerate an increase in preload much better than the LV. The important anatomical and physiological differences in between the left and right ventricles are summarized in Table 15.1.

The concept of volume replacement to treat RV failure is therefore based on the inherent differences in structure and function of the right ventricle compared to the left ventricle. Volume replacement has been used historically to treat RV failure caused by RV infarction. A plethora of studies had validated the usefulness of volume loading to augment RV stroke volume in cases of RV infarction [12–14]. Traditional approaches to the treatment of RV failure have advocated use of fluid boluses in targeting a higher right atrial pressure in patients without concomitant pulmonary congestion [15]. However,

Table 15.1 Important structural and functional differences between right and left ventricles

	Left ventricle	Right ventricle
Shape	Ellipsoid	Crescentic
Wall thickness, mm	7–11	2–5
Mass, g/m^{-2} BSA	17–34	64–109
Coronary blood flow	During diastole	Systole and diastole
Downstream resistance, $dynes.Sec^{-1} cm^{-5}$	High-resistance systemic circulation (800–1600)	Low-resistance pulmonary circulation (40–140)
End-diastolic volume, mm^3	50–100	40–90
Intracavitary pressure, mmHg	Higher (120/10)	Lower (25/5)
Muscle contraction	Primarily longitudinal	Longitudinal, circumferential, and radial
Tolerates better	Pressure overload	Volume overload

subsequent clinical studies failed to replicate the beneficial effect of liberal volume loading in patients with RV infarction and demonstrated that in some instances it might be harmful leading to increased right atrial pressures without an increase in RV stroke volume [16].

In a study of patients with echocardiography-proven RV infarction, the beneficial effect of fluid loading on RV stroke work index was found at a right atrial pressure of 10–14 mmHg. However, volume replacement with right atrial pressure more than 14 mmHg was accompanied by a reduction in the RV stroke index [17]. The harmful effect of overaggressive fluid loading in patients with RV infarction is explained by the interventricular interdependence. The RV and the LV are enclosed by the pericardium and share a common interventricular septum. Overaggressive volume loading of the RV will lead to an increase in RV end-diastolic pressure and shifting of the interventricular septum toward the side of LV, compromising LV filling and resultant cardiac output. This is classically seen in echocardiography in parasternal short axis view as a D-shaped LV with the septum encroaching on the LV cavity (Fig. 15.5).

The degree of septal shift is dependent on the extent in the rise of RV end-diastolic pressure in comparison to the LV end-diastolic pressure. Under normal conditions, an increase in RV end-diastolic pressure due to volume loading leads to an increase in RV stroke volume and subsequent increase in LV end-diastolic pressure so that the relative differences between LV and RV end-diastolic pressures are maintained. However, in conditions associated with an increase in pulmonary vascular resistance or an increase in RV afterload (e.g., pulmonary embolism), the RV fails to increase its forward flow to fluid replacement, leading to an impaired LV filling and harmful effects of fluid resuscitation. In such cases, the therapy should be focused on relieving the cause of increased RV afterload rather than fluid loading to augment preload.

Another harmful effect of excessive fluid loading with compromised RV function is excessive RV wall tension leading to a decreased coronary perfusion of the right ventricle with resultant RV ischemia.

The importance of venous congestion in the development of worsening renal function in advanced decompensated heart failure can possibly explain the greatest improvement of

Fig. 15.5 Displacement of interventricular septum toward left ventricle (D-shaped LV cavity) secondary to RV pressure/volume overload

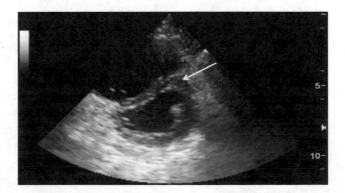

Table 15.2 Grading table for assessment of venous congestion with point-of-care ultrasound VExUS, venous congestion assessment with ultrasound (adapted with permission from Rola P. et al. book "Bedside Ultrasound: a primer for clinical integration."(From Rola et al. Bedside Ultrasound: a primer for clinical integration. Second edition ed. p. 100–7)

	Grade 0	Grade 1	Grade 2	Grade 3	Grade 4
IVC	<5 mm with respiratory variation	5–9 mm with respiratory variation	10–19 mm with respiratory variation	>20 mm with respiratory variation	20 mm with minimal or no respiratory variation
Hepatic vein	Normal S > D	S < D with antegrade S	S flat or inverted or biphasic trace		
Portal vein	< 0.3 pulsatility index	0.3–0.5 pulsatility index	>0.5 pulsatility index		
Renal vein doppler	Continuous monophasic/ pulsatile flow	Discontinuous biphasic flow	Discontinuous monophasic flow (diastole only)		
VExUS score	No congestion IVC grade < 3, HD grade 0, PV grade 0 (RD grade 0)	Mild congestion IVC grade 4, but normal HV/ PV/RV patterns	Moderate congestion IVC grade 4 with mild flow pattern abnormalities in HV/PV/RV	Severe congestion IVC grade 4 with severe flow pattern abnormalities in HV/PV/RV	

PV portal vein, *IVC* inferior vena cava, *RV* renal vein, *HV* hepatic vein

the renal function after medical treatment in patients characterized by echocardiographic signs of the impact of right-ventricular dysfunction on inferior vena cava, portal, hepatic, and renal veins. Recently, a novel grading system was proposed for venous congestion, the Venous Excess Ultrasound (VExUS) grading system based on the combination of multiple ultrasound findings (Table 15.2).

How to Assess Fluid Responsiveness and Titrate Fluids in RV Failure?

Identification of RV failure has classically relied on the well-described clinical signs of an elevated jugular venous pulsation, splitting of the second heart sound, and a prominent tricuspid regurgitation murmur.

Critically ill patients with RV failure need adequate RV preload to maintain optimal RV forward flow. They might often be volume depleted secondary to bleeding, increased vascular permeability, or insensible losses. Positive-pressure ventilation impedes venous return. Sedatives and analgesics can blunt the sympathetic response and venous tone further aggravating the problem. Therefore, careful volume titration is necessary in such patients. The right atrial pressure targets guided by central venous pressure (CVP) should be kept in the high normal range of 8–12 mmHg and titrated further on the basis of hemodynamics and cardiac output (e.g., with the two-to-five rule, Table 15.3) [18].

Table 15.3 The two-to-five rule using dynamic changes in central venous pressure (CVP) [ΔCVP] to guide a fluid challenge. Adapted with permission from Malbrain et al. [19]

1	Measure baseline CVP mmHg)
	(a) CVP <8: give 4 mL/kg bolus over 10 min
	(b) CVP 8–12: give 2 mL/kg bolus over 10 min
	(c) CVP >12: give 1 mL/kg bolus over 10 min
2	Reassess increase in CVP at the end of the bolus (i.e., after 10 min from start at point 1)
	(a) ΔCVP >5: "stop" fluid challenge
	(b) ΔCVP <2: restart with point 1
	(c) ΔCVP 2–5: wait for another 10 min and move to point 3
3	Reassess increase in CVP after another 10 min (i.e., after 20 min from start at point 1)
	(a) ΔCVP >2: "stop" fluid challenge
	(b) ΔCVP <2: restart with 1
4	Repeat until CVP of 14 mmHg or rule broken

Monitoring of pulse pressure variation (PPV) with an arterial catheter in situ has been used as a predictor of fluid responsiveness [20]. The PPV is less reliable in the setting of acute respiratory distress syndrome (ARDS) given poor lung compliance, low tidal volumes, and also when the patient is breathing spontaneously.

However, one must exercise a note of caution when using PPV to predict RV fluid responsiveness. RV is exquisitely sensitive to increase in afterload. Therefore, an increase in PPV above conventionally described thresholds of 12–13% in the setting of RV failure maybe an indicator of RV afterload responsiveness and potential volume overloaded state. Such a patient may potentially decompensate from overzealous fluid administration. Therefore, one should not use PPV in isolation in deciding to fluid challenge a patient with RV failure but look for other signs of potential RV overload (e.g., dilated RV in echocardiography, elevated CVP, distended inferior vena cava). One may also use a PLR maneuver to look for change in PPV in such cases. No change or worsening of PPV post PLR could indicate RV afterload dependence, while decrease in PPV following PLR could indicate fluid responsiveness [21].

Echocardiography can be used to assess RV function more objectively by measurement of tricuspid annular plane systolic excursion in a four-chambered view using tissue Doppler over the tricuspid annulus. Assessment of RV chamber size can also be used to detect RV dilatation. The ratio of RV to LV end-diastolic area between 0.6 and 1 indicates RV dilatation, while a ratio greater than 1 indicates severe RV dilatation. Acute cor pulmonale in echocardiography is indicated by RV–LV size greater than 0.6 in combination with paradoxical septal motion [22]. Along with an assessment of RV function, echocardiography and other modalities should be used to look for the precipitating cause of RV failure (e.g., infarction, embolism, valve disease). This is necessitated by the understanding that RV failure caused by conditions of increased afterload is less likely to respond to fluid resuscitation. Echocardiography is a useful tool to detect features of RV overload such as septal shift toward the LV and thereby guide decisions regarding further fluid therapy. Serial hemodynamic assessment guided by echocardiography is an absolute necessity in titrating fluids in this group of patients. In cases where the RV preload is too high, diuretics and renal replacement therapy to remove excess fluid can be associated with an improvement in cardiac output. The Frank–Starling curve of the RV is flatter and wider than the LV. Hence, a significant amount of fluid needs to be removed before an appreciable increase in cardiac output is achieved in a volume overloaded RV.

A Swan–Ganz pulmonary artery catheter can also be placed to derive reliable, continuous, and objective information about the RV function and response to fluid therapy. The PA catheter allows measurement of cardiac output and mixed venous oxygen saturation, in addition to other static measures such as pulmonary artery occlusion pressure and PA pressure. Measurement of cardiac output using cold saline through PA catheter may underestimate the actual cardiac output, if the patient has significant tricuspid regurgitation, while, the PA catheter continues to be the gold standard in the measurement of cardiac output and systemic and pulmonary vascular resistance. However, it is being used in limited centers worldwide, due to its invasiveness and limited evidence on outcome benefit in the management of cardiac failure. The advanced systems based on the principle of transpulmonary thermodilution have been used to calculate derived indices such as extravascular lung water (EVLW) and pulmonary vascular permeability index (PVPI) to detect pulmonary congestion early in the setting of compromised cardiac function.

Case Vignette

In the case vignette described in the beginning of this chapter, Mr. H appears to be in cardiogenic shock, belonging to wet and cold subtype of the Forrester classification. The patient presents with ischemic chest pain and has risk factors for acute coronary syndrome with past medical history of arterial hypertension, type 2 diabetes mellitus, and chronic smoking. Initial part of his management should focus on stabilizing his ABCs, with supplemental O_2 (escalation to noninvasive ventilation, if required), and starting norepinephrine to support his MAP to ensure adequacy of organ perfusion. Along with blood investigations, an immediate 12-lead electrocardiogram and troponin levels should be performed to rule out a possible ischemic event and manage accordingly. In addition, it would be prudent to look for other precipitating causes. Aggressive fluid resuscitation should be withheld at his stage given his clinical features of volume overload (crackles, gallop rhythm), and any fluid replacement should be guided by a bedside echocardiography and hemodynamic monitoring.

Conclusion

To summarize, fluid management in patients with impaired cardiac function is complex. In the absence of widespread literature, clinicians continue to titrate the fluid therapy based on traditional measures of central venous pressure and clinical examination. There is an overemphasis on restricting fluids in patients with heart failure, but the physician needs to identify the subgroup of patients with cardiogenic shock who might actually benefit from fluid replacement. The fluid boluses need to be titrated to specific end points of end-organ perfusion guided by dynamic measures of fluid responsiveness and frequent echocardiographic assessments. While the PA catheter continues to be the gold standard in assessment of hemodynamics and fluid/vasopressor requirements in these patients, minimally invasive or noninvasive modes have shown potential in providing equivalent information without the attendant risks associated with the placement and maintenance of a PA catheter. One needs to understand the etiology and the type of heart failure that might provide additional information and likelihood of a favorable response to fluid resuscitation.

Take Home Messages
- It is important to identify different subtypes of cardiogenic shock and etiology.
- Not all patients with cardiogenic shock are fluid depleted.
- There is a definitive role of ultrasound and other invasive or noninvasive hemodynamic monitors to guide fluid management.
- Carefully titrated fluid boluses to specific end points are the key in patients with impaired cardiac function.

References

1. Thiele H, Ohman EM, Desch S, Eitel I, De WS. Clinical update management of cardiogenic shock. Eur Heart J. 2015;36:1223–30.
2. Mebazaa A, Gheorghiade M, Piña IL, et al. Practical recommendations for prehospital and early in-hospital management of patients presenting with acute heart failure syndromes. Crit Care Med. 2008;36(1 Suppl):S129–39.
3. Marik PE, Baram M, Vahid B. Does central venous pressure predict fluid responsiveness? A systematic review of the literature and the tale of seven mares. Chest. 2008;134:172–8.
4. Levy B, Bastien O, Bendjelid K, Cariou A, Chouihed T, Combes A, et al. Experts' recommendations for the management of adult patients with cardiogenic shock. Ann Intensive Care. 2015;5:1–10. https://doi.org/10.1186/s13613-015-0052-1.
5. Adler C, Reuter H, Seck C, Hellmich M, Zobel C. Fluid therapy and acute kidney injury in cardiogenic shock after cardiac arrest. Resuscitation. 2013;84(2):194–9.
6. Si X, Cao DY, Chen J, Wu JF, Liu ZM, Xu HL, et al. Effect of systolic cardiac function on passive leg raising for predicting fluid responsiveness: a prospective observational study. Chin Med J. 2018;131(3):253–62.
7. Lichtenstein D. FALLS-protocol: lung ultrasound in hemodynamic assessment of shock. Heart Lung Vessel. 2013;5(3):142–7.

8. Hofer C, Cannesson M. Monitoring fluid responsiveness. Acta Anaesthesiol Taiwan. 2011;49(2):59–65.
9. Lichtenstein D, van Hooland S, Elbers P, Malbrain ML. Ten good reasons to practice ultrasound in critical care. Anaesthesiol Intensive Ther. 2014;46(5):323–335.
10. Bhattacharya J, Staub NC. Direct measurement of microvascular pressures in the isolated perfused dog lung. Science. 1980;210:327–8.
11. Greyson CR. Pathophysiology of right ventricular failure. Crit Care Med. 2008;36(1, Suppl):S57–65.
12. Lopez-Sendon J, Coma-Canella I, Vinuelas AJ. Volume loading in patients with ischemic right ventricular dysfunction. Eur Heart J. 1981;2:329–38.
13. Baigrie RS, Haq A, Morgan CD, et al. The spectrum of right ventricular involvement in inferior wall myocardial infarction: a clinical, hemodynamic and noninvasive study. J Am Coll Cardiol. 1983;1:1396–404.
14. Goldstein JA, Vlahakes GJ, Verrier ED, et al. Volume loading improves low cardiac output in experimental right ventricular infarction. J Am Coll Cardiol. 1983;2:270–8.
15. Siniorakis EE, Nikolaou NI, Sarantopoulos CD, et al. Volume loading in predominant right ventricular infarction: bedside hemodynamics using rapid response thermistors. Eur Heart J. 1994;15:1340–7.
16. Ferrario M, Poli A, Previtali M, et al. Hemodynamics of volume loading compared with dobutamine in severe right ventricular infarction. Am J Cardiol. 1994;74:329–33.
17. Berisha S, Kastrati A, Goda A, et al. Optimal value of filling pressure in the right side of the heart in acute right ventricular infarction. BMJ. 1990;63:98–102.
18. Ventetuolo CE, Klinger JR. Management of acute right ventricular failure in the intensive care unit. Ann Am Thorac Soc. 2014;11(5):811–22.
19. Malbrain ML, Marik PE, Witters I, et al. Fluid overload, de-resuscitation, and outcomes in critically ill or injured patients: a systematic review with suggestions for clinical practice. Anaesthesiol Intensive Ther. 2014;46(5):361–80.
20. Yang X, Du B. Does pulse pressure variation predict fluid responsiveness in critically ill patients? A systematic review and meta-analysis. Crit Care. 2014;18:650.
21. Vieillard-Baron A, Matthay M, Teboul JL, et al. Experts' opinion on management of hemodynamics in ARDS patients: focus on the effects of mechanical ventilation. Intensive Care Med. 2016;42(5):739–49.
22. Vieillard-Baron A, Prin S, Chergui K, Dubourg O, Jardin F. Echo-Doppler demonstration of acute cor pulmonale at the bedside in the medical intensive care unit. Am J Respir Crit Care Med. 2002;166:1310–9.

Fluid Management in Trauma

Kapil Dev Soni and Basant Gauli

Contents

Introduction 332
Goals of Early Resuscitation 332
Initial Choice of Fluid for Trauma Resuscitation 335
Crystalloids 335
Colloids 336
Hypertonic Solutions 337
Penetrating Versus Blunt Injury Versus Head Injuries 337
Initial Trauma Resuscitation Fluid Volume 338
Practical Approach to Initial Fluid Resuscitation and Pattern of Responses 339
Completion of Resuscitation 339
Post-Resuscitation Fluid Management 340
Deresuscitation 340
Conclusion 341
References 342

K. D. Soni (✉)
Critical and Intensive Care, JPN Apex Trauma Center, All India Institute of Medical Sciences, New Delhi, India

B. Gauli
Department of Anaesthesia and Critical Care Medicine, Chitwan Medical College, Bharatpur, Nepal

© The Author(s) 2024
M. L. N. G. Malbrain et al. (eds.), *Rational Use of Intravenous Fluids in Critically Ill Patients*, https://doi.org/10.1007/978-3-031-42205-8_16

IFA Commentary (MLNGM)

Trauma patients require careful management of intravenous fluids, given the complexity of decisions involved, often compounded by blood loss and coagulopathy. This chapter focuses on fluid management in trauma patients, providing guidance and recommendations on specific circumstances. The best fluid for a patient may not always be the one that is readily available, and decisions regarding fluid management must consider the need to provide adequate organ perfusion and oxygen delivery.

To achieve this goal, the principles of initial resuscitation in polytrauma patients should limit the use of crystalloids and prioritize early use of blood products, permissive hypotension in selected patients, and early damage control surgery in patients who do not respond to initial resuscitation. The initial choice of fluid should be normal saline for traumatic brain injury patients and balanced salt solution for other patients. Colloids, albumin, and hypertonic saline are not recommended for resuscitation.

After the initial fluid bolus of 1 L, the patient's response to fluid should be assessed as a rapid responder, transient responder, or minimal/nonresponder. This assessment guides subsequent resuscitation and diagnostic and therapeutic decisions. Overzealous fluid resuscitation in the first 24 h of trauma has been associated with increased mortality, longer duration of mechanical ventilation, and increased risk of intra-abdominal hypertension and abdominal compartment syndrome.

Suggested Reading

1. Wise R, Faurie M, Malbrain MLNG, Hodgson E. Strategies for intravenous fluid resuscitation in trauma patients. World J Surg. 2017;41(5):1170–1183. https://doi.org/10.1007/s00268-016-3865-7. PMID: 28058475; PMCID: PMC5394148.

Learning Objectives

After reading this chapter you will be able to:

1. Describe the principles and evolving strategies of resuscitation in polytrauma patients.
2. Describe the clinical signs of shock and relate them to the degree of blood loss.
3. List the different initial resuscitation fluids and determine the most appropriate type and amount of fluid based on recent evidences.
4. Measure the patient initial responses to fluid resuscitation and different patterns of patient responses and its implication in subsequent therapy.
5. Discuss the basis for further fluid management, organ perfusion, and tissue oxygenation in trauma patients.
6. Explain the adverse effects of fluid overload and outline the steps necessary for preventing and managing the cumulative fluid overload.

Case Vignette

Mr. K, aged 38, is brought in by the ambulance after a high-speed rollover where a car crashed into a pole. Primary survey at the resuscitation area revealed the patient to be confused but following commands. Vitals recorded were blood pressure (BP) of 90/70 mmHg, pulse rate of 121 beats/min, respiratory rate of 28 breaths/min with oxygen saturation being maintained at 94%, and a visible fracture of the right femur. An appropriate size cervical collar was applied, two 16G IV cannulae were inserted, and 2 L/min oxygen was started via nasal prongs.

Questions and Answers

Q1. What is the best fluid type, volume, strategy, and end point of resuscitation?

A1. A point-of-care FAST scan showed free fluid in the right upper quadrant. Shortly afterwards, the patient became hypotensive and there was a transient response to fluid resuscitation. At this point, the patient was taken by the trauma surgery team for damage control surgery. He was then admitted to the intensive care unit (ICU) for further management. He was started on vasopressor. Arterial blood gas showed metabolic acidosis with a lactate of 3.5 mmol/L.

Q2. How should resuscitation proceed so as to restore normal tissue perfusion?

Q3. How would you guide fluid maintenance in this patient group?

A3. On day four, there was an episode of hypotension after stabilization.

Q4. What is your fluid management plan in this patient now?

A4. On day eight, he was conscious, oriented, and hemodynamically stable and given a spontaneous breathing trial but failed. On assessment, the patient was edematous and had a positive cumulative fluid balance of 10 L.

Q5. How will you plan to wean from ventilator and extubate?

Introduction

In the care of critically ill trauma patients, resuscitation from hemorrhagic shock is one of the primary tasks. However, it is surrounded by uncertainties as to the correct approach. The best choice of fluid, volume strategy of fluid resuscitation in varied injuries, monitoring during resuscitation, and appropriate end points for resuscitation are all debatable and unclear. Several recommendations have evolved over recent years incorporating the prevailing uncertainties, yet the resuscitation of these patients remains far from optimal. Recent developments have heralded new approaches which appear promising but need robust studies to establish their benefit. The mortality due to hemorrhagic shock continues to remain unacceptably high in the present era. This chapter focuses on the relevant principles of fluid management in major trauma patients and discusses clinical fluid management in the different phases of trauma care—from early fluid resuscitation to stabilization and deresuscitation.

Goals of Early Resuscitation

Major trauma frequently leads to hemorrhagic shock. The loss of a substantial amount of blood initiates sympathetic compensatory responses to preserve cardiac output. Uncontrolled bleeding causes compensatory responses to be overwhelmed, resulting in a fall in cardiac output and decreased blood pressure. In the presence of continuing bleeding, this affects organ perfusion and often causes multiple-organ dysfunction as well as multi-organ failure. Major trauma is also associated with increased capillary permeability that causes intravascular fluids to shift into the interstitial space, appearing as tissue edema. Therefore, if a decrease in intravascular volume is left uncorrected, it may result in irreversible shock and mortality. Fluid resuscitation primarily aims to attain adequate cardiac output to ensure acceptable oxygen delivery and tissue perfusion until the hemorrhage can be controlled. Major trauma patients commonly have coagulopathy, acidosis, and hypothermia as a result of blood loss and the impact of their injury; this pathophysiological state has been shown to be detrimental to patient outcomes. The traditional concept of early and aggressive fluid administration in severe trauma is associated with increased dilutional coagulopathy, acidosis, and hypothermia (Fig. 16.1), often referred to as the deadly triad that may cause secondary problems such as intra-abdominal hypertension and abdominal compartment syndrome, extremity compartment syndrome, ileus, pulmonary edema, and tissue edema. Therefore, achieving a careful balance between organ perfusion and hemostasis is critical for optimal fluid resuscitation in such patients. The major goal of fluid resuscitation in such scenarios is to maintain an acceptable level of organ perfusion while limiting secondary insults that can occur through an overaggressive approach.

The concept of "damage control resuscitation" (DCR) was developed during recent war conflicts in Afghanistan and Iraq. DCR is a systematic approach to severely injured trauma

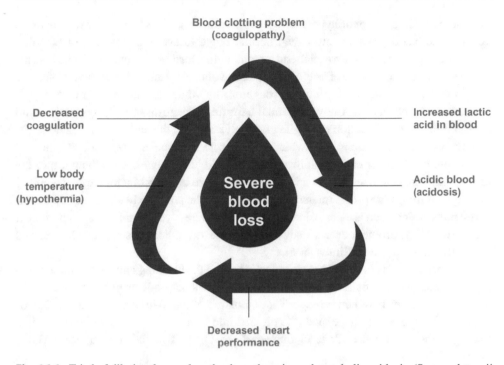

Blood clotting problem
(coagulopathy)

Decreased
coagulation

Increased lactic
acid in blood

Low body
temperature
(hypothermia)

Severe
blood
loss

Acidic blood
(acidosis)

Decreased heart
performance

Fig. 16.1 Triad of dilutional coagulopathy, hypothermia, and metabolic acidosis. (Source: https://www.jems.com/patient-care/trauma-s-lethal-triad-hypothermia-acidos/)

Table 16.1 Components of damage control resuscitation

1 Hemostatic resuscitation
(a) Minimize the use of crystalloid
(b) Use of warm fluid and blood products
(c) Blood product ratios of 1 or 2:1:1 for RBCs, platelet, FFP, respectively
(d) Correction of acidemia
2 Permissive hypotension
(a) In a select population
3 Damage control surgery
(a) Operative
(b) Angiographic
4 Goal-directed correction of coagulopathy

patients and incorporates four major strategies to decrease mortality and morbidity, namely, hemostatic resuscitation, permissive hypotension, damage control surgery, and goal-directed correction of coagulopathy (Table 16.1), to be undertaken simultaneously [1]. Hemostatic resuscitation involves limiting crystalloid use and resuscitation with blood components resembling whole blood as one or two packed red blood cells (PRBCs), one fresh frozen plasma (FFP), and one platelet [2]. The reversal of coagulopathy with hemostatic resuscitation along with prevention of hypothermia and acidosis helps to combat the trauma triad. The concept of hypotensive resuscitation or permissive hypotension involves keeping the blood pressure lower than normal range to avoid aggravation of bleeding while preserving perfusion to vital end organs until bleeding is controlled [3, 4]. This approach avoids the adverse effects of early, large-volume crystalloid resuscitation such as accelerated hemorrhage and dilutional coagulopathy while maintaining circulatory volume and tissue perfusion. A novel potential harmful mechanism of early aggressive fluid resuscitation is the disruption of fragile glycocalyx layer in the endothelium. Endothelial glycocalyx is a thin protein layer which plays a role in vascular integrity and function. Disruption of the layer causes capillary leak of fluid, electrolytes, and albumin into the interstitium that generates edema and evolves to a state of global increased permeability syndrome (GIPS) [3, 5]. This interstitial edema raises the pressure in all major body compartments causing decrease perfusion pressure and progressive organ failure as abdominal compartment syndrome, acute kidney injury, acute respiratory distress syndrome, and compartment syndrome of limbs [5, 6].

The primary focus of initial resuscitation is to stop the bleeding and restore intravascular volume. The initial fluid resuscitation and need of blood products may well depend on the estimated severity of hemorrhage. The estimation of blood loss can be via the physiological effects of hemorrhage, and it is divided into four clinical classes of hemorrhagic shock by the American College of Surgeons' Advanced Trauma Life Support (ATLS) (Table 16.2).

Table 16.2 Signs and symptoms of hemorrhage by class

Parameter	Class I	Class II (mild)	Class III (moderate)	Class IV (severe)
Approximate blood loss	<15%	15–30%	31–40%	>40%
Heart rate	↔	↔/↑	↑	↑/↑↑
Blood pressure	↔	↔	↔/↓	↓
Pulse pressure	↔	↓	↓	↓
Respiratory rate	↔	↔	↔/↑	↑
Urine output	↔	↔	↓	↓↓
Glasgow coma scale score	↔	↔	↓	↓
Base deficit	0 to −2 mEq/L	−2 to −6 mEq/L	−6 to −10 mEq/L	−10 mEq/L or less
Initial resuscitation	Crystalloids	Crystalloids	Crystalloids + albumin (?)	Crystalloids + blood type O neg
Need for blood products	Monitor	Possible	Yes	Massive transfusion protocol

Initial Choice of Fluid for Trauma Resuscitation

The ideal fluid should have a composition similar to that of extracellular fluid; it should be isotonic to avoid intracranial volume variation and should not interfere with blood clotting. The fluid should have high volume expansion properties to prevent excessive fluid resuscitation. There is no single fluid solution with all these properties, and hence the ideal fluid choice for resuscitation of trauma patients remains a subject of debate. Given the paucity of ideal solutions, we believe that it is the rate and amount of fluid which causes secondary problems rather than the type of fluid alone. Balanced crystalloids are the preferred fluid choice during the resuscitation phase.

Crystalloids

In trauma patients with hemodynamic instability, fluid resuscitation with crystalloids is the first-line therapy, of which multiple options are available. Normal saline (0.9% saline), a fluid with its osmolarity approaching that of plasma (slightly higher 308 mM.L^{-1}), is the most common fluid administered during resuscitation. As mentioned in Chap. 9, normal saline is a 0.9% preparation of sodium chloride, equivalent to 154 mmol/L Na and Cl. If sodium chloride completely dissociated in solution, the expected osmolality would be two times 154, or 308 mOsm/kg. Interestingly in vivo measured effective osmolality (tonicity) of 0.9% saline of 286 mOsm/L makes it isotonic to plasma, because a small percentage remains nonionized in water. As such, this fits nicely in the normal range of blood osmolality, of 270–290 mOsm/L. However, the so-called normal saline is an unbuffered, normal saline with supra-physiologic chloride content (154 mEq/L). Balanced salt solutions like lactated Ringer's (Hartmann's solution), Ringer's acetate solution, Plasma-Lyte, and Sterofundin with electrolyte compositions closer to plasma are alternatives to isotonic saline. Crystalloid solutions are discussed in greater detail in Chap. 9.

Large-volume resuscitation with normal saline causes chloride overload and hyperchloremic metabolic acidosis. Chloride overload further reduces renal blood flow by instigating renal vasoconstriction and impaired renal tissue perfusion [7]. Balanced salt solutions, on the other hand, have minimal effect on pH and no effect on renal perfusion; hence, they are presumed to be better options during resuscitation. Their limitations are higher cost, interaction with blood products if mixed, and osmolarity slightly lower than plasma (285–295 mOsm/kg). This can have an impact in traumatic brain injury patients (TBI) as they may increase brain water content aggravating cerebral edema.

There are no large trials comparing normal saline and balanced solutions for trauma resuscitation. Most of the data is extrapolated from trials done in other critically ill patients. In the SPLIT trial that randomized ICU patients to receive either 0.9% saline or Plasma-Lyte, Young and colleagues failed to find any difference in the incidence of acute kidney injury (AKI), need for renal replacement therapy, or mortality between two crystalloid groups [8]. The study has been criticized due to its small sample size, the limited amount of fluids administered (median fluid ~2000 mL), and the fact that a major end point, namely, serum chloride levels, was not monitored. Two large single-center trials, the SMART and the SALT-ED trials, examined the utility of balanced solutions compared with normal saline [9, 10]. The SMART trial found a lower composite outcome of death, new renal replacement therapy, or persistent renal dysfunction among critically ill patients in ICU, but the SALT-ED trial performed in the emergency department failed to show a clear benefit. One of the safest and acceptable approaches to trauma fluid resuscitation is to start with normal saline in TBI patients and balanced salt solution in other hemorrhaging patients.

Colloids

Albumin and synthetic colloids are discussed in further detail in Chaps. 10 and 11, respectively. Colloids were initially proposed as a very effective volume expander with an expansion ratio of 1:2–1:3 in favor of colloids compared to normal saline. However, a recent meta-analysis which included studies in perioperative and critical care settings reported an insignificant gain in volume expansion, a volume ratio varying between 1:1.3 and 1:1.6 [11]. The nationwide trauma registry data from 2002 to 2015 looked at the effects of fluid resuscitation with synthetic colloids in severely injured trauma patients [12]. The analysis of early fluid resuscitation with more than 1 L of colloids was linked with an increased requirement for hemodialysis. Synthetic colloids administered at any dose were associated with an increased rate of multiple-organ failure. Annane and colleagues compared colloids with crystalloids for the resuscitation of critically ill patients presenting with hypovolemic shock. The authors didn't find any difference in 28-day all-cause mortality between the groups and the same was replicated in the trauma subgroup [13].

Hydroxyethyl starch (HES) was one of the most frequently used synthetic colloids. It's use has shown to be associated with significant coagulopathy and adverse kidney effects when compared with balanced salt solution while being used for resuscitation in septic shock states in intensive care units. However, a recent systematic review failed to find any association between the use of starch solutions and acute kidney injury in the perioperative setting of surgical patients [14]. The concerns about the associated renal injury have led to a decline in its use lately. It also affects the function of von Willebrand factor and impedes the polymerization of fibrinogen. Studies that evaluated hemostasis by viscoelastic assays confirmed that starch infusion resulted in weaker blood clot formation and impaired platelet aggregation than crystalloid or albumin [15].

The SAFE study investigators had demonstrated that albumin as a resuscitation fluid does not interfere with kidney function and coagulation. However, in the subgroup of patients with TBI, 28-day mortality was higher in the 4% albumin group compared to

0.9% saline that persisted at the two-year follow-up. This was attributed to exacerbation of cytotoxic or vasogenic cerebral edema induced by albumin [16, 17]. In conclusion, colloids probably do not confer any major advantage, at least in the early resuscitation of trauma patients.

Hypertonic Solutions

Hypertonic saline (HTS) (e.g., 3% or 6% at a dose of 4 mL/kg/15 min, also called small-volume resuscitation) has been considered with significant interest in trauma resuscitation. There are several postulated theoretical benefits of HTS in trauma resuscitation. It provides volume expansion, causes immune modulation, and offers anti-inflammatory properties. It has also been shown to be effective in the reduction of intracranial pressure (ICP). Its ability to achieve a higher degree of plasma expansion with a smaller volume of HTS makes it an attractive option for hemodynamic resuscitation and in achieving optimal hemostasis during periods of initial hemorrhagic shock. However, HTS has failed to improve patient-oriented clinical outcomes when used as a resuscitation fluid in patients with hemorrhagic shock or TBI [18, 19]. Its administration was even associated with higher mortality in the cohort that was not transfused during the initial 24 h [20]. Authors postulated that HTS concealed the clinical signs of hemorrhage, thus delaying transfusions. In contrast, it has shown to decrease the risk of abdominal compartment syndrome and acute kidney injury in patients with severe burns by limiting the use of large-volume resuscitation with the crystalloids [21].

Penetrating Versus Blunt Injury Versus Head Injuries

For most practical purposes of fluid resuscitation, trauma emergency can be divided into three main categories: penetrating injury, blunt injury, and head injuries; and often there are overlaps such as polytrauma. In the case of penetrating injury patients presenting with hypotension, delay in fluid therapy until surgical intervention improves patient outcome [22]. This "scoop and run" policy permits the systolic BP to be maintained between 60 and 70 mmHg until the patient can be taken to the operating room (OR). After controlling the source of bleeding in the OR, a higher BP should be targeted. A similar restrictive policy is acceptable in blunt traumas where slower infusions are favored over rapid boluses with the aim of maintaining a slightly higher systolic BP of 80–90 mmHg. This restrictive policy is thought to minimize intra-abdominal bleeding while maintaining adequate organ perfusion and reducing the risk of complications like coagulopathy, hypothermia, and intra-abdominal hypertension. In the emergency room, clinical presentation is often complicated and target BP goals frequently need to be tailored depending on comorbidities, the patient's physiology, and compensatory mechanisms. However, the restrictive and permissive hypotension strategies should not be applied to patients with TBI and spinal injury. Maintaining a systolic BP between 100 and 110 mmHg is a priority in these patients to preserve adequate cerebral perfusion [23].

Initial Trauma Resuscitation Fluid Volume

The volume of fluid and blood resuscitation required to restore circulating volume and maintain tissue perfusion is difficult to foresee on initial evaluation of a trauma patient. For major trauma patients presenting in hemorrhagic shock, most practice guidelines suggest administration of 1 L of warm crystalloid fluid and 20 mL/kg for pediatric patients weighing less than 40 kilograms as a bolus in initial resuscitation [24]. After the initial fluid bolus, the patient's response to fluid is assessed by vital signs and adequacy of end-organ perfusion and tissue oxygenation. The patient's response can be divided into three groups: rapid responder, transient responder, and minimal or nonresponder. These responses guide subsequent resuscitation and diagnostic and therapeutic decisions as discussed in Table 16.3 [24].

- The rapid responders are a group of patients who have typically lost less than 15% of the blood volume. They quickly respond to the initial fluid bolus and become hemodynamically stable, without signs of impaired tissue perfusion.
- Transient responders have ongoing blood loss or inadequate resuscitation and have lost an estimated 15–40% of their blood volume. They respond to the initial fluid bolus followed by slow deterioration. In most of these patients, transfusion of blood and blood products is indicated. It is of paramount importance to recognize these patients as they often require operative or angiographic control of the hemorrhage.
- Minimal or nonresponders are those patients who fail to respond to bolus crystalloid and blood products administration. This indicates the need for urgent, definitive intervention to control hemorrhage and rule out other causes of shock.

Table 16.3 Patterns of patients responses to initial fluid resuscitation (isotonic crystalloid of 1 L in adults; 20 mL/kg in children)

Parameter	Rapid responder	Transient responder	Minimal or nonresponder
Vital signs	Normalizes rapidly	Transient improvement followed by deterioration	Continues to deteriorate
Estimated blood loss	Low (<15%)	Moderate (15%–40%)	High (>40%)
Crystalloid requirement	Limited	High	High
Blood requirement	Limited	Moderate	Immediate and high
Operative intervention required	Possible	Moderate likelihood	Highly likelihood
Immediate surgical intervention required	No	Variable	Yes/always

The previous recommendation for initial fluid bolus had been two liters, but this was scaled down due to increasing recognition of harms associated with large-volume resuscitation. Studies have shown that overzealous fluid therapy resuscitation in first 24 h of trauma was associated with increased mortality and significantly higher duration of mechanical ventilation and increased risk of abdominal compartment syndrome in polytrauma patients [25, 26]. Further resuscitation is done with use of blood and blood products and damage control surgery as needed. If blood products aren't immediately available, a small boluses of crystalloid fluid (250 cc or 4 mL/kg at a time) for the time being in patients with systolic BP <70 mmHg, altered mental status or loss of peripheral pulses may be attempted to maintain tissue perfusion.

Practical Approach to Initial Fluid Resuscitation and Pattern of Responses

- After initial airway and breathing assessment, two large-caliber (at least 18G) peripheral IV catheters are inserted.
- Blood samples are drawn for crossmatch and sent for appropriate laboratory and blood gas analyses.
- The warmed fluid bolus of isotonic crystalloid fluid is administered. The choice of crystalloid would be isotonic saline if there is coexisting TBI or a balanced solution in remaining cases.
- The usual volume of bolus fluid is 1 L (15 mL/kg) for adults and 20 mL/kg for pediatric patients.
- The response to initial fluid bolus is critical in deciding an appropriate therapeutic strategy in these patients. As defined by the Advanced Trauma Life Support guidelines, the patient response to initial fluid bolus can be divided into three groups: rapid responders, transient responders, and minimal or nonresponders.

Completion of Resuscitation

Once hemostasis is achieved, the goal of resuscitation shifts to the restoration of blood flow, tissue perfusion, and preservation of organ function. Normalization of vital signs does not necessarily reflect adequate resuscitation. This is true especially in younger patients who often maintain their BP even when they are under-resuscitated. They do so with profound vasoconstriction which can result in hypoperfusion. Resuscitation end points should target microcirculation oxygen delivery indices like lactate, base deficit, and ScvO2 to decrease morbidity and mortality [27]. Serial lactate measurement and lactate clearance provide information regarding adequacy of tissue perfusion and guides further resuscitation. Maintaining normal body temperature and adequate pain relief with systemic analgesia will help in reversing vasoconstriction.

Post-Resuscitation Fluid Management

Fluid therapy after completion of resuscitation is needed to compensate for fluid or blood loss due to wounds, drains, continued capillary leak, fever, and the state of hypercatabolism. Deciding on the appropriate amount and choice of fluid is challenging in this phase as there is greater variability among patients. The requirements of fluid may vary considerably in polytrauma patients and those undergoing major emergency surgical procedures. The dose and choice of fluid have to be individualized based on the estimated deficit. Uncorrected hypovolemia may result in tissue hypoperfusion and worsen organ dysfunction. Overzealous fluid dosing may, however, impede oxygen delivery, wound healing, and homeostasis and compromise patient outcome. The general principle is to prevent excessive fluid administration during this phase while maintaining adequate perfusion. Perhaps the best strategy is to look for fluid responsiveness before giving small aliquots of fluid and monitor response to this fluid including its adverse consequences. Methods of fluid responsiveness are further discussed in Chap. 5.

Deresuscitation

Once stabilization is achieved, active removal of fluid with the use of diuretics and ultrafiltration is commonly warranted especially in patients showing signs of tissue edema, compartment syndromes, or pulmonary complications such as edema, ARDS, or contusions. Persistent positive cumulative fluid balance state is implicated in increased morbidity and mortality in terms of prolonged ICU stay, ventilatory requirements, and delayed discharge [25, 26]. The rationale, different methods, and possible consequences of active removal of accumulated fluid, widely known as deresuscitation, is discussed further in Chap. 25.

Case Vignette

For Mr. K, the patient in the vignette, the best fluid and volume for resuscitation should be 1000 mL 0.9% saline till TBI has been ruled out. Once TBI has been ruled out, the fluid of choice should be a balanced crystalloid. Initial resuscitation end point is to target an SBP >110 mmHg till TBI has been ruled out. Once TBI has been ruled out, SBP target of 80–90 mmHg is acceptable as for any other blunt trauma injury. After achievement of hemostasis, the goal of resuscitation is to restore normal tissue perfusion based on serum lactate levels and other markers of microcirculatory flow. The maintenance fluid is estimated along with consideration of fluid loss from wounds leakage, drains and presence of fever, and hypermetabolic state. The need for further fluid boluses or vasopressors during periods of hypotension will be based on the assessment of dynamic indices of fluid responsiveness. Active deresuscitation will be useful in weaning the patient from ventilatory support.

Conclusion

There has been considerable improvement in our understanding of trauma resuscitation and fluid therapy in the past decade. The goal of our therapy should be directed towards improving the patient's physiology and tissue perfusion, maintaining normothermia, and minimizing coagulopathy. The most acceptable fluid for initial resuscitation is a crystalloid, preferably a balanced one unless there is suspicion of TBI or spinal injury. The timely administration of blood and blood products in life-threatening hemorrhagic shock remains the cornerstone of therapy. Initial resuscitation targets are variable depending on the nature of the injury and the patient's response to therapy and needs to be individualized. The current acceptable initial end points of hypotensive resuscitation in the presence of active hemorrhage are target SBP of 60–70 mmHg, 80–90 mmHg, and 100–110 mmHg in penetrating trauma, blunt trauma without head injury, and blunt trauma with head injury, respectively. After initial resuscitation, further fluid therapy should be guided by fluid responsiveness and other physiological parameters. During the recovery phase, a restrictive fluid approach and active removal of accumulated fluid facilitates early extubation and reduces the length of ICU and hospital stay.

Take Home Messages
- The principles of initial resuscitation in polytrauma patients are limiting use of crystalloids and early use of blood products, permissive hypotension in selected patients, and early damage control surgery in patients who don't respond to initial resuscitation.
- The initial choice of fluid is normal saline in traumatic brain injury patients and balanced salt solution in other patients. Colloids, albumin, and hypertonic saline are not recommended for resuscitation.
- After the initial fluid bolus of 1 L, the patient's response to fluid is assessed as rapid responder, transient responder, and minimal or nonresponder, and these responses guide subsequent resuscitation and diagnostic and therapeutic decisions.
- Overzealous fluid resuscitation in the first 24 h of trauma was associated with increased mortality and higher duration of mechanical ventilation and increased risk of ACS.
- Deresuscitation involves the active removal of excess fluid, usually by diuretic therapy, and may be warranted in patients showing signs of tissue edema, compartment syndromes, or pulmonary complications.

References

1. Ball CG. Damage control resuscitation: history, theory and technique. Can J Surg. 2014;57:55–60.
2. Holcomb JB, Tilley BC, Baraniuk S, Fox EE, Wade CE, Podbielski JM, et al. Transfusion of plasma, platelets, and red blood cells in a 1:1:1 vs a 1:1:2 ratio and mortality in patients with severe trauma: the PROPPR randomized clinical trial. JAMA. 2015;313:471–82.
3. Dutton R, Duchesne JC, Kaplan LJ, Balogh ZJ, Malbrain ML. Role of permissive hypotension, hypertonic resuscitation and the global increased permeability syndrome in patients with severe hemorrhage: adjuncts to damage control resuscitation to prevent intra-abdominal hypertension. Anaesthesiol Intensive Ther. 2015;47(2):143–55.
4. Dutton RP. Haemostatic resuscitation. Br J Anaesth. 2012;109:39–46.
5. Regli A, De Keulenaer B, De Laet I, Roberts D, Dabrowski W, et al. Fluid therapy and perfusional considerations during resuscitation in critically ill patients with intra-abdominal hypertension. Anaesthesiol Intensive Ther. 2015;47(1):45–53.
6. Malbrain ML, Marik PE, Witters I, Cordemans C, Kirkpatrick AW, et al. Fluid overload, deresuscitation, and outcomes in critically ill or injured patients: a systematic review with suggestions for clinical practice. Anaesthesiol Intensive Ther. 2014;46(5):361–80.
7. Chowdhury AH, Eleanor F, Francis ST, Lobo DN. A randomized, controlled, double-blind crossover study on the effects of 2-L infusions of 0.9% saline and plasma-lyte 148 on renal blood flow velocity and renal coritcal tissue perfusion in healthy volunteers. Ann Surg. 2012;256:18–24.
8. Young P, Bailey M, Beasley R, Henderson S, Mackle D, Mcarthur C, et al. Effect of a buffered crystalloid solution vs saline on acute kidney injury among patients in the intensive care unit: the SPLIT randomized clinical trial. JAMA. 2015;314:1701–10.
9. Wang L, Byrne DW, Stollings JL, Pharm D, Kumar AB, Hughes CG, et al. Balanced crystalloids versus saline in critically ill adults. N Engl J Med. 2018;378:829–39.
10. Wanderer JP, Wang L, Byrne DW, Collins SP, Slovis CM, Lindsell CJ, et al. Balanced crystalloids versus saline in noncritically ill adults. N Engl J Med. 2018;378:819–28.
11. Barros TG, Njimi H, Vincent J. Crystalloids versus colloids: exploring differences in fluid requirements by systematic review and meta-regression. Anesth Analg. 2015;120:389–402.
12. Hilbert-carius P, Schwarzkopf D, Reinhart K, Hartog CS, Lefering R, Bernhard M, et al. Synthetic colloid resuscitation in severely injured patients : analysis of a nationwide trauma registry (Trauma register DGU). Sci Rep. 2018;8:11567.
13. Annane D, Siami S, Jaber S, Martin C, Elatrous S, Declere AD, et al. Effects of fluid resuscitation with colloids vs crystalloids on mortality in critically ill patients presenting with hypovolemic shock: the CRISTAL randomized trial. JAMA. 2013;310:1809–17.
14. Perner A, Haase N, Guttormsen AB, Tenhunen J, Klemenzson G, et al. 6S trial group; Scandinavian critical care trials group. Hydroxyethyl starch 130/0.42 versus Ringer's acetate in severe sepsis. N Engl J Med. 2012;367(2):124–34.
15. Hartog CS, Bauer M, Reinhart K. The efficacy and safety of colloid resuscitation in the critically ill. Anesth Analg. 2011;112:156–64.
16. Finfer S, Bellomo R, Boyce N, French J, Myburgh J, Norton R. A comparison of albumin and saline for fluid resuscitation in the intensive care unit. N Engl J Med. 2004;350:2247–56.
17. Myburgh J, Cooper DJ, Finfer S, Bellomo R, Norton R, Bishop N, et al. Saline or albumin for fluid fesuscitation in patients with traumatic brain injury. N Engl J Med. 2007;357:874–84.
18. Bulger EM, May S, Brasel KJ, Schreiber M, Kerby JD, Tisherman SA, et al. Out-of-Hospital hypertonic resuscitation following severe traumatic brain injury: a randomized controlled trial. JAMA. 2010;304:1455–64.
19. Bulger EM. 7.5% saline and 7.5% saline/6% dextran for hypovolemic shock. J Trauma. 2011;70:S27–9.

20. Bulger EM, May S, Kerby JD, Emerson S, Stiell IG, Schreiber MA, et al. Out-of-hospital hypertonic resuscitation after traumatic hypovolemic shock: a randomized, controlled trial. Ann Surg.
2011;253:431–41.
21. Noborio M, Ode Y, Aoki Y, Sugimoto H. Hypertonic lactated saline resuscitation reduces the risk
of abdominal compartment syndrome in severely burned patients. J Trauma. 2006;60(1):64–71.
22. Bickell WH, Wall MJ Jr, Pepe PE, Martin RR, Ginger VF, Allen MK, et al. Immediate versus
delayed fluid resuscitation for hypotensive patients with penetrating torso injuries. N Engl J
Med. 1994;331(17):1105–9.
23. Carney N, Totten AM, Reilly CO, Ullman JS, Bell MJ, Bratton SL, et al. Guidelines for the
management of severe traumatic brain injury. Neurosurgery. 2016;80:6.
24. Subcommittee on advanced trauma life support (atls) of the american college of surgeons (acs),
committee on trauma. Advanced Trauma Life Support Course for Physicians. 10th ed. Chicago,
IL: American College of Surgeons; 2018.
25. Jones DG, Nantais J, Rezende-Neto JB, Yazdani S, Vegas P, et al. Crystalloid resuscitation in
trauma patients: deleterious effect of 5L or more in the first 24h. BMC Surg. 2018;18(1):93.
26. Malbrain MLNG, Marik PE, Witters I, Cordemans C, Kirkpatrick AW, Roberts DJ, et al. Fluid
overload, de-resuscitation, and outcomes in critically ill or injured patients: a systematic review
with suggestions for clinical practice. Anaesthesiol Intensive Ther. 2014;46:361–80.
27. Ducrocq N, Kimmoun A, Levy B. Lactate or ScvO2 as an endpoint in resuscitation of shock
states? Minerva Anestesiol. 2013;79(9):1049–58.

Fluid Management in Neurocritical Care

Roop Kishen

CIT: 'The quantity (of fluid) necessary to be injected will probably be found to depend upon quantity of serum lost, the object of the practice being to place the patient in nearly his ordinary state as to the quantity of blood circulating in the vessels'

—*Dr. Robert Lewins,*

Contents

Introduction 348
Physiological Considerations 348
What Kind of Fluid Is Appropriate in NIC Patients? 350
Does Tonicity of the IV Fluids Matter in NIC Patients? 351
Hyperosmolar Therapy in NIC Patients 352
End Points of Fluid Therapy Management in Neurocritical Care: How Much Fluid Is
    Enough? 352
Monitoring Fluid Therapy in NIC Patients 353
A Note on Common Electrolyte Disturbances in NIC Patients 353
    General Considerations 353
    Hyponatraemia 354
    Hypernatremia 356
    Hyperchloraemia 356
    Other Electrolyte Disturbances 356
Fluid Therapy Management in Neurocritical Care: Clinical Practice Recommendations 357
Conclusion 358
References 359

R. Kishen (✉)
Retired Consultant, Intensive Care Medicine & Anaesthesia, Hope Hospital, Salford Royal NHS Foundation Trust, Salford, Manchester, UK

Anaesthesia, Translational Medicine and Neurosciences, Victoria University of Manchester, Manchester, UK

IFA Commentary (MLNGM)

This chapter is a summary of the key learning objectives and take-home messages related to fluid therapy management in patients with neurological injury. The chapter emphasises the importance of understanding the basic physiological and pathological considerations in brain-injured patients and the role of cerebral blood flow in maintaining cerebral homeostasis. It also stresses the need to maintain euvolaemia and avoid both hypovolaemia and hypervolaemia in these patients. The take-home messages highlight the use of isotonic crystalloids as first-line fluids for resuscitation and maintenance, while hypotonic fluids should be avoided due to the risk of brain oedema. Colloids, glucose-containing hypotonic solutions, 4% albumin, and hypertonic 20% albumin are not recommended for resuscitation or maintenance fluids. The use of hypertonic saline (HTS) solutions as resuscitation fluids is also discouraged. The chapter recommends a multimodal approach to monitor fluid therapy, including integration of more than one haemodynamic parameter, arterial blood pressure, and fluid balance. Central venous pressure alone as a fluid management monitoring parameter is discouraged. This chapter also recommends monitoring electrolytes and measured osmolality as safety end points and using mannitol or HTS to reduce intracranial pressure in neuro-intensive care patients. For patients with diffuse cerebral injury, fluid boluses are recommended, and the use of multimodal monitoring of their efficacy is suggested. Overall, this chapter provides a concise and informative overview of the key considerations and recommendations related to fluid therapy management in neurologically injured patients. The emphasis on individualised patient care, multimodal monitoring, and careful evaluation and management of electrolyte abnormalities is particularly notable. The take-home messages provide practical guidance for clinicians involved in the care of these patients.

Suggested Reading

1. Oddo M, Poole D, Helbok R, Meyfroidt G, Stocchetti N, Bouzat P, Cecconi M, Geeraerts T, Martin-Loeches I, Quintard H, Taccone FS, Geocadin RG, Hemphill C, Ichai C, Menon D, Payen JF, Perner A, Smith M, Suarez J, Videtta W, Zanier ER, Citerio G. Fluid therapy in neurointensive care patients: ESICM consensus and clinical practice recommendations. Intensive Care Med. 2018;44(4):449-463. https://doi.org/10.1007/s00134-018-5086-z.

Learning Objectives

After reading this chapter, you will have:

1. Briefly revised the basic physiological and pathological considerations in brain-injured patients.

2. Understood the importance of cerebral blood flow and its role in maintaining cerebral homeostasis.
3. Understood the importance of fluid resuscitation and maintenance of 'normal' intravascular volume status in brain-injured patients as well as understood the important differences between these and non-brain-injured patients as far as the fluid resuscitation is concerned.
4. Have a good knowledge of which fluids to use and which to avoid in these patients with regard to fluid content and fluid osmolality.
5. Understood the principles of monitoring fluid resuscitation and management of further fluid infusion in these patients.
6. Have a knowledge of some specific electrolyte abnormalities encountered in NIC patients and their brief management.
7. Have knowledge of the latest 'clinical practice recommendations' of an expert group of European Society of Intensive Care Medicine.

Case Vignette

Mr. C, aged 38 years, is brought to the emergency department (ED) by an ambulance after being hit by a car on his right side while crossing a busy road. He was thrown about 5 m from the collision site and was found unconscious at the scene by paramedics. His injuries are closed right femoral fracture, pelvic ramus fracture, and bruising over the abdomen. He has been evaluated by emergency physicians, surgeons, and intensivists. His vital observations, at the time of presentation to ED, are BP 85/65 mmHg, HR 123/min, and RR of 24 breaths/min. He has received 3 litres of Plasma-Lyte and two units of blood. His Glasgow Coma Scale (GCS) score was 7 (eyes 2, motor 3, verbal 2) at presentation and has not improved since. He was intubated and ventilated in the ED and reassessed after resuscitation (BP 114/70 mmHg, HR 96/min). He had a full-body computerised tomography (CT) scan that showed a right mid-shaft femoral fracture and base of skull fracture but no mass lesion in the brain except for several small cerebral contusions. No thoracic or internal abdominal injuries were identified on CT. He was transferred to the operating theatre and his femoral fracture was reduced and stabilised with an external fixator. He was transferred to the intensive care unit, where he is now on a ventilator with stable vital signs. He is still unconscious, requiring minimal sedation.

Questions

Q1. What fluids should Mr. C receive now and how should his fluid therapy/balance be monitored?

Introduction

All critically ill patients require fluids during the course of their illness, neurocritical care (NIC) patients being no exception. Fluids are administered orally or intravenously (IV). Orally administered fluids have different systemic effects compared to IV fluids. IV fluids are required during resuscitation of acutely ill patients in shock and in correcting volume deficits, and once normality is established, fluids are necessary for maintenance of volume status. The main objectives of fluid therapy during resuscitation are to maintain organ perfusion by improving cardiac output (CO) and thereby tissue oxygen delivery(DO_2). After achieving stabilisation, oral intake may be adequate in a minority of patients without requiring any further IV fluids; in majority of the patients however, IV fluids will needed for continued volume maintenance, drug carriage, and occasionally parenteral nutrition. As all these fluids contribute to overall fluid intake, and unless care is taken, fluid accumulation can easily occur. Both hypervolaemia and hypovolaemia are detrimental to NIC patients, euvolaemia being the best clinical practice standard [1]. This chapter focuses on the use of IV fluids in NIC patients. This chapter will focus on adult patients, and more information on fluid therapy in children can be found in Chap. 20. Some other chapters will discuss fluids in specific populations: sepsis (Chap. 14), heart failure (Chap. 15), trauma (Chap. 16), perioperative setting (Chap. 18), burns (Chap. 19), liver failure (Chap. 21), abdominal hypertension (Chap. 22), and COVID-19 (Chap. 26).

Physiological Considerations

The objectives of fluid resuscitation in brain-injured patients are to improve and optimise cerebral blood flow (CBF) and cerebral DO_2. Whereas general physiological principles of improving CO and tissue DO_2 with fluid resuscitation apply equally to the central nervous system (CNS) as to other organs, fluid management in NIC patients has some unique features which are different from non-brain-injured patients [1]. These relate to the effects of fluid infusion on CBF, intracranial pressure (ICP), and cerebral perfusion pressure (CPP). Thus, it is essential to understand CBF autoregulation and blood–brain barrier (BBB) physiology, both of which are designed to preserve the integrity of the brain cellular fluid and cerebral interstitial fluid (ISF) composition as well as homeostasis, which is important for proper functioning of the CNS. Both CBF autoregulation and BBB function can be disturbed in the critically ill NIC patients, causing alterations in CBF and ICP and ultimately affecting mortality as well as functional neurological recovery [2].

Under normal physiological conditions, the brain receives about 20% of the CO. CBF, like blood flow to any other organ system in the body, is a function of blood volume, CO, and peripheral vascular resistance and therefore systemic blood pressure(BP). In addition, cerebral vascular resistance (CVR) influenced by cerebral autoregulation also determines CBF [3]. These ensure that, under normal physiological conditions with intact autoregulation, CBF is maintained constant over a wide range of BP (mean arterial pressure [MAP] 60–180 mmHg). Beyond these limits, CBF is pressure dependent. This means that there is a risk of cerebral ischaemia because of low CBF at lower MAP and a risk of cerebral hyperaemia causing possible increase in ICP at higher MAP. Cerebral autoregulation responds to and alters CBF according to the demands of cerebral metabolism and is disrupted by trauma, infarction, brain haemorrhage, both subarachnoid (SAH) as well as intracerebral (ICH), and possibly by local and systemic infections [4].

The BBB is a complex physiological entity resulting from interrelationship between cerebral blood vessels, their endothelium, vascular wall smooth muscle cells, perivascular tissue, and a variety of neuronal cells (e.g. astrocytes, microglia). The endothelial cells have 'tight junctions' allowing movement of gases, water, and nutrients by facilitated diffusion (a type of energy-independent carrier-mediated transport) into the cerebrospinal fluid (CSF) and brain ISF [4, 5]. Evidence is emerging that BBB integrity may also be affected by dysfunction of the endothelial glycocalyx [6]. BBB prevents toxic molecules and electrolytes from entering the brain substance, and its normal physiological 'opening' is regulated by locally mediated molecules [5]. Under pathological processes, such as trauma, ischaemic stroke, haemorrhage (ICH, SAH), infections, and inflammation, the BBB opens with tight junctions becoming more 'permeable' to water, cytokines, electrolytes, etc. [5, 7]

CPP is determined by MAP and ICP, with some minimal contribution from cerebral venous pressure. In simple terms:

$$CPP = MAP - ICP$$

Thus, in hypotensive patients, CPP will be lower despite normal ICP. Conversely, CPP may be inadequate if ICP is high with a 'normal' CBF and MAP. Inadequate CCP is detrimental for brain perfusion and linked to further brain damage, especially in traumatic brain injury (TBI) [8]. Maintenance of optimal CPP, with fluid infusion and inotropes/vasopressors to maintain adequate CO and cerebral DO_2, forms the standard management guideline of the Brain Trauma Foundation (BTF) [9]. It is, therefore, traditional and logical to optimise ' blood pressure to target CPP >70 mmHg [8]. The BTF guidelines suggest maintaining CPP between 50 and 70 mmHg with the caution that lower or higher CPP values are associated with complications [9]. It is also accepted that CPP values need to be individualised for the best outcomes [10].

The effect of fluid management on CBF, CPP, and cerebral oxygenation is complex as illustrated in Fig. 17.1.

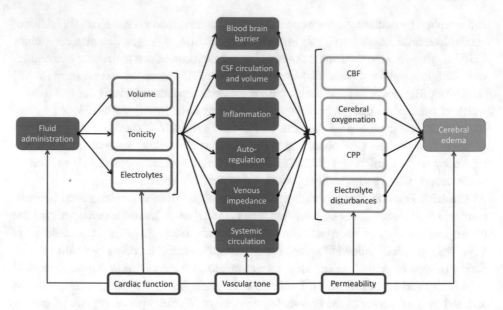

Fig. 17.1 The effect of fluid management on cerebral blood flow (CBF), cerebral perfusion pressure (CPP), and cerebral oxygenation is complex because many intermediate variables exist that should be taken into account to fully appreciate possible cause and effect relationships. (Adapted from Van der Jagt M. under the Open Access CC BY Licence 4.0 [1]) *CBF* cerebral blood flow, *CSF* cerebrospinal fluid, *CPP* cerebral perfusion pressure

What Kind of Fluid Is Appropriate in NIC Patients?

Available literature and major guidelines suggest crystalloids as the primary choice for fluid resuscitation and maintenance in NIC patients; [9, 10] however, the type of crystalloid is not specified. As has been discussed in Chap. 9, some concerns have emerged about excess chloride content of 0.9% saline (NS) resulting in hyperchloraemic metabolic acidosis(HCMA) with potentially increased risk of acute kidney injury, need for renal replacement therapy, increased inflammation, as well as increased mortality. However, randomised control trials in general ICU patients have produced conflicting results when NS is compared with balanced salt solutions, and there is still no definitive consensus for or against using NS versus balanced crystalloids in general ICU patients.

It is difficult to extrapolate these findings to NIC patients because of two major reasons: (1) relatively smaller number of TBI patients were included in these studies (because of the concerns among clinicians that relative hypotonicity of balanced crystalloids may increase ICP) and (2) because of poor understanding of the effects of HCMA on neurological recovery. For example, in the SMART study, a large, single-centre randomised study comparing effects of balanced fluid versus NS, only 17.3% of patients had TBI

(8.8% in balanced crystalloid group and 8.5% in NS group), and clinicians were also free to use NS in TBI group [11]. The concerns about the effects of the tonicity of fluid on ICP are addressed in the next section.

Colloids have been used in the past (and are still being used) with the 'physiological rationale' that their use allows resuscitation with a smaller volume of infused fluid. However, this perceived benefit of colloids has not been proven in randomised studies and meta-analyses [12]. Colloids are discussed in greater detail in Chaps. 10 and 11.

Albumin, a natural colloid, has been the subject of much research and discussion. The SAFE study showed that 4% albumin (compared to NS) had detrimental effects on TBI [13]. In a post hoc analysis of the SAFE study, 460 well-matched patients with TBI, who received albumin, had increased mortality at 24 months after injury when compared to resuscitation with NS [14]. Some researchers have also explored the possible neuroprotective effect of albumin in patients with SAH. In a multicentre dose-ranging study, Suarez and colleagues found that 25% albumin at a dose of 1.25 g/kg/day for 7 days had the best neuroprotective effect in SAH patients with the best clinical outcome at 3 months without producing adverse effects like heart failure or anaphylaxis [15].

Does Tonicity of the IV Fluids Matter in NIC Patients?

BBB is designed to preserve CNS homeostasis. Under normal physiological conditions, osmolalities of plasma and CSF are equal. As BBB is water-permeable, hypotonic fluids can cause water to shift into CSF and brain substance; conversely, hypertonic fluids can cause brain dehydration whether BBB is intact or disrupted [5, 7]. Under normal conditions, neurons maintain their homeostasis by solute depletion and the ability of the BBB and neurovascular unit cells to expel water into the intravascular compartment [16]. Whereas peripheral vascular endothelium is highly permeable to electrolytes, with oedema formation roughly proportional to the infused volume of isotonic fluid, an intact BBB does not allow free passage of electrolytes and thus protects the brain from oedema even when large volumes of isotonic fluids are administered to the patients [16]. This ability to control water and electrolyte homeostasis is locally abolished by disruption of BBB function; fluid shifts become more dependent on the pressure difference between intravascular and extravascular compartments and the prevailing osmolality of the former [5, 7, 16]. Thus, hypo-osmolar fluids, by reducing plasma osmolarity, can cause brain oedema, especially in presence of functional BBB disruption [16].

In a single-centre RCT, 36 patients with SAH were randomised to receive NS and hydroxyethyl starch (HES) in NS or Ringer's lactate (RL) and HES in RL. NS-based fluid therapy was associated with hyperchloraemia, increased tonicity, and more positive fluid balance than balanced fluids. In contrast, the balanced fluids group did not have more hyponatraemia or hypotonicity [17]. However, this is a small study, and the findings need to be validated in a larger trial.

Hyperosmolar Therapy in NIC Patients

Small-volume hypertonic saline (HTS) infusions (usually around 4 mL/kg/15 min) have been used for resuscitation in TBI. In a blinded RCT, 229 severe TBI patients (GCS < 9) with hypotension (systolic BP <100 mmHg) were randomised to receive a 250 ml bolus of either Ringer's lactate or 7.5% HTS in the prehospital phase, in addition to other resuscitation fluids. All patients, regardless of assigned prehospital fluid group, were adequately resuscitated (as judged by normal post-resuscitation BP) upon arrival into the hospital. However, there was no difference in survival to hospital discharge and neurological function as measured by Glasgow Outcome Scale (GOS) at 6 months between the groups [18].

Another indication for hyperosmolar fluid therapy in brain-injured patients is in the management of raised ICP. Mannitol has been popular for a long time as the first-line IV fluid to treat raised ICP in TBI as well as in patients with SAH, ICH, and acute ischaemic stroke (AIS) [19]. Recently, HTS has been gaining popularity over mannitol [19] and a recently published meta-analysis of 12 RCTs showed that HTS was better than mannitol in controlling raised ICP in TBI, though there was no difference in neurological outcome as determined by GOS [20]. Evidence for the beneficial use of hyperosmolar therapies in ICH and AIS is even more sparse. Hyperosmolar therapy does reduce ICP in these conditions; however, its effect on clinical outcome is unclear. A post hoc analysis of the data from one study (Ethnic/Racial Variation of Intracerebral Haemorrhage, ERICH) showed that both mannitol and HTS were associated with unfavourable outcomes at 3 months [21]. It is also worth noting that recently there have been reports of increased in-hospital mortality associated with hyperchloraemia in patients with ICH receiving continuous infusions of 3% HTS and NS [22, 23]. The commonest causes of raised ICP in SAH include hydrocephalus, ICH with intraventricular haemorrhage, and global cerebral oedema. Cerebral oedema can also occur from diffused cerebral injury (DCI) and standard hyperosmolar strategies apply in these patients as well. A systemic review of five observational studies (n = 175) showed that HTS was similar to mannitol in reducing ICP. However, it was unclear if it had any effect on outcome nor could an optimum dose for HTS be recommended in SAH [24].

End Points of Fluid Therapy Management in Neurocritical Care: How Much Fluid Is Enough?

The goal of fluid therapy in NIC patients is to optimise cerebral perfusion and, therefore, cerebral DO_2 while at the same time minimising further/secondary brain injury [6]. Studies have adequately stressed the adverse effects of hypo- as well as hypervolaemia in NIC patients [1]. Unfortunately, achieving euvolaemia in brain-injured patients without sophisticated cardiovascular and brain monitoring is not always possible. Besides, euvolaemia is subject to individual interpretation [1]. Positive fluid balance in NIC patients has been associated with vasospasm (proven on angiography), increased hospital stay, poor

neurological outcome, and adverse cardiovascular side effects [25]. In SAH, hypervolaemia has not been shown to be of benefit in terms of neurological outcome [26]. In another
RCT, SAH patients were randomised to prophylactic triple-H (hypervolaemia, hypertension, and haemodilution) therapy versus normovolaemia [27]. Patients in the normovolae-
mic group received about 3 L/day, while the triple-H group received about 4–5 L/day of
fluids. Clinical outcomes were similar in both groups, while the triple-H group had more
complications like haemorrhagic diathesis, congestive heart failure, arrhythmias, and
extradural haematomata [27]. However, hypovolaemia is also harmful especially in TBI,
despite ICP control [28].

Monitoring Fluid Therapy in NIC Patients

As the dangers of under- or over-resuscitation have been repeatedly emphasised, it is of
utmost importance that fluid management should be carefully monitored. Monitoring of
fluid resuscitation in NIC patients should involve multimodal parameters, [29] which
include non-invasive or invasive blood pressure monitoring, neurological function assessment, invasive haemodynamic monitoring (thermodilution CO measurement, global
end-diastolic volume index [GEDI], stroke volume variation, and other invasive and non-
invasive modalities), CBF assessment (e.g. with transcranial doppler), and measurement
of ICP/CPP and brain tissue oxygenation (jugular venous oximetry). Assessing the middle
cerebral artery mean velocity (MCA MV) in response to fluid infusion, with Transcranial
Doppler, may turn out to be another method to assess fluid management in these patients;
however, larger studies and more robust data are required [30]. Routine monitoring of
brain tissue oxygenation or CBF is not recommended as a standard. Central venous pressure (CVP) monitoring is not useful; fluid management should not be guided by CVP
readings or its response to fluid infusion. Hourly urine output is a time-honoured parameter; it can be used in some patients but cannot be universally applied. Finally, it cannot be
overemphasised that fluid management and its monitoring must be individualised..

A Note on Common Electrolyte Disturbances in NIC Patients

General Considerations

(See Table 17.1).
   Electrolyte disturbances are frequently seen in critically ill patients. Although not a
direct remit of this chapter, a reference is made to these disturbances in NIC patients here,
especially those of sodium (Na^+), as they may affect the type of fluid infused and rate of
its administration. Disturbances of sodium (Na^+) and potassium (K^+) are the commonest
abnormalities seen in NIC patients. Some syndromes are specific to TBI/SAH, with hyponatraemia being more commonly associated with SAH. However, aggressive use of

Table 17.1 Electrolyte disorders in NIC patients at a glance (Please see text for details)

Disorder	Defining parameters (sub-types)	Aetiology	Clinical management
Hyponatraemia	Serum Na$^+$ < 135 mmol/L Mild, moderate, severe Acute or chronic	Diuretics Hyperosmolar fluid use SIADH[a] CSWS[b]	IV 150 mL 3.0% saline over 20 min Recheck serum Na$^+$ Repeat if necessary, till serum Na$^+$ > 130 mmol/L
Hypernatraemia	Serum Na$^+$ > 150 mmol/L Mild, moderate, severe	Hyperosmolar fluid use Hypovolaemia Diabetes insipidus Low intake of H$_2$O	IV balanced electrolyte solutions Careful rehydration
Hyperchloraemia	Serum cl$^-$ > 110 mmol/L	Excessive use of high Cl$^-$ containing fluids (NS, HTS)	IV balanced electrolyte solutions Spontaneous resolution
Hypokalaemia	Serum K$^+$ < 3.5 mmol/L	Diuretics Hyperosmolar fluid use Low K$^+$ containing fluid use	Replacement of K$^+$ with supplements in fluids
Hypomagnesaemia	Serum Mg^{++} < 0.6 mmol/L	Diuretics Hyperosmolar fluids use Poor GI absorption	1–4 g (4–16 mmol) of IV magnesium sulphate over 15–20 min Repeat, if required 5–15 g (20–60 mmol) per hour

[a]SIADH, syndrome of inappropriate secretion of antidiuretic hormone
[b]CSWS, cerebral salt wasting syndrome

osmotically active fluids (e.g. mannitol) and other diuretics, which is one of the common causes of hyponatraemia in these patients to control raised ICP, must not be overlooked. Detailed description of these electrolyte disturbances is outside the scope of this chapter.

Both hypo- and hypernatraemia are common in NIC patients.

Hyponatraemia

Hyponatraemia is defined as a serum Na$^+$ < 135 mmol/L. Depending on serum Na$^+$ levels, hyponatraemia is classified as mild (serum Na$^+$ 134–131 mmol/L), moderate (serum Na$^+$ 130–125 mmol/L), or severe (serum Na$^+$ < 125 mmol/L). Apart from common aetiological factors (e.g. overuse of diuretics), two syndromes resulting in hyponatraemia are specifically associated with NIC patients [31–33]:

(a) Syndrome of Inappropriate secretion of antidiuretic hormone (SIADH).
(b) Cerebral salt wasting syndrome (CSWS).

The distinction between the two can be difficult and requires measurement of several plasma and urine biomarkers and osmolalities [31, 32]. However, which of the two syndromes is responsible for observed hyponatraemia may still not be clear, even after extensive laboratory workup. Some authorities believe that a) CSWS does not exist as a separate entity but is a variant of SIADH with apparent Na^+ loss consequent upon 'unrecognised' volume expansion and/or excessive use of HTS [34], b) is a relatively rare cause of hyponatraemia [33, 35], and c) hyponatraemia in itself is not diagnostic of CSWS [33, 36]. Hyponatraemia can exist as two subtypes: hypotonic hyponatraemia (which can be hypovolaemic, euvolumaeic, or hypervolaemic) and iso- or hypertonic hyponatraemia [31, 32]. For clinical relevance and management, it is also classified as acute (<48 h in development) and chronic (developing over >48 h).

Regardless of aetiology, hyponatraemia needs prompt evaluation and treatment. Clinical management involves careful evaluation of the patient, neurological symptoms, as well as volume status (which usually requires invasive or other cardiovascular monitoring). Chronic hyponatraemic patients can tolerate fairly low levels of serum Na^+, often of the order of <125 mmol/L, because of the adaptive mechanisms to prevent cerebral oedema [33]. However, all NIC patients with hyponatraemia, in whom it is almost always of acute origin (<48 h), should be treated as 'symptomatic, acute hyponatraemic' patients and considered a medical emergency because of a high risk of increasing or worsening cerebral oedema [33]. Suggested treatment is an immediate infusion of 150 mL of 3% hypertonic saline over 20 min. Serum Na^+ must be re-checked and 150 ml of 3% saline may be repeated twice till there is a rise of at least 4–6 mmol/L in serum Na^+ [33, 36, 38, 39], as experience with hypertonic saline, in these situations, has shown that an increase of ≈5 mmol/L in serum Na^+ reduces ICP and risk of cerebral herniation in ≈50% of the patients within 1 h [37]. Once a desired increase in serum Na^+ is achieved, NS should be substituted for 3% saline [33, 38, 39], a search for the underlying cause should be made, and treatment instituted, if possible (e.g. stopping aggressive hyperosmolar therapy). Further correction of serum Na^+ should be slower (10 mmol in the first 24 h and 8 mmol in subsequent 24-h periods, thereafter), till serum Na^+ level is 130 mmol/L. Further infusions of 3% saline may have to be continued, to increase the Na^+ level by 1 mmol/L/h, in patients who are still symptomatic, till there is an improvement in symptoms or serum Na^+ has increased by 10–12 mmol/L or reached 130 mmol/L. Subsequent management is as for mild hyponatraemia [38, 39]. Serum Na^+ corrections of >12 mmol/L in 24 h or > 25 mmol/L in 48 h result in osmotic demyelination syndrome. It is thought to be caused by a rapid swelling of brain tissue and some patients may be more vulnerable to it. However, it is thought that patients with acute hyponatraemia are less prone to develop osmotic demyelination syndrome [33] and immediate treatment should not be withheld in these patients, especially as cerebral herniation is a real concern. It cannot be overemphasised that frequent patient evaluation with respect to volume status and neurological symptoms are of utmost importance in managing these patients. It is also suggested that acute deficiency of glucocorticoids is, in part, responsible for hyponatraemia seen in NIC patients; a trial of glucocorticoids has been suggested, after careful patient evaluation [33].

Hypernatremia

Hypernatraemia is another electrolyte abnormality seen in NIC patients, can adversely affect their mortality and morbidity, as well as prolong their hospital stay. Hypernatremia is defined as a serum Na+ >150 mmol/L and can be mild (serum Na^+ 150–155 mmol/L), moderate (serum Na^+ 155–160 mmol/L, or severe (serum Na^+ > 160 mmol/L). It occurs in ≈50% of NIC patients, consequent upon treatment with hyperosmolar fluids (mannitol, hypertonic saline), hypovolaemia, diabetes insipidus, or low intake of water (because of reduced thirst). Management of hypernatraemia involves careful volume assessment of the patient and replacement of any deficit volume with IV fluids, preferably balanced salt solutions [32]. Care must be taken not to overhydrate the patients and half the fluid deficit should be replaced over 12–24 h and the other half over the next 24 h. Serum Na^+ should be reduced slowly, over 24–48 h to avoid acute osmotic shifts.

Hyperchloraemia

Hyperchloraemia has already been mentioned. It is mostly iatrogenic, caused by infusion of high Cl^- containing fluids (NS, HTS). It is defined as serum chloride level of ≥110 mmol/L. Hyperchloraemia causes HCMA and may adversely affect renal blood flow. Mostly, it needs no treatment and usually corrects itself overtime.

Other Electrolyte Disturbances

Other commonly seen electrolyte abnormality is hypokalaemia (serum K^+ < 3.5 mmol/L). This can, again, be a consequence of diuretic/high osmolar fluid use or replacement with low potassium (K^+) containing fluids. Hypokalaemia can cause arrythmias and is managed simply by adequate replacement of K^+.

A relatively less well-known electrolyte abnormality, hypomagnesaemia, defined as serum magnesium (Mg^{++}) < 0.6 mmol/L (1.5 mg/dL) is probably more common than realised, as Mg^{++} measurements are not routinely performed. Hypomagnesaemia occurs due to reduced absorption of Mg^{++} in gut but in NIC patients is mostly due to use of hyperosmolar solutions (mannitol, HTS) and diuretics (all used in control of ICP) as well as certain antibiotics (aminoglycosides) [40, 41]. Hypomagnesaemia can cause ECG changes (appearance of U waves, prolonged QT interval, ventricular arrhythmias, and *torsade de pointes*) and decreased or impaired responsiveness to inotropes/vasoactive drugs [40–42]. Hypomagnesaemia also causes various neurological symptoms (weakness, paraesthesia, tremors, seizures, etc.). Its management requires careful patient evaluation (particularly with regard to neurological condition, other electrolyte abnormalities, e.g. hypercalcaemia and hypokalaemia, which often accompany it) and replacement therapy. One to 4 g (4–16 mmol) of IV magnesium sulphate over 15–20 min, in repeated doses, or as an infusion of 5–15 g (20–60 mmol) per hour is acceptable standard therapy to keep serum Mg^{++} at 1.0–1.5 mmol/L [40, 41].

Fluid Therapy Management in Neurocritical Care: Clinical Practice Recommendations

A consensus committee of 22 international experts considered various aspects of fluid management in NIC patients. These experts met in 2014 and subsequently deliberated for more than a year in face-to-face meetings and teleconferences, considering various questions about fluid therapy management in NIC patients. They looked at all the available evidence and came up with a consensus and clinical practice recommendations. These recommendations have been published recently as 'Consensus and Clinical Practice Recommendations' (JC-2018) [10]. Their main/broad recommendations for clinical practice are listed at the end under take-home messages (it should be noted that not all recommendations are backed by irrefutable evidence).

Case Vignette
In the case vignette, Mr. C should receive NS in adequate amounts, with monitoring of fluid balance to keep MAP around 80–90 mmHg and UO at about 0.5 mL/kg/h (30–40 mL/h) as these are immediately available parameters in this patient. If available, ultrasound-guided monitoring may be instituted as well to ensure that hypervolaemia does not occur. As there are likely to be no facilities for monitoring ICP in this ICU, it is difficult to make allowances for raised ICP in this patient; a target MAP of 80–90 mmHg will ensure that a CPP of at least 50–60 mmHg is achieved even if ICP begins to rise. Monitoring pupillary size and reaction may warn of impending rise in ICP; however, it should be remembered that pupillary dilatation is rather a late sign of raised ICP. Should there be a suspicion of increased ICP, mannitol or HTS (according to local protocol) can be used to lower it. The best management for this patient is monitoring and care in an appropriate setting.

Conclusion

Fluid therapy management in NIC patients is a complex issue. Whereas the general principles of fluid therapy management in other critically ill patient groups also apply, issues particular to NIC patients require special care. Crystalloids are the first-line fluids for resuscitation as well as maintenance in NIC patients, isotonic crystalloids like NS being in common and frequent use. Concerns are emerging about the effects of high chloride containing fluids on plasma electrolytes, acid–base balance and the possible harmful effect of hyperchloraemia on the injured brain. Hypotonic fluids are not recommended for use in NIC patients as brain oedema is likely to occur. There is a consensus on avoiding colloids in brain-injured patients. Maintaining euvolaemia is the clinical practice standard; both hypovolaemia and hypervolaemia are to be assiduously avoided. Monitoring fluid therapy in NIC patients entails multimodal monitoring parameters and clinicians should not rely on just one individual parameter. Various electrolyte abnormalities are often seen in NIC patients, hypo- and hypernatraemia being common. These electrolyte abnormalities need careful patient evaluation and appropriate fluid management. Finally, as no two patients are similar, fluid management should be individualised.

Take Home Messages
- Isotonic crystalloids should be first-line fluids for resuscitation as well as maintenance. There are no recommendation as yet on balanced crystalloids. In this context, solutions with an osmolality of <260 mosmol/kg are considered hypotonic.
- Colloids, glucose-containing hypotonic solutions, 4% albumin, and high concentration (20–25%) albumin (especially in AIS) are not recommended for resuscitation or as maintenance fluids.
- Hypertonic saline solutions are not recommended as resuscitation fluids either.
- Normovolaemia is suggested as a clinical practice standard.
- For 'achieving' normovolaemia and for general fluid management, a multimodal approach to monitor fluid therapy is strongly recommended. These parameters include, but are not limited to:
  - Integration of more than one haemodynamic parameter.
  - Arterial BP and fluid balance as the main parameters.
  - Other variables like CO, mixed venous oxygen saturation (SvO_2), blood lactate, and urine output should be used/considered.
  - CVP alone as a fluid management monitoring parameter is strongly discouraged.
  - Fluids should not be restricted to achieve a negative fluid balance.
- Negative fluid balance is not recommended in NIC patients.
- Monitoring of electrolytes as well as measured osmolality as a safety end point is recommended.

- Mannitol or HTS can be used as agents to reduce ICP in NIC patients.
  - Serum osmolality and effect of hyperosmolar therapy on BP and fluid balance should be monitored.
- For DCI (Diffused Cerebral Injury) patients, fluid boluses are recommended, as is the use of multimodal monitoring of their efficacy.
  - Transcranial doppler-assessed CBF velocities may be used as secondary end points.

References

1. Van-Der Jagt M. Fluid management of the neurological patient: a concise review. Crit Care. 2016;20:126–37.
2. Mascia L, Sakr Y, Pasero D, et al. Sepsis occurrence in acutely ill patients. I. Extracranial complications in patients with acute brain injury: a post-hoc analysis of SOAP study. Intensive Care Med. 2008;34:720–7.
3. Donnelly J, BudohoskiK P, Smielewski P, et al. Regulation of the cerebral circulation: bedside assessment and clinical implications. Crit Care. 2016;20:129–46.
4. Lawther BK, Kumar S, Krovvidi H. Blood-brain barrier. Cont Edu Anaesth Crit Care Pain. 2011;11:128–32.
5. McCaffery G, Davis TP. Physiology and pathology of blood-brain barrier. J Invest Med. 2012;60:1–17.
6. Ando Y, Okada H, Takemura G, et al. Brain-specific ultrastructure of capillary endothelial glycocalyx and its possible contribution for blood-brain barrier. Sci Rep. 2018;8:17523. https://doi.org/10.1038/s41598-018-35976-2.
7. Banks WA. Characteristics of compounds that cross the blood-brain barrier. BMC Neurol. 2009;9(Suppl.1):S3. https://doi.org/10.1186/1471-2377-9-S1-S3.
8. Rosner MJ, Rosner SD, Johnson AH. Cerebral perfusion pressure: management protocol and clinical results. J Neurosurg. 1995;83:949–62.
9. Bratton S, Chestnut RH, Ghajar J, et al. The brain trauma foundation. The American Association of Neurological Surgeons. The joint section on neurotrauma and critical care. Cerebral perfusion pressure thresholds. J Neurotrauma. 2007;24:S59–64.
10. Oddo M, Poole D, Helbok R, et al. Fluid therapy in neurointensive care patients: ESICM consensus and clinical practice recommendations. Intensive Care Med. 2018;44:449–63.
11. Semler MW, Self WH, Wanderer JP, et al. Balanced crystalloids versus saline in critically ill adults. N Engl J Med. 2018;378:829–39.
12. Perel P, Roberts I, Ker K. Colloids versus crystalloids for fluid resuscitation in critically ill patients. Cochrane Database Syst Rev. 2013;2:CD000567.
13. Finfer S, Bellomo R, Boyce N, et al. A comparison of albumin and saline for fluid resuscitation in the intensive care unit. N Engl J Med. 2004;350:2247–56.
14. Myburgh J, Cooper DJ, Finfer S, et al. Saline or albumin for fluid resuscitation in patients with traumatic brain injury. N Engl J Med. 2007;357:874–84.
15. Suarez JI, Martin RH, Calvillo E, et al. The albumin in subarachnoid haemorrhage (ALISAH) multicentre pilot clinical trial: safety and neurologic outcomes. Stroke. 2012;43:683–90.
16. Ertmer C, Van Aken H. Fluid therapy in patients with brain injury: what does physiology tell us? Crit Care. 2014;18(2):119.

17. Lehman L, Bendel S, Uehlinger DE, et al. Randomised, double-blind trial of the effect of fluid composition on electrolytes, acid-base and fluid homeostasis in patients early after sub-arachnoid haemorrhage. Neurocritic Care. 2013;18:5–12.
18. Cooper DJ, Myles PS, McDermott FT, et al. Prehospital hypertonic saline resuscitation of patients with hypotension and severe traumatic brain injury: a randomised controlled trial. JAMA. 2004;291:1350–7.
19. Farrokh S, Cho S-M, Suarez JI. Fluids and hyperosmolar agents in neurocritical care: an update. Curr Opin Crit Care. 2019;25:105–9. https://doi.org/10.1097/MCC.0000000000005851070.
20. Gu J, Huang H, Huang Y, et al. Hypertonic saline or mannitol for treating elevated intracranial pressure in traumatic brain injury—a metanalysis of randomised controlled trials. Nurosurg Rev. 2019;42:499–509.
21. Shah M, Birnbaum L, Rasmussen J, et al. Effect of hyperosmolar therapy on outcome of spontaneous intracerebral haemorrhage. Ethnic/racial variation of intracerebral Haemorrhage (ERICH) study. J Stroke Cerebrovasc Dis. 2018;27:1061–7.
22. Riha HM, Erdman MJ, Vandigo JE, et al. Impact of moderate hyperchloraemia on clinical outcomes in intracerebral hemorrhage patients treated with continuous infusion hypertonic saline: a pilot study. Crit Care Med. 2017;45:e947–53.
23. Huang K, Hu Y, Wu Y, et al. Hyperchloraemia is associated with poorer outcome in critically ill stroke patients. Front Neurol. 2018;9:485. https://doi.org/10.3389/fneur.2018.00485.
24. Pasarikovski CR, Alotaibi NM, Al-Mufti F, Macdonald RL. Hypertonic saline for increased intracranial pressure after aneurysmal subarachnoid haemorrhage: a systematic review. World Neurosurg. 2017;105:1–6.
25. Kissoon NR, Mandrekar JN, Fugate JE, et al. Positive fluid balance associated with poor outcome in subarachnoid haemorrhage. J Stroke Cerebrovasc Dis. 2015;24:2245–51.
26. Lennihan L, Mayer SA, Fink ME, et al. Effect of hypervolaemic therapy on cerebral blood flow after subarachnoid haemorrhage: a randomised controlled trial. Stroke. 2000;31:383–91.
27. Egge A, Waterloo K, Sjoholm T, et al. Prophylactic hyperdynamic postoperative fluid therapy after aneurysmal subarachnoid haemorrhage: a clinical, prospective, randomised, controlled study. Neurosurgery. 2001;49:593–605.
28. Clifton GL, Miller ER, Choi SC, et al. Fluid thresholds and outcome from severe brain injury. Crit Care Med. 2002;30:739–45.
29. Le Roux P, Menon DK, Citerio G, et al. Consensus summary statement of the international multidisciplinary consensus conference on multimodal monitoring in neurocritical care. Intensive Care Med. 2014;40:1189–209.
30. Chacon-Lozsan F, Pacheco C. Fluid management in neurointensive care patient using transcranial doppler ultrasound: preliminary study. Trends Anaesth Crit Care. 2019;25:21–3.
31. Tenny S, Thorell W. Cerebral salt wasting syndrome. In: StatPearls [Internet]. Treasure Island, FL: StatPearls Publishing; 2021. https://www.ncbi.nlm.nih.gov/books/NBK534855/.
32. Dabrowski W, Wise R, Rzecki Z, et al. Fluid management in neurointensive care. In: Prahakar H, Ali Z, editors. Textbook of neuroanaesthesia and neurocritical care, Vol II neurocritical care. Springer: Singapore; 2019. p. 25–37.
33. Hannon MJ, Thompson CJ. Hyponatraemia in neurosurgical patients. Disorders of fluid and electrolyte metabolism. Focus on hyponatremia. In: Peri A, Thompson CJ, Verbalis JG, editors. Front in hormone research, vol. 52. Basel: Karger; 2019. p. 143–60. https://doi.org/10.1159/000493244.
34. Singh S, Bohn D, Carlotti A, et al. Cerebral salt wasting: truths, fallacies, theories, and challenges. Crit Care Med. 2002;30:2575–9.
35. Hannon MJ, Behan LA, O'Brien MM, et al. Hyponatremia following mild/moderate subarachnoid haemorrhage is due to SIAD and glucocorticoid deficiency and not cerebral salt wasting. J Clin Endocrinol Metab. 2014;99:291–8.

36. Verbalis JG, Goldsmith SR, Greenberg A, et al. Diagnosis, evaluation and treatment of hypona-traemia: expert panel recommendations. Am J Med. 2013;126(10 suppl 1):S1–S42.
37. Koenig MA, Bryan M, Lewin JL 3rd, et al. Reversal of trans-tentorial herniation with hypertonic saline. Neurology. 2008;70:1023–9.
38. Uptodate: https://www.uptodate.com/contents/causes-of-hypotonic-hyponatremia-in-adults?search=cerebral%20salt%20wasting&topicRef=2367&source=see_link
39. Spasovski G, Vanholder R, Allolio B, et al. Clinical practice guideline on diagnosis and treatment of hyponatraemia. Eur J Endocrinol. 2014;170:G1–G47.
40. Hansen B-R, Bruserud Ø. Hypomagnesaemia in critically ill patients. J Intensive Care. 2018;6:21–32. https://doi.org/10.1186/s40560-018-0291-y.
41. Ahmed F, Mohammed A. Magnesium: magnesium: a forgotten electrolyte—a review of hypo-magnesaemia. Med Sci. 2019;7:56–69. https://doi.org/10.3390/medsci7040056.
42. Kishen R Unpublished personal observations. 1999.

Perioperative Fluid Manangement

18

Anirban Hom Choudhuri and Kiranlata Kiro

Contents

Introduction.. 365
Types Fluid... 366
Calculation of Third-Space Loss.. 366
Monitoring Intravascular Volume Status During the Perioperative Period.... 367
Choosing Between Crystalloids and Colloids... 368
'Restrictive' Versus 'Liberal' Strategy.. 369
Fluid Requirements in Special Situations... 371
   Neurosurgery [14].. 371
   Open-Heart Surgery [15]... 372
   Kidney [16] and Liver Transplant Surgery [17]....................................... 372
   Obstetric Surgery.. 373
   Pediatric Surgery [19]... 373
Outpatient and Day-Care Surgery... 375
Conclusion.. 376
References.. 376

A. H. Choudhuri (✉) · K. Kiro
Department of Anesthesiology and Intensive Care, GB Pant Institute of Postgraduate Medical Education and Research, New Delhi, India

© The Author(s) 2024
M. L. N. G. Malbrain et al. (eds.), *Rational Use of Intravenous Fluids in Critically Ill Patients*, https://doi.org/10.1007/978-3-031-42205-8_18

IFA Commentary (MLNGM)

This chapter provides a comprehensive overview of the importance of fluid management in the perioperative period. The authors highlight the significance of fluid regulation in determining the outcome after surgery and emphasizes the importance of understanding the physiology of body fluids and composition of parenteral fluids for perioperative physicians. This chapter outlines the key considerations for fluid management, including calculation of fluid requirement, monitoring of volume status, prevention of hypervolaemia and differences between crystalloid and colloid use. The authors also discuss the use of different fluid administration strategies, including the liberal and restrictive approaches, and note that the choice of strategy will depend on the patient's specific condition. This chapter concludes by highlighting the key take-home messages, including the importance of continuous monitoring of fluid intake and output, the need for individualized approaches to fluid management and the need for special precautions in high-risk patients. Overall, this chapter provides a thorough and informative overview of perioperative fluid management and would be useful for healthcare professionals who are involved in the care of surgical patients. It is well-written and concise and presents information in a clear and organized manner, making it easy to follow and understand.

Learning Objectives

After reading this chapter, you will:

1. Understand the calculation of fluid requirement in the perioperative period based upon the duration of preoperative fasting, type and duration of surgery and extent of blood loss.
2. Learn how to monitor volume status during perioperative period and early detection of hypovolaemia.
3. Study the prevention of hypervolaemia and its associated complications.
4. Appreciate differences between crystalloid and colloid use in the perioperative period.
5. Understand restrictive versus liberal fluid administration strategy.
6. Learn about fluid administration in special situations like elderly, paediatrics and pregnancy.

Case Vignette

Mr. A (aged 50 years, weighing 60 kg) is admitted following subacute intestinal obstruction. The patient has been fasting for the past 24 h. He does not have any comorbid illness. During physical examination, he exhibits signs of hypovolaemia. The plain abdominal X-ray reveals multiple air–fluid levels in the small bowel, and abdominal CT indicates the presence of a jejunal obstruction. He is planned for emergency laparotomy after quick optimization.

Questions

Q1. How should one plan his fluid management during the perioperative period?

Introduction

The outcome after any surgery is dependent on multiple factors among which fluid regulation is an important consideration. The type, amount and rate of fluid administration are primarily determined by the nature of surgery, requirements and losses and coexisting morbidities, if present. Any fluid either too much too little can be of unfavourable consequence. Therefore, knowledge about the physiology of body fluids and the composition of the parenteral fluids is of paramount importance for the perioperative physician. The fluid management in surgical patients is handled jointly by the anaesthetist during surgery and the team monitoring patients' postoperative care.

Rudolph Matas in 1924 first proposed the administration of an intravenous 'drip' during surgery and this has been validated and advanced manifold since then by Moore and Shires in the 1940s and 1950s and by Shoemaker in the 1970s [1, 2]. Classically, perioperative fluid requirement calculations have been practiced according to the '4-2-1 rule' based on the Holliday and Segar method [3]. Over the years, further appreciation of the metabolic stress responses to surgery and physiological principles governing fluid regulation have brought much consistency and conformity to the fluid management protocols. This chapter will focus on adult patients, and more information on fluid therapy in children can be found in Chap. 20. Some other chapters will discuss fluids in specific populations: sepsis (Chap. 14), heart failure (Chap. 15), trauma (Chap. 16), neurocritical care (Chap. 17), burns (Chap. 19), liver failure (Chap. 21), abdominal hypertension (Chap. 22), and COVID-19 (Chap. 26).

Types Fluid

Based upon the patient's requirements, fluids can be of either *replacement* or *maintenance* type. *Replacement* fluids are necessary to treat existing deficits or compensate for ongoing losses during the perioperative period. The common replacement fluids used in the perioperative period include 0.9% sodium chloride (NaCl), Ringer's lactate, balanced salt solution and synthetic colloids. *Maintenance* fluids are those required for optimization of the ongoing losses due to physiological processes in order to maintain homeostasis. The common maintenance fluids are dextrose, dextrose–saline (5%D 0.9% NaCl%), dextrose–hypotonic saline (5%D 0.45%NaCl) and Isolyte solutions. Different crystalloids and synthetic colloids are discussed in more detail elsewhere in the book (see Chaps. 9, 10 and 11).

Calculation of Third-Space Loss

The loss occurring due to fluid shift from the intravascular to the extravascular compartment during surgery is known as third-space loss. This third-space loss follows oedema at the operative site and evaporation from surgical exposure. A lot of formulae are used to calculate third-space loss, although none can be claimed to be superior over the others. The simplest calculation is based upon the type of surgery:

(a) 4 mL/kg/h. for minor and moderate operations (e.g. hernia, hydrocele, cholecystectomy, plating and screwing for limb fractures)
(b) 8 mL/kg/h. for major and supra-major operations (e.g. abdominal hysterectomy, Whipple's procedure, craniotomy)
(c) The calculation may be also based on the amount of tissue handling or trauma during surgery as suggested in the following table (Table 18.1).

Table 18.1 Calculation of surgical third space loss based on tissue handling and/or trauma

Amount of tissue handling or trauma	Fluid requirement (mL/kg/h)
Mild (hernia repair/ophthalmic/otolaryngology procedures)	0–2
Moderate tissue handling (laparoscopic/gynaecologic/orthopaedic/neurosurgical procedures)	2–4
Major tissue handling (open abdominal surgery, e.g. bowel resection anastomosis)	4–8

Monitoring Intravascular Volume Status During the Perioperative Period

Since the purpose of fluid administration is to maintain optimal tissue perfusion, the intravascular volume status should be used to guide fluid therapy. Table 18.2 shows the common parameters (static and dynamic) used to guide fluid administration by determining the volume status.

Table 18.2 Monitoring volume status during the perioperative period with their advantages and disadvantages

Static parameters	CVP, PAOP, LVEDA, GEDV and ITBV
Advantages	**Disadvantages**
• Invaluable parameter in patient care • Marker of cardiac function and pressure gradient of organ perfusion	• Unable to differentiate between fluid responders and non-responders • Unable to predict effect of fluid administration prior to volume expansion • Only extreme values may be of some significance • Factors that increase intramural and transmural pressure (pump failure, valvular heart disease, dysrhythmias, PEEP, pneumothorax, asthma, intra-abdominal hypertension [IAH]) can affect values of CVP and PAOP. Volumetric indices are better in those conditions • Doppler- and echocardiography-mediated parameters need expert training
Dynamic parameters	**SVV, SPV, PPV, ABFV, PWV amplitude, SVC collapsibility and IVC distensibility index, EEO, tidal volume challenge**
Advantages	**Disadvantages**
• Useful indicators with high sensitivity and specificity in patients with stable cardiac rhythms having regular RR interval and undergoing elective mechanical ventilation with 8–10 mL/kg • Precede changes in cardiac output and blood pressure leading to earlier intervention	• Only reliable with tidal volume > 8 mL/kg because of non-linear relationship between chest wall compliance and intra thoracic pressure at lower tidal volumes • Increasing the number of breaths over which the dynamic indices are calculated can increase the values. This may be erroneous in many clinical devices that employs software to sample a defined time interval without identifying the number of breaths • Influenced by the presence of cardiac arrhythmias, viz. atrial fibrillation, premature ventricular contractions • Doppler- and echocardiography-mediated parameters need expert training

CVP central venous pressure, *PAOP* pulmonary artery occlusion pressure, *LVEDA* left-ventricular end-diastolic area, *GEDV* global end-diastolic volume, *ITBV* intrathoracic blood volume, *SVV* stroke volume variability, *SPV* systolic pressure variation, *PPV* pulse pressure variation, *ABFV* aortic blood flow variation, *PWV* plethysomographic waveform variation amplitude, *SVC* superior vena cava, *IVC* inferior vena cava, *EEO* end-expiratory occlusion test

Choosing Between Crystalloids and Colloids

Extracellular fluid (ECF) replacement is better replenished by crystalloids. The distribution of crystalloids in the extracellular (interstitial) space is theoretically three times that of the intravascular space. Hence, after administration of 1 L of crystalloid and after checking the volumes after 1 h, about 250 mL will be present in the intravascular compartment and about 750 mL in the extravascular compartment (interstitial space). Only a negligible amount of isotonic fluid fills up the intracellular compartment. However, excessive crystalloids can dilute the plasma proteins thereby reducing plasma oncotic pressure causing fluid filtration from the intravascular to the interstitial compartment. This can lead to complications like interstitial pulmonary oedema.

Colloids on the contrary, being larger in size have difficulty crossing the capillary membrane and are returned easily via the lymphatics. They stay much longer in the intravascular compartment, exert colloid oncotic pressure (COP) and are needed in much smaller volumes. But if the vascular permeability is increased due to any cause, they can reach the interstitial space and produce interstitial COP. This can exacerbate pulmonary oedema. They can also cause allergic reactions and are costlier than crystalloids. Therefore, a good option in perioperative patients is to administer the maximum amount of fluid as crystalloids until there is any risk of overload. However, the choice is best decided by the physician on an individual basis (Table 18.3).

Table 18.3 Theoretical distribution after 1 h of 1 L of different types of fluid administered

	Intracellular space	Interstitial space	Intravascular space
1 L of (ab)normal saline (0.9% NaCl) or isotonic (balanced) crystalloid	0	750	250
1 L of 5% dextrose (hypotonic)	667	250	83
1 L of 3% hypertonic saline	Decrease	>750	>250
1 L of colloid	0	0	1000

'Restrictive' Versus 'Liberal' Strategy

The choice between restrictive and liberal strategies for fluid administration is blurred with discrepancies and disparities in the definition, methodology and outcome variables. However, it is generally accepted that when total administered fluid exceeds 5 L/day, there is a trend towards increased mortality and morbidity, especially in patients undergoing high-risk surgery. Whenever possible, fixed fluid regimens of varying composition not exceeding 3 L/day can be safe. The actual amounts can vary depending on the volume status and response to incremental boluses. In surgical procedures where the risk of oedema is high, e.g. lobectomy and pneumonectomy, restrictive fluid regimes are strongly advocated. Table 18.4 shows findings of the landmark studies on restrictive and liberal fluid administration during the perioperative period.

Table 18.4 Important studies comparing liberal versus restrictive fluid administration during the perioperative period

Author and year	Design	Population	Intervention	Conclusion
Lobo et al. 2002 [4]	RCT	20 colon cancer	LG ≥3 L fluid +154 mmol Na/ day; RG <2 L fluid +77 mmol Na/day	↑weight gain, delayed recovery and ↑LOS in LG
Brandstrup et al. 2003 [5]	Multicentric RCT	172 elective colorectal surgery	LG: Preload 6% HES 500 mL; third space 7, 5, 3 mL/kg/h for the first, second and third hours, respectively. Fasting 500 mL NS. Blood loss 500 mL; 1:3 crystalloid and thereby vol to vol colloid. >1.5 L blood component depending on HCT RG: No preload/ third-space adjustment. Fasting 5%D 500 mL Blood loss vol to vol 6% HES thereby for >1.5 L blood loss; blood component based on HCT	Reduced complications after elective colorectal resection in RG
MacKay et al. 2006 [6]	RCT	80 colorectal surgery	Median IV fluid intake LG–RG = 8.75:4.5 L	Gastrointestinal recovery and duration of stay in the hospital was similar in the groups

(continued)

Table 18.4 (continued)

Author and year	Design	Population	Intervention	Conclusion
Holte et al. 2007 [7]	RCT	32 colonic surgery	Preload: LG 10 mL/kg/h, RG none Fluid protocol: LG 18 mL/kg RL in first hour followed by starch 7 mg/kg; PACU 10 mL/kg/h RL RG 7 mL/kg RL first hour followed by 5 mL/kg in subsequent hours; starch 7 mg/kg; PACU no fluids	Significant improvement in pulmonary function and postoperative hypoxaemia in RG group
Holte et al. 2007 [8]	RCT	48 knee arthroplasty	Preload: LG 10 mL/kg/h, RG none Fluid protocol: LG 30 mL/kg, RG 10 mL/kg with similar colloid and postoperative fluid orders	Significant weight gain, reduced incidence of nausea and hypercoagulability were observed in LG
Kabon et al. 2005 [9]	RCT	256 colonic resection	LG 16–18 mL/kg RG 8 mL/kg	No correlation with wound infection
Nisanevich et al. 2005 [10]	RCT	152 abdominal surgery	LG 10–12 mL/kg/h, RG 4 mL/kg/h RL	Episodes of hypotension > in RG treated by fluid bolus Weight gain observed in LG Delayed postoperative recovery and ↑ duration of stay in hospital in LG
Holte 2004 [11]	RCT	48 laparoscopic cholycystectomy	LG 40 mL/kg RL RG 15 mL/kg RL	Better pulmonary function, exercise capacity, reduced stress response, low nausea dizziness, fatigue, thirst and early discharge were observed in LG
Maharaj 2005 [12]	RCT	80 diagnostic laparoscopy	LG 2 mL/kg/h RG 3 mL/kg	Frequency of mild moderate or severe PONV was significantly less in LG Mean postop pain scores was less in LG

Table 18.4 (continued)

Author and year	Design	Population	Intervention	Conclusion
RELIEF trial 2018 [13]	RCT	3000 major abdominal surgery	LG–RG = 6100 mL: 3700 mL LG crystalloid 10 mL/kg followed by 8 mL/kg/h (may be reduced further after 4 h if required), 1.5 mL/kg/h for 24 h postoperative period RG ≤5 mL/kg at induction, followed by 5 mL/kg/h (esophageal Doppler or pulse wave analyser for fluid bolus in hypotension) and 0.8 mL/kg/h in first 24 h postoperative period preference of inotrope over fluids to treat hypotension if no evidence of hypovolaemia	No difference in rate of one-yr disability free survival between groups Higher rate AKI in RG (8.6% vs. 5%) Septic complication RRT similar in both groups Surgical site infection and RRT more in RG

RCT randomised control trial, *LG* liberal fluid group, *RG* restrictive fluid group, *PONV* postoperative nausea and vomiting, *AKI* acute kidney injury, *PACU* post-anaesthesia care unit, *RRT* renal replacement therapy, *HCT* haematocrit, *RL* Ringer's lactate, *NS* 0.9%sodium chloride, *5%D* 5% dextrose

Fluid Requirements in Special Situations

Neurosurgery [14]

Neurosurgical patients frequently receive diuretics in the preoperative period for reduction of intracranial pressure (ICP) and often have hypovolaemia intraoperatively following blood loss. All hypo-osmolar fluids like 0.45% saline or 5% glucose in water cause a reduction in plasma osmolality and water movement across the blood–brain barrier (BBB) into the brain tissue. Besides, glucose administration increases local and global ischaemia leading to neurological damage. Therefore, salt-free solutions containing glucose are best avoided in patients with brain and spinal cord injuries. During resuscitation of traumatic brain-injured (TBI) patients, hypertonic saline solutions are useful in reducing ICP and maintain cerebral perfusion pressure without producing an osmotic diuresis. This is discussed more into detail in Chap. 17.

Open-Heart Surgery [15]

Cardiac surgery, particularly procedures involving cardiopulmonary bypass (CPB), is associated with the activation of many complex physiological and biochemical pathways, making volume replacement complicated. The patient's underlying electrolyte status must be reviewed before choosing the fluid; potassium-containing fluids must be avoided in presence of hyperkalaemia. Excessive crystalloid administration is associated with volume overload and pulmonary oedema which are more likely in patients with a low ejection fraction. Colloids with the exception of albumin have the disadvantage of causing coagulation abnormalities (which is already deranged in CPB patients) and anaphylactic reactions and are only used in the pre-bypass period. In infants and children undergoing cardiac surgery, blood volume replacements are preferred over non-blood volume replacement regimens. Some studies have shown benefits in priming the CPB pump with colloids (plasma, albumin) to elevate the colloid oncotic pressure (COP).

Kidney [16] and Liver Transplant Surgery [17]

The determination of volume status in patients undergoing kidney transplant is a challenge and the conventional monitors can be misleading. The compensatory mechanisms that maintain effective vascular volume and tissue perfusion are obtunded in patients with end-stage kidney disease. The mean arterial pressure which adequately preserves the renal microcirculation is also difficult to ascertain. One approach is to follow the 'goal-directed therapy' (GDT) based upon dynamic indices. Another approach is the administration of fluid based on 'triggers' and is known as 'flow-directed theray' (FDT). In both cases, the change in cardiac output (CO) is used as an indicator to assess the effectiveness of therapy. After a given volume is administered, usually 500 ml of crystalloid, the CO response is checked; a 15% increase in CO with a CVP rise of at least 2 mmHg constitutes a positive response. When there is no positive response, other therapies can be tried (i.e. vasopressor and/or inotropic therapy to treat hypotension) (See also Chap. 14).

The patient undergoing liver transplant surgery has end-stage liver disease (ESLD) which is associated with low systemic vascular resistance (SVR) causing sodium and water retention by the kidneys. This increases the amount of total body fluid. But the presence of portal hypertension expands the splanchnic circulation leading to a fall in the relative amount of fluid in the systemic circulation. There is movement of protein-rich fluid into the body cavities causing ascites and pleural effusions. Moreover, the cross-clamping of inferior vena cava during surgery contributes to hypotension and renal dysfunction. Preoperative coagulopathy is common and haemorrhage can occur at any stage of the operation. Therefore, any excess of fluid administration should be avoided during surgery and a low CVP is desirable. The use of fresh frozen plasma, platelets and cryoprecipitate is commonly advocated to prevent coagulopathy and reduce risk of volume overload (See also Chap. 21).

Obstetric Surgery

Perioperative maintenance of adequate intravascular volume status is very important in pregnant patients. Usually, these patients are exposed to rapid volume fluctuations during caesarean section. Since spinal anaesthesia is commonly chosen for its rapid onset, minimal patient risk and negligible risk of fetal drug transfer, preloading is particularly important. Wollman and Marx [18] first described the concept of preloading, by administering 10–20 mL/kg of intravenous crystalloids in pregnant females around 15–20 min prior to spinal anaesthesia. But later studies showed that preloading can induce the release of atrial natriuretic peptide (ANP) which can damage the endothelial glycocalyx and lead to increased excretion of preload fluid from the intravascular compartment. To address these inconsistencies, the concept of co-loading gained acceptance. Co-loading is more appropriate physiologically as fluid administration coincides exactly with the time of maximal vasodilatory effect of spinal anaesthesia.

Pediatric Surgery [19]

Since children are very sensitive to even minor fluctuations in volume status, the clinical assessment is of greater significance. The losses in paediatrics can range from 1 mL/kg/h for a minor surgical procedure to as high as 15–20 mL/kg/h for major abdominal procedures. It may even go up to 50 mL/kg/h for surgery for necrotizing enterocolitis in premature infants. The younger the child, the greater is the relative proportion of losses because of the large ECF volume when compared with older children and adults. Third-space losses should be replaced with crystalloids (0.9% NaCL or LR). Box 18.1 shows the guidelines for administration of balanced salt solutions according to the child's age and extent of tissue trauma (See also Chap. 20).

Box 18.1 Guidelines for Fluid Administration in Children According to Age and Extent of Tissue Trauma

First hour (*plus* item 3 if applicable)

- 25 mL/kg in children ≤3 years.
- 15 mL/kg in children ≥4 years.

All other hours (*plus* item 3)

- Maintenance plus extent of tissue trauma (as per item 3).

Maintenance volume = 4 mL/kg/h.

Item 3

Mild tissue trauma (e.g. hernia, hydrocele, circumcision, tonsillectomy) → 2 mL/kg/h.

Moderate tissue trauma (appendicectomy, obstructed inguinal hernia, etc.) → 4 mL/kg/h.

Severe tissue trauma (tracheo-esophageal fistula, congenital diaphragmatic hernia, etc.) → 6 mL/kg/h.

Both hypo- and hyperglycaemia can have serious adverse effects in paediatric patients and the general consensus is to selectively administer dextrose only in children at high risk for hypoglycaemia and to even consider the use of lower dextrose-containing fluids. The highest risk of hypoglycaemia is in neonates, children receiving hyper alimentation and those with endocrinopathies, in whom monitoring blood glucose levels and adjusting the rate of infusion are also important. The rate of glucose infusion can start at 120–300 mg/kg/h (compared to adults 1–1.5 g/kg/day) to maintain an acceptable blood glucose level after which it can be titrated as per need. The idea is also to prevent lipid mobilization in hypoglycaemia-prone infants.

As compared to adults, children are more susceptible to hospital acquired hyponatraemia which has been attributed to use of hypotonic IVFs (0.2%/0.45% NaCl) in elevated AVP situation: acutely ill patients, postsurgical state, hypovolaemia, medications, pneumonia, meningitis. A suspicion of hyponatraemia in paediatric patients can be difficult due to very nonspecific symptoms like headache, nausea, vomiting, confusion, lethargy and muscle cramps often confused with the generalized irritability frequently observed in a hospitalized child. With larger brain/skull size ratio and with rapid fall in sodium levels, a child's brain gets very little time to adapt and may precipitate hyponatraemic encephalopathy as seen in high-risk patients [20]. Dysnatremia-induced neurological complications following minor surgical procedures in apparently healthy children raise serious concerns regarding safety of hyponatraemic IVFs in paediatric patients [21]. Evidence-based guidelines now recommend isotonic fluids (sodium concentration similar to Plasma-Lyte or 0.9% saline) in children who are acutely ill or require maintenance IVFs [22, 23] (barring neonates <28 days, cases like DI, severe diarrhoea, burns, congenital or acquired renal, hepatic or cardiac diseases, traumatic brain injury where fluid requirements have been attended more specifically). Concerns of hypernatraemia, fluid overload with oedema and hypertension and hyperchloraemic acidosis have been raised with use of isotonic fluids in paediatric patients, but there is no available data of higher risk with use of isotonic in comparison to hypotonic IVFs in patients aged 28 days to 18 years.

Outpatient and Day-Care Surgery

The choice of fluid in outpatient and day-care surgery is highly variable depending on the nature of surgery. Some procedures like liposuction are associated with considerable fluid shifts, while some dental procedures may have minimal fluid loss. However, administration of 'liberal' doses of fluid minimizes certain undesirable effects like postoperative nausea and vomiting (PONV), pain and dizziness. Some advocate early feeding during the postoperative period to minimize the risk of unwarranted hypovolaemia.

Case Vignette

Box 18.2 shows the maintenance and replacement fluid requirements of the patient in the case vignette.

Box 18.2 Calculation of Fluid Requirements

Hourly maintenance requirement M (mL) = (A+ B + C).

A (mL) = 4 × first 10 kg body weight.

B (mL) = 2 × next 10 kg of body weight.

C (mL) = remaining kg of body weight.

Fasting requirement F (mL) = (A+ B + C) × h (where h is the number of hours of fasting).

Half of the calculated fasting requirement is administered in the first hour and the remaining half is administered in the second and third hours.

Our case vignette mentions a 50-year-old patient of 60 kg body weight with 24 h of fasting.

Hourly maintenance requirement M(mL) in our patient = (40 mL + 20 mL +40 mL),i.e. 100 mL.

Fasting requirement (mL) = 100 × 24 i.e. 2400 mL.

Third space loss (mL) = 8 × 60 i.e. 480 mL/h.

First hour fluid requirement =100 mL + (50% of 2400) mL + 480 mL i.e. 100 + 1200 + 480 mL = 1780 mL + F.

Second hour fluid requirement = 100+ (25% of 2400) + 480 i.e. 100 + 600 + 480 = 1180 mL + F.

Third hour fluid requirement = 100+ (25% of 2400) + 480 i.e. 100 + 660 + 480 = 1180 mL + F.

Subsequent hours = 480 mL + F.

Where F is the surgical loss (*surgical blood loss to be replaced by crystalloid 1:3, Colloid/blood – 1:1 ratio*).

Conclusion

There has been an increase in the use of a highly individualized and goal-directed approach for restoring near-normal fluid balance in the perioperative period. It is appreciated that the static parameters (CVP, heart rate, etc.) are not reliable in accurately assessing volume status and 'fluid responsiveness' guided by dynamic parameters is a better option. However, the suitability of a parameter is linked to its availability and comfort of use in the operative setting to expect the desired benefits.

Both 'liberal' and 'restrictive' approaches have been found to be useful in different conditions, the former in low-risk and ambulatory patients and the latter in high-risk patients. Crystalloids have been found to be reliable and safe, and the use of balanced salt solutions along with the older fluids has been found to be better than colloids in patients with kidney diseases without much difference in outcome.

Take Home Messages
- Fluid administration during the perioperative period is both an art and science.
- The predicted calculations are based upon body weight, duration of fasting, extent of blood loss, etc., but such calculations may be inadequate and imprecise.
- It is necessary to continuously monitor the fluid intake and output with help of appropriate monitoring tools. There is no single monitor that performs best in all circumstances.
- Both 'restrictive' and 'liberal' strategies for fluid administration are useful in specific conditions.
- Both crystalloids and colloids can be used although the former is preferred over the latter as the first choice.
- Special precautions should be adopted in high-risk patients with reduced threshold for tolerating hypo- or hypervolaemia especially the paediatric age group, elderly, those with accompanying kidney diseases, etc.

References

1. Matas R. The continued intravenous "drip" with remarks on the value of continued gastric drainage and irrigation by nasal intubation with a gastroduodenal tube (Jutte) in surgical practice. Ann Surg. 1924;79:643–61.
2. Srinivasa S, Hill AG. Perioperative fluid administration: historical highlights and implications for practice. Ann Surg. 2012;256:1113–8.
3. Holiday MA, Segar WE. The maintenance need for water in parenteral fluid therapy. Pediatrics. 1957;19:823–32.

4. Lobo DN, Bostock KA, Neal KR, Perkins AC, Rowlands BJ, Allison SP. Effect of salt and water balance on recovery of gastrointestinal function after elective colonic resection: a randomised controlled trial. Lancet. 2002;25: 359(9320):1812–8.
5. Brandstrup B, Tonnesen H, Beier-Holgersen R, et al. Effects of intravenous fluid restriction on postoperative complications: comparison of two perioperative fluid regimens: a randomized assessor-blinded multicenter trial. Ann Surg. 2003;238:641–8.
6. MacKay G, Fearon K, McConnachie A, Serpell MG, Molloy RG, O'Dwyer PJ. Randomized clinical trial of the effect of postoperative intravenous fluid restriction on recovery after elective colorectal surgery. Br J Surg. 2006;93(12):1469–74.
7. Holte K, Foss NB, Andersen J, Valentiner L, Lund C, Bie P, Kehlet H. Liberal or restrictive fluid administration in fast-track colonic surgery: a randomized, double-blind study. Br J Anaesth. 2007;99(4):500–8.
8. Holte K, Kristensen BB, Valentiner L, Foss NB, Husted H, Kehlet H. Liberal versus restrictive fluid management in knee arthroplasty: a randomized, double-blind study. Anesth Analg. 2007;105(2):465–74.
9. Kabon B, Akça O, Taguchi A, Nagele A, Jebadurai R, Arkilic CF, Sharma N, Ahluwalia A, Galandiuk S, Fleshman J, Sessler DI, Kurz A. Supplemental intravenous crystalloid administration does not reduce the risk of surgical wound infection. Anesth Analg. 2005;101(5):1546–53.
10. Nisanevich V, Felsenstein I, Almogy G, Weissman C, Einav S, Matot I. Effect of intraoperative fluid management on outcome after intraabdominal surgery. Anesthesiology. 2005;103(1):25–32.
11. Holte K, Klarskov B, Christensen DS, Lund C, Nielsen KG, Bie P, Kehlet H. Liberal versus restrictive fluid administration to improve recovery after laparoscopic cholecystectomy: a randomized, double-blind study. Ann Surg. 2004;240(5):892–9.
12. Maharaj CH, Kallam SR, Malik A, Hassett P, Grady D, Laffey JG. Preoperative intravenous fluid therapy decreases postoperative nausea and pain in high risk patients. Anesth Analg. 2005;100(3):675–82.
13. Myles PS, Bellomo R, Corcoran T, Forbes A, Peyton P, Story D, Christophi C, Leslie K, McGuinness S, Parke R, Serpell J, Chan MTV, Painter T, McCluskey S, Minto G, Wallace S. Australian and New Zealand College of Anaesthetists clinical trials network and the Australian and New Zealand Intensive Care Society clinical trials group. Restrictive versus liberal fluid therapy for major abdominal surgery. N Engl J Med. 2018;378(24):2263–74.
14. Oddo M, Poole D, Helbok R, et al. Fluid therapy in neurointensive care patients: ESICM consensus and clinical practice recommendations. Intensive Care Med. 2018;44:449–63.
15. Young R. Perioperative fluid and electrolyte management in cardiac surgery: a review. J Extra Corpor Technol. 2012;44:20–6.
16. Calixto Fernandes MH, Schricker T, Magder S, Hatzakorzian R. Perioperative fluid management in kidney transplantation: a black box. Crit Care. 2018;22(1):14.
17. Fayed NA, Yassen KA, Abdulla AR. Comparison between 2 strategies of fluid management on blood loss and transfusion requirements during liver transplantation. J Cardiothorac Vasc Anesth. 2017;31(5):1741–50. https://doi.org/10.1053/j.jvca.2017.02.177. Epub 2017 Feb 22. PMID: 28552297.
18. Wollman S, Marx C. Acute hydration for prevention of hypotension of spinal anesthesia in parturients. Anesthesiology. 1968;29:374–80.
19. Langer T, Limuti R, Tommasino C, van Regenmortel N, Duval E, Caironi P, et al. Anaesthesiol Intensive Ther. 2018;50:49–58.
20. Moritz ML, Ayus JC. Prevention of hospital-acquired hyponatremia: a case for using isotonic saline. Pediatrics. 2003;111(2):227–30.

21. Langer T, Malbrain L, Van Regenmortel N. Hypotonic or isotonic maintenance fluids for paediatric patients: the never-ending story. Anaesthesiol Intensive Ther. 2020;52(5):357–8.
22. Feld LG, Neuspiel DR, Foster BA, et al. Clinical practice guideline: maintenance intravenous fluids in children. Pediatrics. 2018;142(6):e20183083.
23. National Institute for Health and Care Excellence. Intravenous fluid therapy in children and young people in hospital. London: National Institute for Health and Care Excellence; 2020. (NICE Guideline, No. 29). https://www.ncbi.nlm.nih.gov/books/NBK563449

Fluid Management in Major Burns

19

Aditya Lyall and Abhay Singh Bhadauria

Contents

Introduction 386
Pathophysiology 387
Fluid Estimation and Administration 388
Choice of Fluid and Monitoring 389
Conclusion 391
References 392

> **IFA Commentary (MLNGM)**
> Burn care has greatly improved over the past few decades, thanks to better understanding of burn shock pathophysiology and the development of targeted burns resuscitation. While inadequate fluid resuscitation shock is now rare in clinical practice due to early aggressive intervention, attention has shifted to the morbidity and mortality related to post-resuscitation oedema and fluid creep in burns care. Severe burns cause systemic inflammation and fluid extravasation due to transendothelial hyperfiltration, with patients with more than 20% total burn surface area at the greatest risk. The disruption of large areas of normal skin results in both sustained heat

A. Lyall (✉)
Department of Critical Care Medicine Fortis-Escorts Hospital, Faridabad, Haryana, India

A. S. Bhadauria
Department of Critical Care Medicine, Apollomedics Hospital, Lucknow, UP, India

© The Author(s) 2024
M. L. N. G. Malbrain et al. (eds.), *Rational Use of Intravenous Fluids in Critically Ill Patients*, https://doi.org/10.1007/978-3-031-42205-8_19

and fluid loss, complicating temperature regulation. In the absence of adequate fluid resuscitation immediately following the burn, a patient would rapidly develop intravascular hypovolaemia due to elevated capillary transendothelial pressure and hyperfiltration across the injured endothelium, resulting in low-output shock. While adequate fluid resuscitation is essential in preventing critically low cardiac output, the presence of elevated transendothelial pressure means there is significant extravasation of resuscitation fluid and oedema formation. This oedema can develop in both burned and unburned tissue, occurring within minutes after the injury and peaking at 12–24 h after injury. Endothelial dysfunction and capillary leak are present within 2 h post-burn. There is no consensus on the ideal resuscitation fluid and strategy, nor on how to achieve adequate resuscitation while avoiding the adverse effects of excessive resuscitation. Significant variability exists in fluid strategies and haemodynamic monitoring during burn care by clinicians. The latest evidence regarding the choice of fluids, adjunctive treatments, the role of abdominal hypertension, and the end points used to guide fluid resuscitation in burn patients are summarised in Table 19.1. The IFA suggests a novel, holistic, and dynamic resuscitation protocol with targets and end points for the more challenging burn cases that includes an active de-resuscitation phase according to the ROSE concept and based on newly available physiologic parameters from transpulmonary thermodilution [1, 2].

Suggested Reading

1. Peeters Y, Lebeer M, Wise R, Malbrain M. An overview on fluid resuscitation and resuscitation endpoints in burns: past, present and future. Part 2—avoiding complications by using the right endpoints with a new personalized protocolized approach. Anaesthesiol Intensive Ther. 2015; 47:S15–26.
2. Peeters Y, Vandervelden S, Wise R, Malbrain M. An overview on fluid resuscitation and resuscitation endpoints in burns: past, present and future. Part 1—historical background, resuscitation fluid and adjunctive treatment. Anaesthesiol Intensive Ther. 2015; 47:S6–S14.

Table 19.1 Recommendations regarding fluid resuscitation and resuscitation end points in severe burn patients

Fluids	
1. Normal saline	Given the fact that fluid resuscitation in burn management requires large volumes, the use of saline cannot be recommended in a burn resuscitation protocol
2. Balanced crystalloid	Based on the available evidence, balanced crystalloid solutions are a pragmatic initial resuscitation fluid in the majority of acutely ill (and burn) patients

Table 19.1   (continued)

Fluids	
3. Semi-synthetic colloids	Given the recent data concerning the use of semi-synthetic colloids (and starches in particular), their use in critically ill patients including burn patients cannot be recommended
4. Albumin	Based on the available evidence, the use of albumin 20% can be recommended in severe burns, especially in the de-resuscitation phase guided by indices of capillary leak, body weight, (cumulative) fluid balance, fluid overload, extravascular lung water, and intra-abdominal pressure
5. Hypertonic solutions	To this day, there is insufficient evidence to reach consensus regarding the safety of hypertonic saline in burn resuscitation. Whenever using hypertonic saline in clinical practice however, close monitoring of sodium levels is highly advised
Adjunctive therapy	
6. Vitamin C	Vitamin C prevents intra-abdominal hypertension in burns patients. However the current level of evidence for Vitamin C means that it cannot be recommended routinely
7. Plasmapheresis	The benefit of plasmapheresis on outcome in burn patients still needs to be validated in large prospective, randomised trials. As such, its use cannot be recommended
8. Other therapy Hydrocortisone Oxygen Hydroxocobalamin Sedation	In case of use of etomidate for intubation, the secretion of cortisone could be suppressed for up to 18 h as for patients regularly taking corticoids High levels of oxygen (100%) for up to 6–18 h are required for CO intoxication and smoke inhalation trauma Severely burn casualties can suffer a very early refractory shock – Most of the time outright on scene – During house fire with smoke inhalation injury and cyanide intoxication. The antidote consists of intravenous hydroxocobalamin 70 mg/kg of body weight Avoid hypotensive and cardiodepressive sedation
Abdominal hypertension	
9. Intra-abdominal pressure (IAP)	During the resuscitation phase as well as the recovery phase, intra-abdominal pressure (IAP) needs to be measured in burn patients at least four to six times per day
10. Medical treatment	Medical management (improvement of abdominal compliance, evacuation of intra-abdominal contents, evacuation of intra-luminal contents, limitation of fluid intake, optimisation of organ perfusion) comes first and should be initiated whenever IAP increases above 12 mmHg
11. Surgical treatment	Escharotomies should be performed in case of circular thoracic or abdominal eschars, while surgical decompressive laparotomy is only a last resort in case medical management fails

(continued)

Table 19.1 (continued)

Fluids	
Resuscitation end points	
12. Monitoring	Every severely burned patient (>20% TBSA in adults or > 15% TBSA in children) should be adequately monitored with regard to fluid status, fluid responsiveness, and organ perfusion
13. Urine output	Diuresis is a poor end point in the complex cases (many recent articles still recommend UO as the criteria with the other classical haemodynamic parameters) that may lead to over- or underestimation of fluid resuscitation and as such can no longer be recommended; however, in situations with limited monitoring techniques, it can still be used to guide fluid resuscitation (see further under urine output algorithm)
14. Barometric preload	Barometric preload indicators like central venous pressure (CVP) or pulmonary artery occlusion pressure (PAOP) should not be used to guide fluid resuscitation in burn patients. It can still be used or least the trend of the CVP in situations without modern monitoring
15. Volumetric preload	Volumetric preload indicators (like right ventricular or global end-diastolic volume) are superior compared to barometric ones and are recommended to guide fluid resuscitation, especially in burn patients with increased IAP. (see further under GEDVI algorithm.)
16. Lung water	The use of extravascular lung water is recommended to guide de-resuscitation in burn patients not transgressing spontaneously from ebb to flow phase
17. Fluid responsiveness	Fluid resuscitation in burn patients should be guided by physiological parameters or tests that are able to predict fluid responsiveness. (see further under PPV algorithm.)
18. Perfusion	Fluid resuscitation should only be given/increased in case of evidence of tissue hypoperfusion (base deficit, lactate, etc.)
Stepwise approach	
19. PPV algorithm	If a patient is sedated and mechanically ventilated, an algorithm based on pulse pressure variation (PPV) can be used in severe burns, under the condition that PPV measurements are reliable with an experienced staff (Fig. 19.1)
20. GEDVI algorithm	If PPV is unreliable, volumetric parameters obtained with transpulmonary thermodilution can be used to guide fluid resuscitation in severe burns. Here, the GEDVI is interpreted as a measure of preload and EVLWI as a safety parameter warning for pending pulmonary oedema (Fig. 19.2). If the GEDVI is high, the measurement needs to be corrected with the global ejection fraction as this leads to a more accurate estimation of preload
21. Urine output algorithm	If PPV or volumetric parameters are unreliable, or when monitoring possibilities are limited, urine output can be used to guide fluid resuscitation in severe burns (Fig. 19.3)

CVP central venous pressure, *EVLWI* extravascular lung water index, *GEDVI* global end-diastolic volume index, *IAP* intra-abdominal pressure, IVIG: intravenous immunoglobulins, PAOP: pulmonary artery occlusion pressure, TBSA: total burned surface area

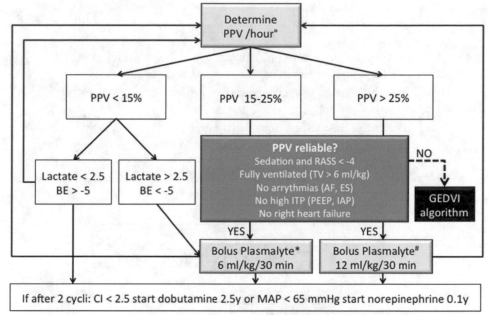

Fig. 19.1 Pulse pressure variation algorithm to guide resuscitation in severely burned patients. If the patient is mechanically ventilated and PPV is reliable, fluid resuscitation is guided by the PPV algorithm [14, 15]. *AF* atrial fibrillation, *BE* base excess, *CI* cardiac index, *ES* extrasystole, *GEDVI* global end-diastolic volume index, *IAP* intra-abdominal pressure, *ITP* intrathoracic pressure, *MAP* mean arterial pressure, *PEEP* positive end-expiratory pressure, *PPV* pulse pressure variation, *TV* tidal volume

Learning Objectives

After reading this chapter, you will:

1. Understand the pathophysiology of burn shock and the development of targeted burn resuscitation.
2. Identify the risk factors for post-resuscitation oedema in burn patients.
3. Evaluate the evidence regarding the choice of fluids and adjunctive treatments for burn patients.
4. Describe the role of abdominal hypertension in burn patients and its implications for fluid resuscitation.
5. Analyse the end points used to guide fluid resuscitation in burn patients and their appropriateness in different clinical scenarios.
6. Discuss the principles of a holistic resuscitation protocol for burn patients, including targets and end points for the more challenging cases.

7. Explain the concept of transendothelial hyperfiltration and its role in the generation of tissue oedema in burn patients.
8. Assess the importance of avoiding capillary hypertension in preventing transendothelial hyperfiltration and associated complications in burn patients.
9. Identify the biomarkers and techniques that can be used to track the development of burn injury and guide resuscitation.
10. Recognise the adverse effects of excessive fluid resuscitation, including intra-abdominal hypertension and compartment syndromes, and strategies to mitigate these risks.

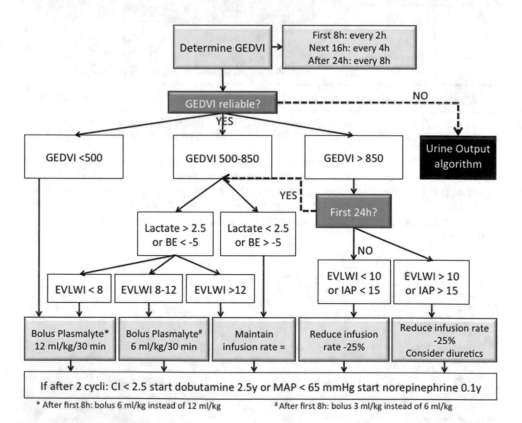

Fig. 19.2 Global end-diastolic volume index algorithm to guide resuscitation in severely burned patients. If PPV is unreliable and the patient has a PiCCO catheter and GEDVI is reliable, fluid resuscitation is guided by the GEDVI algorithm [14, 15]. *BE* base excess, *CI* cardiac index, *EVLWI* extravascular lung water index, *GEDVI* global end-diastolic volume index, *IAP* intra-abdominal pressure, *MAP* mean arterial pressure

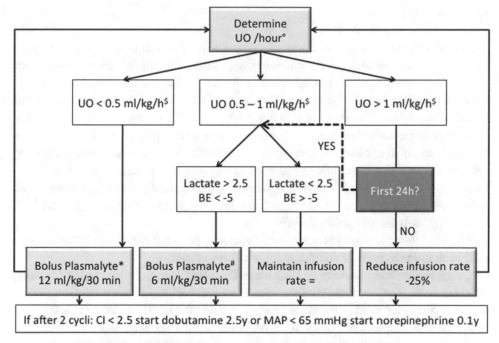

Fig. 19.3 Urine output algorithm to guide resuscitation in severely burned patients. If the patient has no PiCCO catheter (or GEDVI is not reliable) and PPV is not reliable, fluid resuscitation is guided by the UO algorithm [14, 15]. *BE* base excess, *CI* cardiac index, *IAP* intra-abdominal pressure, *MAP* mean arterial pressure, *UO* urine output

Case Vignette:

Mr. S, a 42-year-old male, was brought to the emergency department with second-degree burns covering 25% of his total body surface area. He was in pain and hypotensive with a blood pressure of 90/60 mmHg, heart rate of 120 beats per minute, and a urine output of 20 mL/h. He had no significant medical history, and his initial labs showed elevated serum lactate levels. The medical team initiated fluid resuscitation using intravenous fluids.

Questions

Q1. Why is intravenous fluid resuscitation essential for burn patients?

Q2. What is the goal of fluid resuscitation in burn patients?

Introduction

Burn management has undergone a lot of changes with advancements in the medical field over the past few decades. As our understanding of the pathophysiological consequences of burns has evolved, so has our approach in the daily management of the burn patients. Early resuscitation is essential as hypovolaemia sets in rapidly, with compromised cardiac function leading to what has been called as burn shock. If left untreated, burn shock can cause 58% of deaths within 72 h of major thermal injury [1]. Appropriate and timely resuscitation is essential to offset the development of burn shock and has been clearly shown to reduce mortality. However, fluid management in this subset of patients is based on formulae and concepts elucidated decades ago, with no clear consensus on the ideal resuscitation fluid. Colloid use in burns remains mired in controversy; resuscitation targets and ideal monitoring tools are still poorly defined.

The ideal fluid for burns resuscitation is debatable, though there appears to have been a shift back towards usage of colloids along with crystalloids.

Colloids were used as early as 1942 when Cope and Moore, following the Cocoanut Grove disaster [2]. Over time, with the knowledge that capillary leakage led to accumulation of sodium-rich fluid in the burned tissues and that the intravascular volume could be corrected with balanced salt solutions, crystalloids became favoured over colloid use during the first 24 h. Resuscitation formulae utilising crystalloids include the Baxter and Shires Parkland formula and modified Brooke formula by Pruitt, both using Ringer's lactate for resuscitation during the first 24 h [3]. There was also increased recognition that over-resuscitation is as dangerous as under-resuscitation and leads to a vast array of complication ranging from kidney injury, worsening of oedema, ARDS, airway oedema, and loss of skin grafts secondary to tissue oedema, a concept known as "fluid creep" as proposed by Pruitt [4].

Early and rapid resuscitation of the burn patient is a priority, as hypovolaemia and burn shock sets in rapidly especially in patients with major burns, generally defined as burns involving more than 20% total body surface area. Shock in burns has features of distributive, hypovolaemic, and cardiogenic shock; fluid administration needs to be tailored to the characteristics of the patient, as the rapid sequestration of the intravascular volume into the second and third space needs to be counterbalanced to maintain adequate tissue perfusion and prevent organ damage. This chapter will focus on adult patients, and more information on fluid therapy in children can be found in Chap. 20. Some other chapters will discuss fluids in specific populations: sepsis (Chap. 14), heart failure (Chap. 15), trauma (Chap. 16), neurocritical care (Chap. 17), perioperative setting (Chap. 18), liver failure (Chap. 21), abdominal hypertension (Chap. 22), and COVID-19 (Chap. 26).

Pathophysiology

Burns to a large surface area cause extensive damage, not only directly but also by causing a cascade of changes which ultimately increases the morbidity and mortality. Burns to more than 15–20% of total body surface area are a major cause of mortality unless they receive prompt and adequate resuscitation.

Injury to the tissue in and around the burns area causes disruption of sodium ATPase, leading to intracellular accumulation of sodium and fluid shift resulting in cellular oedema and intravascular depletion.

There is disruption of the collagen and hyaluronic acid scaffolding which normally maintains the integrity of the interstitial space, leading to loss of fluid in the extravascular spaces. Furthermore, the loss of intravascular proteins to the interstitial spaces reduces plasma oncotic pressure; these changes are profound in the injured area but also occur in the non-injured areas. This reduced plasma oncotic pressure leads to intense oedema formation especially once fluid resuscitation starts [5].

In addition, thermal injury results in the release of inflammatory mediators and vasoactive products like histamines, prostaglandins, and leukotrienes along with activation of complement system; these have a twofold effect. Firstly, they contribute to increased vascular permeability leading to extensive fluid shifts from the intravascular compartment resulting in oedema, hypovolaemia, and haemoconcentration. Secondly, these mediators appear to cause cardiac dysfunction – the intense local vasoconstriction coupled with systemic vasodilatation result in increased afterload and reduced preload. Tumour necrosis factor alpha and IL-1 have been found to be elevated in burn patients with apoptotic cells detected in left ventricular tissue; these changes are hypothesised to be contributors to the cardiac dysfunction. Cardiac output is not fully restored with fluid resuscitation as the preload improves and the complete resolution may take 48–72 h [5].

Burn shock is a combination of hypovolaemic, cardiogenic, and distributive shock. These changes become evident as early as within first five to 6 h post injury, more so in the injured area; therefore, prompt adequate fluid resuscitation and maintaining the intravascular volume in the face of ongoing third spacing are extremely important while managing a patient with burns especially during the first 24 h. Over-resuscitation leads to a whole set of different complications and should be avoided. Capillary integrity in non-injured tissue gradually recovers in 12–24 h, beyond which intravascular losses decrease and aggressive fluid management can be tailored down to maintain adequate tissue and organ perfusion (Fig. 19.4).

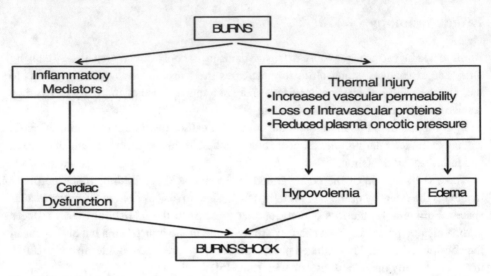

Fig. 19.4 Pathophysiology of burn shock

Fluid Estimation and Administration

Estimation of percentage of body surface area (BSA) burnt is the first step when managing a patient. The Wallace rule of nines, the Lund and Browder chart (in paediatric patients), and the rule of palm (using the patient's palm without fingers and wrist as 1%) can all be used to estimate the BSA. During BSA estimation, only deep partial-thickness burns (previously called second-degree burns) and full-thickness burns (previously called third- and fourth-degree burns) are calculated for fluid administration; superficial partial-thickness burns (previously called first-degree burns) are not included.

Numerous formulae for fluid resuscitation have been proposed; however, the formula given by Baxter and Shires at the Parkland Hospital (referred to as the Parkland formula) is the most commonly followed universally, using Ringer's lactate up to 4 mL/kg/% TBSA (total burned surface area) in the first 24 h, half during the first 8 h and the rest over the next 16 h. It is important to remember that time is estimated from the time of injury, and in cases of delayed presentation a more rapid fluid administration may be required.

The intravenous route of fluid resuscitation is preferred, although oral or enteral routes can also be used in cases of limited resources. Vomiting and gastric ileus may however make it difficult to deliver large amounts of fluids orally. Intraosseous lines can be used in emergencies or if intravenous access is difficult.

IV cannulae need to be properly secured as the developing oedema may dislodge the cannulae or make further access difficult; a central venous catheter may be prudent in cases of significant torso and limbs burns.

Arterial catheterisation can be helpful especially for blood pressure monitoring and repeated sampling and also in cases where the burns make it difficult to place the cuffs or electrodes.

Early and adequate resuscitation is important to prevent renal failure, organ dysfunction, and death. Hypovolaemia and shock rapidly develop in the absence of timely fluid administration, and inadequate fluid resuscitation leads to worsening of burns shock. On the contrary, overzealous and unchecked fluid administration results in "fluid creep" [4]—this tends to occur when the total volume of resuscitation exceeds 6 mL/kg/% TBSA, or the Ivy index of 250 mL/kg. Fluid creep causes worsening of oedema in the injured and uninjured area, intra-abdominal hypertension, ARDS, intraocular hypertension, conversion of superficial to deep burns due to impaired vascularity, and organ failure. Fluid administration needs to be initiated timely especially during the initial hours, as ongoing third spacing of fluid causes intense intravascular losses and maintenance of adequate intravascular volume is paramount to ensure adequate tissue perfusion. Care should be taken while assessing patients, as patients presenting with shock probably have some other underlying injury causing hypotension since burn shock generally sets in gradually.

Choice of Fluid and Monitoring

Colloids were initially the fluid of choice for burn resuscitation, earlier formulae advocated plasma as the replacement fluid, e.g. Harkins, or body weight burn budget, Evans formulae. Gradually, it was observed that the fluid lost in burn tissue was rich in sodium and proteins, and the volume could be replaced with balanced solutions only, whereas (ab) normal saline (NaCl 0.9%) given in large amounts more rapidly results in hyperchloraemic metabolic acidosis.

Currently, most patients receive Ringer's lactate or Plasma-Lyte during initial resuscitation, as per the Parkland formula and modified Brooke formula. Ringer's lactate while hypotonic tends to correct the volume status and electrolyte imbalance and also avoids hyperchloraemic acidosis that occurs with the use of normal saline. The problem with lactate containing buffered solutions is that when they are given in vast amounts as is the case in severe burns, plasma lactate levels may increase due to exogenous lactate accumulation in combination with diminished metabolisation especially in shock and liver failure.

The problem with crystalloid resuscitation is the large volume of fluids involved, which is recognised to result in worsening oedema, renal dysfunction, airway complications including ARDS, abdominal compartment syndrome, and intraocular hypertension. This has led to renewed interest in colloids, especially human albumin. Colloid use reduces the volume required for resuscitation especially in cases of anticipated larger volume losses including delayed presentation, large burn area, and inhalational injuries [6]. Post major burns, there is generalised increase in capillary permeability even in the unburned tissues with loss of albumin and smaller proteins molecules; this is however transient lasting for up to 12 h. Oedema and further third spacing are nonetheless persistent due to hypoproteinaemia and reduction in plasma oncotic pressures; increased lung water also occurs as a result. Colloids maintain the intravascular volume by maintaining the plasma oncotic pressure and decreasing third spacing [7]. Various formulae utilise colloids early or late as rescue therapy; Slater and Haifa formulae utilise FFP and plasma immediately post-injury. Goodwin et al. used albumin early in resuscitation and found reduced volume requirement and improved cardiac function [8]. Others have used albumin 8–12 h later as rescue fluid in cases of high projected volume losses and have shown a trend towards reduced volume of resuscitation and mortality reduction[6, 9]. However, data regarding timing and dose are still lacking – a meta-analysis by Navickis et al. [10] found no significant effect on mortality when albumin was used during the first 24 h; but when they excluded two studies with high risk of bias, there was in fact a reduction in mortality with albumin as well as marked reduction in the development of a compartment syndrome.

Hydroxyethyl starch (HES) is associated with increased risk of renal dysfunction and their use in burn resuscitation remains controversial and should be abandoned.

Hypertonic saline has been used for resuscitation keeping in mind that large-volume crystalloids will result in more severe oedema and complications including acute kidney injury [11].

Fresh frozen plasma (FFP) is not without its own problems, namely, infection risk and TRALI; hence, it is not the first choice of colloid for burns resuscitation.

Urine output monitoring guides fluid resuscitation, with a target urine output of 0.5 mL/kg to 1 mL/kg, although this parameter is unreliable in renal dysfunction. There is a danger of increasing the volume of infusion to offset low urine output without appropriate subsequent de-escalation. Goal-directed fluid therapy has been studied in burns including transpulmonary thermodilution [12]. However, there is insufficient data to support its use; these devices are also unavailable in many centres.

Lactate and base deficit as monitoring tools have been studied but their role in the face of ongoing third spacing is not well established. B-type natriuretic peptide (BNP) and proteinuria have also been studied as potential monitoring tools during resuscitation; a high BNP level with low proteinuria was associated with better outcomes [13]. We refer to the IFA commentary and some recent papers looking more in detail at the different monitoring targets and goals [14, 15].

Case Vignette
- Why is intravenous fluid resuscitation essential for burn patients?

    Answer: Intravenous fluid resuscitation is essential for burn patients to prevent hypovolaemic shock and acute kidney injury. Burn injuries cause the loss of intravascular volume, leading to hypovolaemia, hypotension, and inadequate tissue perfusion. IV fluids are given to restore intravascular volume, correct electrolyte imbalances, and improve organ perfusion.

- What is the goal of fluid resuscitation in burn patients?

  Answer: The goal of fluid resuscitation in burn patients is to maintain adequate organ perfusion and treat shock. The Parkland formula can be used to determine the initial volume of fluid needed for resuscitation, which involves giving of lactated Ringer's solution/Plasma-Lyte 4 mL/kg/body weight/percentage of the total body surface area (TBSA) burned. Half of the calculated volume is given in the first 8 h post-burn, with the remaining half given in the next 16 h. The goal is to maintain a urine output of 0.5–1 mL/kg/h, which indicates adequate organ perfusion.

  Fluid management should be tailored to the patient's condition, urine output, etc., and strict adherence to resuscitation formula is not recommended.

Conclusion

Burn resuscitation poses a unique challenge, as progressive intravascular depletion leads to burn shock; early and appropriate therapy aims to minimise or prevent burns shock, tissue hypoperfusion, and organ dysfunction. Under-resuscitation increases morbidity and mortality, whereas overzealous fluid administration is equally harmful and causes fluid creep. Fluid administration needs to be tailored to the patient's condition and strict adherence to resuscitation formulae may not be prudent; physicians need to tailor their resuscitation strategy to the evolving targets. Colloids have a place later on in the resuscitation process particularly in cases of anticipated larger fluid volume requirement including deeper burns, inhalational injuries, and late presentation.

Take Home Messages
- Estimation of the percentage of body surface area (BSA) burnt is the first step when managing a patient, and there are several methods to estimate BSA.
- During BSA estimation, only deep partial-thickness and full-thickness burns are calculated for fluid administration; superficial partial-thickness burns are not included.
- The most commonly followed formula for fluid resuscitation is the Parkland formula, which uses Ringer's lactate up to 4 mL/kg/%TBSA in the first 24 h, half during the first 8 h and the rest over the next 16 h.
- Time is estimated from the time of injury, and in cases of delayed presentation a more rapid fluid administration may be required.
- Early and adequate resuscitation is important to prevent renal failure, organ dysfunction, and death.

- Care should be taken while assessing patients, as patients presenting with shock probably have some other underlying injury causing hypotension since burn shock generally sets in gradually.
- Most patients receive Ringer's lactate or Plasma-Lyte during initial resuscitation, as per the Parkland formula and modified Brooke formula; however, fluids should be tailored on the patient's individual needs following the ROSE concept.
- Crystalloid resuscitation results in worsening oedema, renal dysfunction, airway complications including ARDS, abdominal compartment syndrome, and intra-ocular hypertension.
- Colloid use reduces the volume required for resuscitation, especially in cases of anticipated larger volume losses including delayed presentation, large burn area, and inhalational injuries.
- Clear data on the type timing and dose of colloids early or late as rescue therapy are still lacking.

References

1. Swanson JW, Otto AM, Gibran NS, Klein MB, Kramer CB, Heimbach DM, et al. Trajectories to death in patients with burn injury. J Trauma Acute Care Surg. 2013;74(1):282–8.
2. Cope O, Moore FD. The redistribution of body water and the fluid therapy of the burned patient. Ann Surg. 1947;126(6):1010–45.
3. Cartotto R, Greenhalgh D. Colloids in acute burn resuscitation. Crit Care Clin. 2016;32:507–23.
4. Pruitt BA Jr. Protection from excessive resuscitation:"pushing the pendulum back". J Trauma. 2000;49(3):567–8.
5. Rae L, Fidler P, Gibran N. The physiologic basis of burn shock and the need for aggressive fluid resuscitation. Crit Care Clin. 2016;32(4):491–505.
6. Park SH, Hemmila MR, Wahl WL. Early albumin use improves mortality in difficult to resuscitate burn patients. J Trauma Acute Care Surg. 2012;73(5):1294–7.
7. Demling RH, Kramer G, Harms B. Role of thermal injury induced hypoproteinemia on fluid flux and protein permeability in burned and nonburned tissue. Surgery. 1984;95(2):136–44.
8. Goodwin CW, Dorethy J, Lam V, Pruitt BA. Randomized trial of efficacy of crystalloid and colloid resuscitation on hemodynamic response and lung water following thermal injury. Ann Surg. 1983;197(5):520–31.
9. Cochran A, Morris SE, Edelman LS, Saffle JR. Burn patient characteristics and outcome following resuscitation with albumin. Burns. 2007;33(1):25–30.
10. Navickis RJ, Greenhalgh DG, Wilkes MM. Albumin in Burn Shock resuscitation: a meta analysis of controlled clinical studies. J Burns Care Res. 2016;37(3):268–78.
11. Huang PP, Stucky FS, Dimick AR, Treat RC, Bessey PQ, Rue LW. Hypertonic sodium resuscitation is associated with renal failure and death. Ann Surg. 1995;221:543–57.
12. Holm C, Mayr M, Tegeler J, Horbrand F, Henckel von Donnersmarck G, Muhlbauer W, et al. A clinical randomized studyon the effects of invasive monitoring on burn shock resuscitation. Burns. 2004;30(8):798–807.

13. de Leeuw K, Nieuwenhuis MK, Niemeijer AS, Eshuis H, Beerthuizen GI, Janssen WM. Increased B-type natriuretic peptide and decreased proteinuria might reflect decreased capillary leakage and is associated with a better outcome in patients with severe burns. Crit Care. 2011;15(4):R161.
14. Peeters Y, Lebeer M, Wise R, Malbrain M. An overview on fluid resuscitation and resuscitation endpoints in burns: past, present and future. Part 2—avoiding complications by using the right endpoints with a new personalized protocolized approach. Anaesthesiol Intensive Ther. 2015;47:S15–26.
15. Peeters Y, Vandervelden S, Wise R, Malbrain M. An overview on fluid resuscitation and resuscitation endpoints in burns: past, present and future. Part 1 - historical background, resuscitation fluid and adjunctive treatment. Anaesthesiol Intensive Ther. 2015;47:S6–S14.

Fluid Management in Paediatric Patients

20

Sonali Ghosh

Contents

Introduction 399
Physiology of Body Fluid in Children 399
    Fluids for the Paediatric Population: Resuscitation, Replacement and Maintenance 400
Individual Clinical Scenarios 403
    Children with Dehydration 403
Sepsis and Septic Shock 405
Diabetic Ketoacidosis 406
Conclusion 408
References 408

IFA Commentary (MLNGM)

In critically ill children, the administration of fluids is a crucial aspect of their management. The type and amount of fluid given to a critically ill child depends on their clinical condition and fluid status. Resuscitation fluids are used to treat hypovolemia and hypotension in critically ill children in shock. The aim of resuscitation is to restore and maintain adequate tissue perfusion, oxygenation, and organ function. Commonly used fluids include crystalloids (such as normal saline, lactated Ringer's solution, and balanced salt solutions) and colloids (such as albumin). The choice of resuscitation fluid depends on the underlying condition of the child, the degree of

---

S. Ghosh (✉)
PICU, MarengoAsia Hospital, Faridabad, Haryana, India

M. L. N. G. Malbrain et al. (eds.), *Rational Use of Intravenous Fluids in Critically Ill Patients*, https://doi.org/10.1007/978-3-031-42205-8_20

hypovolemia, and the presence of any comorbidities. It is important to monitor the child's response to resuscitation fluids closely and adjust the type and amount of fluid as needed. Replacement fluids are used to correct fluid and electrolyte imbalances in critically ill children. The aim of replacement therapy is to maintain homeostasis and prevent complications associated with fluid and electrolyte disturbances. Replacement fluids are usually isotonic solutions such as normal saline, lactated Ringer's solution, and balanced salt solutions. In some cases, hypotonic solutions, such as 0.45% saline, may be used to correct hypernatremia or hypertonic dehydration. The amount and composition of replacement fluids depend on the child's clinical condition and fluid status. Maintenance fluids are used to maintain hydration and electrolyte balance in critically ill children who are unable to take fluids orally. The aim of maintenance fluid therapy is to replace ongoing losses and prevent dehydration and electrolyte disturbances. The amount and composition of maintenance fluids depend on the child's age, weight, and clinical condition. The most commonly used fluids for maintenance therapy are isotonic solutions such as normal saline, lactated Ringer's solution, and balanced salt solutions. The rate of maintenance fluid administration should be adjusted according to the child's ongoing fluid losses and response to therapy. In contrast to adults where there is a shift towards hypotonic intravenous maintenance fluid therapy (IV-MFT), in children isotonic maintenance is still preferred because of the risk for hyponatremia. The recently published ESPNIC guidelines propose 16 recommendations based on a literature search and expert consensus (Table 20.1) [1]. Although there is a high level of consensus, the level of evidence for most recommendations is low. The recommendations are consistent with previous guidelines, including the use of isotonic fluids, reduced infusion volumes, and the use of the enteral route when possible. However, the researchers note that the reporting of key outcomes was inconsistent, which prevented further meta-analyses. The study raises several implications for practice, including highlighting the importance of IV fluid composition, glucose and plasma electrolyte monitoring, and the potential harm of excessive fluids and volume overload. The authors acknowledge the challenge of implementing these recommendations, particularly due to the lack of availability of ready-to-use IV-MFT solutions in some countries. In summary, resuscitation, replacement, and maintenance fluids are used in the management of critically ill children to restore and maintain fluid and electrolyte balance, correct imbalances, and prevent complications associated with fluid and electrolyte disturbances. The choice of fluid, amount, and composition of fluids depends on the underlying condition and clinical status of the child, and should be closely monitored and adjusted as needed.

Suggested Reading
1. Brossier DW, Tume LN, Briant AR, Jotterand Chaparro C, Moullet C, Rooze S, Verbruggen S, Marino LV, Alsohime F, Beldjilali S et al: ESPNIC clinical practice guidelines: intravenous maintenance fluid therapy in acute and critically ill children—a systematic review and meta-analysis. Intensive Care Med. 2022;48(12):1691–708.

Table 20.1 ESPNIC recommendations on IV maintenance fluids in critically ill children

Recommendations	Level of evidence	Consensus
PiCO 1: IV-MFT indications	–	–
In acutely ill children, the enteral or oral route for the delivery of maintenance fluid therapy should be considered, if tolerated, to reduce the failure rate of hydration access and costs	C	Strong consensus
In critically ill children with improving hemodynamic state, the enteral or oral route for the delivery of maintenance fluid therapy should be considered, if tolerated, to reduce length of stay in term neonates	GCP	Strong consensus
PiCO 2: Use of isotonic fluids		
In acutely and critically ill children, isotonic maintenance fluid should be used to reduce the risk of hyponatremia	A	Strong consensus
PiCO 3: Use of balanced solutions		
In critically ill children, balanced solutions should be favoured when prescribing intravenous maintenance fluid therapy to slightly reduce length of stay	B	Strong consensus
In acutely ill children, balanced solutions should be used when prescribing intravenous maintenance fluid therapy to slightly reduce length of stay	A	Strong consensus
In acutely and critically ill children, lactate buffer solution should not be considered in the case of severe liver dysfunction to avoid lactic acidosis	D	Consensus
PiCO 4: IV-MFT fluid composition (Ca, Mg, P, micronutrients, glucose)	–	–
In acutely and critically ill children, glucose provision in intravenous maintenance fluid therapy should be considered in sufficient amounts and guided by blood glucose monitoring (at least daily) to prevent hypoglycaemia	GCP	Consensus
In critically ill children, glucose provision in intravenous maintenance fluid therapy should not be excessive and guided by blood glucose monitoring (at least daily) to prevent hyperglycaemia	B	Consensus
In acutely and critically ill children, there is insufficient evidence to recommend routine supplementation of magnesium, calcium and phosphate in intravenous maintenance fluid therapy	GCP	Strong consensus
In acutely and critically ill children, an appropriate amount of potassium should be considered and added to intravenous maintenance fluid therapy, based on the child's clinical status and regular potassium level monitoring to avoid hypokalemia	GCP	Consensus

(continued)

Table 20.1 (continued)

Recommendations	Level of evidence	Consensus
In acutely and critically ill children, there is insufficient evidence to recommend routine supplementation of vitamins and trace elements in intravenous maintenance fluid therapy, in the absence of signs of deficiency	GCP	Strong consensus
PiCO 5: Volume of IV-MFT administered	–	–
In acutely and critically ill children, in order to prevent fluid creep and reduce fluid intake, the total daily amount of maintenance fluid therapy should be considered including IV fluids, blood products, all IV medications (both infusions and bolus drugs), arterial and venous line flush solutions and enteral intake, but does not include replacement fluids and massive transfusion	D	Strong consensus
In acutely and critically ill children, avoidance of fluid overload and cumulative positive fluid balance should be considered, to avoid prolonged mechanical ventilation and length of stay	D	Strong consensus
In acutely and critically ill children, who are at risk of increased endogenous secretion of ADH, restriction of total intravenous maintenance fluid therapy volume (calculated by Holliday and Segar formula) should be considered to some extent, to avoid a decrease in natremia but the amount and duration of this restriction is uncertain	C	Strong consensus
In acutely and critically ill children who are at risk of increased endogenous secretion of ADH, restricting maintenance fluid therapy volume to between 65% and 80% of the volume calculated by the Holliday and Segar formula should be considered to avoid fluid overload In children at greater risk of oedematous states, e.g., heart failure, renal failure or hepatic failure, restricting maintenance fluid therapy volume to between 50% and 60% of the volume calculated with the Holliday and Segar formula should be considered to avoid fluid overload	GCP	Strong consensus
Whilst receiving intravenous maintenance fluid therapy, re-assessment of acutely and critically ill children should be considered at least daily in terms of fluid balance and clinical status and regularly regarding electrolytes, especially sodium level	D	Consensus

ADH anti-diuretic hormone, *GCP* good clinical practice, *IV-MFT* intravenous maintenance fluid therapy; Consensus (expert votes): 90% <agreement <95%; Strong consensus:>95% agreement

Learning Objectives

After reading this chapter, you will:

1. To learn about the physiology of body fluids in children.
2. The difference in distribution of body fluids at different stages of paediatric age group.
3. Evidence-based approach for choosing the type of fluid for resuscitation, replacement and maintenance fluid.
4. To learn about the fluid management in various common clinical scenarios in paediatric age group.

> **Case Vignette**
>
> A 2-year-old boy presented to the emergency department with a 2-day history of watery loose stools. His oral intake was poor, and he had passed urine once since morning. His eyes appeared sunken and had a weak cry. On examination his peripheral pulses were very feeble, peripheries were cool, capillary filling time was prolonged (>3 s) and blood pressure was at fifth centile for his age.
>
> **Question**
>
> Q1. What are the clinical considerations while managing this child?

Introduction

Children are more prone to water and electrolyte imbalances compared to adults for a number of reasons: (a) higher total body water content [1], (b) relatively higher insensible losses due to a higher surface area to body mass ratio [2, 3] and (c) possible presence of immature regulatory mechanisms [4, 5]. Hence fluid therapy in children should be considered challenging in all respects and should be treated as a pharmacological intervention with precise indications, contraindications and adverse effects.

Physiology of Body Fluid in Children

In children, the relative amount of body water varies considerably with age [6]. Total body water (TBW) is 90% of the body weight in the fetus, predominantly in the extracellular compartment (ECF represents ~65% of TBW). In a full-term newborn baby, TBW constitutes 75–80% of body weight; the intracellular fluid (ICF) increases to ~45% of TBW and consequently, the proportion of ECF undergoes a relative decrease to ~55% of TBW. In the first year of life due to an increase in fat, TBW reduces to around 60%. The ratio of ECF to ICF continues to change, with increase in ICF to 60% of TBW at the end of the first year and ECF accounting for the remaining 40%. The relative drop in ECF is mainly due to a reduction in interstitial fluid, while the percentage of intravascular fluid appears to be fairly constant. In a child, TBW is ≈60% with ICF being 35% of TBW. A similar ratio is seen in adults (Table 20.2).

The composition of intra-/extracellular fluids and regulation of body water in children is not different from that of normal adults and is detailed in Chaps. 2 and 3. The composition of different intravenous fluids is described in Chap. 9. Briefly, isotonic fluids have a composition similar to ECF, whereas hypotonic fluids are lower in tonicity and potassium

Table 20.2 Composition of body fluid in paediatric and adult groups (adapted from Langer et al. [21])

	Fetus	Baby	Child	Adult
Total body water (TBW)	85%	65%	60%	60%
Intracellular water (ICW)	25%	35%	35%	40%
Extracellular water (ECW)	60%	30%	25%	20%

concentration compared to plasma (Table 20.3). Isotonic fluids are used for fluid resuscitation, to correct an acute intravascular fluid deficit and for the replacement of extracellular fluid losses. Most intravenous fluids employed in the paediatric population contain glucose, ranging between 5% and 10%.

Fluids for the Paediatric Population: Resuscitation, Replacement and Maintenance

There is a strong consensus in favour of using isotonic, possibly balanced fluids perioperatively and for resuscitation and replacement in the paediatric intensive care unit [7] although there remains significant heterogeneity in clinical practice. In a survey by Way et al., about 10% of anesthesiologists reported a prescription practice of using a bolus of hypotonic dextrose saline to treat intraoperative hypovolemia in the paediatric population [8].

The ideal tonicity of maintenance fluids in the paediatric population is still debated [9–12]. The physiological rationale is to prescribe maintenance fluids in children to replace fluids lost through urinary output and insensible losses when oral or enteral intake is not possible. In theory, at least, the composition of maintenance fluids should be similar to that of lost fluids. Additionally, maintenance fluids should be able to hydrate both the extracellular and the intracellular compartments. Table 20.4 gives an overview of the composition of the different compartments. Since fluids lost through skin, lung and stool (insensible loss) or through urine are hypotonic, a number of experts argue that maintenance fluids should be hypotonic. They believe that hypotonic fluid will reduce plasma osmolarity, generate osmotic driving pressure and allow water movement from the extra- to the intracellular compartment, hydrating both compartments.

Reduction in plasma osmolarity should suppress anti diuretic hormone (ADH) secretion. Hence in physiologic conditions, there will be excretion of electrolyte-free water

Table 20.3 Characteristics of intravenous fluids employed in the paediatric population

	Hypotonic					Isotonic						Enteral	
	Dextrose 5%	Paediatric solution	NaCl 0.3%	D 5% in NaCl 0.45%	Glucion 5%	Lactated Ringer's	Acetated Ringer's	D 1% in Balanced solution	Plasma Lyte	NaCl 0.9%	Sterofundin ISO	Water	Human milk
Na$^+$ [mEq/L]	–	23	51	77	54	130	132	140	140	154	145	<1	10
K$^+$ [mEq/L]	–	20	–	–	26	4	4	4	5	–	4	<0.1	15
Ca^{2+} [mEq/L]	–	–	–	–	–	3	3	2	–	–	5	2.5	12.5
Mg^{2+} [mEq/L]	–	3	–	–	5	–	–	2	3	–	2	2.5	25
Cl$^-$ [mEq/L]	–	20	51	77	55	109	110	118	98	154	127	<0.1	13
Lactate [mEq/L]	–	–	–	–	25	28	–	–	–	–	–	–	–
Acetate [mEq/L]	–	23	–	–	–	–	29	30	27	–	24	–	–
Phosphate [mEq/L]	–	3	–	–	6	–	–	–	–	–	–	–	1.3
Malate [mEq/L]	–	–	–	–	–	–	–	–	–	–	5	–	–
Gluconate [mEq/L]	–	–	–	–	–	–	–	–	23	–	–	–	–
Dextrose [mmol/L]	278	278	–	278	278	–	–	56	–	–	–	–	200[a]
In-vivo SID [mEq/L]	–	26	–	–	30	28	29	30	50	–	29	–	1.3
Tonicity [mOsm/L]	0	92	102	154	170	274	278	296	296	308	312	10	125

Intravenous fluids have been divided into *hypotonic* and *isotonic* and listed according to increasing tonicity. For comparison, the composition of drinking water and human milk has been added (*enteral*)

In-vivo SID all organic molecules contained in balanced solutions are strong anions. The resulting calculated SID (in-vitro SID) is equal to 0 mE/L. Once infused, the organic molecules are metabolized to CO_2 and water; the resulting in-vivo SID corresponds to the amount of organic anions metabolized. Tonicity = number of solutes to which cell membranes are impermeable. In this context glucose, which rapidly crosses cell membranes, is not included in the calculation

Adapted from Langer et al. [21] with permission according to the Open Access CC BY Licence 4.0

[a] 200 refers to mmol/L of lactose, in case of human milk

Table 20.4 Fluid compartments and their composition

	ECF			ICF		
	Plasma	ISF	CSF	ICF_{ST}	ICF_{RBC}	TBW
% of body weight	4.7	20	0.3	31.5	3.5	60
Na^+ [mEq/L]	143	137	145	10	19	64
K^+ [mEq/L]	4	3	3	155	95	88
Ca^{2+} [mEq/L]	2	2	2	<0.1	<0.1	0.8
Mg^{2+} [mEq/L]	2	2	2	10	5	6
Cl^- [mEq/L]	107	111	125	10	52	54
Lac^- [mEq/L]	1	1	1.5	1	1	1
Other anions [mEq/L]	–	–	–	34	9	18
HCO_3^- [mEq/L]	25	31	24	11	15	19
Albumin [g/dL]	5	< 1	<0.1	<0.1	<0.1	<1
A^- [mEq/L]	16	< 1	1	118	42	66
SID [mEq/L]	42	31	24	130	57	85

Table summarizes the simplified composition of different body fluid compartments of a child aged 12 months or more, schematically divided into extracellular (ECF) and intracellular (ICF). In addition, the theoretical average composition of total body water (TBW), resulting from the mixing of ICF and ECF, was calculated and reported in Table. *ISF* interstitial fluid, *CSF* cerebrospinal fluid, *ICF* "standard" intracellular fluid, ICF_{RBC} red blood cells fluid, Na^+ sodium concentration, K^+ potassium concentration, Ca^{2+} ionized calcium concentration, Mg^{2+} ionized magnesium concentration, Cl^- chloride concentration, Lac^- lactate concentration, *other anions* sum of the concentration of other anions, HCO_3^- bicarbonate concentration, A^- dissociated, electrically charged part of 'non carbonic buffers' (A_{TOT}), *SID* strong ion difference. All concentrations, except for Albumin, are expressed in mEq/L
Adapted from Langer et al. [21] with permission according to the Open Access CC BY Licence 4.0

through diluted urine. However, in critically ill or hospitalized children, ADH secretion is stimulated by the presence of several non-osmotic stimuli, resulting in an inability to excrete free water. In the presence of inappropriately high ADH levels, administration of hypotonic fluid in critically ill children is likely to result in positive water balance and may increase the risk of water intoxication and hyponatremia with consequent neurologic disorders. For these reasons, another group of experts advocates the use of isotonic instead of hypotonic fluids for maintenance therapy in hospitalized children.

In a single-centre study from Canada, 258 post-operative patients from 6 months to 16 years of age were randomized to receive either isotonic (0.9% saline) or hypotonic (0.45% saline) as maintenance solution for 48 h. Hypotonic fluids significantly increased the risk of hyponatremia, compared to isotonic saline (40.8% vs 22.7%), but 0.9% saline was not associated with increased risk of hypernatremia. Interestingly, ADH levels and risk of adverse events were not different between the two groups [13].

The risk of developing hyponatremia in the paediatric population was recognized by the American Academy of Pediatrics (AAP). AAP recommends that paediatric patients in the age group between 28 days and 18 years requiring intravenous maintenance fluid should receive isotonic solutions with appropriate potassium and dextrose [14].

In acutely ill children there is limited evidence regarding the optimal fluid therapy. In a recent trial by Lehtiranta et al. to evaluate the risk of electrolyte disorders and fluid retention in a group of acutely ill children receiving plasma-like isotonic fluid therapy. It was conducted at Oulu University Hospital, Finland, from October 2016 to April 2019. A total of 614 children were randomized to receive commercially available plasma-like isotonic fluid (140 mmol/L of sodium and 5 mmol/L potassium in 5% dextrose) or moderately hypotonic fluid (80 mmol/L sodium and 20 mmol/L potassium in 5% sextrose). It was found that the risk of electrolyte disorders was 6.7 times greater in children who received isotonic fluids compared to hypotonic fluids. Hypokalemia was found to be a significant electrolyte disorder [22].

Individual Clinical Scenarios

Children with Dehydration

Dehydration is the most common cause of fluid and electrolyte disturbance-related critical illness in children globally. The first step in management is to assess the degree of dehydration. Table 20.5 describes the assessment criteria for degree of dehydration.

After the initial assessment, the patient must be regularly re-evaluated during treatment. A good history can reveal the cause of dehydration. It may also help to predict isotonic, hypotonic or hypertonic dehydration. A neonate having poor intake of breast milk or a child with plenty of watery stools and poor oral intake often develop hypernatremic dehydration. On the other hand, a child with watery diarrhea who is only drinking large quantities of plain water or low-salt fluid will have hyponatremic dehydration. Physical examination can determine the degree of dehydration but it may be difficult to assess the skin pinch in premature infants or severely malnourished children.

Table 20.5 Clinical assessment of degree of dehydration

	Mild dehydration	Moderate dehydration	Severe dehydration
Degree of dehydration	<5% in infant; <3% in older child	5–10% in infant; 3–6% in older child	>10% in infant; >6% in older child
Look	Well and alert	Restless	Lethargic
Eyes	Normal	Sunken	Sunken
Skin pinch	Goes back normally	Goes back slowly	Goes back very slowly
Thirst	Drinks normally	Increased thirst	Drinks poorly
Mucosa	Moist	Dry	Parched
Pulse/HR	Normal or increased pulse	Tachycardia	Peripheral pulses weak with rapid pulse
Capillary filling time	<2 s	Delayed	Prolonged
Skin touch	Warm	Cool and pale	Cold and mottled

Calculation of Fluid Deficit Assess the degree of dehydration and multiply the percentage of dehydration with patient's weight (converting the unit to litre). For example, a 10 kg child with 10% dehydration has a fluid deficit of 1 L.

Fluid Management A child with severe dehydration needs acute intervention in the form of adequate fluid resuscitation. The resuscitation phase ensures rapid restoration of intravascular volume. Initial fluid choices are crystalloids e.g. 0.9% saline or Ringer's lactate. Colloids like 5% albumin, blood and FFP are not the initial choice but can be considered if the patient has bleeding manifestations with underlying coagulopathy. The initial fluid bolus is 20 mL/kg of crystalloids, given within 10–20 min. Children with severe dehydration may require multiple fluid boluses for adequate restoration of intravascular volume.

After initial resuscitation, the maintenance plus deficit is to be calculated for 24 h. After deducting the fluid boluses, the rest of the calculated fluid needs to be administered over 24 h. Let us now take an example of a 10 kg child with 10% dehydration:

- Total deficit volume = 1000 mL (by multiplying the percentage of dehydration with body weight of the child in litre).
- Maintenance fluid requirement = 1000 mL (by applying is Holiday Segar formula, 100 mL/kg for first 10 kg i.e. 1000 mL).
- Fluid bolus given once = 200 mL (20 mL/kg).
- The remaining deficit plus maintenance fluid volume of 1800 mL (1000 mL + 1000 mL − 200 mL) is to be given over 24 h.

Potassium is added to the maintenance fluid once the child passes urine. Children in whom significant ongoing losses are present need to receive replacement solutions.

Holliday-Segar formula for maintenance fluid requirements by weight			
	Water		Electrolytes (mEq/L
Weight (kg)	mL/day	mL/h	H_2O and mmol/L H_2O)
0–10	100/kg	4/kg	Sodium 30
			Potassium 20
11–20	1000 + 50/kg for each kg >10	40 + 2/kg for each kg >10	Sodium 30
			Potassium 20
>20	1500 + 20/kg for each kg >20	60 + 1/kg for each kg >20	Sodium 30
			Potassium 20

Hypernatremic Dehydration is dangerous due to complications of hypernatremia as well as its therapy. The child is usually lethargic and irritable and can manifest with neurologic symptoms. In hypernatremia, the movement of water from intracellular to extracellular space helps to preserve intravascular volume. By the time they receive medical attention, they would already be profoundly intracellularly dehydrated. Initial fluid resuscitation for hypernatremic dehydration should be with 0.9% saline with the aim of restoring intravascular volume. Ringer's lactate should be avoided as it may lead to a rapid reduction of sodium levels. To minimize the risk of cerebral edema, serum Na should not decrease by >12 mEq/L in 24 h. The rate of correction will depend on the initial sodium level.

Once the intravascular volume is restored, further correction of dehydration can be achieved with 5% dextrose with ½ normal saline that has a higher content (50% more) of free water than 0.9% saline. The sodium concentration of the IV fluids should be adjusted according to serum sodium levels. One way of achieving the target is to use two different fluids with varying sodium concentrations e.g. 5% Dextrose with 1/4 normal saline and 5% Dextrose with normal saline. If serum sodium levels decrease rapidly, the rate of 5% Dextrose with normal saline may be increased with a simultaneous decrease in the rate of 5% Dextrose with 1/4 normal saline. Rapid reduction in serum sodium may precipitate seizures as a manifestation of cerebral edema, requiring acute correction with an infusion of 3% saline at a dose of 4 mL/kg. When the child is conscious and ready to accept oral fluids, plain water or hypotonic fluids should be avoided.

Hyponatremic Dehydration involves loss of both sodium and water in stools with a higher loss of sodium relative to water. Also, volume depletion stimulates ADH synthesis resulting in a reduction of renal excretion of free water. The initial goal is to correct intravascular volume losses with isotonic fluids; most patients respond well to basic management as outlined for dehydration. Care should be taken to avoid overly rapid correction of Na > 12 mEq/L in 24 h as this can be associated with the risk of central pontine myelinolysis. Serum sodium should be monitored closely; if the patient presents with neurologic symptoms as a result of hyponatremia, 3% saline should be given to raise serum sodium rapidly.

Sepsis and Septic Shock

There is no specific recommendation regarding the optimal type of resuscitation fluid in the management of paediatric sepsis. Isotonic crystalloids are recommended as the initial fluid of choice [15]. Fluid boluses of 20 mL/kg over 5 min up to 60 mL/kg can be given till perfusion improves; these can be given by push or pressure bag devices while simultaneously observing for signs of fluid overload i.e. rales, gallop rhythm, hepatomegaly [15] .

However, the concept of administering fluid boluses in paediatric septic shock has recently been challenged following the landmark FEAST study [16]. In this study, Maitland and colleagues randomized 3170 children with evidence of hypoperfusion into three groups: (a) albumin-bolus group that received 20–40 mL of 5% albumin solution per kg of body weight, (b) saline-bolus group receiving 20–40 mL of 0.9% saline solution per kg of body weight and (c) control group, which received no fluid bolus. All three groups received maintenance fluids at a rate of 2.5–4 mL/kg/h. Compared to the control group, mortality rate was significantly higher in both bolus groups at 48 h and also at 4 weeks; mortality was related mostly to cardiovascular failure. Interestingly, mortality rates were not significantly different between the bolus groups. However, criticisms of the study include its external validity in high- and middle-income countries (the study was conducted in sub-Saharan Africa), large number of children with malaria being enrolled and possibility of worsening pre-existing anemia by hemodilution in bolus groups.

Fish Trial (Fluids in Shock) It was a pilot RCT conducted across 13 hospitals in England from July 2016 to April 2017. It aimed to evaluate whether a restricted fluid bolus of 10 ml/kg compared with the current recommendation of 20 mL/kg is associated with improved outcomes in children presenting to UK emergency departments with presumed septic shock. Seventy-five participants were randomized. The volume of study bolus fluid after 4 h was 44% lower in the 10 mL/kg group. Length of hospital stay, PICU free days at 30 days did not differ significantly between the groups. It was observed that severity of illness in participants in the trial group was less than expected.

Further fluid administration after the initial resuscitation should be guided with hemodynamic variables and must be re-evaluated periodically.

Diabetic Ketoacidosis

In diabetic ketoacidosis (DKA) extracellular fluid deficit is usually in the range of 5–10%. In moderate DKA ECF volume deficit is 5–7% and in severe DKA 7–10%. Unfortunately, clinical estimation of volume depletion is often inaccurate. Some simple means of diagnosing ECF contraction are increases in urea nitrogen and hemoglobin concentration. Serum sodium concentration, an otherwise important marker for extracellular volume status, becomes unreliable in DKA, as osmotic effects of hyperglycemia cause a shift of water from intracellular to extracellular space, leading to dilutional hyponatremia. A simple formula can be utilized to calculate expected sodium, correcting the sodium level for hyperglycemia. In contrast, serum sodium should increase following correction of hyperglycemia with fluid infusion and insulin. Failure of serum sodium to rise or a paradoxical fall in sodium level following correction of glucose levels can be a sign of impending cerebral edema.

The goals of fluid therapy in DKA are:

- Restoration of circulating volume.
- Replacement of extracellular and intracellular fluid deficit.
- Replacement of Na, K, Mg, PO4 and other electrolytes.

Fluid Therapy Despite large overall volume deficits, patients in DKA rarely present in shock as their intravascular volume is usually preserved. Traditionally 0.9% saline is considered the fluid of choice for initial resuscitation and replacement of volume deficit. Current guidelines still recommend 0.9% saline over other fluids [17], though recent studies support the use of balanced salt solutions as the initial resuscitation fluid of choice for DKA in both adults and children because balanced salt solutions can restore the pH faster and avoid the risk of dilutional hyperchloremic metabolic acidosis [18, 19]. In a double-blind randomized control trial of 77 children with diabetic ketoacidosis, Yung and colleagues compared the effect of Hartman's solution and 0.9% saline in achieving serum bicarbonate level >15 mmol/L [19]. In the overall population, the time to reach the primary end-point and time to normalize pH were not different between the two groups. However, in sicker patients, Hartman's solution was able to normalize pH more quickly. Patients in the Hartman's solution group also received less total fluid per kg [19]. There is no data to support the use of colloids in managing DKA.

- Deficit replacement is calculated according to the percentage of dehydration. Maintenance fluid is calculated using the Holliday Segar formula. The daily maintenance requirement plus the deficit fluid is given over 24–48 h.
- Initially, isotonic fluid may be administered at 10 mL/kg over 30–60 min.
- If the peripheral perfusion is poor, a fluid bolus may be given more rapidly over 15–30 min and may be repeated till perfusion is restored. The bolus fluid is not calculated in the total fluid requirement.
- Once the peripheral perfusion is restored, recent guidelines suggest using 0.45–0.9% saline to restore total body volume deficit [17].
- Once RBS is below 250 mg/dL, 5% dextrose is added to fluids.
- Clinical assessment of hydration status and effective osmolality are used to guide fluid therapy. Repeated measurements of electrolytes are also essential.
- Rapid correction of hyperglycemia and high-volume fluid resuscitation in the first few hours are associated with an increased risk of cerebral edema. The risk of cerebral edema is also related to initial low sodium levels [20].
- The use of chloride-rich fluids like isotonic saline leads to the development of hyperchloremia and dilutional hyperchloremic acidosis that may mask the resolution of ketoacidosis. To avoid this confusion, measurement of beta hydroxyl butyrate can be performed.

Case Vignette
In the vignette at the start of this chapter, this child is in moderate dehydration due to acute gastroenteritis. A fluid bolus of 0.9% normal saline at 20 mL/kg needs to be given as tissue perfusion is poor. The child needs to be reassessed for perfusion parameters and the possible need for a repeated bolus. If no further boluses are required, considering 10% dehydration, the deficit needs to be calculated by multiplying the percentage of dehydration by weight. This along with the maintenance fluid needs to be given over 24 h.

Conclusion

The decisions surrounding resuscitation with intravenous fluids vary according to disease states in sick children. Fluid therapy should be guided according to fluid status, electrolyte and glucose levels. If the initial assessment shows a poor peripheral perfusion, fluid boluses need to be given. Fluid therapy in cases of dehydration includes calculating the deficit volume and the maintenance volume. Sodium levels should be monitored as the type of fluid will change accordingly. In paediatric septic shock, the initial fluid bolus is still 20 mL/kg which can be given at a rapid rate up to 40–60 mL/kg, but signs of fluid overload must be monitored for. In DKA, if patient is in a volume-depleted state, the initial fluid bolus is 10 mL/kg which needs to be given slowly. Isotonic saline is still the fluid of choice for resuscitation. There is some evidence supporting balanced salt solutions in resuscitation but more studies are needed.

> **Take Home Messages**
> - Fluid therapy should be guided according to the initial clinical assessment of the patient.
> - Children are more prone to fluid and electrolyte disturbances.
> - The type and rate of fluid administration will depend upon whether we use it for resuscitation, replacement or as maintenance fluid.
> - There is a strong consensus for using isotonic fluid as resuscitation and replacement fluid.
> - The ideal tonicity of maintenance fluid is still debated.

References

1. Friis-Hansen BJ, Holiday M, Stapleton T, et al. Total body water in children. Pediatrics. 1951;7(3):321–7.
2. Darrow DC, Pratt EL, Darrow DC, et al. Fluid therapy; relation to tissue composition and the expenditure of water and electrolyte. J Am Med Assoc. 1950;143(4):432–9.
3. Heeley AM, Talbot NB. Insensible water losses per day by hospitalized infants and children. AMA Am J Dis Child. 1955;90(3):251–5.
4. O'Brien F, Walker IA. Fluid homeostasis in the neonate. Paediatr Anaesth. 2014;24(1): 49–59.
5. Mårild S, Jodal U, Jonasson G, et al. Reference values for renal concentrating capacity in children by the desmopressin test. Pediatr Nephrol. 1992;6(3):254–7.

6. Friis-Hansen B. Body water compartments in children: changes during growth and related changes in body composition. Pediatrics. 1961;28:169–81.
7. Sümpelmann R, Becke K, Crean P, et al. German Scientific Working Group for Paediatric Anaesthesia. European consensus statement for intraoperative fluid therapy in children. Eur J Anaesthesiol. 2011;28(9):637–9.
8. Way C, Dhamrait R, Wade A, et al. Perioperative fluid therapy in children: a survey of current prescribing practice. Br J Anaesth. 2006;97(3):371–9.
9. Duke T, Molyneux EM. Intravenous fluids for seriously ill children: time to reconsider. Lancet. 2003;362(9392):1320–3.
10. Moritz ML, Ayus JC. Prevention of hospital-acquired hyponatremia: a case for using isotonic saline. Pediatrics. 2003;111(2):227–30.
11. Holliday MA. Isotonic saline expands extracellular fluid and is inappropriate for maintenance therapy. Pediatrics. 2005;115(1):193–4.
12. Mattheij M, Van Regenmortel N. Maintenance fluids for children: hypotonic fluids are still the best choice. Pediatr Emerg Care. 2016;32(2):e4.
13. Choong K, Arora S, Ji C, et al. Hypotonic versus isotonic maintenance fluids after surgery for children: a randomized controlled trial. Pediatrics. 2011;128(5):857–66.
14. Feld LG, Neuspiel DR, Foster BA, Leu MG, Garber MD, Austin K, et al. Clinical practice guideline: maintenance intravenous fluids in children. Pediatrics. 2018;142(6):e20183083.
15. Davis AL, Carcillo JA, Aneja RK, Deymann AJ, Lin JC, Nguyen TC, et al. American College of Critical Care Medicine clinical practice parameters for hemodynamic support of pediatric and neonatal septic shock. Crit Care Med. 2017;45:1061–93.
16. Maitland K, Kiguli S, Opoka RO, Engoru C, Olupot P, Akech SO, et al. Mortality after fluid bolus in African children with severe infection. N Engl J Med. 2011;364:2483–95.
17. Wolfsdorf JI, Glaser N, Agus M, Fritsch M, Hanas R, Rewers A, Sperling MA, Codner E. ISPAD clinical practice consensus guidelines 2018: diabetic ketoacidosis and the hyperglycemic hyperosmolar state. Pediatr Diabetes. 2018;19(Suppl 27):155–77.
18. Chua HR, Venkatesh B, Stachowski E, Schneider AG, Perkins K, Ladanyi S, Kruger P, Bellomo R. Plasma-Lyte 148 vs 0.9% saline for fluid resuscitation in diabetic ketoacidosis. J Crit Care. 2012;27:138–45.
19. Yung M, Letton G, Keeley S. Controlled trial of Hartmann's solution versus 0.9% saline for diabetic ketoacidosis. J Paediatr Child Health. 2017;53:12–7.
20. Edge JA, Jakes RW, Roy Y, Hawkins M, Winter D, Ford-Adams ME, Murphy NP, Bergomi A, Widmer B, Dunger DB. The UK case-control study of cerebral oedema complicating diabetic ketoacidosis in children. Diabetologia. 2006;49:2002–9.
21. Langer T, Limuti R, Tommasino C, van Regenmortel N, Duval ELIM, Caironi P, Malbrain MLNG, Pesenti A. Intravenous fluid therapy for hospitalized and critically ill children: rationale, available drugs and possible side effects. Anaesthesiol Intensive Ther. 2018;50(1):49–58. https://doi.org/10.5603/AIT.a2017.0058. Epub 2017 Nov 18. PMID: 29151001.
22. Lehtiranta S, Honkila M, Kallio M, et al. Risk of electrolyte disorders in acutely ill children receiving commercially available plasmalike isotonic fluids: a randomized clinical trial. JAMA Pediatr. 2021;175(1):28–35. https://doi.org/10.1001/jamapediatrics.2020.3383.

Fluid Management in Liver Failure

21

Michaël Mekeirele and Alexander Wilmer

Contents

Introduction 413
Acute-On-Chronic Liver Failure (ACLF) 414
  Pathophysiology of Circulatory Dysfunction in Patients with Cirrhosis 414
  Hemodynamic Approach During Decompensation 415
    General Background 415
    Special Considerations During Resuscitation 416
    Supcrimposcd Shock Syndromcs 417
    Choosing the Right Fluid 418
  Acute Liver Failure (ALF) 419
    Special Considerations During Resuscitation 419
    Superimposed Shock Syndromes 420
    Choosing the Right Fluid 420
Conclusion 421
References 423

M. Mekeirele (✉)
Department of Critical Care, Vrije Universiteit Brussel (VUB), Universitair Ziekenhuis Brussel (UZB), Jette, Belgium
e-mail: Michael.Mekeirele@uzbrussel.be

A. Wilmer
Medical Intensive Care Unit, Katholieke Universiteit Leuven (KUL), Universitair Ziekenhuis Gasthuisberg, Leuven, Belgium
e-mail: alexander.wilmer@uzleuven.be

© The Author(s) 2024
M. L. N. G. Malbrain et al. (eds.), *Rational Use of Intravenous Fluids in Critically Ill Patients*, https://doi.org/10.1007/978-3-031-42205-8_21

IFA Commentary (PN)

Critically ill patients with liver disease are known to experience hemodynamic alterations, which can lead to systemic hypotension, reduced cardiac output, and altered vascular resistance. These changes can be due to a variety of factors such as changes in the hepatic vasculature, reduced synthesis of vasodilatory and vasoconstrictive factors, and alterations in the activity of the renin-angiotensin-aldosterone system. Fluid therapy is a vital component of managing critically ill patients with liver disease, as these patients are prone to developing complications such as fluid and electrolyte imbalances, bleeding, and hypotension. The goals of fluid therapy in these patients are to restore effective circulating volume, improve organ perfusion, and prevent complications such as acute kidney injury. The best monitoring tools to guide fluid therapy depend on the patient's individual circumstances, but some commonly used tools include: first, hemodynamic monitoring that involves the use of various methods to directly measure cardiovascular parameters such as cardiac output, systemic vascular resistance, and central venous pressure. Commonly used techniques include pulmonary artery catheterization, echocardiography, and arterial waveform analysis. Second, fluid responsiveness assessment that involves assessing the patient's response to fluid administration, which can help guide further therapy. Various methods can be used to assess fluid responsiveness, such as dynamic variables (such as pulse pressure variation) and passive leg raising. Finally, serum biomarkers that measure serum markers such as lactate, central venous oxygen saturation, and hepatic venous pressure gradient can help assess the patient's hemodynamic status and guide fluid therapy. One key consideration in fluid therapy for liver disease patients is the potential for fluid (hypovolemia and hypervolemia) and electrolyte imbalances. This can be exacerbated by the presence of ascites, which may require treatment with diuretics or paracentesis. Additionally, patients with liver disease may have impaired renal function, making careful monitoring of fluid balance and renal function essential. In terms of the type of fluid given, there is ongoing debate about the optimal fluid, with some studies suggesting that balanced crystalloids (without lactate buffer) may be preferable to saline in reducing the risk of kidney injury and other complications. However, individual patient factors must be considered when selecting a fluid type. The type, dose, and use of albumin is a subject of ongoing research and debate. Some studies suggest that albumin can improve hemodynamics and reduce mortality in patients with liver disease, while others have found no significant benefit. Overall, fluid therapy in critically ill patients with liver disease is a complex and dynamic process that requires careful monitoring and individualized management to avoid potential complications and optimize patient outcomes.

Learning Objectives
After reading this chapter, you will:

1. Be able to describe the hemodynamic alterations specific to cirrhosis.
2. Be able to integrate the hemodynamic parameters of a patient with liver failure.
3. Be able to choose the right tools to guide fluid therapy in liver failure.

Case Vignette
A 45-year-old male with CHILD C liver cirrhosis is admitted to the ICU following a variceal hemorrhage. During stabilization, he received 1 L of balanced crystalloids. The bleeding was stopped after variceal ligations. High-dose PPI and Terlipressin were initiated. At this time, he is still hypotensive 80/35 mmHg (MAP 50 mmHg) and has marked peripheral edema, ascites, and an $S_{cv}O_2$ of 75%. He feels cold peripherally and has a mottled skin. When applying a passive leg raise, his blood pressure increases to 90/40 (MAP 59 mmHg). The lactate level is 15 mmol/L.

Questions
Q1. Would you administer this patient an extra fluid bolus?
Q2. What could help you decide between the administration of fluids or the application of either inotropes or vasopressors.
Q3. What would you do if the lactate level decreased to only 10 mmol/L after 6 h despite your best efforts?

Introduction

The general concepts of fluid management also apply to patients with liver failure. However, both acute liver failure (ALF) and acute-on-chronic liver failure (ACLF) are associated with marked hemodynamic changes due to inflammation, portal hypertension, and diminished clearing capacity of the liver for vasoactive substances. These hemodynamic changes are characterized by decreased systemic vascular resistance, increased cardiac output, central functional hypovolemia, increased arterial compliance, and peripheral vasodilatation. It is important to take these changes into account to determine the timing and volume of fluid administration and/or application of vasopressors and when interpreting the results obtained by hemodynamic monitoring devices. Although complex, the importance of adequate fluid management in liver failure cannot be overstressed since both hypervolemia and hypovolemia can further compromise residual liver function [1]. The choice of fluids in liver failure is relevant and perhaps more specific given the undeniable beneficial effects of albumin in certain indications. Particularly in acute on chronic liver failure, the advantages of albumin exceed those of mere volume expansion [1–5].

In this chapter, we will first discuss fluid management in acute on chronic liver failure. This syndrome is characterized as an acute liver decompensation in patients with a chronic underlying liver disease (mostly cirrhosis) with a high short-term mortality due to multiple organ failure. Second, we will discuss the scarce data on fluid management in patients with acute liver failure without underlying liver disease. This chapter will focus on adult patients, and more information on fluid therapy in children can be found in Chap. 20. Some other chapters will discuss fluids in specific populations: sepsis (Chap. 14), heart failure (Chap. 15), trauma (Chap. 16), neurocritical care (Chap. 17), perioperative setting (Chap. 18), burns (Chap. 19), abdominal hypertension (Chap. 22), and COVID-19 (Chap. 26).

Acute-On-Chronic Liver Failure (ACLF)

Pathophysiology of Circulatory Dysfunction in Patients with Cirrhosis

While the changes in hemodynamics of patients with cirrhosis have been described for years, a paradigm shift has occurred recently concerning the pathogenesis of these hemodynamic alterations. The "classical" view is that cirrhosis obstructs portal flow leading to portal hypertension which in turn induces splanchnic and systemic vasodilatation (Fig. 21.1). This vasodilatation leads to a state of functional hypovolemia with three important aspects. First, this activates the renin-angiotensin-aldosterone (RAAS) cascade leading to ascites formation via the retention of sodium and water. Second, this functional hypovolemia activates vasoconstrictor systems, including renal vasoconstriction. This can lead to renal failure although the patient will remain in a functional hypovolemic state

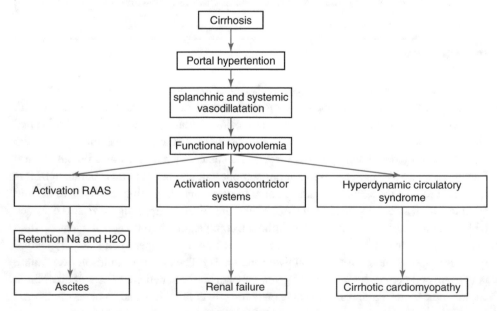

Fig. 21.1 Classical view on hemodynamic alterations due to cirrhosis

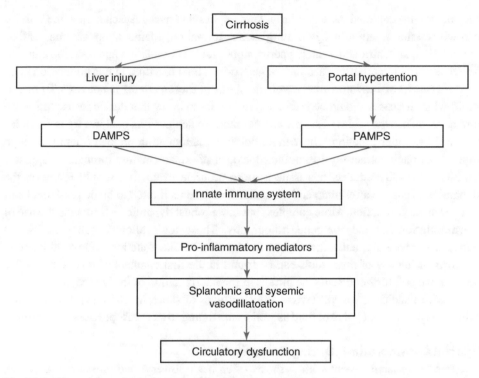

Fig. 21.2 New view on hemodynamic alterations due to cirrhosis

despite the activation of RAAS. Third, this hypovolemic state can induce a hyperdynamic circulatory syndrome potentially leading to a cirrhotic cardiomyopathy. The latter, in its milder form, blunts the contractile responsiveness to stress and alters diastolic relaxation [1, 6, 7]. The new view on the pathogenesis of the hemodynamic alterations emphasizes the importance of inflammation in cirrhosis (Fig. 21.2). In this hypothesis, cirrhosis leads to both liver injury and portal hypertension increasing plasma concentrations of damage associated molecular patterns (DAMPS) and pathogen associated molecular patterns (PAMPS). These DAMPS and PAMPS activate the innate immune system, causing the release of proinflammatory mediators which in turn cause splanchnic and systemic vasodilatation and circulatory dysfunction [1, 8]. It is important to recognize that due to fluid retention the average circulating blood volume in patients with cirrhosis is higher than in healthy persons [7]. However, the volume is unevenly distributed between central and abdominal compartment [9, 10]. With increasing severity of cirrhosis, this uneven distribution is magnified and becomes relevant for fluid administration [7].

Hemodynamic Approach During Decompensation

General Background
Classical signs of decompensated liver failure include ascites and edema. Large volumes of extracellular fluid may accumulate in the form of ascites and edema, while the patient

may be volume depleted intravascularly. This implies that over-resuscitation with IV fluids can worsen the situation by aggravating ascites formation, edema, hyponatremia, cardiac dysfunction, and intra-abdominal hypertension. Fluid accumulation and overload can also increase portal hypertension and induce gastro-intestinal bleeding in this population [1].

Assessment of the intravascular volume status in these patients is not easy. To understand what measures should be taken, it is important to know that during resuscitation we aim to rebalance the scales of supply and demand. To achieve this goal, we try to optimize the cardiovascular function. This can be done by manipulating preload (mainly through fluids), cardiac contractility (using inotropes), or afterload (mainly through vasopressor titration). To fully address this issue a more accurate evaluation should focus on the dynamics of change after interventions rather than on data limited to blood pressure, heart rate, or urine production. More complex, but more robust dynamic tests include the use of thermodilution methods or echocardiography. These tools allow a better distinction between intravascular and extravascular fluid status, cardiac function, and vasodilatation. A thorough review of these tools can be found in the first chapters of this book. In this section, we will further discuss the pitfalls in the interpretation of the hemodynamic status in ACLF. In addition, we will review different types of shock in ACLF since these determine the appropriate choice of fluid as well as the timing to start vasopressors or inotropes.

Special Considerations During Resuscitation

The decompensated patient with cirrhosis often has a lower blood pressure at baseline. Some authors state that a mean arterial pressure of 60 mmHg could suffice during resuscitation, while others stress the importance of mean arterial pressure (MAP) above 65 mmHg given the high incidence of renal failure in cirrhosis [11]. We prefer a MAP above 65 mmHg. Beyond the monitoring of blood pressure and heart rate, successful resuscitation in intensive care is frequently evaluated by changes in central venous oxygen saturation ($S_{cv}O_2$) and lactate clearance. $S_{cv}O_2$ is used as a surrogate marker for cardiac output. Since patients with ACLF are generally hyperdynamic, $S_{cv}O_2$ is usually normal or slightly elevated even in the presence of hypovolemia. An approach to volume resuscitation based on lactate clearance should consider that a damaged liver will clear lactate at a slower pace. This implies that in patients with cirrhosis, the evolution of lactate over time is more important than the absolute value [12].

In patients with cirrhosis, the normal values of dynamic preload indices such as pulse pressure variation (PPV) and stroke volume variation (SVV) can be altered [13]. On the one hand, a low systemic vascular resistance can theoretically alter the aortic compliance and in this way alter the PPV [14, 15]. On the other hand, some authors warn that due to ascites intra-abdominal hypertension could influence these values [13]. However, in our experience this is rarely the case. When aware of these additional limitations, changes in PPV during resuscitation in ACLF remain a useful tool.

More informative tests include thermodilution methods (static) or echocardiography (dynamic). Invasive "calibrated" monitoring devices like PICCO (Getinge, Solna, Sweden) or a Swan Ganz catheter cannot be completely replaced by noninvasive or "uncalibrated"-derived measurements [16, 17]. Only transthoracic echocardiography offers a completely noninvasive alternative for holistic hemodynamic monitoring [1]. In the absence of adequate transthoracic imaging, some authors advocate the use of transesophageal echocardiography claiming a good safety profile in patients with varices up to grade 2 without recent upper gastro-intestinal bleeding [18]. We would however suggest being prudent in this population and would opt for a calibrated intravascular monitoring device in this situation such as PICCO.

Superimposed Shock Syndromes

The two most prevalent types of shock in patients with cirrhosis are septic shock and hemorrhagic/hypovolemic shock [19, 20]. The correct differentiation guides the choice of fluid and timing for the introduction of vasopressors.

Sepsis is the most prevalent reason for admission to ICU of patients with cirrhosis and the index of suspicion of septic shock should always be high [19, 20]. Given the impaired immunity of these patients, early start of antibiotics is suggested when an infection is suspected. Antibiotic prophylaxis in variceal bleeds is highly recommended to avoid spontaneous bacterial peritonitis and subsequent deterioration of ACLF [21]. Fluid resuscitation remains a cornerstone in the management of septic shock as well as in patients with cirrhosis. However, with increasing severity of liver disease, a larger amount of the administered volume will pool in the splanchnic compartment [7]. Therefore, the impact on improved circulatory function will be less than in noncirrhotic patient populations with septic shock. Earlier start of vasopressors to restore perfusion pressure and avoid fluid overload seems appropriate.

Variceal bleeding is the second most common cause of ICU admission in this population, often presenting as a hemorrhagic shock [19, 20]. Aside from attaining source control, correction of coagulation and hemoglobin levels take priority. Red blood cell transfusion above a target of 7 g/dL and platelet transfusion above 50,000 platelets per microliter is recommended [22, 23]. More controversial and more relevant to fluid management is the optimization of coagulation.

While fresh frozen plasma contains all clotting factors, it takes 1 mL/kg of plasma to correct the PT for 1% [24]. This implies that generally a huge volume would be required to normalize coagulation, potentially fueling the variceal bleeding. Given this fact, we would recommend the administration of a much smaller volume of concentrated clotting factors. One should however be aware that specific concentrates lack several clotting factors and consider administration of some fresh frozen plasma to supplement these missing factors.

At the time of writing, there is no validated endpoint for restoration of coagulation. In cirrhosis production of both pro- and antithrombotic, fibrinogenic, and fibrinolytic factors are impaired due to liver injury. During compensated cirrhosis, a new equilibrium is established while PT and aPTT remain impaired [25]. The role of functional testing like TEG or ROTEM in this population during decompensation is still to be determined [26, 27].

Choosing the Right Fluid

As in the general population crystalloids should be used as a first-line treatment in resuscitation. In particular balanced solutions should be preferred to "normal" saline given the known risk of acidosis and kidney failure due to hyperchloremic metabolic acidosis [28].

Although little data exist studying specifically patients with cirrhosis, it seems even more reasonable to opt for balanced solutions in this population given the fact that patients with cirrhosis are prone to developing additional renal failure. It is also known that "normal" saline worsens the formation of ascites and induces other extra-vascular fluid accumulation. It should be noted though that some authors advise against the use of specific balanced solutions such as Ringer lactate or acetate-containing solutions given the decreased metabolic clearance in patients with cirrhosis. Only limited data support these concerns and they appear to be only true for Ringer lactate [29].

As stated in previous chapters there is no place for starches anymore aside from perhaps a perioperative surgical bleed in a non-infectious patient. Resuscitation with starches in septic shock or during variceal bleeding is known to be associated with worsening of hepatic function and renal failure potentially increasing mortality [21].

Albumin has always been a molecule of interest in cirrhosis (Table 21.1). It is produced by the liver and has numerous functions including influencing oncotic pressure, binding, and transport of endogenous and exogeneous substances, antioxidant, antithrombotic, immunomodulatory, anti-inflammatory properties, and endothelial stabilization [3]. Albumin is not recommended as a nutritional support. It should also not be administered to correct hypo-albuminemia per se in the absence of hypovolemia [3]. There are two well-established evidence-based indications for albumin in cirrhosis. First, in the prevention of postparacentesis circulatory dysfunction and prevention of renal vasoconstriction [4, 12]. The AASLD guidelines of 2012 suggest 6–8 g albumin per liter of ascites for paracentesis above 5 L [30]. Second, as part of the treatment of hepatorenal syndrome. A dose of 1 g/kg albumin for 2 days is advised [8]. To limit the fluid load, albumin 20% is preferred to lower concentrations.

The role of albumin during resuscitation is still heavily debated. The ALBIOS trial did not show a mortality benefit at 28 and 90 days after a resuscitation strategy including Albumin 20% administration in a general ICU population to correct serum albumin levels up to 30 g/L. On the other hand, post hoc subgroup analysis in patients with septic shock at enrollment did show a survival advantage in the group treated with albumin at 90 days

Table 21.1 Common reasons for applying albumin. Well-studied indications are in green, indications with soft or conflicting evidence in orange, and wrongful indications in red

Indication albumin	Recommendation
Prevention post paracentesis renal vasoconstriction and circulatory dysfunction	6–8 g albumin per liter of ascites for paracentesis above 5 L
Treatment of a hepatorenal syndrome	1g/kg albumin for 2 days using albumin 20%
Spontaneous bacterial peritonitis to decrease renal impairment	1.5 g/kg on day one and 1 g/kg on day three
Volume resuscitation with albumin 4%	Potential mortality benefit in septic shock compared to saline 0.9%
Aiming at a serum albumin >30 g/L during resuscitation by applying Albumine 20%	Potential mortality benefit in septic shock
Scavenging bacterial products	Evidence is lacking
Keep albumin above 30 g/L in decompensated liver cirrhosis patients with persistent ascites despite diuretic therapy	Mortality benefit in ANSWER trial, but not in MACHT and ATTIRE
Nutritional support to keep albumine >30 g/L	Not recommended for this indication

[31]. The SAFE study compared the administration of fluid boluses of either saline 0.9% or albumin 4% in patients with sepsis. Again at first no difference was observed while a post hoc analysis again showed a trend toward mortality benefit in the subgroup with septic shock. However, all patients in the SAFE study were included after the initial resuscitation phase [32]. This implies there is currently still no evidence supporting the unique use of albumin as a resuscitation fluid.

Recent studies also suggest three potential additional indications for albumin infusion. First, it is claimed that albumin administration can restore the capacity of scavenging bacterial products [4]. Second, albumin administration decreased renal impairment and mortality in patients with spontaneous bacterial peritonitis. A dose of 1.5 g/kg on day one and 1 g/kg on day three is suggested [5]. Finally, the ANSWER trial showed a decreased 18-month mortality in decompensated patients with liver cirrhosis with persistent ascites despite diuretic therapy who were treated with IV albumin on a weekly basis [33]. However, the data of this ANSWER trial were not confirmed by the MACHT study that used lower albumin doses [34]. Furthermore, the recently published ATTIRE study showed no additional benefit of increasing the albumin level above 30 g/L using albumin 20% compared to usual care in patients hospitalized on the normal ward with decompensated liver cirrhosis [35].

At the time of writing a lot of promising studies are awaited. The PRECIOSA study tries to answer the question of which patients can benefit most from long term administration of albumin. This is an unanswered question given the conflicting evidence of the ASNWER trial, the MACHT study, and the ATTIRE study. Furthermore addition of plasmapheresis and DIALIVE (a new device aimed at removing damage associated molecular patterns (DAMPS) and pathogen associated molecular patterns (PAMPS)) are studied and could extend the appropriate indications of albumin [2].

Acute Liver Failure (ALF)

Special Considerations During Resuscitation

Many patients with acute liver failure are admitted to the ICU with intravascular volume depletion due to impaired oral intake caused by vomiting and/or encephalopathy. On the other hand, similar to the patient with ACLF, both volume depletion and liver congestion can lead to hypoxic hepatitis worsening residual liver function or inducing multiple organ failure. Specific to ALF, fluid overload can also increase intracranial hypertension and lead to brain edema and death [36].

As is the case with cirrhotic patients' PT and aPTT values correlate poorly with the bleeding risk given the fact that both procoagulant and anticoagulant factors are impaired. Also in ALF a new equilibrium is often attained [37, 38]. Usually, there is no need for aggressive correction of the deranged coagulation with blood products in order to reduce the bleeding risk. In addition, in the cases listed for liver transplant, the administration of plasma might compromise the eligibility of the patient for transplantation.

For similar reasons as in patients with ACLF, the diagnostic value of $S_{cv}O_2$ or lactate clearance is diminished in ALF. Due to the hyperdynamic circulation, the $S_{cv}O_2$ can be normal or slightly elevated in the presence of hypovolemia [12]. Given the decreased liver function, lactate clearance can be slower and could be more useful as a marker for liver injury [1].

More reliable for fluid management are dynamic maneuvers such as the passive leg raising test, thermodilution methods, pulse contour analysis, or echocardiography. However, during dynamic maneuvers one should be aware of the potential risk of increasing intracranial hypertension [1].

In a cohort study including 35 ALF patients SVV (obtained by PICCO), PPV, and respiratory change in peak left ventricular outflow tract velocity were evaluated for their accuracy to predict fluid responsiveness. In this study, SVV and echocardiographic parameters (inferior vena cava distensibility and LVOT) were poor predictors while PPV using a cutoff of 9% predicted fluid responsiveness with moderate accuracy (area under the receiver operating characteristics AUROC curve 0.75). Of note is that the accuracy of PPV was decreased (AUROC 0.72) in the presence of intra-abdominal hypertension (intra-abdominal pressure above 12 mmHg), which was present in 12 of the 15 patients in whom the abdominal pressure was measured [39]. Before transplantation for ALF, monitoring for intra-abdominal pressure seems to be indicated as rapid formation of ascites can occur with further compromise of the renal function. After transplantation, intra-abdominal hypertension has been described as an independent risk factor for renal failure [40].

Superimposed Shock Syndromes

Patients with acute liver failure are often admitted in a dehydrated state due to impaired oral intake caused by vomiting and encephalopathy [36]. In addition, these patients develop an inflammatory response that is associated with systemic vasodilatation, capillary leak, and increase in insensible fluid loss aggravating this hypovolemia [1]. Given the immune dysfunction in acute liver failure, patients with ALF are at a high risk of combined septic/hypovolemic shock [1]. However, unmasking an infection can be daunting, since patients with acute liver failure are often hyperdynamic at baseline. In this case, it is preferred to introduce a vasopressor at an early stage rather than administering only fluids.

Choosing the Right Fluid

An important complication in ALF is intracranial hypertension. Although hard data are lacking this implies hypotonic fluids could be harmful. To sustain sufficient cerebral perfusion pressure crystalloids are preferred above colloids. Given the decreased metabolizing capacity some authors warn also in ALF against the use of Ringers lactate and acetate-containing balanced solutions. Only limited data support these concerns and they appear to be only true for Ringer lactate [29]. The role of albumin has not been studied in ALF.

> **Case Vignette**
>
> A 45-year-old male with a CHILD C liver cirrhosis is admitted to the ICU following a variceal hemorrhage. During stabilization, he received 1 L of balanced crystalloids. The bleeding was stopped after variceal ligations. High-dose PPI and Terlipressin were initiated. At this time he is still hypotensive 80/35 mmHg (MAP 50 mmHg), and has marked peripheral edema, ascites, and an $S_{cv}O_2$ of 75%. He feels peripheral cold and has mottled skin. When applying a passive leg raise his blood pressure increases to 90/40 (MAP 59 mmHg). The lactate level is 15 mmol/L.

Conclusion

Acute liver failure and acute on chronic liver failure are characterized by decreased systemic vascular resistance, increased cardiac output, central functional hypovolemia, increased arterial compliance, and peripheral vasodilatation. The importance of adequate fluid management in liver failure cannot be overstressed since both hypervolemia and hypovolemia can further compromise the residual liver function.

In cirrhosis, the average circulating blood volume is higher than in a healthy person and it is more unevenly distributed between the central and abdominal compartments with increasing severity of cirrhosis. Assessment of the intravascular volume status in these patients is not simple. Focus on the dynamics of change is important. Resuscitation techniques based on changes in lactate and $S_{cv}O_2$ are less useful in patients with liver failure. The most robust dynamic tests include the use of thermodilution methods or echocardiography. The two most prevalent types of shock in patients with cirrhosis are septic shock and hemorrhagic shock. The correct differentiation guides the choice of fluid and timing for the introduction of vasopressors. Generally, strategies that reduce the need for large fluid volume administration via the earlier start of vasopressors or by administration of clotting factor concentrates seem more appropriate. As in the general population, balanced crystalloids should be used as a first-line treatment in resuscitation. There is some evidence suggesting against the use of ringer lactate. Albumin should also not be administered to correct hypo-albuminemia per se. The benefits of albumin are undeniable when applied in the setting of paracentesis or treatment of hepatorenal syndrome. The role of albumin during resuscitation is still heavily debated. At the time of writing promising studies are performed that will further impact the indications for albumin use in this population.

In acute liver failure many patients are admitted to the ICU with intravascular volume depletion due to impaired oral intake caused by vomiting and/or encephalopathy. Specific in ALF fluid overload can also increase intracranial hypertension and lead to brain edema and death. Dynamic maneuvers such as the passive leg raising test, thermodilution methods, pulse contour analysis, and echocardiography are most suitable to evaluate the fluid status and fluid responsiveness. Of these tests, the passive leg raising test could increase intracranial pressure. Although hard data are lacking hypotonic fluids could theoretically increase intracranial pressure in ALF and might be better avoided. Balanced crystalloids are generally the fluid of choice in ALF.

Questions and Answers

Q1. Would you administer this patient an extra fluid bolus?

A1. Yes, the hypotensive state with positive passive leg raising test and cold mottled skin suggest an unresolved functional hypovolemia and fluid responsiveness. The high $S_{cv}O_2$ can be attributed to the hyperdynamic circulation due to cirrhosis. Patients with cirrhosis can be intravascularly volume-depleted while showing signs of edema and ascites. However, the effect after fluid administration should be evaluated since administering too much fluid can aggravate ascites formation, edema, cardiac dysfunction, and even increase portal hypertension and restart gastro-intestinal bleeding.

Q2. What could help you decide between the administration of fluids or application of either inotropes or vasopressors.

A2. Advanced hemodynamic monitoring can be applied when in doubt. As a non-invasive technique, an echocardiography can be performed. Alternatively, calibrated invasive techniques such as PICCO or Swann Ganz can be applied.

Q3. What would you do if the lactate level decreased to only 10 mmol/L after 6 h despite your best efforts?

A3. Continue surveilling the patient, but wait patiently as long as lactate is decreasing and there are no signs of evolving end organ failure. Lactate could be a marker for the severity of liver disease rather than a marker of unresolved shock. A slowly decreasing lactate level should not necessarily lead to continued aggressive administration of fluids.

Take Home Messages

- Liver cirrhosis is characterized by decreased systemic vascular resistance, increased cardiac output, central functional hypovolemia, increased arterial compliance, and peripheral vasodilatation.
- Over-resuscitation with IV fluids can aggravate ascites formation, edema, hyponatremia, cardiac dysfunction, and intra-abdominal hypertension. Fluid accumulation and overload can also increase portal hypertension and induce gastrointestinal bleeding in this population.
- Most static parameters are less useful in cirrhosis. Given the generally hyperdynamic state of cirrhotic patients $S_{cv}O_2$ is less useful to assess cardiac output in cirrhosis. Likewise lactate clearance is often impaired due to liver damage.
- Advanced hemodynamic monitoring techniques favoring dynamics of change are valuable tools to optimize fluid therapy. These include the "calibrated" PICCO and Swann Ganz as well as transthoracic echocardiography.

References

1. Weiss E, Paugam-Burtz C, Jaber S. Shock etiologies and fluid management in liver failure. Semin Respir Crit Care Med. 2018;39(5):538–45.
2. Bernardi M, Angeli P, Claria J, Moreau R, Gines P, Jalan R, et al. Albumin in decompensated cirrhosis: new concepts and perspectives. Gut. 2020;69(6):1127–38.
3. Caraceni P, Domenicali M, Tovoli A, Napoli L, Ricci CS, Tufoni M, et al. Clinical indications for the albumin use: still a controversial issue. Eur J Intern Med. 2013;24(8):721–8.
4. Jalan R, Schnurr K, Mookerjee RP, Sen S, Cheshire L, Hodges S, et al. Alterations in the functional capacity of albumin in patients with decompensated cirrhosis is associated with increased mortality. Hepatology. 2009;50(2):555–64.
5. Thévenot T, Bureau C, Oberti F, Anty R, Louvet A, Plessier A, et al. Effect of albumin in cirrhotic patients with infection other than spontaneous bacterial peritonitis. A randomized trial. J Hepatol. 2015;62(4):822–30.
6. Schrier RW, Arroyo V, Bernardi M, Epstein M, Henriksen JH, Rodés J. Peripheral arterial vasodilation hypothesis: a proposal for the initiation of renal sodium and water retention in cirrhosis. Hepatology. 1988;8(5):1151–7.
7. Møller S, Bendtsen F, Henriksen JH. Effect of volume expansion on systemic hemodynamics and central and arterial blood volume in cirrhosis. Gastroenterology. 1995;109(6):1917–25.
8. easloffice@easloffice.eu, European Association for the Study of the Liver. EASL clinical practice guidelines for the management of patients with decompensated cirrhosis. J Hepatol. 2018;69(2):406–60.
9. Kiszka-Kanowitz M, Henriksen JH, Møller S, Bendtsen F. Blood volume distribution in patients with cirrhosis: aspects of the dual-head gamma-camera technique. J Hepatol. 2001;35(5):605–12.
10. Henriksen JH, Bendtsen F, Sørensen TI, Stadeager C, Ring-Larsen H. Reduced central blood volume in cirrhosis. Gastroenterology. 1989;97(6):1506–13.
11. Nadim MK, Durand F, Kellum JA, Levitsky J, O'Leary JG, Karvellas CJ, et al. Management of the critically ill patient with cirrhosis: a multidisciplinary perspective. J Hepatol. 2016;64(3):717–35.
12. Canabal JM, Kramer DJ. Management of sepsis in patients with liver failure. Curr Opin Crit Care. 2008;14(2):189–97.
13. Feltracco P, Biancofiore G, Ori C, Saner FH, Della Rocca G. Limits and pitfalls of haemodynamic monitoring systems in liver transplantation surgery. Minerva Anestesiol. 2012;78(12):1372–84.
14. Biancofiore G, Critchley LA, Lee A, Yang XX, Bindi LM, Esposito M, et al. Evaluation of a new software version of the FloTrac/Vigileo (version 3.02) and a comparison with previous data in cirrhotic patients undergoing liver transplant surgery. Anesth Analg. 2011;113(3):515–22.
15. Gouvêa G, Diaz R, Auler L, Toledo R, Martinho JM. Evaluation of the pulse pressure variation index as a predictor of fluid responsiveness during orthotopic liver transplantation. Br J Anaesth. 2009;103(2):238–43.
16. Bernards J, Mekeirele M, Hoffmann B, Peeters Y, De Raes M, Malbrain ML. Hemodynamic monitoring: to calibrate or not to calibrate? Part 2—non-calibrated techniques. Anaesthesiol Intensive Ther. 2015;47(5):501–16.
17. Peeters Y, Bernards J, Mekeirele M, Hoffmann B, De Raes M, Malbrain ML. Hemodynamic monitoring: to calibrate or not to calibrate? Part 1—calibrated techniques. Anaesthesiol Intensive Ther. 2015;47(5):487–500.
18. Dalia AA, Flores A, Chitilian H, Fitzsimons MG. A comprehensive review of transesophageal echocardiography during orthotopic liver transplantation. J Cardiothorac Vasc Anesth. 2018;32(4):1815–24.

19. Das V, Boelle PY, Galbois A, Guidet B, Maury E, Carbonell N, et al. Cirrhotic patients in the medical intensive care unit: early prognosis and long-term survival. Crit Care Med. 2010;38(11):2108–16.
20. Moreau R, Jalan R, Gines P, Pavesi M, Angeli P, Cordoba J, et al. Acute-on-chronic liver failure is a distinct syndrome that develops in patients with acute decompensation of cirrhosis. Gastroenterology. 2013;144(7):1426–37, 37.e1–9.
21. Li Y, Zhang CQ. Management of variceal hemorrhage. Gastroenterology Res. 2009;2(1):8–19.
22. Villanueva C, Colomo A, Bosch A, Concepción M, Hernandez-Gea V, Aracil C, et al. Transfusion strategies for acute upper gastrointestinal bleeding. N Engl J Med. 2013;368(1):11–21.
23. (UK) NCGC. Acute upper gastrointestinal bleeding: management. 2012.
24. Puetz J. Fresh frozen plasma: the most commonly prescribed hemostatic agent. J Thromb Haemost. 2013;11(10):1794–9.
25. Lisman T, Porte RJ. Rebalanced hemostasis in patients with liver disease: evidence and clinical consequences. Blood. 2010;116(6):878–85.
26. Kumar M, Ahmad J, Maiwall R, Choudhury A, Bajpai M, Mitra LG, et al. Thromboelastography-guided blood component use in patients with cirrhosis with nonvariceal bleeding: a randomized controlled trial. Hepatology. 2020;71(1):235–46.
27. Lentschener C, Flaujac C, Ibrahim F, Gouin-Thibault I, Bazin M, Sogni P, et al. Assessment of haemostasis in patients with cirrhosis: relevance of the ROTEM tests?: a prospective, cross-sectional study. Eur J Anaesthesiol. 2016;33(2):126–33.
28. Semler MW, Self WH, Rice TW. Balanced crystalloids versus saline in critically ill adults. N Engl J Med. 2018;378(20):1951.
29. Ergin B, Kapucu A, Guerci P, Ince C. The role of bicarbonate precursors in balanced fluids during haemorrhagic shock with and without compromised liver function. Br J Anaesth. 2016;117(4):521–8.
30. Runyon BA, AASLD. Introduction to the revised American Association for the Study of Liver Diseases practice guideline management of adult patients with ascites due to cirrhosis 2012. Hepatology. 2013;57(4):1651–3.
31. Caironi P, Tognoni G, Gattinoni L. Albumin replacement in severe sepsis or septic shock. N Engl J Med. 2014;371(1):84.
32. Finfer S, Bellomo R, Boyce N, French J, Myburgh J, Norton R, et al. A comparison of albumin and saline for fluid resuscitation in the intensive care unit. N Engl J Med. 2004;350(22):2247–56.
33. Caraceni P, Riggio O, Angeli P, Alessandria C, Neri S, Foschi FG, et al. Long-term albumin administration in decompensated cirrhosis (ANSWER): an open-label randomised trial. Lancet. 2018;391(10138):2417–29.
34. Solà E, Solé C, Simón-Talero M, Martín-Llahí M, Castellote J, Garcia-Martínez R, et al. Midodrine and albumin for prevention of complications in patients with cirrhosis awaiting liver transplantation. A randomized placebo-controlled trial. J Hepatol. 2018;69(6):1250–9.
35. China L, Freemantle N, Forrest E, Kallis Y, Ryder SD, Wright G, et al. A randomized trial of albumin infusions in hospitalized patients with cirrhosis. N Engl J Med. 2021;384(9):808–17.
36. Trotter JF. Practical management of acute liver failure in the intensive care unit. Curr Opin Crit Care. 2009;15(2):163–7.
37. Hugenholtz GC, Adelmeijer J, Meijers JC, Porte RJ, Stravitz RT, Lisman T. An unbalance between von Willebrand factor and ADAMTS13 in acute liver failure: implications for hemostasis and clinical outcome. Hepatology. 2013;58(2):752–61.
38. Lisman T, Bakhtiari K, Adelmeijer J, Meijers JC, Porte RJ, Stravitz RT. Intact thrombin generation and decreased fibrinolytic capacity in patients with acute liver injury or acute liver failure. J Thromb Haemost. 2012;10(7):1312–9.

39. Audimoolam VK, McPhail MJ, Willars C, Bernal W, Wendon JA, Cecconi M, et al. Predicting fluid responsiveness in acute liver failure: a prospective study. Anesth Analg. 2017;124(2):480–6.

40. Shu M, Peng C, Chen H, Shen B, Zhou G, Shen C, et al. Intra-abdominal hypertension is an independent cause of acute renal failure after orthotopic liver transplantation. Front Med China. 2007;1(2):167–72.

Fluid Management in Intra-abdominal Hypertension

22

Manu L. N. G. Malbrain [ID], Prashant Nasa, Inneke De laet,
Jan De Waele, Rita Jacobs, Robert Wise, Luca Malbrain,
Wojciech Dabrowski, and Adrian Wong

Manu L. N. G. Malbrain (✉) · W. Dabrowski
First Department of Anaesthesiology and Intensive Therapy, Medical University of Lublin,
Lublin, Poland
e-mail: wojciech.dabrowski@umlub.pl

P. Nasa
Critical Care Medicine, Prevention and Infection Control, NMC Specialty Hospital,
Dubai, United Arab Emirates
e-mail: dr.prashantnasa@hotmail.com

I. De laet
Intensive Care Unit, Ziekenhuis Netwerk Antwerpen, ZNA Stuivenberg, Antwerp, Belgium
e-mail: inneke.delaet@zna.be

J. De Waele
Intensive Care Unit, Universitair Ziekenhuis Gent, Ghent, Belgium
e-mail: jan.dewaele@ugent.be

R. Jacobs
Intensive Care Unit, Universitair Ziekenhuis Antwerpen, Antwerp, Belgium

R. Wise
Discipline of Anaesthesia and Critical Care, School of Clinical Medicine, University of
KwaZulu-Natal, Durban, South Africa

Intensive Care Department, Oxford University Trust Hospitals, John Radcliffe Hospital,
Oxford, UK

L. Malbrain
University School of Medicine, Katholieke Universiteit Leuven (KUL), Leuven, Belgium

A. Wong
Intensive Care and Anaesthesia, King's College Hospital NHS Foundation Trust, London, UK
e-mail: adrian.wong@nhs.net

Contents

Introduction.. 430
Definitions... 431
   Intra-abdominal Pressure.. 431
   Intra-abdominal Hypertension and Abdominal Compartment Syndrome....................... 431
   Hemodynamic Effects and Impact on End-Organ Function.. 432
   Globally Increased Permeability Syndrome... 432
Fluids and IAH... 433
   Why Do We Like Fluids in IAH?.. 433
   Understanding the Linkage Between Over Fluids and IAH?... 434
   Do Patients with IAH Have a More Positive Fluid Balance?... 436
      Relation Between Fluids and IAH in Severe Burn Patients...................................... 436
      Relation Between Fluids and IAH in Severe Acute Pancreatitis............................... 437
      Relation Between Fluids and IAH in Trauma Patients... 438
      Relation Between Fluids and IAH in Mixed ICU Patients....................................... 438
   Does IAP Improve with Interventions Acting on Reducing Fluid Balance?................... 442
Conclusion... 451
References.. 452

IFA Commentary

There is a relationship between fluid resuscitation, fluid accumulation and secondary intrabdominal hypertension (IAH). Evidence supports this relationship in patients with sepsis, acute pancreatitis, severe burn injury, emergency surgery and severe trauma. Among the fluids, crystalloids are more likely to contribute to a cumulative positive balance and IAH, compared to colloids and hypertonic solutions. IAP should be measured during fluid resuscitation using a bladder catheter with an infusion of no more than 25 mL 0.9% saline. Overzealous fluid administration can lead to secondary IAH and venous congestion and may affect any organ of the body. The effect of IAH on the gut includes intestinal edema, mesenteric vein compression, decreased perfusion, bacterial translocation and disruption of the gut microbiome. The development of IAH is usually associated with worse patient outcomes. Fluid stewardship is recommended for the use of IV fluids during different phases based on the ROSE model. The IAH can be managed with medical management. De-resuscitation with active fluid removal may require diuretics or ultrafiltration in a few cases. However, the timing of renal replacement therapy during resuscitation is currently unclear. Surgical decompression or escharotomy may be required in case of (primary) abdominal compartment syndrome.

Learning Objectives

After reading this chapter, you will:

1. Understand the pathophysiology of intra-abdominal hypertension (IAH) and abdominal compartment syndrome (ACS).
2. Understanding the terminology, primary and secondary IAH, ACS, and discussing global increased permeability syndrome (GIPS) and capillary leak.
3. Recognize fluid resuscitation as one of the major risk factors leading to increased intra-abdominal pressure (IAP) and secondary IAH and ACS.
4. Comprehend that as venous return is already impeded in IAH the combination of positive pressure ventilation and PEEP may lead to dramatic effects on cardiovascular and kidney function.
5. Learn that fluids should initially be titrated based on volumetric preload indicators and functional hemodynamic parameters and they should be tapered when IAP increases.
6. Understand that during the deresuscitation phase, in selected patients there may be a potential place for hypertonic solutions (like hypertonic lactated saline or albumin 20%) together with a combination treatment of diuretics or ultrafiltration via renal replacement therapy.
7. Learn that patients treated with an open abdomen may lose substantial amounts of fluids and nitrogen (hypercatabolic) which needs to be substituted with isotonic replacement fluids and nutritional support.

Case Vignette

A 42-year-old male with a body mass index of 23 kg/m^2 and no relevant past medical history was admitted to the surgical intensive care unit (ICU) after a pneumonectomy, pericardectomy and partial thoracic wall resection for invasive pulmonary cancer. After admission to the ICU, the patient remained in refractory shock. A surgical revision was performed on the first postoperative day (POD 1) where diffuse oozing was found but no significant bleeding. Over the next 5 postoperative days, the patient developed a significant capillary leak syndrome with intravascular underfilling and extravascular (interstitial) fluid accumulation. There was increased pulse pressure variation (PPV) above 20%, a positive passive leg raising test, fluid responsive hypotension (after a bolus of 4 mL/kg intravenous fluid), need for inotropes (dobutamine) and vasopressors (norepinephrine at a dose of 0.4 μg/kg/min), and worsening renal function.

Questions

Q1. What fluids should be administered?

Intravenous fluids were given liberally (mainly balanced crystalloids but in the operating room 2 L of saline was given over 30 min) and the cumulative fluid balance reached on POD 7 was in excess of 10 L. During the first postoperative week, intra-abdominal pressure (IAP) increased daily from 14 mmHg until it reached 29 mmHg on POD 8, confirming the diagnosis of secondary abdominal compartment syndrome (, i.e., IAP >20 mmHg with new or deteriorating organ dysfunction, caused by pathology outside the abdominal cavity).

Q2. How do you interpret the increased PPV in the setting of ACS?

The clinical condition of the patient deteriorated further with impaired oxygenation despite lung protective ventilation and a continuous infusion of neuromuscular blockade (cisatracurium). Nitric oxide ventilation was attempted (because of pulmonary hypertension on transesophageal echocardiography) with only partial success and the patient progressed to anuria. At this time, a decompressive laparotomy (DL) was performed at the bedside in the ICU, which revealed no intra-abdominal abnormalities. Immediately after opening the peritoneum, a dramatic improvement in ventilation parameters and oxygenation was observed, and diuresis resumed.

Q3. Were all medical management options used before DL?

A Bogota bag was used for temporary abdominal closure, followed by placement of a vacuum-assisted closure (VAC) dressing 2 days later. Each day, around 4 L of fluid were drained via the VAC system.

Q4. Do you have any concerns regarding the interstitial (third) space fluid losses?

Despite the initial improvement after decompressive laparotomy, renal function deteriorated again and continuous venovenous hemofiltration (CVVH) with ultrafiltration was started at POD 13. The vasopressor dose remained at a low level (0.05 μg/kg/min norepinephrine), and ventilator support could be kept at low levels throughout the remainder of the patient's clinical course.

Q5. Is there a role for hypertonic solutions and diuretics in this patient?

Introduction

Intra-abdominal hypertension (IAH) occurs in 25% of critically ill patients on admission and it is an independent risk factor for morbidity and mortality. About one patient in two will develop IAH at some point within the first week of ICU stay while 5% will develop full-blown abdominal compartment syndrome (ACS) as will be discussed further. Different risk factors for IAH have been identified and studied and fluid resuscitation is one of them. This paper will look at the relationship between overzealous fluid administration and the development of secondary IAH and ACS. Chap. 25 will discuss fluid accumulation syndrome and deresuscitation.

This chapter will focus on adult patients, and more information on fluid therapy in children can be found in Chap. 20. Some other chapters will discuss fluids in specific populations: sepsis (Chap. 14), heart failure (Chap. 15), trauma (Chap. 16), neurocritical care (Chap. 17), perioperative setting (Chap. 18), burns (Chap. 19), liver failure (Chap. 21), and COVID-19 (Chap. 26).

Definitions

Intra-abdominal Pressure

The IAP is the steady-state pressure concealed within the abdominal cavity [1]. The IAP can be directly measured via the intraperitoneal cavity either via a Verres needle connected to a pressure transducer during laparoscopy, during chronic ambulatory peritoneal dialysis or in the case of paracentesis for tense ascites. However, the gold standard for intermittent IAP estimation is via the bladder with a maximal instillation of 20–25 mL (1 mL/kg in children up to 10 kg) of sterile saline through a urinary catheter. The transducer should be zeroed at the level where the midaxillary line crosses the iliac crest and IAP should be expressed in mmHg (conversion factor from mmHg to cmH_2O is 1.36). IAP should be measured at end-expiration in the supine position whilst abdominal muscle contractions are absent. Normal IAP is approximately 5–7 mmHg in adults, and around 10 mmHg in critically ill patients, but depends on body weight and level of obesity [2]. After abdominal surgery, IAP is usually around 12–14 mmHg.

Intra-abdominal Hypertension and Abdominal Compartment Syndrome

According to the Abdominal Compartment Society (WSACS, www.wsacs.org), intra-abdominal hypertension (IAH) is defined as a sustained increase in IAP equal to or greater than 12 mmHg [1]. IAH can be further classified into primary, secondary or tertiary IAH [1]. Primary IAH originates from injury or disease within the abdominopelvic cavity (e.g., a ruptured abdominal aortic aneurysm, bowel perforation and spleen rupture), whereas secondary IAH results from conditions that have an extra-abdominal origin (e.g., sepsis, major burns or other conditions requiring massive fluid resuscitation) [3]. Tertiary IAH refers to the more chronic condition of an open and frozen abdomen after initial treatment for either primary or secondary IAH. IAH is graded as follows: grade I between 12 and 15 mmHg, grade II between 15 and 20 mmHg, grade III between 20 and 25 mmHg, and grade IV are IAP values above 25 mmHg. Abdominal compartment syndrome (ACS) is defined as a sustained increase in IAP above 20 mmHg that is associated with new organ dysfunction/failure. The abdominal perfusion pressure (APP), ideally a value higher than 60 mmHg, is calculated by subtracting the IAP from the mean arterial pressure (MAP).

Hemodynamic Effects and Impact on End-Organ Function

The presence of IAH leads to elevation of the diaphragm, which increases intrathoracic pressure and compromises cardiac function by decreasing preload and cardiac output and increasing afterload [4]. Moreover, the rise in intrathoracic pressure also affects pulmonary function [5] and may lead to intracranial hypertension due to functional obstruction of cerebral venous outflow [6]. The development of renal dysfunction due to increased IAP is attributed to compression of the renal veins and arteries, decreased renal arterial blood flow, venous congestion and reduced cardiac output. The gut seems to be particularly vulnerable to increases in IAP. Besides a reduction in arterial perfusion of intra-abdominal organs, IAH leads to a compression of mesenteric veins causing venous hypertension, intestinal edema and ileus (Fig. 22.1).

The pathophysiological impact of elevated IAP on the various organ systems mimics a state similar to sepsis. To restore hemodynamic stability, fluid resuscitation is often the first choice. However, administering large amounts of fluids may result in secondary IAH and ACS. The increased IAP stimulates anti-diuretic hormone (ADH), further promoting fluid retention [7] as well as renin-angiotensin-aldosterone release [8]. Besides the main impact on cardiorespiratory function, IAH affects all organ functions within and outside the abdominal cavity [9].

Globally Increased Permeability Syndrome

As a result of the pathological changes associated with injury, capillary permeability increases, causing a loss of colloid oncotic pressure and net extravasation of fluid to the

Fig. 22.1 The vicious pathophysiological cycle of fluid overload leads to intra-abdominal hypertension and abdominal compartment syndrome with subsequent kidney dysfunction. *ACS* abdominal compartment syndrome, *CO* cardiac output, *IAH* intra-abdominal hypertension, *MOF* multiple organ failure, *VCI* vena cava inferior

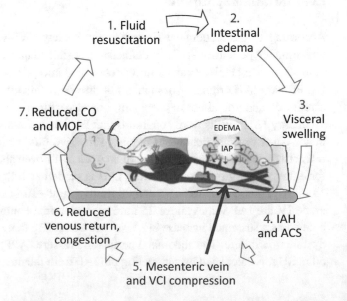

interstitial and intracellular spaces [10]. Isotonic, hypotonic and small molecular weight (colloid) solutions (including albumin) have been shown to leak across the capillary bed causing edema. These fluid shifts are magnified by conventional fluid resuscitation protocols and may lead to visceral edema. In the lungs, fluid extravasation and increased permeability of the pulmonary capillaries can lead to pulmonary edema and increased extravascular lung water. In the GI tract, splanchnic edema can increase IAP and cause a decrease in tissue oxygenation, increased gut susceptibility to infection, impaired wound healing and ileus. Therefore administering intravenous fluids potentially induces a vicious cycle, where interstitial edema induces organ dysfunction that contributes to fluid accumulation (Fig. 22.1). Peripheral and generalized edema is not only of cosmetic concern, as believed by some, but it is harmful to the patient as a whole and can cause organ edema and deterioration in organ function. Some patients will not progress to the "flow" phase spontaneously and will remain in a persistent state of global increased permeability syndrome and ongoing fluid accumulation. The global increased permeability syndrome can hence be defined as fluid overload in combination with new-onset organ failure. This is referred to as "the third hit of shock" [11]. The percentage of fluid accumulation is calculated by dividing the cumulative fluid balance in litres by the patient's baseline body weight and multiplying it by 100. Fluid overload is defined at any stage of illness as greater than 10% fluid accumulation and is associated with worse outcomes [12]. Studies demonstrate an association between fluid overload, illustrated by the increase in the cumulative fluid balance and worse outcomes in critically ill patients with septic shock.

Fluids and IAH

Why Do We Like Fluids in IAH?

Fluids are a double-edged sword, especially in patients with IAH. The importance of increasing circulating blood volume in patients with IAH and ACS has been known for decades, and the implementation of guidelines and protocols for fluid management in sepsis has saved countless lives. However, is this really always the case? Burn resuscitation is a well-known example, where mortality was significantly decreased using aggressive crystalloid resuscitation. In recent years the pendulum has swung back toward a more cautious approach to fluid resuscitation as the deleterious effects of fluid accumulation became apparent. In fact, most burn resuscitation guidelines are still based on the Parkland formula published in the 1960s and guided by crude static markers such as arterial pressure, central venous pressure or urine output. In another example, septic shock is managed with fluid resuscitation at a dose of 30 mL/kg that can be started within the first hour. This is the first and foremost therapeutic action recommended in the Surviving Sepsis Campaign Guidelines [13]. The problem is not in the fluid per se but in the dose, timing and protocols that guide our treatment. Understanding of the pathophysiology has improved and more sophisticated and reliable devices for monitoring have recently been developed, challenging previous concepts of fluid resuscitation and responsiveness.

Recently, the phenomenon of 'fluid creep' has also been described in critically ill patients [14]. In their study of 14,654 patients during their cumulative ICU stay of 103,098 days, Van Regenmortel et al. found that maintenance and replacement fluids accounted for 24.7% of the mean daily total fluid volume, far exceeding resuscitation fluids (6.5%) and were the most important sources of sodium and chloride overload. Fluid creep represented 32.6% of the mean daily total fluid volume. Therefore, in septic patients, non-resuscitation fluids had a larger absolute impact on cumulative fluid balance than resuscitation fluids. Recently, more attention is being paid to the different phases of IV fluid management (and the ROSE concept). However, we must pay attention that the pendulum is not swinging back toward more restrictive fluid management and the use of early vasopressors [15–17]. The final results of the ongoing RADAR-2 and CLASSIC trials will shed more light on this topic [16, 18].

Understanding the Linkage Between Over Fluids and IAH?

The dangers of under-resuscitation in terms of the amount or timing of fluid administration are clear, but the adverse effects of over-resuscitation, especially using crystalloids, are only recently being recognized. There is increasing evidence that IAH may be the missing link between over-resuscitation, multi-organ failure and death [19, 20]. Risk factors for the development of IAH and definitions related to IAH and ACS as published by the World Society for the abdominal compartment syndrome are listed in Table 22.1 [3].

Secondary ACS has been described in trauma, burns and sepsis. The multi-centre studies on the prevalence and incidence of IAH in mixed ICU patients also showed that a positive net fluid balance as well as a positive cumulative fluid balance were predictors for poor outcomes, whereas non-survivors had a positive cumulative fluid balance [21, 22]. Similar results have also been found by Alsous where at least 1 day of negative fluid balance ($\leq$−500 mL) achieved by the third day of treatment was a good independent

Table 22.1 Risk factors for intra-abdominal hypertension

A. Related to diminished abdominal wall compliance
– Mechanical ventilation, especially dyssynchrony with the ventilator and the use of accessory muscles
– Use of positive end expiratory pressure (PEEP) or the presence of auto-PEEP
– Basal pleuropneumonia
– High body mass index
– Pneumoperitoneum
– Abdominal (vascular) surgery, especially with tight abdominal closures
– Pneumatic anti-shock garments
– Prone and other body positioning
– Abdominal wall bleeding or rectus sheath hematomas
– Correction of large hernias, gastroschisis or omphalocele
– Burns with abdominal eschars

Table 22.1 (continued)

B. Related to increased intra-abdominal contents

- Gastroparesis
- Gastric distention
- Ileus
- Volvulus
- Colonic pseudo-obstruction
- Abdominal tumour
- Retroperitoneal/abdominal wall hematoma
- Enteral feeding
- Intra-abdominal or retroperitoneal tumor
- Damage control laparotomy

C. Related to abdominal collections of fluid, air or blood

- Liver dysfunction with ascites
- Abdominal infection (pancreatitis, peritonitis, abscess,…)
- Haemoperitoneum
- Pneumoperitoneum
- Laparoscopy with excessive inflation pressures
- Major trauma
- Peritoneal dialysis

D. Related to capillary leak and fluid resuscitation

- Acidosis[a] (pH below 7.2)
- Hypothermia[a] (core temperature below 33 °C)
- Coagulopathy[a] (platelet count below 50,000/mm³ OR an activated partial thromboplastin time (APTT) more than two times normal OR a prothrombin time (PTT) below 50% OR an international standardized ratio (INR) more than 1.5)
- Polytransfusion / trauma (>10 units of packed red cells/24 h)
- Sepsis (as defined by the American-European Consensus Conference definitions)
- Severe sepsis or bacteraemia
- Septic shock
- Massive fluid resuscitation (> 5 L of colloid or >10 L of crystalloid/24 h with capillary leak and positive fluid balance)
- Major burns

Adapted with permission from Kirkpatrick et al. [1]

[a] The combination of acidosis, hypothermia and coagulopathy has been called the deadly triad of trauma

predictor of survival in patients with septic shock [23]. However, one must be aware of potential confounders (pre-resuscitation status, ongoing (abdominal) sepsis, comorbidities, etc.) as this was a retrospective observational study. In light of this increasing body of evidence regarding the association between massive fluid resuscitation, intra-abdominal hypertension, organ dysfunction and mortality, it seems wise to at least incorporate IAP as a parameter in all future studies regarding fluid management and to question current clinical practice guidelines, not in terms of whether to administer intravenous fluids at all, but in terms of the parameters we use to guide our treatment.

Do Patients with IAH Have a More Positive Fluid Balance?

A recent systematic review combining pooled data was available from 1517 patients obtained from an individual patient meta-analysis and seven cohort or case-controlled studies [12]. The pooled results revealed that the 597 patients with IAH (incidence being 39.4%) had a more positive fluid balance than those without IAH (7777.9 ± 3803 mL versus 4389.3 ± 1996.4 mL) (Fig. 22.2). The cumulative fluid balance after 1 week of ICU stay was on average 3388.6 ± 2324.2 mL more positive. The Forest plot is shown in Fig. 22.3.

An extensive review of the literature (between 1999 and 2020) identified 32 prospective studies investigating the relationship between intravenous fluids and IAH. We will briefly discuss the data obtained from the literature review in relation to different patient populations.

Relation Between Fluids and IAH in Severe Burn Patients

O' Mara et al. compared crystalloid and colloid resuscitation regimens in patients with massive burns [24]. Patients in the crystalloid group received more fluids per kilogram body weight, both in the first 24 h and during the whole course of resuscitation. This led to a significantly higher increase in IAP. Ruiz-Castilla et al., studied 25 severely burned

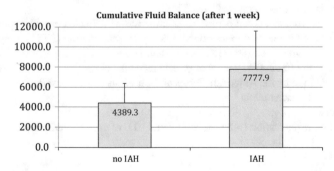

Fig. 22.2 Bar graph showing mean cumulative fluid balance after 1 week of intensive care unit (ICU) stay. Light grey bars showing data in patients without intra-abdominal hypertension, IAH (left) vs those with IAH (right). (Adapted from Malbrain et al. with permission [12])

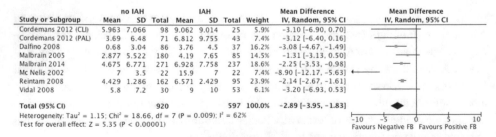

Study or Subgroup	no IAH Mean	SD	Total	IAH Mean	SD	Total	Weight	Mean Difference IV, Random, 95% CI
Cordemans 2012 (CLI)	5.963	7.066	98	9.062	9.014	25	5.9%	-3.10 [-6.90, 0.70]
Cordemans 2012 (PAL)	3.69	6.48	71	6.812	9.755	43	7.4%	-3.12 [-6.40, 0.16]
Dalfino 2008	0.68	3.04	86	3.76	4.5	37	16.2%	-3.08 [-4.67, -1.49]
Malbrain 2005	2.877	5.522	180	4.19	7.65	85	14.5%	-1.31 [-3.13, 0.50]
Malbrain 2014	4.675	6.771	271	6.928	7.758	237	18.6%	-2.25 [-3.53, -0.98]
Mc Nelis 2002	7	3.5	22	15.9	7	22	7.4%	-8.90 [-12.17, -5.63]
Reintam 2008	4.429	1.286	162	6.571	2.429	95	23.9%	-2.14 [-2.67, -1.61]
Vidal 2008	5.8	7.2	30	9	10	53	6.1%	-3.20 [-6.93, 0.53]
Total (95% CI)			920			597	100.0%	-2.89 [-3.95, -1.83]

Heterogeneity: Tau² = 1.15; Chi² = 18.66, df = 7 (P = 0.009); I² = 62%
Test for overall effect: Z = 5.35 (P < 0.00001)

Favours Negative FB   Favours Positive FB

Fig. 22.3 Forest plot looking at cumulative fluid balance after 1 week of ICU stay in patients with and without intra-abdominal hypertension (IAH). (Updated and adapted from Malbrain et al. [12])

Table 22.2 Summary of studies in burn patients examining the relation between fluid resuscitation and IAH

Author, year	Patients	Findings
O'Mara et al., 2005 [24]	$n = 31$ Crystalloid ($n = 15$) vs. plasma ($n = 16$) resuscitation group	More resuscitation fluids administered (ml/kg), more IAH and more end-organ damage in crystalloid group
Ruiz-Castilla et al., 2014 [25]	n = 25 (>20% TBSA)	More IV fluids are given in IAH patients in the first 24 h after burns unit admission
Oda et al., 2006 [26]	n = 36 (≥40% TBSA) Hypertonic lactated saline (n = 14) Ringer's lactate (n = 22)	Hypertonic lactated saline resuscitation can reduce the risk of secondary ACS with lower fluid load in burn shock than with Ringer's lactate solution
Mbiine et al., 2017 [29]	n = 64 (adults and children)	More IAH among the fluid-overloaded patients; difference not significant, probably due to small sample size
Wise et al., 2016 [30]	n = 56 severely burned adults	Higher incidence of IAH, with positive cumulative fluid balance in non-survivors
Küntscher et al., 2006 [28]	n = 16	Poor correlation between IAP and total blood volume index. This was not primarily investigated and was one of the secondary endpoints.
Oda et al., 2006 [27]	n = 48	Extensively burned patients who required large volumes of fluid, especially when in excess of 300 mL/kg/24 h, show a high incidence of complication with ACS

adult patients and found that the prevalence of IAH was higher in patients with >20% TBSA burned. Also, the patients with IAH received significantly more crystalloids in the first 24 h after admission [25]. Similarly, Oda and co-workers found that in shock associated with burn, fluid resuscitation with low-volume hypertonic lactated saline can reduce the risk of secondary ACS compared to resuscitation with Ringers' lactate solution [26]. In another study by Oda et al., a significant correlation between IAP and resuscitation volume was found, and most patients with ACS received more than 300 mL/kg/24 h [27]. Kuntscher found that the CVP is more influenced by IAP than by the actual intravascular volume status of the patient, however, there was a poor correlation between IAP and total blood volume [28]. Mbiine et al., also found a higher incidence of IAH among burn patients who were fluid overloaded, albeit not significant [29]. In the work of Wise et al., a group of 56 adult burn patients were examined and patients who developed ACS had higher cumulative fluid balances [30] (Table 22.2).

Relation Between Fluids and IAH in Severe Acute Pancreatitis

Zhao et al. studied 120 patients with severe acute pancreatitis (SAP) receiving three different resuscitation solutions [31]. Incidence of IAH and ACS were significantly lower in subgroups with lower fluid resuscitation volume. Similarly, Mao et al. found in a group of 76 patients

Table 22.3 Summary of studies in severe acute pancreatitis examining the relation between fluid resuscitation and IAH

Author, year	Patients	Findings
Zhao et al., 2013 [31]	$n = 120$	Incidence of IAH and ACS is significantly lower in subgroups with lower fluid resuscitation volume
Mao et al., 2009 [32]	$n = 76$	More ACS in rapid fluid expansion group with more fluid (crystalloid and colloid) on ICU admission
Du et al., 2011 [33]	$n = 41$	Less IAH in hydroxy-ethyl starch group. However, it is not clear the total amount of fluids administered and conflicting statements are there in the article ("no other colloids in Ringer's lactate group "in the methods, however, "larger amounts of other colloids in Ringer's lactate group" reported in the results)
Ke et al., 2012 [34]	$n = 58$	24-h fluid balance (first day) is a significant risk factor for IAH

with SAP that the incidence of ACS was significantly lower in patients with lower initial fluid resuscitation [32]. In the study of Du et al. involving 41 patients with SAP, colloid resuscitation correlated with less IAH, while the total amount of IV fluid did not differ significantly between colloid and crystalloid groups [33]. This has pointed to the possibility that not only the amount but also the type of fluid used is important in the prevention of IAH. Ke and co-workers studied 56 patients with SAP and found that the fluid balance during the first day of ICU admission was an independent predictor for the development of IAH [34] (Table 22.3).

Relation Between Fluids and IAH in Trauma Patients

Balogh et al., found that trauma patients who developed ACS, either primary or secondary, had more fluids infused than patients without ACS [35]. Similarly, Mahmood et al. showed in a group of 117 trauma patients that those with higher IAP received significantly more blood transfusions as well as more crystalloids during the first 2 h of hospitalization [36]. In the recent study by Vatankhah et al. patients with blunt abdominal trauma who developed ACS received significantly more intravenous fluids, both crystalloids and blood products, in the first 24 h of their hospital stay [37]. Raeburn et al. studied 77 trauma patients requiring post-injury damage control laparotomy and were divided into two groups according to the development of ACS [38]. The patients with ACS received more intravenous fluids, however, this difference did not reach significance, which was contrary to the previously published work in the field (Table 22.4).

Relation Between Fluids and IAH in Mixed ICU Patients

The incidence of IAH and ACS in a group of 40 medical ICU patients with a positive fluid balance of more than 5 L/24 h was high, with 85% developing IAH and 25% developing ACS [39]. Cordemans et al. had similar findings where the average positive cumulative fluid balance after 1 week was higher in critically ill patients developing IAH [40].

Table 22.4 Summary of studies in trauma patients examining the relation between fluid resuscitation and IAH

Author, year	Patients	Findings
Balogh et al., 2003 [35]	$n = 188$	More fluids (crystalloid and packed RBC) in both primary and secondary ACS than in non-ACS patients. More than 3 L of crystalloid infusion in the emergency room predicts both primary and secondary ACS. More than 7.5 L of crystalloid infusion before ICU admission strongly predicts secondary ACS
Mahmood et al., 2014 [36]	$n = 117$	Blood transfusion and IV fluids showed significant correlation with IAP >20 mmHg using univariate analysis
Vatankhan et al., 2018 [37]	$n = 100$	The mean volume of the IV fluids was significantly higher in the patients with ACS
Raeburn et al., 2001 [38]	$n = 77$	24 h IV fluids volume was not predictive of the development of ACS

Moreover, increased mean IAP was determined as an independent risk factor for not achieving conservative late fluid management (defined as even-to-negative fluid balance on at least two consecutive days during the first week of ICU stay). Dalfino et al. studied a group of 69 patients undergoing elective cardiac surgery [41]. Twenty-two patients (31.8%) developed IAH. In this subgroup, baseline values of IAP, although normal, were significantly higher. The duration of surgery was also longer and fluid balance was higher. In the subsequent analysis, the positive fluid balance comprised one of three independent predictors for developing IAH, with baseline IAP and central venous pressure. Similarly, Muturi et al. in their work involving 113 surgical ICU patients, found that large volume intravenous fluid administration over 24 h and a positive fluid balance were significantly associated with the development of IAH [42]. Moreover, among IAH patients, those who subsequently developed ACS had a higher fluid balance and received more intravenous fluids in 24 h. In the recent work of Kotlińska-Hasiec et al. [43], patients undergoing hip or knee replacement were divided into liberal or restrictive fluid therapy subgroups. A rise in IAP after surgery was seen in both subgroups, but it was significantly greater in the liberal subgroup. Furthermore, a strong correlation between IAP and extra-cellular water content was noticed in the liberal subgroup, which is in keeping with the theory of fluid extravasation being one of the important mechanisms in the development of IAH. Šerpytis and Ivaškevičius studied 77 patients after abdominal surgery and found a significant positive correlation between the daily changes in IAP and the daily changes in fluid balance during all three postoperative days, i.e. IAP increased with a positive fluid balance and decreased with a negative one [44]. Biancofiore and co-workers studied 108 patients after orthotopic liver transplantation. They found that patients with IAH (31%) received a significantly higher amount of IV fluids than those with a normal IAP [45].

Acute renal failure developed in 17 recipients (16%), 11 (65%) of whom had IAH ($p < 0.01$), with a mean IAP of 27.9 ± 9.9 mmHg vs 18.6 ± 5.2 mmHg in those without acute renal failure ($p < 0.001$). Intraoperative transfusions of more than 15 units packed RBC, respiratory failure and IAH ($p < 0.01$) were independent risk factors for renal failure.

Iyer et al. also found that patients who developed IAH received significantly more intravenous fluids in the first 24 h of admission (4.24 L vs 2.75 L in non-IAH patients, $p < 0.001$), and their fluid balance was significantly more positive after 24 h (2.47 L vs 1.23 L, $p < 0.001$) [46]. Dalfino and co-authors recruited a group of 123 patients admitted to a general ICU [47]. The primary end-point of the study was the relationship between intra-abdominal hypertension (IAH) and acute renal failure. IAH was detected in 30.1% of patients. This study showed that the cumulative fluid intake in the first 72 h after admission was higher in IAH patients, although this difference was not significant. On the contrary, cumulative fluid balance in the first 72 h was significantly higher in IAH patients (3.76 L vs 0.68 L, $p < 0.001$). Consequently, a positive fluid balance was found to be an independent risk factor of IAH ($p = 0.002$). Vidal et al. observed that patients with IAH had consistently higher daily and cumulative fluid balances [48]. Malbrain et al. showed that among six etiological factors and ten predisposing conditions possibly correlated with IAH, only two were significantly associated, namely fluid resuscitation (OR 3.3; 95% CI 1.2–9.2) and polytransfusion (transfusion of >6 units of packed red blood cells in the 24 h before the study entry) [21].

In a multi-centre, prospective epidemiologic study, patients with IAH had significantly higher rates of massive fluid resuscitation (>3.5 L of colloids or crystalloids in the 24 h before the study) [49]. Fluid resuscitation was one of four independent predictors of IAH (OR, 1.88; 95%CI 1.04–3.42; $p = 0.04$), including independent of admission type (medical or surgical). The occurrence of IAH during the ICU stay was also an independent predictor of mortality (relative risk of 1.85; 95%CI1.12–3.06; $p = 0.01$). Patients with IAH on admission had significantly higher SOFA scores during their stay than patients without IAH. Blaser et al. investigated independent risk factors for IAH in a group of 563 mechanically ventilated ICU patients [50]. Patients with IAH received significantly more large volume fluid resuscitation (>5 L/24 h). However, fluid resuscitation was not considered an independent risk factor. In a more recent study by the same group, the prevalence, risk factors and outcomes of intra-abdominal hypertension in a mixed multicentre ICU population of 491 patients were investigated [51]. Nearly half of all patients ($n = 240$; 48.9%) developed IAH during the observation period, and nearly half (46.3%) had primary IAH. One of the independent risk factors for the development of IAH was a positive daily fluid balance (OR 1.1638, $p = 0.001$). Dabrowski et al. found a strong correlation between IAP and total body water, extracellular water content and volume excess in critically ill patients and between IAP and extracellular water content in surgical patients [52].

Finally, a meta-analysis combining individual patient databases of different studies including 1669 patients showed that the only independent predictors for IAH were SOFA score and fluid balance on the day of admission [53] (Table 22.5).

Table 22.5 Summary of studies examining the relation between fluid resuscitation and IAH

Author, year	Patients	Findings
Blaser et al., 2011 [50]	$n = 563$, medical ICU patients	Patients with IAH more frequently received massive fluid resuscitation (>5 L/24 h)
Daugherty et al., 2007 [39]	$n = 40$, medical ICU patients with positive fluid balance >5 L/24 h	Incidence of IAH was 85% and ACS was 25% among patients receiving large-volume resuscitation (net positive fluid balance of 5 L within the preceding 24 h)
Cordemans et al., 2012 [40]	$n = 123$, medical ICU patients	Higher average positive cumulative fluid balance after 1 week in patients developing IAH
Dalfino et al., 2008 [47]	$n = 123$, medical ICU patients	Cumulative fluid balance higher in IAH group ($p < 0.001$)
Iyer et al., 2014 [46]	$n = 403$, mixed ICU patients	Intravenous fluid received >2.3 L is an independent predictor of IAH
Vidal et al., 2008 [48]	$n = 83$, mixed ICU patients	Fluid resuscitation is a risk factor for development of IAH with relative risk (RR) 2.5 and p = 0.04
Malbrain et al., 2005 [49]	$n = 265$, mixed ICU patients	Massive fluid resuscitation (>3.5 L/24 h prior to admission) is an independent predictor for IAH
Blaser et al., 2019 [51]	$n = 491$, mixed ICU patients	Mcdian fluid balance was higher in IAH patients. Daily positive fluid balance was an independent predictor for IAH
Malbrain et al., 2004 [21]	$n = 97$, mixed ICU patients	Fluid resuscitation was at the limit of statistical significance as a predictor of IAH
Malbrain et al. 2014 [53]	$n = 1669$, mixed ICU patients	Thc only independent predictors for IAH were SOFA score and fluid balance on the day of admission
Dalfino et al., 2013 [41]	$n = 69$, surgical ICU patients	Positive fluid balance was an independent risk factor for IAH
Dąbrowski et al., 2015 [52]	$n = 120$, surgical ICU patients	IAP strongly correlated with extracellular water
Biancofiore et al., 2003 [45]	$n = 108$, surgical ICU patients	The patients with IAH needed a significantly higher amount of IV fluids than those with a normal IAP
Muturi et al., 2017 [42]	$n = 113$, surgical ICU patients	The amount of IV fluids over 24 h was a significant risk factor for IAH
Kotlińska-Hasiec et al., 2017 [43]	$n = 63$, surgical ICU patients	Significantly higher IAP in patients receiving liberal crystalloid therapy. Correlation between IAP and extracellular water
Šerpytis and Ivaškevičius, 2008 [44]	$n = 77$, surgical ICU patients	Significant positive correlation between the daily changes in IAP and the daily changes in fluid balance

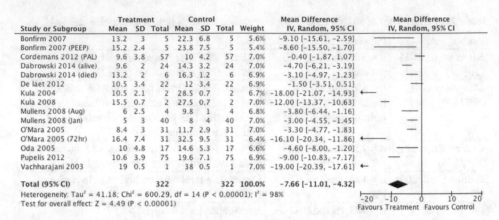

Study or Subgroup	Treatment			Control			Weight	Mean Difference IV, Random, 95% CI	Mean Difference IV, Random, 95% CI
	Mean	SD	Total	Mean	SD	Total			
Bonfirm 2007	13.2	3	5	22.3	6.8	5	5.6%	−9.10 [−15.61, −2.59]	
Bonfirm 2007 (PEEP)	15.2	2.4	5	23.8	7.5	5	5.4%	−8.60 [−15.50, −1.70]	
Cordemans 2012 (PAL)	9.6	3.8	57	10	4.2	57	7.0%	−0.40 [−1.87, 1.07]	
Dabrowski 2014 (alive)	9.6	2	24	14.3	3.2	24	7.0%	−4.70 [−6.21, −3.19]	
Dabrowski 2014 (died)	13.2	2	6	16.3	1.2	6	6.9%	−3.10 [−4.97, −1.23]	
De laet 2012	10.5	3.4	22	12	3.4	22	6.9%	−1.50 [−3.51, 0.51]	
Kula 2004	10.5	2.1	2	28.5	0.7	2	6.7%	−18.00 [−21.07, −14.93]	
Kula 2008	15.5	0.7	2	27.5	0.7	2	7.0%	−12.00 [−13.37, −10.63]	
Mullens 2008 (Aug)	6	2.5	4	9.8	1	4	6.8%	−3.80 [−6.44, −1.16]	
Mullens 2008 (Jan)	5	3	40	8	4	40	7.0%	−3.00 [−4.55, −1.45]	
O'Mara 2005	8.4	3	31	11.7	2.9	31	7.0%	−3.30 [−4.77, −1.83]	
O'Mara 2005 (72hr)	16.4	7.4	31	32.5	9.5	31	6.4%	−16.10 [−20.34, −11.86]	
Oda 2005	10	4.8	17	14.6	5.3	17	6.6%	−4.60 [−8.00, −1.20]	
Pupelis 2012	10.6	3.9	75	19.6	7.1	75	6.9%	−9.00 [−10.83, −7.17]	
Vachharajani 2003	19	0.5	1	38	0.5	1	7.0%	−19.00 [−20.39, −17.61]	
Total (95% CI)			322			322	100.0%	−7.66 [−11.01, −4.32]	

Heterogeneity: Tau² = 41.18; Chi² = 600.29, df = 14 (P < 0.00001); I² = 98%
Test for overall effect: Z = 4.49 (P < 0.00001)

Favours Treatment Favours Control

Fig. 22.4 Forest plot looking at the effect of fluid removal on intra-abdominal pressure. (Updated and adapted from Malbrain et al. [12])

Does IAP Improve with Interventions Acting on Reducing Fluid Balance?

Thirteen studies investigated the effects of fluid removal (use of furosemide or renal replacement therapy with net ultrafiltration) on IAP (Fig. 22.4). These were case studies or small series [24, 40, 44, 54–62]. A total fluid removal of 4876.3 ± 4178.5 mL resulted in a drop in IAP from 19.3 ± 9.1 to 11.5 ± 3.9 mmHg (Fig. 22.5). A dose-related effect was observed: the more negative the net fluid balance or fluid removal the greater the decrease in IAP (Fig. 22.6). Although difficult if not impossible to prove, many of these studies were done in patients who were over-resuscitated. The impact of diuretics or fluid removal may be variable when applied as a general strategy. The use of diuretics is preferred but this should be done in a targeted approach, where one looks at the different contributors to IAH, and acts accordingly. The different medical management strategies are summarized in Fig. 22.7.

Fig. 22.5 Boxplot showing the effect of fluid removal (after) on intra-abdominal pressure (IAP, mmHg). Solid line indicates median IAP with interquartile range. (Adapted from Malbrain et al. with permission [12])

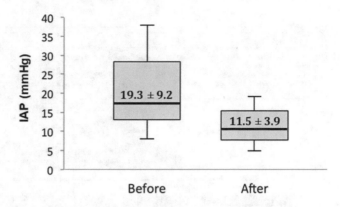

Fig. 22.6 Pearson correlation graph showing the change in intra-abdominal pressure (ΔIAP) in relation to the amount of fluid removed (ΔFluid Balance). (Adapted from Malbrain et al. with permission [12])

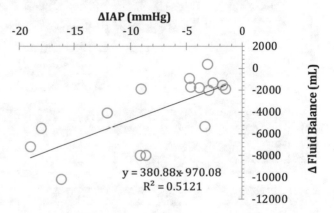

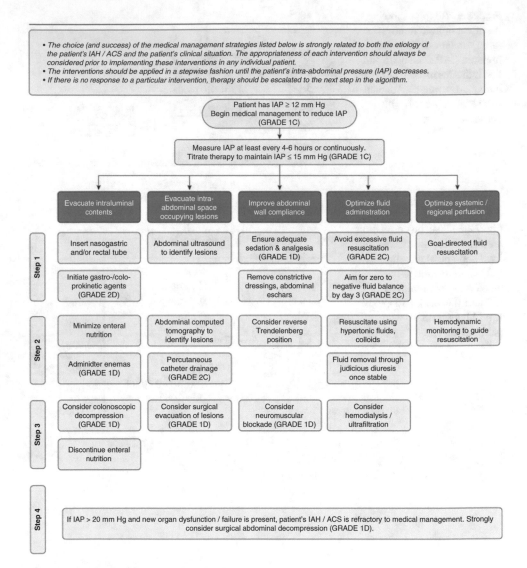

Fig. 22.7 WSACS 2013 intra-abdominal hypertension/abdominal compartment syndrome medical management algorithm. (Figure reproduced and adapted with permission from Kirkpatrick et al. according to the Open Access CC BY Licence 4.0 [1])

Recommendations for Fluid Management in Secondary IAH

Note: This section presents some recommendations and suggestions for prevention and treatment of fluid accumulation in patients with or at risk for IAH, based on personal experience of the co-authors. It does not aim to provide an exhaustive, graded and concise overview of the literature as current evidence is mostly limited to observational, retrospective or small clinical studies and more randomized trials are needed to better establish a personalized approach to fluid management in IAH.

Question 1. Is There Evidence to Prefer Albumin (Any Tonicity) or Hypertonic Solutions to Crystalloids During General Management?

Several studies evaluated the use of albumin as a resuscitation fluid. Except for patients with traumatic brain injury, current evidence suggests that albumin is well tolerated as a resuscitation fluid. However, there is no evidence suggesting that albumin offers outcome benefits over crystalloid solutions. A retrospective study in 114 patients showed that the use of PAL (PEEP set at level of IAP followed by albumin 20% followed by furosemide) treatment was able to keep cumulative fluid balance 'in check' with a significant drop in IAP and EVLWI and a rise in P/F ratio [63]. This also resulted in faster weaning and improved survival when compared to a matched control group.

- We *recommend against* the use of high-dose (20–25%) albumin as resuscitation fluid in early phase of IAH patients.
- We *recommend against* the use of low-dose (4%) albumin as resuscitation fluid in IAH patients with low blood pressure.
- We *recommend using* hypertonic albumin 20% only in selected patients, in the late phase of septic shock and during deresuscitation of patients with secondary IAH.
- We *suggest against* the use of hypertonic saline solutions as resuscitation fluids in IAH patients with low blood pressure.

Question 2. Is There Evidence to Prefer Colloids to Crystalloids During General Management?

In a randomized controlled trial involving 41 patients with SAP, hydroxyethyl starch resuscitation resulted in a decrease in IAP, and reduced need for mechanical ventilation compared to cases where Ringer's lactate was used. HES resuscitation led to a decrease in the IAP and reduced the use of mechanical ventilation, achieving a negative fluid balance before such a balance was achieved by a Ringer's lactate solution [33]. However, from randomized controlled trials there is no evidence that resuscitation with colloids reduces the risk of death, compared to resuscitation with crystalloids, in patients with trauma, burns or following surgery [64].

- We *suggest against* the use of synthetic colloids as resuscitation fluids in IAH patients with low blood pressure.
- We *recommend against* the use of starch solutions in patients with sepsis-associated secondary IAH and low blood pressure.
- We *suggest using* crystalloids as first-line resuscitation fluids in IAH patients with low blood pressure.
- We *recommend against* the use of glucose-containing hypotonic solutions and other hypotonic solutions (osmolality <260 mosm/L) as resuscitation fluids in general and IAH patients.

Question 3. Is There Evidence to Prefer Using Buffered Crystalloids During General Management?

Wu et al. conducted a randomized controlled trial in 40 patients with SAP comparing resuscitation with 0.9% saline to Ringer's lactate solution and found that patients who were resuscitated with Ringer's lactate solution had reduced systemic inflammation compared with those who received saline. There was, however, no difference in outcome between study groups [65]. A recent meta-analysis from 2018 confirmed the anti-inflammatory effects of Ringer's lactate and showed that it tended to have lower mortality rates compared to 0.9% saline [66].

A RCT involving 60 patients with acute pancreatitis, but without systemic inflammatory response syndrome or organ failure, received either aggressive vs. standard resuscitation with Ringer's lactate solution. There was a greater rate of clinical improvement with aggressive hydration vs. standard practice [67].

According to the Working Group IAP/APA Acute Pancreatitis Guidelines Ringer's lactate is the recommended fluid for initial resuscitation in acute pancreatitis [68].

Balanced solutions have been shown to be superior to unbalanced solutions for fluid replacement [69]. Ringer's acetate seems to be the most appropriate choice for large replacements [70].

The recently conducted pragmatic SMART study confirmed the superiority of buffered (so-called balanced) solutions over (ab)normal saline (NaCl 0.9%) [71]. Among 15,802 critically ill adults, the use of balanced crystalloids for intravenous fluid administration resulted in a lower rate of the composite outcome of death from any cause, new renal-replacement therapy, or persistent renal dysfunction than the use of saline.

- We *recommend using* buffered (or balanced) crystalloids as first-line resuscitation fluids in IAH patients with low blood pressure.

Question 4. Is There Evidence Regarding the Best Maintenance Solution in IAH?
In a large retrospective study, Van Regenmortel found that maintenance fluid accounted for volume, sodium and chloride overload exceeding resuscitation fluids. This burden can be avoided by adopting a hypotonic (and balanced) maintenance strategy [14]. Similar results were found when comparing glucose 5% plus Na154 (0.9% saline) vs Na54 as maintenance solution in patients undergoing thoracic surgery [72].

- We *recommend* the use of crystalloids as preferred maintenance fluids in IAH patients.
- We *recommend against* the use of colloids, glucose- and salt- containing isotonic solutions, or albumin as maintenance fluids in IAH patients.
- We *recommend* the use of hypotonic and balanced crystalloids as preferred maintenance fluids in IAH patients.
- We *suggest* monitoring electrolytes (Na^+, Cl^-) and osmolality as a safety endpoint for fluid therapy in IAH patients.

Question 5. Is There Evidence to Prefer Hypertonic Solutions for the Management of Acute Rise in IAP?
Several animal studies proved that hypertonic saline (HTS) resuscitation improves hemodynamics [73–76]. HTS treatment allows smaller fluid volume resuscitation in the burn shock period and reduces the risk of low abdominal perfusion and secondary ACS [26]. The American Burn Association evaluated the efficacy of HTS in burn patients, but currently has not found clear evidence in favour of, or against them. Additional studies are required to define the correct dosage and timing [77].

- We *recommend against* the use of mannitol solution for reducing increased IAP.
- We *recommend* the use of hypertonic saline solution for reducing increased IAP in selected patients.
- We *suggest* using a predefined trigger for starting osmotherapy to treat elevated IAP.
- We *suggest* using a combination of clinical, laboratory and worsening organ function variables (defined as a SOFA score equal to or greater than 3) in combination with IAP >20 mmHg for starting osmotherapy to treat elevated IAP.
- We *suggest* using an IAP threshold >25 mmHg, independent of other variables, as a trigger for starting osmotherapy to reduce IAP.
- We *recommend against* the use of an IAP threshold below 15 mmHg independent of other variables as a trigger for starting osmotherapy to reduce IAP.
- We *suggest* monitoring measured serum osmolarity and electrolytes to limit the side effects of osmotherapy.
- We *suggest* monitoring IAP response to hyperosmolar fluids to limit the side effects of osmotherapy.

Question 6. Is There Evidence for the Best Management in Case of ACS and Intestinal Ischemia?

- We *recommend* assessing the efficacy of fluid infusion in ACS patients with suspicion of intestinal ischemia using a multimodal approach that includes arterial blood pressure, cardiac output and reversal of IAP-related hypoperfusion as the main endpoints.
- We *suggest* that an increase in the plasma disappearance rate of indocyanine green, and improvements in renal resistive index should be used as secondary endpoints when assessing the efficacy of fluids for the reversal of intestinal ischemia in ACS patients.

Question 7. Is There Evidence Regarding Impact of Fluid Load on IAH?
Two RCTs in 76 and 115 patients with SAP show that rapid, uncontrolled fluid resuscitation (10–15 mL/kg/h or until a haematocrit <35% within 48 h) significantly worsened the rates of infections, abdominal compartment syndrome, the need for mechanical ventilation and even mortality. Hematocrit should be maintained between 30% and 40% in the acute response stage [32].

- We *suggest* monitoring the effects of any fluids administered on IAP, arterial blood pressure and fluid balance as secondary variables to limit the side effects.
- We *suggest* that clinicians consider targeting normovolaemia during fluid replacement in IAH patients.
- We *recommend* the use of a multimodal approach, guided by the integration of more than a single hemodynamic variable, to optimize fluid therapy in IAH patients.
- We recommend considering using IAP, arterial blood pressure and fluid balance as the main endpoints to optimize fluid therapy in IAH patients.
- We *suggest* integrating other variables (such as cardiac output, functional haemodynamics, $S(c)vO_2$, blood lactate, base deficit, urinary output, extravascular lung water, bio-electrical impedance analysis, capillary leak index, pulmonary vascular permeability index) to optimize fluid therapy in IAH patients.
- We *recommend against* the use of central venous pressure alone (as CVP may be erroneously increased) as an (safety) endpoint for guiding fluid therapy in IAH patients.
- We *suggest* the use of restrictive fluid strategies (aiming for an overall neutral to negative fluid balance within the first week) in IAH patients.

- We *suggest* using body weight, daily and cumulative fluid balance as a safety endpoint for fluid therapy in IAH patients.
- We *suggest* monitoring measured osmolarity, total protein levels, haematocrit levels and colloid oncotic pressure as a safety endpoint for fluid therapy in IAH patients.

Question 8. Is There Evidence Regarding Resuscitation with Fresh Frozen Plasma?
Wang et al. conducted a RCT in 132 patients with SAP concerning the effect of fluid resuscitation with fresh frozen plasma. FFP shortens the duration of positive fluid balance, decreases the amount of positive fluid balance within 72 h, reduces the duration of mechanical ventilation and admissions to the ICU and improves PaO_2/FiO_2 and mortality in SAP [78].

- We *recommend against* the use of fresh frozen plasma as resuscitation fluid in IAH patients.

Question 9. Is There Evidence Regarding Adjunctive Use of High-Dose Vitamin C?
In the 1990s, Matsuda et al. were able to reduce fluid requirements and edema formation during burn resuscitation in dogs and guinea pigs by using high-dose ascorbic acid therapy [79, 80].

A few years later they reproduced the beneficial effects of high-dose ascorbic acid in humans in a prospective, randomized study [81].

During the first 24 h, resuscitation fluid volume requirements were significantly reduced. Ascorbic acid has an apparent (osmotic) diuretic effect that may lead to hypovolemia. The decreased insensible fluid losses may also lead to a reduced inflammatory response and earlier mobilization of fluid.

- We *recommend against* the use of adjunctive high-dose ascorbic acid in the treatment of IAH patients.

Case Vignette

Questions and Answers

Going back to the clinical vignette the patient was in profound septic shock and capillary leak with intravascular underfilling and extravascular fluid overload.

Q1. What fluids should be administered?

A1. Fluids should be administered, however, a combination of balanced crystalloids (e.g. PlasmaLyte) with hypertonic solutions (like albumin 20%) guided by plasma albumin levels, osmolality and serum colloid oncotic pressure. The combination of vasopressors should allow fluids to be limited. Source control must be checked and adequate. It must be noted that traditional filling pressures like CVP may be erroneously increased and volumetric preload parameters may better reflect the true filling status in IAH.

The patient was fluid responsive as shown by the high PPV and the positive passive leg raising test.

Q2. How do you interpret the increased PPV in the setting of ACS?

A2. The clinician must be aware that IAP can falsely increase PPV and SVV, for instance when IAP goes up from 10 to 20 mmHg this may result in an increase of PPV from 12% to 24%. Therefore, our traditional thresholds identifying fluid responsiveness must be adapted when IAP is increased.

The clinical condition of the patient deteriorated further and a decompressive laparotomy was performed at the bedside in the ICU, which revealed no intra-abdominal abnormalities.

Q3. Were all medical management options used before DL?

A3. Before DL is chosen all medical management options must be tried and evaluated. In this case, it would have been an option (in view of the positive cumulative fluid balance) to mobilize the excess fluids with albumin 20% in combination with diuretics or CVVH and aggressive ultrafiltration. Only when all medical options fail should surgery be undertaken.

Each day, around 4 L of fluid were drained via the VAC system.

Q4. Do you have any concerns regarding the interstitial (third) space fluid losses?

A4. Third space fluid losses can be substantial in patients with open abdomen and TAC with VAC. These fluid and nitrogen losses need to be taken into account and replaced when indicated.

Despite the initial improvement after decompressive laparotomy renal function deteriorated again and continuous venovenous hemofiltration (CVVH) with ultrafiltration was started.

Q5. Is there a role for hypertonic solutions and diuretics in this patient?

A5. As stated above hypertonic solutions can be an option in selected cases, and can be used at the later deresuscitation phase in combination with diuretics or CVVH and UF.

Conclusion

Intravenous fluid administration plays an important role in the development of secondary IAH and ACS. Multiple pathophysiological mechanisms have been described. Fluid resuscitation in IAH is a double-edged sword, that can improve cardiac output initially, but overzealous ongoing fluid administration can further increase IAP, leading to fluid accumulation, and organ dysfunction including AKI. Daily and cumulative fluid balance has been identified as an independent risk factor in several clinical studies and can contribute to the development of IAH, and a vicious cycle leading to venous congestion, gut oedema with diminished gut contractility and organ failure. Evidence identifying the best resuscitation targets and management strategies regarding type, timing and amountof fluids in patients with IAH is scarce and further research is required.

Take Home Messages
- There is a clear relationship between amount and dose of (crystalloid) fluid resuscitation, fluid accumulation and secondary IAH.
- Development of IAH is more likely in the setting of sepsis (capillary leak), severe burn injury, severe acute pancreatitis, emergency surgery and trauma and the presence of the deadly triad (coagulopathy, acidosis, hypothermia).
- Fluid resuscitation in IAH may preserve cardiac output, however, it does not prevent organ damage (vicious cycle and double-edged sword).
- Fluid resuscitation leads also to venous congestion (or venous hypertension), which in turn results in gut edema and diminished gut contractility.
- Fluid removal with diuretics or CVVH may restore cumulative fluid balance and lower IAP.
- Medical management comes first and surgical decompression can be used as a last resort, also in secondary ACS.
- Elevated vascular permeability due to a stress-related inflammatory response associated with positive fluid balance leads to extravascular fluid accumulation, which is likely to result in gastrointestinal tract edema and increased IAP.
- Development of ACS in burns is associated with the total burned surface area TBSA (>20%) and the total amount of administered fluid volume (>300 mL/kg)
- In cases of SAP, the less fluids patients receive after the initial resuscitation, the lower the risk of developing secondary IAH and/or ACS.
- Crystalloids are associated with more positive fluid balance and a greater likelihood of developing IAH compared to colloids or hypertonic solutions.

References

1. Kirkpatrick AW, Roberts DJ, Jaeschke R, De Waele JJ, De Keulenaer BL, Duchesne J, Bjorck M, Leppaniemi A, Ejike JC, Sugrue M et al. Methodological background and strategy for the 2012–2013 updated consensus definitions and clinical practice guidelines from the abdominal compartment society. Anaesthesiol Intensive Ther. 2015;47 Spec No:63–77.
2. De Keulenaer BL, De Waele JJ, Powell B, Malbrain ML. What is normal intra-abdominal pressure and how is it affected by positioning, body mass and positive end-expiratory pressure? Intensive Care Med. 2009;35(6):969–76.
3. Malbrain ML, Cheatham ML, Kirkpatrick A, Sugrue M, Parr M, De Waele J, Balogh Z, Leppaniemi A, Olvera C, Ivatury R, et al. Results from the international conference of experts on intra-abdominal hypertension and abdominal compartment syndrome. I. Definitions. Intensive Care Med. 2006;32(11):1722–32.
4. Malbrain ML, De Waele JJ, De Keulenaer BL. What every ICU clinician needs to know about the cardiovascular effects caused by abdominal hypertension. Anaesthesiol Intensive Ther. 2015;47(4):388–99.
5. Regli A, Pelosi P, Malbrain M. Ventilation in patients with intra-abdominal hypertension: what every critical care physician needs to know. Ann Intensive Care. 2019;9(1):52.
6. De Laet I, Citerio G, Malbrain MLNG. The influence of intra-abdominal hypertension on the central nervous system: current insights and clinical recommendations, is it all in the head? Acta Clin Belg. 2007;62(Suppl. 1):89–97.
7. Holte K, Sharrock NE, Kehlet H. Pathophysiology and clinical implications of perioperative fluid excess. Br J Anaesth. 2002;89(4):622–32.
8. Bloomfield GL, Blocher CR, Fakhry IF, Sica DA, Sugerman HJ. Elevated intra-abdominal pressure increases plasma renin activity and aldosterone levels. J Trauma. 1997;42(6):997–1004; discussion 1004–1005.
9. Malbrain MLNG, Roberts DJ, Sugrue M, De Keulenaer BL, Ivatury R, Pelosi P, Verbrugge F, Wise R, Maes H, Mullens W. The polycompartment syndrome: a concise state-of-the-art review. Anaesthesiol Intensive Ther. 2014;46(5):433–50.
10. Duchesne JC, Kaplan LJ, Balogh ZJ, Malbrain ML. Role of permissive hypotension, hypertonic resuscitation and the global increased permeability syndrome in patients with severe hemorrhage: adjuncts to damage control resuscitation to prevent intra-abdominal hypertension. Anaesthesiol Intensive Ther. 2015;47(2):143–55.
11. Malbrain MLNG, Van Regenmortel N, Saugel B, De Tavernier B, Van Gaal P-J, Joannes-Boyau O, Teboul J-L, Rice TW, Mythen M, Monnet X. Principles of fluid management and stewardship in septic shock: it is time to consider the four D's and the four phases of fluid therapy. Ann Intensive Care. 2018;8(1):66.
12. Malbrain ML, Marik PE, Witters I, Cordemans C, Kirkpatrick AW, Roberts DJ, Van Regenmortel N. Fluid overload, de-resuscitation, and outcomes in critically ill or injured patients: a systematic review with suggestions for clinical practice. Anaesthesiol Intensive Ther. 2014;46(5):361–80.
13. Dellinger RP, Carlet JM, Masur H, Gerlach H, Calandra T, Cohen J, Gea-Banacloche J, Keh D, Marshall JC, Parker MM, et al. Surviving Sepsis Campaign guidelines for management of severe sepsis and septic shock. Crit Care Med. 2004;32(3):858–73.
14. Van Regenmortel N, Verbrugghe W, Roelant E, Van den Wyngaert T, Jorens PG. Maintenance fluid therapy and fluid creep impose more significant fluid, sodium, and chloride burdens than

resuscitation fluids in critically ill patients: a retrospective study in a tertiary mixed ICU population. Intensive Care Med. 2018;44(4):409–17.

15. Malbrain ML, Van Regenmortel N, Owczuk R. It is time to consider the four D's of fluid management. Anaesthesiol Intensive Ther. 2015;47 Spec No:1–5.

16. Silversides JA, Perner A, Malbrain M. Liberal versus restrictive fluid therapy in critically ill patients. Intensive Care Med. 2019;45(10):1440–2.

17. Jacobs R, Lochy S, Malbrain M. Phenylephrine-induced recruitable preload from the venous side. J Clin Monit Comput. 2018;33:373–6.

18. Meyhoff TS, Hjortrup PB, Moller MH, Wetterslev J, Lange T, Kjaer MN, Jonsson AB, Hjortso CJS, Cronhjort M, Laake JH, et al. Conservative vs liberal fluid therapy in septic shock (CLASSIC) trial-protocol and statistical analysis plan. Acta Anaesthesiol Scand. 2019;63(9):1262–71.

19. Kirkpatrick AW, Colistro R, Laupland KB, Fox DL, Konkin DE, Kock V, Mayo JR, Nicolaou S. Renal arterial resistive index response to intraabdominal hypertension in a porcine model. Crit Care Med. 2007;35(1):207–13.

20. Kirkpatrick AW, Laupland KB. "The higher the abdominal pressure, the less the secretion of urine": another target disease for renal ultrasonography? Crit Care Med. 2007;35(5 Suppl):S206–7.

21. Malbrain ML, Chiumello D, Pelosi P, Wilmer A, Brienza N, Malcangi V, Bihari D, Innes R, Cohen J, Singer P, et al. Prevalence of intra-abdominal hypertension in critically ill patients: a multicentre epidemiological study. Intensive Care Med. 2004;30(5):822–9.

22. Malbrain ML, Chiumello D, Pelosi P, Bihari D, Innes R, Ranieri VM, Del Turco M, Wilmer A, Brienza N, Malcangi V, et al. Incidence and prognosis of intraabdominal hypertension in a mixed population of critically ill patients: a multiple-center epidemiological study. Crit Care Med. 2005;33(2):315–22.

23. Alsous F, Khamiees M, DeGirolamo A, Amoateng-Adjepong Y, Manthous CA. Negative fluid balance predicts survival in patients with septic shock: a retrospective pilot study. Chest. 2000;117(6):1749–54.

24. O'Mara MS, Slater H, Goldfarb IW, Caushaj PF. A prospective, randomized evaluation of intra-abdominal pressures with crystalloid and colloid resuscitation in burn patients. J Trauma. 2005;58(5):1011–8.

25. Ruiz-Castilla M, Barret JP, Sanz D, Aguilera J, Serracanta J, Garcia V, Collado JM. Analysis of intra-abdominal hypertension in severe burned patients: the Vall d'Hebron experience. Burns. 2014;40(4):719–24.

26. Oda J, Ueyama M, Yamashita K, Inoue T, Noborio M, Ode Y, Aoki Y, Sugimoto H. Hypertonic lactated saline resuscitation reduces the risk of abdominal compartment syndrome in severely burned patients. J Trauma. 2006;60(1):64–71.

27. Oda J, Yamashita K, Inoue T, Harunari N, Ode Y, Mega K, Aoki Y, Noborio M, Ueyama M. Resuscitation fluid volume and abdominal compartment syndrome in patients with major burns. Burns. 2006;32(2):151–4.

28. Kuntscher MV, Germann G, Hartmann B. Correlations between cardiac output, stroke volume, central venous pressure, intra-abdominal pressure and total circulating blood volume in resuscitation of major burns. Resuscitation. 2006;70(1):37–43.

29. Mbiine R, Alenyo R, Kobusingye O, Kuteesa J, Nakanwagi C, Lekuya HM, Kituuka O, Galukande M. Intra-abdominal hypertension in severe burns: prevalence, incidence and mortality in a sub-Saharan African hospital. Int J Burns Trauma. 2017;7(6):80–7.

30. Wise R, Jacobs J, Pilate S, Jacobs A, Peeters Y, Vandervelden S, Van Regenmortel N, De Laet I, Schoonheydt K, Dits H, et al. Incidence and prognosis of intra-abdominal hypertension and abdominal compartment syndrome in severely burned patients: pilot study and review of the literature. Anaesthesiol Intensive Ther. 2016;48(2):95–109.

31. Zhao G, Zhang JG, Wu HS, Tao J, Qin Q, Deng SC, Liu Y, Liu L, Wang B, Tian K, et al. Effects of different resuscitation fluid on severe acute pancreatitis. World J Gastroenterol. 2013;19(13):2044–52.

32. Mao EQ, Tang YQ, Fei J, Qin S, Wu J, Li L, Min D, Zhang SD. Fluid therapy for severe acute pancreatitis in acute response stage. Chin Med J. 2009;122(2):169–73.

33. Du XJ, Hu WM, Xia Q, Huang ZW, Chen GY, Jin XD, Xue P, Lu HM, Ke NW, Zhang ZD, et al. Hydroxyethyl starch resuscitation reduces the risk of intra-abdominal hypertension in severe acute pancreatitis. Pancreas. 2011;40(8):1220–5.

34. Ke L, Ni HB, Sun JK, Tong ZH, Li WQ, Li N, Li JS. Risk factors and outcome of intra-abdominal hypertension in patients with severe acute pancreatitis. World J Surg. 2012;36(1):171–8.

35. Balogh Z, McKinley BA, Holcomb JB, Miller CC, Cocanour CS, Kozar RA, Valdivia A, Ware DN, Moore FA. Both primary and secondary abdominal compartment syndrome can be predicted early and are harbingers of multiple organ failure. J Trauma. 2003;54(5):848–59. discussion 859-861.

36. Mahmood I, Mahmood S, Parchani A, Kumar S, El-Menyar A, Zarour A, Al-Thani H, Latifi R. Intra-abdominal hypertension in the current era of modern trauma resuscitation. ANZ J Surg. 2014;84(3):166–71.

37. Vatankhah S, Sheikhi RA, Heidari M, Moradimajd P. The relationship between fluid resuscitation and intra-abdominal hypertension in patients with blunt abdominal trauma. Int J Crit Illn Inj Sci. 2018;8(3):149–53.

38. Raeburn CD, Moore EE, Biffl WL, Johnson JL, Meldrum DR, Offner PJ, Franciose RJ, Burch JM. The abdominal compartment syndrome is a morbid complication of postinjury damage control surgery. Am J Surg. 2001;182(6):542–6.

39. Daugherty EL, Hongyan L, Taichman D, Hansen-Flaschen J, Fuchs BD. Abdominal compartment syndrome is common in medical intensive care unit patients receiving large-volume resuscitation. J Intensive Care Med. 2007;22(5):294–9.

40. Cordemans C, de Iaet I, van Regenmortel N, Schoonheydt K, Dits H, Huber W, Malbrain ML. Fluid management in critically ill patients: the role of extravascualr lung water, abdominal hypertension, capillary leak and fluid balance. Ann Intensive Care. 2012;2(Suppl 1):S1.

41. Dalfino L, Sicolo A, Paparella D, Mongelli M, Rubino G, Brienza N. Intra-abdominal hypertension in cardiac surgery. Interact Cardiovasc Thorac Surg. 2013;17(4):644–51.

42. Muturi A, Ndaguatha P, Ojuka D, Kibet A. Prevalence and predictors of intra-abdominal hypertension and compartment syndrome in surgical patients in critical care units at Kenyatta National Hospital. BMC Emerg Med. 2017;17(1):10.

43. Kotlinska-Hasiec E, Rutyna RR, Rzecki Z, Czarko-Wicha K, Gagala J, Pawlik P, Zaluska A, Jaroszynski A, Zaluska W, Dabrowski W. The effect of crystalloid infusion on body water content and intra-abdominal pressure in patients undergoing orthopedic surgery under spinal anesthesia. Adv Clin Exp Med. 2017;26(8):1189–96.

44. Serpytis M, Ivaskevicius J. The influence of fluid balance on intra-abdominal pressure after major abdominal surgery. Medicina (Kaunas). 2008;44(6):421–7.

45. Biancofiore G, Bindi ML, Romanelli AM, Boldrini A, Consani G, Bisa M, Filipponi F, Vagelli A, Mosca F. Intra-abdominal pressure monitoring in liver transplant recipients: a prospective study. Intensive Care Med. 2003;29(1):30–6.
46. Iyer D, Rastogi P, Aneman A, D'Amours S. Early screening to identify patients at risk of developing intra-abdominal hypertension and abdominal compartment syndrome. Acta Anaesthesiol Scand. 2014;58(10):1267–75.
47. Dalfino L, Tullo L, Donadio I, Malcangi V, Brienza N. Intra-abdominal hypertension and acute renal failure in critically ill patients. Intensive Care Med. 2008;34(4):707–13.
48. Vidal MG, Ruiz Weisser J, Gonzalez F, Toro MA, Loudet C, Balasini C, Canales H, Reina R, Estenssoro E. Incidence and clinical effects of intra-abdominal hypertension in critically ill patients. Crit Care Med. 2008;36(6):1823–31.
49. Malbrain M, Chiumello D, Pelosi P, Bihari D, Innes R, Ranieri VM, Del Turco M, Wilmer A, Brienza N, Malcangi V, et al. Incidence and pyognosis of intyaabdominal hypeytension in a mixed population of critically ill patients: a multiple-center epidemiological study. Crit Care Med. 2005;33(2):315–22.
50. Reintam Blaser A, Parm P, Kitus R, Starkopf J. Risk factors for intra-abdominal hypertension in mechanically ventilated patients. Acta Anaesthesiol Scand. 2011;55(5):607–14.
51. Reintam Blaser A, Regli A, De Keulenaer B, Kimball EJ, Starkopf L, Davis WA, Greiffenstein P, Starkopf J, Incidence RF. Outcomes of intra-abdominal study I: incidence, risk factors, and outcomes of intra-abdominal hypertension in critically ill patients—a prospective multicenter study (IROI study). Crit Care Med. 2019;47(4):535–42.
52. Dabrowski W, Kotlinska-Hasiec E, Jaroszynski A, Zadora P, Pilat J, Rzecki Z, Zaluska W, Schneditz D. Intra-abdominal pressure correlates with extracellular water content. PLoS One. 2015;10(4):e0122193.
53. Malbrain M, Chiumello D, Cesana BM, Blaser AR, Starkopf J, Sugrue M, Pelosi P, Severgnini P, Hernandez G, Brienza N, et al. A systematic review and individual patient data meta-analysis on intra-abdominal hypertension in critically ill patients: the wake-up project World initiative on Abdominal Hypertension Epidemiology, a Unifying Project (WAKE-Up!). Minerva Anestesiol. 2014;80(3):293–306.
54. Bonfim RF, Goulart AG, Fu C, Torquato JA. Effect of hemodialysis on intra-abdominal pressure. Clinics. 2007;62(2) https://doi.org/10.1590/S1807-59322007000200009.
55. Dabrowski W, Kotlinska-Hasiec E, Schneditz D, Zaluska W, Rzecki Z, De Keulenaer B, Malbrain M. Continuous veno-venous hemofiltration to adjust fluid volume excess in septic shock patients reduces intra-abdominal pressure. Clin Nephrol. 2014;82(1):41–50.
56. De Laet I, Deeren D, Schoonheydt K, Van Regenmortel N, Dits H, Malbrain M. Renal replacement therapy with net fluid removal lowers intra-abdominal pressure and volumetric indices in critically ill patients. Ann Intensive Care. 2012;2
57. Kula R, Szturz P, Sklienka P, Neiser J, Jahoda J. A role for negative fluid balance in septic patients with abdominal compartment syndrome? Intensive Care Med. 2004;30(11):2138–9.
58. Kula R, Szturz P, Sklienka P, Neiser J. Negative fluid balance in patients with abdominal compartment syndrome—case reports. Acta Chir Belg. 2008;108(3):346–9.
59. Mullens W, Abrahams Z, Skouri HN, Francis GS, Taylor DO, Starling RC, Paganini E, Tang WH. Elevated intra-abdominal pressure in acute decompensated heart failure: a potential contributor to worsening renal function? J Am Coll Cardiol. 2008;51(3):300–6.

60. Mullens W, Abrahams Z, Francis GS, Taylor DO, Starling RC, Tang WH. Prompt reduction in intra-abdominal pressure following large-volume mechanical fluid removal improves renal insufficiency in refractory decompensated heart failure. J Card Fail. 2008;14(6):508–14.

61. Pupelis G, Plaudis H, Zeiza K, Drozdova N, Mukans M, Kazaka I. Early continuous veno-venous haemofiltration in the management of severe acute pancreatitis complicated with intra-abdominal hypertension: retrospective review of 10 years' experience. Ann Intensive Care. 2012;2(Suppl 1):S21.

62. Vachharajani V, Scott LK, Grier L, Conrad S. Medical management of severe intra-abdominal hypertension with aggressive diuresis and continuous ultra-filtration. Int J Emerg Intensive Care Med. 2003;6(2)

63. Cordemans C, De Laet I, Van Regenmortel N, Schoonheydt K, Dits H, Martin G, Huber W, Malbrain ML. Aiming for a negative fluid balance in patients with acute lung injury and increased intra-abdominal pressure: a pilot study looking at the effects of PAL-treatment. Ann Intensive Care. 2012;2(Suppl 1):S15.

64. Perel P, Roberts I. Colloids versus crystalloids for fluid resuscitation in critically ill patients. Cochrane Database Syst Rev. 2007;(4):CD000567.

65. Wu BU, Hwang JQ, Gardner TH, Repas K, Delee R, Yu S, Smith B, Banks PA, Conwell DL. Lactated Ringer's solution reduces systemic inflammation compared with saline in patients with acute pancreatitis. Clin Gastroenterol Hepatol. 2011;9(8):710–17.e711.

66. Iqbal U, Anwar H, Scribani M. Ringer's lactate versus normal saline in acute pancreatitis: a systematic review and meta-analysis. J Dig Dis. 2018;19(6):335–41.

67. Buxbaum JL, Quezada M, Da B, Jani N, Lane C, Mwengela D, Kelly T, Jhun P, Dhanireddy K, Laine L. Early aggressive hydration hastens clinical improvement in mild acute pancreatitis. Am J Gastroenterol. 2017;112(5):797–803.

68. Working Group IAPAPAAPG. IAP/APA evidence-based guidelines for the management of acute pancreatitis. Pancreatology. 2013;13(4 Suppl 2):e1–15.

69. Powell-Tuck J, Gosling P, Lobo D, Allison S, Carlson G, Gore M, Lewington A, Pearse R, Mythen M. Summary of the British consensus guidelines on intravenous fluid therapy for adult surgical patients (GIFTASUP). J Intensive Care Soc. 2009;10(1):13–5.

70. Guilabert P, Usua G, Martin N, Abarca L, Barret JP, Colomina MJ. Fluid resuscitation management in patients with burns: update. Br J Anaesth. 2016;117(3):284–96.

71. Semler MW, Self WH, Wanderer JP, Ehrenfeld JM, Wang L, Byrne DW, Stollings JL, Kumar AB, Hughes CG, Hernandez A, et al. Balanced crystalloids versus saline in critically ill adults. N Engl J Med. 2018;378(9):829–39.

72. Van Regenmortel N, Hendrickx S, Roelant E, Baar I, Dams K, Van Vlimmeren K, Embrecht B, Wittock A, Hendriks JM, Lauwers P, et al. 154 compared to 54 mmol per liter of sodium in intravenous maintenance fluid therapy for adult patients undergoing major thoracic surgery (TOPMAST): a single-center randomized controlled double-blind trial. Intensive Care Med. 2019;45(10):1422–32.

73. Ni HB, Ke L, Sun JK, Tong ZH, Ding WW, Li WQ, Li N, Li JS. Beneficial effect of hypertonic saline resuscitation in a porcine model of severe acute pancreatitis. Pancreas. 2012;41(2):310–6.

74. Machado MC, Coelho AM, Pontieri V, Sampietre SN, Molan NA, Soriano F, Matheus AS, Patzina RA, Cunha JE, Velasco IT. Local and systemic effects of hypertonic solution (NaCl 7.5%) in experimental acute pancreatitis. Pancreas. 2006;32(1):80–6.

75. Shields CJ, Winter DC, Sookhai S, Ryan L, Kirwan WO, Redmond HP. Hypertonic saline attenuates end-organ damage in an experimental model of acute pancreatitis. Br J Surg. 2000;87(10):1336–40.

76. Horton JW, Dunn CW, Burnweit CA, Walker PB. Hypertonic saline-dextran resuscitation of acute canine bile-induced pancreatitis. Am J Surg. 1989;158(1):48–56.

77. Pham TN, Cancio LC, Gibran NS, American Burn A. American Burn Association practice guidelines burn shock resuscitation. J Burn Care Res. 2008;29(1):257–66.
78. Wang MD, Ji Y, Xu J, Jiang DH, Luo L, Huang SW. Early goal-directed fluid therapy with fresh frozen plasma reduces severe acute pancreatitis mortality in the intensive care unit. Chin Med J. 2013;126(10):1987–8.
79. Matsuda T, Tanaka H, Hanumadass M, Gayle R, Yuasa H, Abcarian H, Matsuda H, Reyes H. Effects of high-dose vitamin C administration on postburn microvascular fluid and protein flux. J Burn Care Rehabil. 1992;13(5):560–6.
80. Matsuda T, Tanaka H, Williams S, Hanumadass M, Abcarian H, Reyes H. Reduced fluid volume requirement for resuscitation of third-degree burns with high-dose vitamin C. J Burn Care Rehabil. 1991;12(6):525–32.
81. Tanaka H, Matsuda T, Miyagantani Y, Yukioka T, Matsuda H, Shimazaki S. Reduction of resuscitation fluid volumes in severely burned patients using ascorbic acid administration: a randomized, prospective study. Arch Surg. 2000;135(3):326–31.

Sodium and Chloride Balance in Critically Ill Patients

23

Ranajit Chatterjee and Ashutosh Kumar Garg

Contents

Introduction 461
   Water and Sodium Balance 462
Management of Hyponatremia 466
Management of Hypernatremia 470
Chloride Balance 471
   Introduction 471
   Chloride Distribution and Measurement 472
Chloride Physiology 473
   Chloride and the Stewart Approach 473
   Disorders of Chloraemia and Manipulation of Chloride in the ICU 474
   Clinical Approach to Dyschloremia 475
      Hypochloremia 475
      Hyperchloremia 476
Critical Analysis of Crystalloids on the Basis of above Discussion 477
Chloride in the ICU: The Research Agenda 478
Conclusions 479
References 479

R. Chatterjee (✉)
Critical care, Swami Dayanand Hospital, Delhi, India

A. K. Garg
Kailash Deepak Hospital, Karkardooma, New Delhi, India

© The Author(s) 2024
M. L. N. G. Malbrain et al. (eds.), *Rational Use of Intravenous Fluids in Critically Ill Patients*, https://doi.org/10.1007/978-3-031-42205-8_23

IFA Commentary (MLNGM)

The administration of excessive amounts of sodium during intravenous fluid therapy in the hospital can lead to iatrogenic fluid overload, which is a potential side effect that has received little attention [1]. While excessive fluid volume has traditionally been considered the primary cause of this condition, a recent review suggests that the sodium that is administered is also a significant factor in causing harm to hospitalized patients [2]. Intravenous fluid therapy is associated with a range of detrimental effects, including clinical problems related to specific colloid solutions (e.g. hydroxyethyl starches) and NaCl 0.9%. The most serious side effect of fluid therapy is fluid overload, which is an independent risk factor for morbidity and mortality in critically ill and surgical patients. While the root cause of iatrogenic fluid overload has been attributed to excessive fluid volume, the amount of sodium administered has been largely neglected. The largest source of sodium in the ICU comes from maintenance fluid therapy, which is prescribed to meet patients' daily needs for fluids and electrolytes. Additionally, a significant amount of sodium is obtained through fluid creep, where large amounts of fluids are administered as a vehicle for intravenous medication or to keep intravenous lines open, often using NaCl 0.9%. Attention should be drawn to the significant amounts of sodium administered to hospitalized patients and how it contributes to fluid retention. The amount of sodium administered during typical hospital stays exceeds regular dietary sodium intake and the kidneys only have limited capacity handling of an acute sodium load. Moreover, the retention of water associated with sodium overload is energy-demanding and catabolic. The review quantifies the effect size of sodium-induced fluid retention and discusss its potential clinical impact, proposing various preventive and therapeutic options, including low-sodium maintenance fluid therapy and avoiding NaCl 0.9% as the diluent for medication. While caution should be exercised to avoid hyponatremia and hypovolemia, we believe that addressing sodium-induced fluid overload is the next logical step after addressing iatrogenic volume overload. In summary, unphysiological amounts of sodium administered to hospitalized patients through maintenance fluid therapy and fluid creep can lead to harmful fluid retention.

Suggested Reading

1. Van Regenmortel N, Langer T, De Weerdt T, Roelant E, Malbrain M, Van den Wyngaert T, Jorens P: Effect of sodium administration on fluid balance and sodium balance in health and the perioperative setting. Extended summary with additional insights from the MIHMoSA and TOPMAST studies. *J Crit Care*; 2022, 67:157–165.
2. Van Regenmortel N, Moers L, Langer T, Roelant E, De Weerdt T, Caironi P, Malbrain M, Elbers P, Van den Wyngaert T, Jorens PG: Fluid-induced harm in the hospital: look beyond volume and start considering sodium. From physiology towards recommendations for daily practice in hospitalized adults. *Ann Intensive Care*; 2021, 11(1):79.

Learning Objectives
After reading this chapter, you will:

1. ICU patients receive large amounts of sodium and chloride during treatment, which can lead to hypernatremia and hyperchloremia.
2. Infusion of high amounts of chloride can cause hyperchloremic metabolic acidosis.
3. The proportions of sodium and chloride in 0.9% sodium chloride are equal, resulting in a SID of zero, so administration of large volumes can result in a rise in serum sodium and chloride.
4. In brain-injured patients, large volumes of hypotonic solutions must be avoided to prevent cerebral swelling and intracranial hypertension.
5. The use of 'balanced' solutions for maintenance and resuscitation can reduce the development of hyperchloremic acidosis in sepsis patients.
6. Chloride is the major strong anion in blood and plays an important role in the pathogenesis of metabolic acidosis.
7. Alterations in the chloride balance and chloraemia can alter the acid-base status, cell biology, renal function, and haemostasis, and may have negative implications.

Case Vignette
An 18-year-old male was brought to ER in an unconscious state. He had an alcoholic smell on his breath and his blood pressure (BP) was 110/60 mmHg. Physical examination was unremarkable except for him being drowsy. Preliminary laboratory results were as follows: Serum sodium 139 meq/L, potassium 5 meq/L, bicarbonate 22 meq/L, chloride 87 meq/L and glucose of 90 mg/ dL. Blood alcohol level was undetectable and urine microscopy was significant for oxalate crystals. A diagnosis of poisoning with antifreeze (ethylene glycol) was made.

Questions
Q1: Analyse the acid-base status?

Introduction

Patients admitted to the intensive care unit (ICU) typically receive large amounts of sodium and chloride during their ICU treatment [1]. Both hypernatremia and hyperchloremia are frequent complications in critically ill patients and are associated with adverse outcomes [2, 3]. The infusion of high amounts of chloride is also recognized as a cause of hyperchloremic acidosis [4, 5]. The problem with 0.9% sodium chloride is that the proportions of sodium and chloride are equal in solution, and administration of large volumes will result in a rise in serum chloride. Hyperchloremia (relative to serum sodium) results in a metabolic acidosis because of the decrease in strong-ion difference (SID), first described by Stewart in 1983.

The lactate, acetate, and gluconate anions that replace chloride in balanced solutions are removed rapidly from the plasma by the liver (which is faster than renal chloride elimination); this widens the plasma SID and are alkalinizing.

The choice of fluid for resuscitation has been ongoing debate for long, and the 'ideal' resuscitation fluid has yet to be identified. In patients with brain injury, large volumes of hypotonic solutions must be avoided because of the risk of cerebral swelling and intracranial hypertension. Traditionally, 0.9% sodium chloride has been used in patients at risk of intracranial hypertension, but there is increasing recognition that 0.9% sodium chloride is not without its problems.

Roquilly et al. [6] showed a reduction in the development of hyperchloremic acidosis in brain-injured patients when given 'balanced' solutions for maintenance and resuscitation compared with 0.9% sodium chloride. Balanced solutions will be discussed in Chap. 24.

Water and Sodium Balance

Disorders of water and sodium balance are common, but the pathophysiology is frequently misunderstood. As an example, the plasma sodium concentration is regulated by changes in water intake and excretion, not by changes in sodium balance. Hyponatremia primarily reflects water excess, while hypernatremia is a free water deficit state. Hypovolemia represents the loss of sodium and water, and edema is primarily due to sodium and water retention.

It has to be understood that both hyponatremia and hypernatremia are frequently iatrogenic and associated with adverse patient outcomes, especially in the elderly. Hyponatremia occurs more commonly than hypernatremia and is usually in acute hospital care rather than community care; both conditions are more common in the elderly.

Disorders of Sodium Balance The two disorders of sodium balance are hyponatremia and hypernatremia.

Determinants of Plasma Sodium Concentration Sodium and accompanying anions (mostly chloride and bicarbonate) are the main determinants of the plasma and extracellular fluid (ECF) osmolality. By contrast, intracellular potassium and accompanying anions are the main determinant of the intracellular osmolality.

Since water freely crosses most cells, the osmolality is the same in the extracellular and intracellular fluids. Thus, the plasma sodium concentration reflects the osmolality in both compartments even though potassium is the major intracellular cation.

Theoretically, hypernatremia is caused by a disturbance in water homeostasis and sodium content [7]. These mechanisms are derived from the Edelman equation, which in simplified form is as follows [8]:

$$\text{Plasma sodium} = \frac{\left(\text{Total exchangeable Na}^+ + \text{total exchangeable K}^+\right)}{\text{Total body water}}$$

It should be noted that approximately 30% of total body sodium and a smaller fraction of total body potassium are bound in areas such as bone where they are nonexchangeable and osmotically inactive.

Hyponatremia Hyponatremia is almost always due to the oral or intravenous intake of water that cannot be completely excreted. Normal individuals can excrete more than 10 L of urine per day (and more than 400 mL per hour) and therefore will not develop hyponatremia unless water intake exceeds this value, which occurs most often in psychotic patients with primary polydipsia. Hyponatremia caused by massive water intake rapidly resolves as soon as water intake stops, provided that the ability to dilute the urine is intact.

Persistent hyponatremia is associated with impaired water excretion, which is most often due to an inability to suppress the release of antidiuretic hormone (ADH) or to advanced renal failure. The two major causes of persistent ADH secretion are the syndrome of inappropriate ADH secretion (SIADH) and reduced effective arterial blood volume. The latter can occur due to true volume depletion (e.g., diuretics, vomiting, or diarrhea) or decreased tissue perfusion in heart failure or cirrhosis. In the last two disorders, severity of the hyponatremia parallels that of the underlying disease.

Although water is retained in patients with hyponatremia, the degree of ECF volume expansion is not clinically important. The cell membranes are permeable to water, and approximately two-thirds of the excess fluid moves into the cells.

Hyponatremia due to water retention, is typically associated with a reduction in plasma osmolality and tonicity. This creates an osmotic gradient that favours water movement from the ECF into cells and the brain. Water movement into the brain can lead to cerebral edema and potentially severe neurologic symptoms, particularly if hyponatremia is acute. In addition, overly rapid correction of severe chronic hyponatremia can lead to potentially irreversible neurologic injury (central pontine myelinolysis).

True hyponatremia is always a **hypoosmolar** condition. The aberration to this rule is illustrated by the following examples:

Hyponatremia can be caused by osmotic water movement out of the cells, which increases the extracellular volume and, by dilution, lowers the plasma sodium concentration. This phenomenon can occur when hyperosmolality is induced by hyperglycemia or the administration of hypertonic mannitol. Because plasma tonicity is increased, these patients do not experience an increase in intracellular and brain volume caused by water movement into the cells. On the contrary, hypertonicity results in water movement out of the cells and the brain. The movement of water out of the brain with hypertonic mannitol provides the rationale for its use in the treatment of cerebral edema and increased intracranial pressure. The plasma sodium rises towards its baseline value as the hyperglycemia is treated or mannitol is excreted in the urine. This condition, where hyponatremia is associated with an increase in plasma osmolality, is called **redistributive or translocational hyponatremia**.

Hyponatremia may occur in the presence of normal plasma osmolality. Extreme elevations in plasma lipids or proteins will increase the volume of the non-aqueous phase of plasma. In this situation, the measured plasma sodium concentration can be significantly lower than the actual (aqueous phase) sodium concentration. This condition is called *pseudohyponatremia.*

Hyponatremia may be associated with a normal or high plasma osmolality in patients with **renal failure** in whom the osmotic effect of urea retention counterbalances the reduction in plasma osmolality induced by hyponatremia. However, urea readily diffuses into cells and is considered an ineffective osmole. The plasma tonicity (i.e., effective plasma osmolality) is equal to the plasma osmolality minus the contribution of urea and is reduced in proportion to the reduction in plasma sodium. Thus, these patients can develop the manifestations of hyponatremia.

Hypernatremia Hypernatremia is most often the result of failure to replace water losses due to impaired thirst or lack of access to water. It can also be induced by the intake of salt in excess of water or the administration of a hypertonic salt solution.

In contrast to hyponatremia in which water moves into the cells, the increase in plasma tonicity in hypernatremia usually pulls water out of the cells, resulting in a decrease in intracellular volume.

Disorders of Water Balance The two disorders of water balance are hypovolemia and edema.

Hypovolemia Hypovolemia refers to any condition in which the ECF volume is reduced and, when severe, can lead to hypotension or shock. Hypovolemia is usually induced by salt and water losses that are not replaced (e.g., vomiting, diarrhea, diuretic therapy, bleeding, or third-space sequestration). By contrast, unreplaced primary water loss, due to insensible loss by evaporation from the skin and respiratory tract or to increased urinary water loss due to diabetes insipidus, does not usually lead to hypovolemia, because water is lost disproportionately from the intracellular fluid compartment which contains approximately two-thirds of the total body water.

True hypovolemia due to fluid losses should be distinguished from decreased tissue perfusion in heart failure and cirrhosis in which cardiac dysfunction and systemic vasodilation, respectively, are the major hemodynamic abnormalities.

Concurrent Changes in Plasma Sodium Concentration The plasma sodium concentration in hypovolemic patients may be normal, low (most often due to hypovolemia-induced release of ADH, which limits urinary water excretion), or high (if water intake is impaired). The effect on the plasma sodium concentration depends upon both the composition of the fluid that is lost and fluid intake.

In true hypovolemia due to vomiting, diarrhea, or diuretic therapy, the direct effect of fluid loss on the plasma sodium concentration depends upon the concentration of sodium plus potassium in the fluid that is lost. The rationale for including the potassium concentration is discussed above.

If, as occurs in most cases of vomiting and diarrhea, the sodium plus potassium concentration in the fluid that is lost is less than the plasma sodium concentration, water is lost in excess of sodium plus potassium which will tend to increase the plasma sodium concentration. As an example, suppose that 1 L of diarrheal fluid has a sodium plus potassium concentration of 75 mEq/L. This represents the electrolytes contained in 500 mL of isotonic saline (sodium concentration 154 mEq/L). The loss of 500 mL of isotonic electrolytes will have no effect on the plasma sodium concentration. In addition, 500 mL of electrolyte-free water is excreted, which will raise the plasma sodium concentration.

If the sodium plus potassium concentration is the same as the plasma sodium concentration (as with bleeding), there will be no change in plasma sodium concentration induced by the fluid loss.

If the sodium plus potassium concentration lost is greater than the plasma sodium concentration, as can occur with thiazide diuretics, the plasma sodium concentration will fall. The high urine sodium plus potassium concentration (which exceeds the sodium concentration of the plasma) is produced because thiazide diuretics act in the distal tubule and therefore do not interfere with urinary concentrating ability, which depends upon sodium chloride reabsorption in the loop of Henle. The high ADH levels induced by hypovolemia result in water reabsorption, high urine osmolality, and high urine electrolyte concentrations.

The changes in plasma sodium concentration directly induced by fluid loss do not necessarily represent the final outcome. Hypovolemia stimulates nonosmotic release of ADH, which will promote retention of ingested water or infused electrolyte-free water, which will lower the plasma sodium concentration, independent of the composition of the fluid lost.

Edema Edema (including ascites) is a manifestation of sodium excess and an expanded ECF volume. Movement of fluid out of the vascular space into the interstitium is most often mediated by an increase in capillary hydraulic pressure. Tissue perfusion is variable in these disorders, depending upon the cause of edema.

When due to renal failure or glomerulonephritis, tissue perfusion may be increased if cardiac function is intact.

When due to heart failure or cirrhosis, tissue perfusion is often reduced due to decreased cardiac function and vasodilation, respectively.

When due to nephrotic syndrome, tissue perfusion may be reduced due to hypoalbuminemia or edema due to primary renal sodium retention.

Effect on Plasma Sodium Concentration Sodium retention in edematous patients is not associated with hypernatremia, since a proportionate amount of water is retained. However, hyponatremia can occur if there is a concurrent reduction in the ability to excrete water. As an example, hyponatremia is common in patients with heart failure and cirrhosis because the reduction in tissue perfusion increases the secretion of ADH, thereby limiting the excretion of ingested water. In these disorders, the severity of hyponatremia is directly related to the severity of the underlying disease and is therefore a predictor of an adverse prognosis.

Management of Hyponatremia

The spectrum of hyponatremia ranges from hypovolemic, normovolemic to hypervolemic state. Therefore the estimation of volume status is of paramount importance since the treatment protocol in these three situations differ vastly. See Figure 23.1.

The diagnosis of hyponatremia should be carried out systematically. It consists of five components- osmolality(hypo/normo/hyper), serum sodium, acute/chronic, symptomatic/asymptomatic and hypo/normo/hypervolemia status. So a patient with acute diarrhoea may have an acute, symptomatic, hypovolemic, hypoosmolar hyponatremia, whereas a patient with pneumonitis and SIADH may have a chronic, asymptomatic, normovolemic, hypoosmolar hyponatremia.

Hypovolemic hyponatremia may be due to non-renal sodium losses e.g. GI losses (diarrhoea, vomiting), skin losses (burns) or dietary sodium restriction. Typically, the UNa < 20 mEq/L, UOsm >400 mOsm/kg H_2O, FE UA < 8% (indicating hypovolaemia), FE Na < 1% or FE Urea<35%. The latter is used in preference to FENa if prior diuretics have been used.

Hypovolaemic hyponatremia may also occur due to predominantly renal losses, the culprits being diuretic excess, renal failure (tubular disease), mineralo-corticoid deficiency

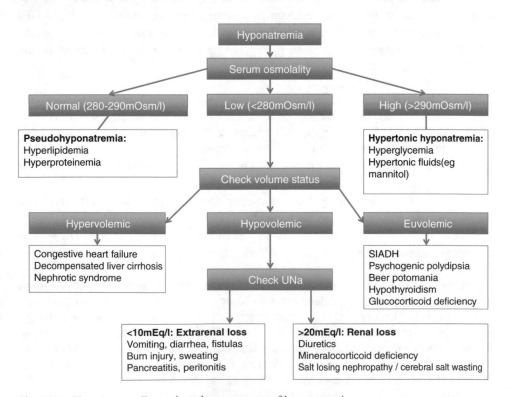

Fig. 23.1 Flowchart on diagnosis and management of hyponatremia

and cerebral salt wasting syndrome. Typically, the UNa > 20 mEq/L, UOsm < 300–400 mOsm/kg H_2O, FE UA < 8%.

Euvolaemic hyponatremia is the most common form seen in hospitalized patients, who may have a slight increase or decrease in volume, but it is not clinically evident, and they do not have oedema. Examples include:

- SIADH (syndrome of inappropriate ADH).
- Glucocorticoid deficiency.
- Hypothyroidism.
- Impaired water excretion.
- Hypotonic fluid replacement post surgery.

The essential features of diagnosis of SIADH are as follows:

- Decreased serum osmolality.
- High urine osmolality (>300 mOsm/L).
- Clinical euvolumia.
- Urinary sodium >40 mEq/L.
- Serum uric acid <4 mg/ dl.
- FE UA >12%.
- Normal thyroid and adrenal function.
- No recent diuretic use.

The common causes of SIADH are malignancy, pulmonary disorders, CNS disorders and various drugs.

Hypervolaemic hyponatremia is characterized by both sodium and water retention, with proportionately more water. Therefore, these patients have an increased amount of total body sodium but as water retention is more significant, there is relative hyponatremia. Examples include:

- CCF.
- Nephrotic syndrome.
- Cirrhosis.
- Acute or chronic renal failure.

Clinical manifestations depend on the severity and acuity.

Chronic hyponatremia can be severe (sodium concentration less than 110 mEq/L), yet remarkably asymptomatic because the brain has adapted by decreasing its tonicity over weeks to months.

Acute hyponatremia that has developed over hours to days can be severely symptomatic with relatively moderate hyponatremia.

Mild hyponatremia (sodium concentrations of 130–135 mEq/L) is usually asymptomatic.

Clinical presentations include nausea, malaise, headache, lethargy, disorientation, respiratory arrest, seizure, coma, permanent brain damage, brainstem herniation and death. Patients may exhibit signs of hypovolemia or hypervolemia.

Treatment: Four aspects must be considered:
1. Asymptomatic vs. symptomatic.
2. Acute (within 48 h).
3. Chronic (>48 h).
4. Volume status.

Correction of serum sodium:
Acute symptomatic hyponatremia

- more rapid correction may be possible,
- 1–2 mEq/L to a total 4–6 mEq.

Chronic hyponatremia

- slower rate of correction advised,
- 12 mEq in 24 h
- < 18 mEq in first 48 h.

Hemodynamic monitoring distinguishes hypovolemic from euvolaemic and hypervolaemic hyponatremia in cases where formulae may give deceptive results.

There are different formulae to calculate the sodium deficit in critically ill patients; these are popular amongst intensive care unit residents.

Hypovolaemic hyponatremia not only needs sodium correction, but also replacement of lost water. Euvolaemic and hypervolaemic hyponatremia needs water restriction.

Treatment of symptomatic hyponatremia
- Initial bolus 2 ml/kg 3% saline.
- Repeat at 5 min interval > max 3 boluses.
- Thereafter 100-200 ml 3% saline over 1–2 hours (rule of thumb: 1 ml/kg increases serum sodium by 1 mEq/L).
- Cerebral symptoms subside with increase in serum sodium by 4–6 mEq/L.

Management of euvolaemic hyponatremia
- Cornerstone of sodium correction in SIADH is correction of the cause (e.g. tumor, pain, nausea, stress).
- Free water restriction.
- Replacement of water loss with normal saline or 3% saline.
- Loop diuretics like furosemide to decrease the concentrating ability of kidneys.
- Drugs.
  - Democlocycline.
  - ADH antagonists e.g. tolvaptan, conivaptan.

Expect a rapid increase in serum sodium with increasing urine output when non-osmotic ADH release subsides after volume repletion. This is the time when desmopressin has to be added to avoid over rapid correction.

Vaptans   These are nonpeptide competitive ADH antagonists, which act by inhibiting the action of vasopressin on its receptors V1a/V2 and enhancing free water excretion without increasing renal sodium and potassium excretion (Aquaretics).

- Indication.
  - Refractory case of euvolemic and hypervolemic moderate-to-severe hyponatremia.
- Contraindication.
  - Hypovolemic hyponatremia.
  - Anuria.
- Dosage.
  - Loading dose: 20 mg IV over 30 minutes.
  - Continuous infusion 20 mg/day over 24 hr., maximum duration 4 days.
- Adverse reaction.
  - Pyrexia.
  - Hypokalemia.
  - Headache.
  - Orthostatic hypotension.
- Specific consideration.
  - Hepatic impairment.
        decrease the dose,
  - Renal impairment.
        decrease the dose,
  - Pregnancy.
        can cause harm to fetus,
  - Pediatric use.
        no studies.

Osmotic demyelination syndrome

- Rapid correction of sodium in hyponatremia would cause the extracellular fluid to be relatively hypertonic.
- Free water would then move out of the cells to decrease this relative hypertonicity, leading to a central pontine myelinolysis.
- Central pontine myelinolysis is a concentrated, frequently symmetric, noninflammatory demyelination within the central basis ponts.
- In at least 10% of patients with central pontine myelinolysis, demyelination also occurs in extrapontine regions, including the midbrain, thalamus, basal nuclei and cerebellum.

Clinical presentation of osmotic demyelination syndrome (ODS) is heterogeneous and depend on the regions of the brain involved:

- Seizures.
- Disturbed consciousness.
- Gait changes.
- Respiratory depression or arrest.
- Spastic quadriparesis.
- Dysphagia.
- Dysarthria.
- Diplopia.
- Risk factors of ODM includes alcoholism, malnutrition, hypokalemia, liver failure and malignancy.

Management of Hypernatremia

The incidence of hypernatremia is much less common than hyponatremia. Hypernatremia can be divided again into three subtypes in the same fashion as hyponatremia -hypovolaemic, euvolaemic and hypervolaemic. The attached flowchart describes the different types and treatment of this disorder. See Figure 23.2.

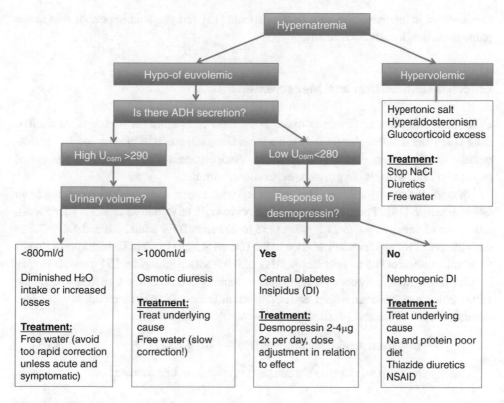

Fig. 23.2 Flowchart on diagnosis and management of hypernatremia

Chloride Balance

Introduction

Chloride is the major strong anion in blood, accounting for approximately one-third of plasma tonicity, for 97 to 98% of all strong anionic charges and for two-thirds of all negative charges in plasma [9]. Sodium and chloride ions were once termed the 'king and queen of electrolytes' respectively [10]; over the years, chloride has become the forgotten ion. With progress in our understanding of acid–base and chloride channel physiology, the chloride ion is regaining its prominence.

In the 1990s, hyperchloraemic acidosis became more intently studied [11] as the physicochemical approach (Stewart approach) to acid–base analysis [12] received wider acceptance.

Within the Stewart approach, chloride is the dominant negative strong ion in plasma and a key contributor to the strong ion difference (SID), one of three independent variables that determine the hydrogen ion concentration. Hyperchloraemia is quite commonly encountered in intensive care unit (ICU) patients [13] and plays an important role in the pathogenesis of metabolic acidosis.

Chloride Distribution and Measurement

Chloride distribution in the three major body fluid compartments – plasma, interstitial fluid (ISF) and intracellular fluid. It is the most abundant anion in plasma and ISF (extracellular fluid); its concentration in these two compartments differ slightly as a result of capillary impermeability to proteins, especially albumin.

Chloride is the predominant extracellular ion with a normal concentration ranging from 94–111 meq/L [14]. The main source of chloride is dietary sodium chloride (table salt), the intake of which is 7.8 to 11.8 g/day (133 to 202 mmol) for adult men and 5.8 to 7.8 g/day (99 to 133 mmol) for adult women in the United States [15]. This intake approximates to administration of 0.5 to 1.3 litres per day of 0.9% saline (chloride, 154 mmol/l).

Chloride significantly contributes to plasma tonicity and is used in formulae to estimate serum anion gap, urine anion gap, and strong ion difference (Stewart method) which is less popular for use in clinical practice due to its complex interpretations.

$$\text{Serum Anion Gap} = \text{serum} \left[Na^+ - \left[Cl^- + HCO3^- \right] \right] \tag{23.1}$$

$$\text{Delta gap} = \left(\text{change in anion gap} \right) - \left(\text{change in bicarbonate} \right) \tag{23.2}$$

(The normal anion gap is assumed to be 12, and the normal HCO_3 is assumed to be 24.)

Interpretation of the generated ratio:
- −6 = Mixed high and normal anion gap acidosis
- −6 to 6 = Only a high anion gap acidosis exists
- over 6 = Mixed high anion gap acidosis and metabolic alkalosis

$$\text{Delta ratio} = \left(\text{change in anion gap} \right) / \left(\text{change in bicarbonate} \right) \tag{23.3}$$

(The normal anion gap is assumed to be 12, and the normal HCO_3 is assumed to be 24.)

Interpretation of the generated ratio:
- 0.4 = normal anion gap metabolic acidosis
- 0.4–0.8 = mixed high and normal anion gap acidosis exists.
- 0.8–2.0 = purely due to a high anion gap metabolic acidosis
- Over 2.0 = high anion gap acidosis with pre-existing metabolic alkalosis.

$$\text{Urine Anion Gap} = \text{urine} \left[Na^+ + K^+ \right] - Cl^- \tag{23.4}$$

$$\text{Strong ion difference (SID)} = \left(\text{Na}^+ + \text{K}^+ + \text{Mg}^{++} + \text{Ca}^{++}\right)$$
$$-\left(\text{Cl}^- + \text{lactate} + \text{other strong anions}\right) \quad (23.5)$$

$$\text{Na+, K+, Cl–, HCO3 – in meq / L}$$

The role of chloride in urine anion gap measurements is unique and indirect as chloride here serves as a surrogate marker of NH4 + excretion in urine. A positive urine anion gap in the presence of metabolic acidosis is often abnormal and points towards low urinary NH4 + excretion, thus impaired urinary acid excretion.

Chloride Physiology

Approximately 21,000 mEq of chloride is filtered everyday, of which >99% is absorbed (55% in the proximal tubule, 25–35% in the thick ascending loop (TAL) of Henle and the remainder in the distal tubule) and only 100–250 meq is excreted every day [16].

Once in the proximal tubular lumen, chloride is reabsorbed actively via anion exchangers [SLC26A6] (chloride-formate, chloride-hydroxyl, chloride-oxalate exchanger) on luminal side and leaves the cell via a K + Cl- co-transporter and chloride selective channels.

In the TAL, chloride is reabsorbed via luminal Na-K-2Cl co-transporter and leaves the cell via ClC-Ka channel co-localized with Barttin protein. Reabsorption of sodium chloride in the TAL is essential for generation of medullary osmotic gradient, a pre-requisite for excreting concentrated urine. Once tubular fluid reaches the macula densa, its activity is modulated by chloride concentration such that low chloride concentration activates macula densa cells, thereby stimulating renin release.

In the distal convoluted tubule, chloride is actively reabsorbed via luminal Na-Cl co-transporters and leaves the cell via basolateral chloride channels.

Chloride and the Stewart Approach

An understanding of Stewart's approach may help to understand how chloride might affect the hydrogen ion concentration [H+] [12].

In the traditional approach, bicarbonate independently determines pH as reflected by the Henderson–Hasselbalch equation:

$$pH = pK + \log\left(\left[\text{HCO3}-\right]/\left[\text{CO2}\right]\right)$$

With the Stewart approach however, bicarbonate is just one of the various dependent ions. Together with other completely dissociated strong ions, chloride determines the SID:

$$SID = \left(\text{Na} + \text{K} + \text{Mg} + \text{Ca}\right) - \left(\text{Cl} + \text{lactate}\right)$$

Determination of [H+] depends on three independent variables:

- the SID.
- the partial pressure of carbon dioxide.
- total weak acid concentration.

A change in any of these three variables, and not in bicarbonate, will change the acid–base balance. Bicarbonate becomes a marker and not a mechanism, a major difference between the Stewart approach and the traditional Henderson–Hasselbalch approach.

Quantitatively, a change in the strong ion composition leading to lower SID will increase [H+] while an increase in SID will decrease [H+].

Hyperchloremic acidosis therefore causes acidosis by decreasing SID and not through hyperchloremia alone. This notion is supported by data demonstrating a stronger association between SID and bicarbonate than that between chloride and bicarbonate [31]. Hyperchloraemic acidosis is now increasingly described in terms of its SID nature, including the contribution of the strong ion gap or unmeasured anions [19, 20].

At the other end of the spectrum, alkalosis may thus occur with both hypochloraemia and hyperchloraemia, with the latter occurring in the presence of greater hypernatraemia (greater SID) [21]. This again highlights the importance of relative rather than absolute chloraemia.

In a study of patients with chronic obstructive pulmonary disease, subjects were found to have hypochloraemia without significant changes in plasma sodium, resulting in a higher SID and subsequent alkalosis [22]. This interestingly concurs with an animal study showing increased renal chloride excretion during hypochloraemia of respiratory acidosis.

Disorders of Chloraemia and Manipulation of Chloride in the ICU

Hyperchloraemia or hypochloraemia, resulting from disease processes or clinical manipulations, is common in the ICU and should always be considered in relation to sodium.

Hyperchloraemia with hypernatraemia, or hypochloraemia with hyponatraemia, will not change the SID and thus will not affect the acid–base balance. Intravenous administration of chloride-rich fluids is probably the most common and modifiable cause of hyperchloraemia in the ICU.

Chloride is also an essential component of intravenous fluids used in daily clinical practice and its concentration in different replacement fluids (mmol/L) is as follows [14]:

4% Albumin = 128; Normal saline (0.9%) = 154; Half normal saline (0.45%) = 77; Ringers lactate = 111,; PlasmaLyte = 98; Hydroxyethyl starch = range 110–154.

The chloride content of these fluids, from 0.9% saline to the various colloids suspended in saline is supraphysiologic [23], with significant hyperchloraemia following the administration of such fluids in volunteers, intraoperatively or as cardiopulmonary bypass priming fluid.

Whilst saline was a life-saving measure when first introduced during the cholera pandemic of Europe in the 1830s [24], it should be noted that the saline used then was of a different composition. A reconstitution of the Thomas Latta solution revealed a sodium concentration of 134 mmol/l, chloride 118 mmol/l and bicarbonate 16 mmol/l. The historical or scientific basis of the present-day 0.9% composition of saline remains a mystery, even when traced to those cholera pandemic days that marked the beginning of the intravenous fluid therapy and its various solutions [25].

Finally, the role of chloride-rich fluids and resulting acidosis in causing inferior outcomes in sepsis [17], renal vasoconstriction [17] and acute kidney injury [18] has been debated. Chloride-rich fluids result in acidosis, and evidence from animal studies particularly in sepsis point to a possible association with negative outcomes.

Clinical Approach to Dyschloremia

Symptoms related to derangement in chloride levels usually depend upon underlying cause and hence treatment also widely varies.

Hypochloremia

Hypochloremia can occur due to various reasons (Table 23.1), most commonly due to gastrointestinal or renal loss of chloride ions and also following administration of hypotonic fluids or water gain in excess of chloride (dilutional hypochloremia).

Chloride levels are inversely proportional to bicarbonate levels so to maintain electroneutrality, hence hypochloremia is usually associated with alkalosis due to increased bicarbonate reabsorption.

Patient with hypochloremia may present with following clinical features which may be due to concomitant metabolic alkalosis, rather than hypochloremia per se.

Table 23.1 Causes of hypochloremia

Mechanism	Loss location	Example
Chloride loss	Gastrointestinal	Vomiting
		Gastric fluid drainage
		High-volume ileostomy drainage
	Renal	Diuretic use
		Bartter syndrome
		Gitelman syndrome
Excess water gain (compared with chloride)	Congestive heart failure	Infusion of hypotonic solutions
	Syndrome of inappropriate antidiuretic hormone	
Excess sodium gain (compared with chloride)		Infusion of sodium bicarbonate

- Confusion/stupor/coma.
- Dizziness.
- Neuromuscular irritability - muscle twitching, numbness or tingling in the face and extremities.
- Arrhythmias.
- Nausea, vomiting.
- Tetany.

The initial diagnostic step in patients with hypochloremia and metabolic alkalosis is to assess urinary chloride which if >40 meq/L (chloride resistant metabolic alkalosis) suggests either salt wasting nephropathy such as Bartter or Gitelman syndrome (distinguished by urinary calcium excretion) or volume overload states such as congestive heart failure, hyperaldosteronism or apparent mineralocorticoid excess (differentiated through clinical history, physical exam, echocardiogram and measurement of serum aldosterone level along with plasma renin activity or concentration).

If hypochloremia exists with metabolic acidosis, the prevalent acid-base abnormality is usually normal AG metabolic acidosis. The urine AG can be used to differentiate between GI or renal loss.

In a patient with hypochloremia with normonatremia and normal or low serum bicarbonate, serum anion gap (Eq. 23.1) and delta gap (Eq. (23.2)) or delta ratio (Eq. 23.3) should be routinely measured which will uncover the mixed acid–base disorders as seen in case 1.

If poisoning with alcohol is suspected, serum osmolar gap (Eqs. 23.6 and 23.7) should be calculated. However, in patients with hypochloremia and hyponatremia, the primary focus should be shifted towards hyponatremia management.

$$\text{Serum Osmolar Gap} = \text{Calculated Serum Osmolarity}$$
$$- \text{measured serum osmolarity} \qquad (23.6)$$

$$\text{Calculated S. Osmolarity} (\text{mosm}/\text{kg}) = 2[\text{Na}+] + \text{BUN}/2.8$$
$$+ \text{Glucose}/18 + \text{Ethanol}/4.6 \qquad (23.7)$$

$$\text{Na} + (\text{meq}/\text{L}), \text{BUN, glucose and ethanol} (\text{mg}/\text{dL})$$

Hyperchloremia

The most common modifiable etiology of hyperchloremia is excessive infusion of chloride-rich solutions e.g. saline especially during fluid resuscitation or total parenteral nutrition. It may also be secondary to water loss relative to chloride loss which may be related to renal or extra renal causes, the most common in ICU being diarrhoea. Another mechanism is an increase in tubular chloride reabsorption as seen in renal tubular acidosis (RTA) (Table 23.2).

In patients with hyperchloremia, metabolic acidosis and high anion gap metabolic acidosis, poisoning with toluene and isopropyl alcohol should be suspected. Urine osmolar gap (Eqs. 23.8 and 23.9) should be calculated.

Table 23.2 Causes of hyperchloremia

Mechanism	Loss location	Example
Chloride administration		Chloride-rich intravenous fluids
		Total parenteral nutrition
Water loss (true water loss or relative to chloride)	Renal	Diabetes insipidus
		Diuretic use
		Osmotic diuresis
		Postobstructive diuresis
	Extrarenal	Fever
		Hypermetabolic state
		Diarrhea
		Burns
		Exercise and severe dehydration
Definitive or relative increase in tubular chloride reabsorption		Renal tubular acidosis
		Renal failure
		Acetazolamide use
		Ureteral diversion procedure
		Post-hypocapnia

In those with **hyperchloremia, metabolic acidosis and negative serum anion gap, pseudohyperchloremia** should be suspected. Hypertriglyceridemia, multiple myeloma and toxicity with salicylate or bromide must be considered and their levels checked [16, 17].

$$\text{Urine Osmolar Gap} = \text{Calculated Urine osmolarity} - \text{measured urine osmolarity} \quad (23.8)$$

$$\text{Calculated Urine Osmolarity}\left(\text{mosm} / \text{kg}\right) = 2\left[Na^+ + K^+\right]$$
$$+ BUN / 2.8 + Glucose / 18 \quad (23.9)$$

With the following units used in the formula

$$Na^+, K^+\left(\text{meq} / L\right), BUN \,\&\, glucose\left(\text{mg} / dL\right)$$

In patients with hyperchloremia and metabolic acidosis, patients usually have normal-anion gap metabolic acidosis (NAGMA) that could be either due to gastrointestinal losses or renal loss of HCO3 or renal inability to acidify urine. This can be differentiated using urine anion gap (Eq. 23.4) and urine osmolar gap (Eqs. 23.8 and 23.9).

Critical Analysis of Crystalloids on the Basis of above Discussion

Numerous crystalloids are commercially available; clinicians are often perturbed as to the appropriate use of these fluids. A wrong choice can lead to deterioration in critically ill patients.

The commonest fluid used in clinical practice is normal saline. Unfortunately, the terminology itself is a misnomer as it is not normal because it has a higher sodium and chloride content relative to plasma and it is also slightly hyperosmolar. As already explained, hyperchloremia is harmful. There is a significant increase in mortality if the plasma chloride level exceeds 110 meq/L. Moreover, the high sodium load is detrimental to a failing kidney. The SID of normal saline is 0, and as we know the lower the SID, the higher the possibility of metabolic acidosis. Thus normal saline has the propensity to cause metabolic acidosis. However, being slightly hyperosmolar, it is an ideal solution for head trauma patients.

Ringer's lactate on the other hand has less sodium and chloride content. However, the lactate that is present is converted into bicarbonate, and glucose is produced by the gluconeogenetic pathway. In patients with impaired hepatic function, lactic acidosis might occur and in diabetic patients, hyperglycemia is a possibility. However, the SID of Ringer's lactate is close to that of plasma, which adds to its advantage.

Balanced salt solutions replace lactate with acetate and gluconate, which has an extrahepatic mechanism of conversion to bicarbonate. The level of acetate is too low to cause cardiovascular instability. The SID of most of the balanced salt solutions exceeds 40; their alkaline state makes them a near ideal solution in metabolic acidosis.

Chloride in the ICU: The Research Agenda

Clinically, there is a need to re-evaluate our intravenous fluid practice - the patient's main source of external chloride. The evidence that the choice of fluids affects acid–base balance and could cause the undesirable physiological alterations described above cannot be ignored.

More importantly, all of this preliminary evidence leads to a number of research questions that are pertinent to chloride and the care of ICU patients:

How common is hyperchloraemia in the ICU?

Is hyperchloraemia an independent predictor of death or other adverse outcomes?

Does hyperchloraemia only matter when associated with SID changes or acidaemia?

Can the elimination of chloride-rich fluids lead to clinical benefits?

These questions need urgent attention because millions of litres of saline and millions of millimoles of excess chloride are being administered to patients worldwide every day.

Case Vignette

In this patient, most of the laboratory values appear normal, and it is possible to easily overlook the serious acid-base disorder if attention is not given towards the remarkably low chloride value which suggests a complex acid–base disorder with high anion gap metabolic acidosis (serum anion gap of 30) and superimposed metabolic alkalosis (delta gap of 18 and delta ratio of 10). The high anion gap points towards unmeasured anions, later found to be oxalic acid, the metabolite of ethylene glycol.

Conclusions

Chloride has been neglected for too long. Alterations in the chloride balance and chlorae-mia, both absolute and relative to natraemia, can alter the acid–base status, cell biology, renal function, and haemostasis but the clinical consequences of these biological and physiological alterations remain unclear. Most of these alterations appear to have negative implications so there is an urgent need to conduct trials & research into the epidemiology and outcome implications of disorders of chloride balance and chloride concentration.

Take Home Messages
- Avoid using large volumes of 0.9% sodium chloride in ICU patients, except those at risk of intracranial hypertension.
- Consider using 'balanced' solutions for maintenance and resuscitation in sepsis patients.
- Hyperchloremic acidosis can be caused by the infusion of high amounts of chloride.
- Chloride is an important ion in blood and should not be neglected in acid-base analysis.
- Further research is needed to fully understand the clinical implications of altera-tions in sodium and chloride balance and concentration.

References

1. Hessels L, Oude Lansink A, Renes MH, van der Horst IC, Hoekstra M, Touw DJ, et al. Postoperative fluid retention after heart surgery is accompanied by a strongly positive sodium balance and a negative potassium balance. Physiol Rep. 2016;4:e12807.
2. Waite MD, Fuhrman SA, Badawi O, Zuckerman IH, Franey CS. Inten-sive care unit-acquired hypernatremia is an independent predictor of increased mortality and length of stay. J Crit Care. 2013;28:405–12.
3. Oude Lansink-Hartgring A, Hessels L, Weigel J, de Smet AMGA, GommersD PPVN, et al. Long-term changes in dysnatremia incidence in the ICU: a shift from hyponatremia to hyperna-tremia. Ann Intensive Care. 2016;6:22.
4. Shaw AD, Raghunathan K, Peyerl FW, Munson SH, Paluskiewicz SM, Scher-mer CR. Association between intravenous chloride load during resuscita-tion and in-hospital mor-tality among patients with SIRS. Intensive Care Med. 2014;40:1897–905.
5. Yunos NM, Bellomo R, Story D, Kellum J. Bench-to-bedside review: chlo- ride in critical illness. Crit Care. 2010;14:226.
6. Roquilly A, Loutrel O, Cinotti R, Rosenczweig E, Flet L, Mahe PJ, Dumont R, Chupin AM, Peneaux C, Lejus C, Blanloeil Y, Volteau C, Asehnoune K. Balanced versus chloride-rich solu-tions for fluid resuscitation in braininjured patients: a randomized double-blind pilot study. Crit Care. 2013;17:R77.
7. van de Louw A, Shaffer C, Schaefer E. Early intensive care unit-acquired hypernatremia in severe sepsis patient receiving 0.9% saline fluid resuscitation. Acta Anaesthesiol Scand. 2014;58(8):1007–14.

8. Edelman IS, Leibman J, O'meara MP, Birkenfeld LW. Interrelations between serum sodium concentration, serum osmolarity and total exchangeable sodium, total exchangeable potassium and total body water. J Clin Investig. 1958;37(9):1236–56.

9. Ganong WF. Review of medical physiology. 22nd ed. New York: McGraw Hill; 2005.

10. Berend K, Vanhulsteijn LH, Gans ROB. Chloride: the queen of electrolytes? Euro J Intern Med. 2012;23:203–11.

11. Waters JH, Gottlieb A, Schoenwald P, Popovic MJ, Sprung J, Nelson DR. Normal saline versus lactated Ringer's solution for intraoperative fluid management in patients undergoing abdominal aortic aneurysm repair: an outcome study. Anesth Analg. 2001;93:817–22.

12. Stewart PA. How to understand acid–base. In: A quantitative primer for biology and medicine. New York: Elsevier; 1981.

13. Klemtz K, Ho L, Bellomo R. Daily intravenous chloride load and the acid– base and biochemical status of intensive care unit patients. J Pharm Pract Res. 2008;38:296–9.

14. Myburgh JA, Mythen MG. Resuscitation fluids. N Engl J Med. 2013;369:1243–51.

15. Food and Nutrition Board. Institute of Medicine of the National Academies: dietary reference intakes for water, potassium, sodium, chloride, and sulfate. Washington, DC: National Academies Press; 2004.

16. Rose BD, Post TW. Introduction to renal function: clinical physiology of acid-base and electrolyte disorders. 5th ed. McGraw-Hill; 2001.

17. Yunos NM, Bellomo R, Story D, Kellum J. Bench-to-bedside review: chloride in critical illness. Crit Care. 2010;14:226.

18. Yunos NM, Bellomo R, Hegarty C, Story D, Ho L, et al. Association between a chloride-liberal vs chloride-restrictive intravenous fluid administration strategy and kidney injury in critically ill adults. JAMA. 2012;308:1566–72.

19. Rocktaeschel J, Morimatsu H, Uchino S, Bellomo R. Unmeasured anions in critically ill patients: can they predict mortality? Crit Care Med. 2003;31:2131–6.

20. Antinoni B, Piva S, Paltenghi M, Candiani A, Latronico N. The early phase of critical illness is a progressive acidic state due to unmeasured anions. Eur JAnaesthesiol. 2008;25:566–72.

21. Story DA. Hyperchloraemic acidosis: another misnomer? Crit Care Resusc. 2004;6:188–92.

22. Alfaro V, Torras R, Ibanez J, Palacios L. A physical–chemical analysis of the acid–base response to chronic obstructive pulmonary disease. Can JPhysiolPharmacol. 1996;74:1229–35.

23. Wakim KG. 'Normal' 0.9% salt solution is neither 'normal' nor physiological [letter]. JAMA. 1970;214:1710.

24. Latta T. Malignant cholera. Lancet. 1831–1832(ii):274–7.

25. Awad S, Allison SP, Lobo DN. The history of 0.9% saline. ClinNutr. 2008;27:179–88.

Balanced Solutions: Choice of Buffer

24

Suneel Kumar Garg

"Each time new experiments are observed to agree with the predictions, the theory survives and our confidence in it is increased; but if ever new observation is found to disagree, we have to abandon or modify the theory"

—*Stephen Hawking,*

Contents

Introduction 483
Buffered/Balanced Crystalloids 483
Sodium Lactate vs Sodium Acetate Solution 485
Acetate and Gluconate Buffered Solutions 487
Acetate and Malate Buffered Solutions 489
Conclusion 490
References 490

IFA Commentary (MLNGM)

Buffered solutions are commonly used in medical settings to help maintain acid–base balance in patients. The choice of buffer can impact the effectiveness and safety of the solution. The ideal solution to maintain pH should have a strong ion difference (SID) of around 24–28 mmol/L, whereas abnormal saline has a SID of zero and hereby can induce hyperchloremic metabolic acidosis. Lactate, malate, acetate, gluconate and pyruvate are all potential buffer choices for balanced solutions (Figure). The selection of a particular buffer is influenced by several factors, including pH, the desired buffering capacity and the safety profile of the buffer. Lactate is a commonly

S. K. Garg (✉)
Saiman Healthcare, Delhi, India

© The Author(s) 2024
M. L. N. G. Malbrain et al. (eds.), *Rational Use of Intravenous Fluids in Critically Ill Patients*, https://doi.org/10.1007/978-3-031-42205-8_24

used buffer in balanced solutions. It has a pKa of 3.9, which allows it to buffer acidic conditions effectively. Lactate is also metabolized to bicarbonate in the liver, providing an additional mechanism for regulating acid–base balance. Malate is another buffer option with a pKa of 3.2. It can buffer both acidic and basic conditions effectively and is metabolized in the liver to bicarbonate. However, malate can also increase aluminum absorption, which may be a concern for some patients. Acetate has a pKa of 4.8 and can buffer acidic conditions effectively. It is also metabolized in the liver to bicarbonate. Acetate is generally considered safe, but large doses may cause metabolic acidosis. Gluconate has a pKa of 4.4 and can buffer both acidic and basic conditions. It is metabolized to CO_2 and water and is generally considered safe. However, gluconate can increase potassium levels, which may be a concern in patients with renal impairment. Pyruvate has a pKa of 2.5 and can buffer acidic conditions effectively. It is metabolized to bicarbonate in the liver and has been investigated for use in resuscitation fluids. However, high doses of pyruvate have been associated with hemodynamic instability and metabolic acidosis. Overall, the choice of buffer in balanced solutions should be based on the individual patient's needs and safety profile.

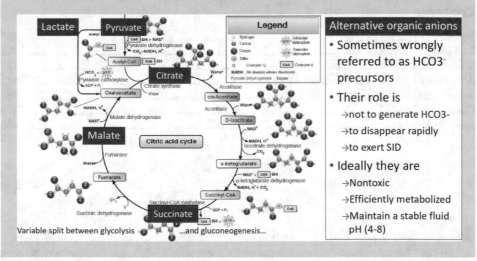

Learning Objectives

After reading this chapter, you will:

1. Understand the importance of buffers in balanced solutions.
2. Understand the role of different types of buffers in maintaining acid–base balance.
3. Understand the potential benefits and drawbacks of different buffers in clinical settings.

> **Case Vignette**
>
> Mr. X, aged 47 years, is admitted from the ED for the management of sepsis. He was resuscitated with 30 mL/kg of 0.9% normal saline. He was started on norepinephrine infusion as he was poorly responsive to fluids. Estimation of his right atrial pressure via inferior vena cava triggers many more liters of intravenous saline. His morning blood analysis results: Cl-120 mEq/L, HCO3–12 mEq/L, lactate-5.5 mEq/L. He was anuric, hypoxemic, acidemic and on high-flow oxygen via nasal cannulae.
>
> What are the possible reasons for his metabolic acidosis? Are balanced solutions better than normal saline? Which balanced solution is preferable amongst those available?

Introduction

The 2021 Surviving Sepsis Guidelines suggested an immediate resuscitation in a shocked patient, to maintain perfusion of tissues. Intravenous fluids are integral to the multimodal strategy used in resuscitation. Despite their widespread usage, there remains uncertainty about the relative safety of various intravenous fluids. "Normal" saline, i.e. 0.9% sodium chloride (NaCl) was developed by Dutch physiologist Dr. Hartog Jacob Hamburger around the 1900s and is classified as an unbuffered/unbalanced crystalloid [1, 2]. Despite its name, it is not physiologically normal due to its higher chloride concentration, and zero strong ion difference (SID) compared to plasma. The SID of the plasma is approximately 40 mEq/l. As per the Stewart physiochemical approach, there is a net decrease in the plasma SID, after boluses of 0.9% NaCl, resulting in a non-anion gap metabolic acidosis. Non-anion gap acidosis engendered by 0.9% NaCl may lead to hyperkalemia, diminished renal perfusion and increased mortality. Sodium and chloride balance will be discussed in Chap. 23.

Buffered/Balanced Crystalloids

Buffered/balanced crystalloids are designed to mimic the composition of human plasma. The key differences between 0.9% NaCl and buffered/balanced crystalloid solutions are the presence of physiological or near-physiological amounts of chloride, a nearly physiological SID and also the presence of additional anions, such as lactate, acetate, malate and gluconate. These anions act as physiological buffers by generating bicarbonate on metabolism. Despite physiological similarities of these solutions to human plasma, presently there is no ideal balanced or physiologically "normal" crystalloid (Table 24.1).

Table 24.1 Composition of human plasma compared to various available buffered/balanced crystalloids solutions

	Human Plasma	0.9% Saline	Ringer's Lactate/ Sodium Lactate	Ringer's Acetate/ Sodium Acetate	Acetate and Malate based Buffered Solution (Sterofundin)	Acetate and Gluconate based Buffered Solution (Plasma-Lyte 148)
Sodium (mmol/l)	136–145	154	130	130	145	140
Chloride (mmol/l)	98–106	154	109	112	127	98
Potassium (mmol/l)	3.5–5.5	Nil	4	5	4	5
Magnesium (mmol/l)	0.8–1.0	Nil	Nil	1	1	1.5
Calcium (mmol/l)	2.2–2.6	Nil	2.7	1	2.5	Nil
Acetate (mmol/l)	Nil	Nil	Nil	27	24	27
Gluconate (mmol/l)	Nil	Nil	Nil	Nil	Nil	23
Lactate (mmol/l)	Nil	Nil	28	Nil	Nil	Nil
Malate (mmol/l)	Nil	Nil	Nil	Nil	5	Nil
eSID (mEq/l)	42	0	27		25.5	50
Theoretical osmolarity (mosmol/l)	291	308	273	276	309	294
Ph	7.35–7.45	4.5–7.0	6.0–7.5	6.0–8.0	5.1–5.9	6.5–8.0

Buffered/balanced crystalloids are commonly used as both resuscitation and maintenance fluid in the emergency room, intensive care units and during elective and emergency surgery. Various buffered solutions are not biologically equivalent due to a variable concentration of ancillary cations (sodium, potassium, calcium, magnesium) in addition to differences in buffering agents. Furthermore, a difference in osmolarity of various solutions is also an important practical consideration. As shown in Table-1, Ringer's lactate (RL) and Ringer's acetate (RA) are hypotonic solutions that can lead to post-resuscitation positive fluid balance, edema, weight gain and increase in intracranial pressure when used in larger volumes [3].

Sodium Lactate *vs* Sodium Acetate Solution

In the 1880s, British physiologist Dr. Sydney Ringer demonstrated the influence of crystalloids on the ex vivo beating of a frog's heart [4, 5]. This fluid was known as Ringer's solution. Ringer's solution was modified in 1932 by American pediatrician Dr. Alexis Hartmann by adding sodium lactate to act as a buffering agent in an effort to combat acidosis [6, 7]. This fluid was popularized as sodium lactate or RL or Hartmann's solution and may be considered the first balanced crystalloid. Lactated solution contains 2.7 mmol/l of calcium and and should not be mixed with blood or blood-related products. In fact, mixing calcium containing solutions with some antibiotics like ceftriaxone can cause the precipitation asinsoluble ceftriaxone calcium salt [8]. Use this recent reference for compatibility of various solutions with balanced crystalloids. PMID: 32401743.

There is an abundance of human studies comparing 0.9% saline with balanced solutions but data is scarce for the comparison of various balanced solutions. To compare acetate with lactate: acetate is metabolized widely and more rapidly than lactate and is not entirely dependent on hepatic metabolism and patient age [9]. Also, acetate solutions are less liable to bacterial contamination when compared with lactate in peritoneal dialysate solutions [10]. In contrast to lactate metabolism, acetate metabolism is preserved in severe shock [11]. Acetate is also more alkalinizing than lactate, which may confer benefits in treating acidemic patients requiring fluid resuscitation. Acetate does not affect glucose or insulin concentration unlike lactate, which is converted to glucose via gluconeogenesis and can cause significant hyperglycemia especially in patients undergoing major surgery [12, 13].

Hypoxia and hypotension can occur in patients with chronic kidney disease dialyzed with solutions containing acetate because of increased nitric oxide synthesis [14–16]. Kirkendol RL et al., first reported that sodium acetate produced a dose-related decrease in cardiac contractility and blood pressure in dogs [17]. Initial reports by Kirkendol RL et al. conflicted with his own research showing that a slow infusion of acetate failed to cause adverse haemodynamic effects [18]. Two decades later, Jacob et al., also examined the effect of acetate on myocardial energy metabolism on isolated perfused rat heart and reported a negative effect on cardiac contractility [19].

There were no human studies to support these findings until Schrander-vd Meer AM, demonstrated the haemodynamic effects of acetate in patients undergoing high-volume renal replacement therapy (RRT) [20]. He concluded that acetate-associated vasodilatation and negative inotropic effect led to haemodynamic instability in these patients.

In another crossover study on humans involving 12 patients undergoing hemodiafiltration, Selby et al. demonstrated that exposure to acetate-free dialysate was associated with less deterioration in systemic haemodynamics, and less suppression of myocardial contractility [21].

In a recent study, RL and RA infusions were compared with regard to acid–base balance and haemodynamic stability in patients undergoing abdominal gynecologic surgery. Patients received a mean dose of 4054 ± 450 ml of either one or the other; there was no difference in terms of mean arterial blood pressure and norepinephrine requirements between the study groups. pH and serum HCO3- concentration decreased slightly but significantly only with RL [22].

Patients with liver disease pose a challenge to anaesthesiologists and intensivists; the fluid choice for resuscitation and maintenance is an important consideration. In a study of patients with cirrhosis undergoing general anaesthetic for elective surgery by Hatem A Attalla et al., RA was associated with significantly higher pyruvate levels and ketone bodies while lactate was higher in the RL group. pH, HCO3, base excess, liver function, blood glucose level and haemodynamic parameters were similar in both groups. These findings suggest that RA decreased the metabolic load to the liver and improved hepatic energy status in patients with liver dysfunction, so it may be more beneficial than RL as an intraoperative fluid [23].

In another study, Nakayama et al. studied the effect of RA and RL on intraoperative and postoperative haemodynamics, metabolism, blood gas and renal as well as liver function in patients undergoing hepatectomy. Intraoperative serum lactate levels increased significantly in both groups however, postoperatively, lactate levels were significantly higher in the RL group [24].

In another interesting study, RA was compared with RL to find its usefulness in patients with liver dysfunction. Acid–base balance, electrolytes and liver function showed no significant changes in any group. It was concluded that the status of liver dysfunction did not affect the metabolism of lactic acid and either RA or RL can be used as intraoperative maintenance fluid [25].

Hyperglycemia in the perioperative period results in increased morbidity and mortality [26]. Precipitating factors for hyperglycemia are stress response to surgery and anesthesia, intraoperative use of drugs, tissue damage and bleeding. There is a fear of using RL in the perioperative period because of the risk of lactate being converted to glucose especially in diabetic patients. A recent prospective, parallel group, observational study assessed the incidence of hyperglycemia, lactatemia and metabolic acidosis with the use of RL and RA in non-diabetic patients undergoing major head and neck free flap or abdominal surgery [27]. Intraoperative hyperglycemia was more frequent in RL group compared to RA group. RA group patients undergoing major abdominal surgery showed higher blood sugar compared to free flap surgery. When the duration of surgery exceeded 6 h, acetate-based solutions resulted in significantly higher lactate levels with progressive metabolic acidosis.

In conclusion, RL and RA are comparable in terms of haemodynamic stability and acid–base status. Longer surgery duration resulted in significantly higher lactate levels with progressive metabolic acidosis when using acetate-based fluids. RL and RA can both be used as intraoperative maintenance fluid in patients with liver dysfunction. Hyperglycemia was variable with different types of surgical procedures.

Acetate and Gluconate Buffered Solutions

This is an isotonic, buffered intravenous crystalloid solution with a physiochemical composition that closely reflects human plasma. Unlike RL, which contains calcium; acetate and gluconate-based buffered solution are calcium-free and therefore compatible with blood and blood components.

These solutions contain 23 mmol/L of gluconate. Little is known about the clinical significance of gluconate. Approximately 80% of gluconate is eliminated via renal mechanisms. As gluconate plays a role in the galactomannan antigenicity, patients receiving Plasma-Lyte®-148 (PL-148) may test false positive for the galactomannan antigen lasting up to 24 h [28, 29].

It is unclear if PL-148 will lead to an increase in unmeasured anions when given in large quantities. In an Australian study, TJ Morgan compared bicarbonate-based balanced fluid with PL-148 for cardiopulmonary bypass circuit priming. With the trial fluid, metabolic acid–base status was normal, whereas PL-148 triggered a surge of unmeasured anions persisting throughout bypass, and produced a slight metabolic acidosis without a clear clinical significance [30].

In a similar study by Davies et al, it was observed that when PL-148 was administered as a cardiopulmonary bypass pump-prime fluid, there were supra-physiologic plasma levels of acetate and gluconate when compared to a bicarbonate pump priming solution. The implications of supra-physiological gluconate and acetate levels remain undetermined [31].

The development of metabolic acidosis is well recognized during cardiopulmonary bypass. It is postulated that PL-148 will not lead to acidosis compared to RL as a priming fluid. In a prospective, double blind, randomized control trial on 22 patients undergoing cardiopulmonary bypass for coronary artery bypass surgery, Liskaser et al. compared Haemaccel-Ringer's and PL-148 as a priming fluid for the development of acidosis [32]. All patients developed a metabolic acidosis and the decrease in base excess was the same for both primers, although with different mechanisms of acidosis viz hyperchloremic with Haemaccel-Ringer's and increase in unmeasured anions (most probably acetate and gluconate) with PL-148.

For patients undergoing major liver surgery, use of lactate-free solutions may be beneficial. Shin WJ et al., compared the effects of RL and PL-148 on liver functions and serum lactate in living donors undergoing right hepatectomy. The lactate concentrations was significantly higher in the RL group than in the PL-148 group, 1 h postoperatively. In addition, albumin levels were significantly lower and the peak total bilirubin concentration and prothrombin time were significantly higher in the RL group. However, these changes did not persist beyond the first or second postoperative days [33].

A similar multicenter, prospective, double-blind randomized controlled trial by Weinberg L et al compared the effects of Hartman solution (HS) with PL-148 in patients undergoing major liver resection. Patients treated with HS were more hyperchloremic, hyperlactatemic and also lost more blood. Mean PT and aPTT were significantly lower and haemoglobin was higher, immediately after surgery in the PL-148 group. There were no significant differences in pH, bicarbonate, albumin and phosphate levels [34].

There is little data to compare various buffered solutions peri-operatively for renal transplantation. Normal saline is widely advocated as it is potassium free, however recent evidence suggests that balanced solutions may be more appropriate. In a double-blind study, the effect of different crystalloids on acid–base balance and early kidney function postrenal transplant was studied by Hadimioglu et al. Patients were randomized to three groups to receive either normal saline, RL or PL-148. There was a statistically significant decrease in pH and base excess and a significant increase in serum chloride in patients receiving saline during surgery. Lactate levels increased significantly in patients who received RL. No significant changes in acid-base balance or lactate levels occurred in patients who received PL-148 [35].

There are few studies that have monitored changes in cognitive functioning as a result of infusion of different buffered solutions. In a recent Indian study, Jigyasa Shahani et al. compared the cerebral-protective effects of RL and gluconate-based buffered solution (Kabilyte) in patients undergoing cardiopulmonary bypass. There was no significant difference between the preoperative and postoperative cognitive test scores in both groups [36].

In conclusion, RL and gluconate-based buffered solutions are comparable in terms of metabolic acid–base status and cognitive function in patients undergoing cardiopulmonary bypass. The surge of unmeasured anions remains clinically non-relevant. Use of gluconate-based buffered solutions does not appear to be of benefit in patients undergoing liver surgery.

Whether the use of balanced multi-electrolyte solution (PL-148) in preference to 0.9% sodium chloride solution (saline) in critically ill patients reduces the risk of acute kidney injury or death is uncertain. Simon Finfer et al compared the efficacy of PL-148 with saline as fluid therapy in the intensive care unit (ICU) for 90 days in a multicenter, prospective, doubleblind randomized controlled trial. Death within 90 days after randomization occurred in 21.8% in the PL-148 group versus 22.0% in the saline group (P=0.90), which was statistically non-significant. New renal-replacement therapy was initiated in 12.7% in the PL-148 group versus 12.9% in the saline group, which was also non-significant. The mean (±SD) maximum increase in serum creatinine level was 0.41±1.06 mg per deciliter (36.6±94.0 µmol per liter) in the PL-148 group and 0.41±1.02 mg per deciliter (36.1±90.0 µmol per liter) in the saline group, for a difference of 0.01 mg per deciliter. The number of adverse and serious adverse events did not differ meaningfully between the groups. Authors found no evidence that the risk of death or acute kidney injury among critically ill adults in the ICU was lower with the use of PL-148 than with saline [37].

Acetate and Malate Buffered Solutions

Malate is a citric acid cycle intermediate. It is a standard component in resuscitation and maintenance fluid therapy for a wide range of patients, e.g. sepsis, trauma, perioperative and critically ill patients. Data is insufficient regarding its plasma distribution, renal excretion and metabolism after intravenous injection except from a small number of animal studies. The liver is an important consumer of malate [38]; the kidneys also play an important role in malate metabolism.

Intraoperative fluid management continues to be a daily challenge in anesthetic practice. Various buffered solutions have different effects on acid–base status, electrolyte levels, coagulation and renal and hepatic function. A recent study by Morgan TJ et al., compared the influence of RL and malate buffered solution (Sterofundin) on acid–base changes, haemodynamics and readiness for extubation on 30 consecutive children undergoing scoliosis surgery. There was no statistically significant difference in the volume of infused fluid and changes in pH. The strong ion difference was decreased in both groups, though it normalized earlier with Sterofundin [39]. What about other primary outcomes?

In another recent study on children, RL was compared with Sterofundin in terms of intraoperative acid-base and electrolytes status. A total of 30 children aged between 1 and 13 years were randomized. In the RL group, the mean difference in pH between the baseline and end of surgery was statistically significant. The mean difference in base excess was similar in both groups [40].

A prospective, randomized, controlled trial assessed the effects of using Sterofundin or RL as the intraoperative fluid in patients undergoing major head and neck surgery with free flap reconstruction. Intraoperative lactate levels were significantly high in the RL group at 2, 4, 6, and 8 h. The pH was comparable between groups except at 8 h where the RL group had a significantly lower pH than the Sterofundin group. There was no significant difference between both groups in terms of sodium, potassium, chloride, bicarbonate and $pCO2$ levels [41].

In conclusion, RL and Sterofundin are comparable in terms of acid–base physiology and electrolytes in adults but Sterofundin is better in pediatric patients undergoing major surgery. Also, use of Sterofundin reduced lactate levels in comparison with RL in patients undergoing prolonged surgery.

There are no human studies comparing the four balanced crystalloids as resuscitation fluid; a single large study in animals was performed in the late 80 s. This compared the ability of four balanced crystalloid solutions (normal saline, RL, Plasma Lyte-A and Plasma Lyte-R) to prevent death after a fatal haemorrhage to simulate human exsanguination in unanesthetized swine. Swine were randomized to receive crystalloids at different percentages of replacement. The percentages of blood lost were replaced with 14% normal saline in 5 minutes, 100% normal saline in 20 minutes, and 300% normal saline, RL, Plasma Lyte-A and Plasma Lyte-R [42]. RL provided the best survival rate of 67% compared to 30% with Plasma-Lyte-A. After an analysis of arterial blood gas, lactate, acid-base, heart rate and aortic pressure measurements, it was concluded that RL is the superior crystalloid because of its decreased chloride load (compared to normal saline) and the absence of acetate or magnesium (compared to Plasma-Lyte-14).

Case Vignette

Mr. X, the patient in the vignette shows clinical signs of septic shock and the purpose of resuscitation is to improve tissue perfusion. The choice of fluid should be based on clinician preference. It is reasonable to resuscitate Mr. X with normal saline if the volume used is not large (1 to 2 L) otherwise balanced solutions are preferred.

Conclusion

It is unlikely that one balanced solution is better than another in this situation. Ideally, the choice of fluid for resuscitation/maintenance should be individualized qualitatively, e.g. a particular fluid for a specific type of surgery and quantitatively, e.g. an appropriate amount at the appropriate time and at the appropriate rate. Results from single-center studies should be viewed with caution before making any clinical decision based on these. There is a strong need for multi-center trials comparing various balanced solutions such as resuscitation and /or maintenance fluid.

Take Home Message
- Buffers play a crucial role in maintaining acid–base balance in the body.
- Different buffers have different characteristics and can be used in balanced solutions for different purposes.
- Lactate, acetate, gluconate and malate are the most commonly used buffers in balanced solutions and can help prevent the development of hyperchloremic metabolic acidosis.
- The choice of buffer in balanced solutions should be tailored to the patient's specific clinical needs and conditions.
- The optimal buffer for balanced solutions is still under debate, and further research is needed to determine the best choice in different clinical scenarios.

References

1. Hamburger HJ. Osmotischer Druck und Ionenlehre in den medicinischen Wissenschaften: Zugleich Lehrbuch physikalischchemischer Methoden. Wiesbaden: J. F. Bergmann; 1902.
2. Awad S, Allison SP, Lobo DN. The history of 0.9% saline. Clin Nutr. 2008;27(2):179–88.
3. Tommasino C, Moore S, Todd MM. Cerebral effects of isovolemic hemodilution with crystalloid or colloid solutions. Crit Care Med. 1988;16:862–8.
4. Miller DJ. Sydney Ringer; physiological saline, calcium and the contraction of the heart. J Physiol. 2004;555(Pt 3):585–7.

5. Ringer S. Regarding the action of the hydrate of soda, hydrate of ammonia, and the hydrate of potash on the ventricle of the frog's heart. J Physiol (London). 1880/82;3:195–202.
6. Lee JA. Sydney Ringer (1834–1910) and Alexis Hartmann (1898–1964). Anaesthesia. 1981;36(12):1115–21.
7. Hartmann AF, Senn MJ. Studies in the metabolism of sodium R-lactate. I. Response of normal human subjects to the intravenous injection of sodium R-lactate. J Clin Invest. 1932;11(2):327–35.
8. Murney P. To mix or not to mix – compatibilities of parenteral drug solutions. Aust Prescr. 2008;31:98–101.
9. Skutches CL, Holroyde CP, Myers RN, Paul P, Reichard GA. Plasma acetate turnover and oxidation. J Clin Invest. 1979;64:708–13.
10. Richardson JA, Borchardt KA. Br Med J. 1969;3:749.
11. Kveim M, Nesbakken R. Utilization of exogenous acetate during canine haemorrhagic shock. Scand J Clin Lab Invest. 1979;39:653–8.
12. Akanji AO, Hockaday TD. Acetate tolerance and the kinetics of acetate utilization in diabetic and nondiabetic subjects. Am J Clin Nutr. 1990;51:112–8.
13. Arai K, Kawamoto M, Yuge O, Shiraki H, Mukaida K, Horibe M, Morio M. A comparative study of lactated Ringer and acetated Ringer solution as intraoperative fluids in patients with liver dysfunction. Masui. 1986;35:793–9.
14. Veech RL, Gitomer WL. The medical and metabolic consequences of administration of sodium acetate. Adv Enzym Regul. 1988;27:313–43.
15. Quebbeman EJ, Maierhofer WJ, Piering WF. Mechanisms producing hypoxemia during hemodialysis. Crit Care Med. 1984;12:359–63.
16. Amore A, Cirina P, Mitola S, Peruzzi L, Bonaudo R, Gianoglio B, Coppo R. Acetate intolerance is mediated by enhanced synthesis of nitric oxide by endothelial cells. J Am Soc Nephrol. 1997;8:1431–6.
17. Kirkendol RL, Pearson JE, Bower JD, Holbert RD. Myocardial depressant effects of sodium acetate. Cardiovasc Res. 1978;12:127–36.
18. Kirkendol PL, Robie NW, Gonzalez FM, Devia CJ. Cardiac and vascular effects of infused sodium acetate in dogs. Trans Am Soc Artif Intern Organs. 1978;24:714–8.
19. Jacob AD, Elkins N, Reiss OK, Chan L, Shapiro JI. Effects of acetate on energy metabolism and function in the isolated perfused rat heart. Kidney Int. 1997;52:755–60.
20. Schrander-vd Meer AM, Ter Wee PM, Kan G, et al. Improved cardiovascular variables during acetate free biofiltration. Clin Nephrol. 1999;51:304–9.
21. Selby NM, Fluck RJ, Taal MW, McIntyre CW. Effects of acetate-free double-chamber hemodiafiltration and standard dialysis on systemic hemodynamics and troponin T levels. ASAIO J. 2006;52:62–9.
22. Klaus F, Hofmann-Kiefer DC, Kammerer T, Jacob M, Paptistella M, Conzen P, Rehm M. Influence of an acetate- and a lactate-based balanced infusion solution on acid base physiology and hemodynamics: an observational pilot study. Eur J Med Res. 2012;17:21.
23. Hatem A, Attalla MD, Montaser S, Abulkassem MD, Khaled M, Abo Elenine MD. Alexandria J Anaesthesia Intensive Care. 2005;8(2)
24. Nakayama M, Kawana S, Yamauchi M, Tsuchida H, Iwasaki H, Namiki A. Utility of acetated Ringer solution as intraoperative fluids during hepatectomy. Masui Jpn J Anesthesiol. 1995;44:1654–60.
25. Isosu T, Akama Y, Tase C, Fujii M, Okuaki A. Clinical examination of acetated Ringer solution in patients with normal liver function and those with liver dysfunction. Masui Jpn J Anesthesiol. 1992;41:1707–13.
26. Tilak V, Schoenberg C, Castro AF 3rd, Sant M. Factors associated with increases in glucose levels in the perioperative period in non-diabetic patients. Open J Anaesth. 2013;3:176–85.

27. Balakrishnan S, Kannan M, Rajan S, Purushothaman SS, Kesavan R, Kumar L. Evaluation of the metabolic profile of ringer lactate versus ringer acetate in nondiabetic patients undergoing major surgeries. Anesth Essays Res. 2018;12:719–23.
28. Petraitiene R, Petraitis V, Witt JR, Durkin MM, Bacher JD, Wheat LJ, Walsh TJ. Galactomannan antigenemia after infusion of gluconate-containing plasma-Lyte. J Clin Microbiol. 2011;49:4330–2.
29. Hage CA, Reynolds JM, Durkin M, Wheat LJ, Knox KS. Plasmalyte as a cause of false-positive results for aspergillus galactomannan in bronchoalveolar lavage fluid. J Clin Microbiol. 2007;45:676–7.
30. Morgan TJ, Power G, Venkatesh B, Jones MA. Acid-base effects of a bicarbonate-balanced priming fluid during cardiopulmonary bypass: comparison with plasma-Lyte 148. A randomised single-blinded study. Anaesth Intensive Care. 2008;36:822–9.
31. Davies PG, Venkatesh B, Morgan TJ, Presneill JJ, Kruger PS, Thomas BJ, Roberts MS, Mundy J. Plasma acetate, gluconate and interleukin-6 profiles during and after cardiopulmonary bypass: a comparison of plasma-Lyte 148 with a bicarbonate-balanced solution. Crit Care. 2011;15:R21.
32. Liskaser FJ, Bellomo R, Hayhoe M, Story D, Poustie S, Smith B, Letis A, Bennett M. Role of pump prime in the etiology and pathogenesis of cardiopulmonary bypass-associated acidosis. Anesthesiology. 2000;93:1170–3.
33. Shin WJ, Kim YK, Bang JY, Cho SK, Han SM, Hwang GS. Lactate and liver function tests after living donor right hepatectomy: a comparison of solutions with and without lactate. Acta Anaesthesiol Scand. 2011;55:558–64.
34. Weinberg L, Pearce B, Sullivan R, Siu L, Scurrah N, Tan C, Backstrom M, Nikfarjam M, McNicol L, Story D, Christophi C, Bellomo R. The effects of plasmalyte-148 vs. Hartmann's solution during major liver resection: a multicentre, double-blind, randomized controlled trial. Minerva Anestesiol. 2015;81:1288–97.
35. Hadimioglu N, Saadawy I, Saglam T, Ertug Z, Dinckan A. The effect of different crystalloid solutions on acid-base balance and early kidney function after kidney transplantation. Anesth Analg. 2008;107:264.
36. Shahani J, Saiyyed A. Comparison of Kabilyte® and Ringer lactate as prime solution on cognitive functions in patients undergoing cardiopulmonary bypass. Int J Sci Res(IJSR). 2017;6(7):1754–6.
37. Simon Finfer, Sharon Micallef, Naomi Hammond, et al. For the plus study investigators and the australian and new zealand intensive care society clinical trials group. Balanced multielectrolyte solution versus saline in critically ill adults. NEJM 2022;386(9):815–26.
38. Zander R. Fluid Management. 2nd ed. Melsungen: Bibliomed-Medizinische Verlagsgesellschaft mbH; 2009.
39. Sharma A, Monu Yadav B, Rajesh Kumar P, Lakshman S, Iyenger R, Ramchandran G. A comparative study of Sterofundin and Ringer lactate based infusion protocol in scoliosis correction surgery. Anaesth Essays Res. 2016;10(3):532–7.
40. Shariffuddin BAPP, Adeline C, Chinna K, Lucy C. A comparison of Sterofundin and Ringer's lactate on intraoperative acid base and electrolytes status in children: a randomized controlled trial. Anaesth Critic Care Med J. 2018;3(1):000128.
41. Rajan S, Srikumar S, Tosh P, Kumar L. Effect of lactate versus acetate-based intravenous fluids on acid-base balance in patients undergoing free flap reconstructive surgeries. J Anaesthesiol Clin Pharmacol. 2017;33:514–9.
42. Traverso LW, Lee WP, Langford MJ. Fluid resuscitation after an otherwise fatal hemorrhage: I. Crystalloid solutions. J Trauma. 1986;26:168–75.

Fluid Accumulation and Deresuscitation

25

Manu L. N. G. Malbrain ⓘ, Jonny Wilkinson, Luca Malbrain, Prashant Nasa, and Adrian Wong

Contents

Introduction 502
Definitions 504
Pathophysiology 506
Liberal Versus Restrictive Fluid Regimens 508
Monitoring Hypervolemia and Guiding Deresuscitation 511
    Clinical Signs of Hypervolemia 511
    Laboratory Signs and Biomarkers 513
    Radiological and Imaging Signs 515
    Advanced Hemodynamic Monitoring 517
How to Perform Deresuscitation? 518
Conclusions 521
References 523

Manu L. N. G. Malbrain (✉)
First Department of Anaesthesiology, Medical University of Lublin, Lublin, Poland

J. Wilkinson
ITU and Anaesthesia and NICE IV Fluid Lead, Northampton, UK

L. Malbrain
University School of Medicine, Katholieke Universiteit Leuven (KUL), Leuven, Belgium

P. Nasa
Critical Care Medicine, NMC Specialty Hospital, Dubai, Dubai, UAE
e-mail: dr.prashantnasa@hotmail.com

A. Wong
Intensive Care and Anaesthesia, King's College Hospital NHS Foundation Trust, London, UK

© The Author(s) 2024
M. L. N. G. Malbrain et al. (eds.), *Rational Use of Intravenous Fluids in Critically Ill Patients*, https://doi.org/10.1007/978-3-031-42205-8_25

IFA Commentary (SG)

Fluid accumulation of more than 10% is associated with higher morbidity and mortality. However, fluid accumulation is a continuum, and a single threshold value does not encompass everyone. It is a state of pathological overhydration with worse patient outcomes. Organ dysfunction with fluid accumulation is defined as fluid accumulation syndrome. IV fluids should be regarded as drugs, and stewardship focusing on 4D's (Drug, dose, duration, and de-escalation) is recommended to mitigate the problem of fluid accumulation. IV fluid prescription should consider four indications (resuscitation, maintenance, replacement, and nutrition) and the conceptual model of ROSE (resuscitation, optimization, stabilization, and evacuation). De-escalation and de-resuscitation are strategies to avoid fluid accumulation. Recent evidence supports the feasibility of fluid restriction during resuscitation. De-escalation means discontinuation or reducing IV fluids to prevent fluid accumulation. De-resuscitation is an active fluid removal to treat fluid accumulation causing organ dysfunction. Tools such as negative passive leg raising test, extravascular lung water and bioelectrical impedance, and venous congestion on point-of-care ultrasound are promising to guide de-resuscitation. Diuretics with or without hyperoncotic albumin are the first step in de-resuscitation. Mechanical fluid removal (ultrafiltration) can be considered in case of diuretic failure or contraindication. The end-point of de-resuscitation are either goal-based (fluid balance, physiological or clinical improvement) or safety concerns.

The goal of fluid resuscitation is to improve tissue perfusion. However, overzealous resuscitation measures may lead to fluid overload and tissue edema, further worsening tissue and organ damage. The fluid overload state is compounded further by poorly planned maintenance fluid therapy and often avoidable 'fluid creep'. Pathophysiology and clinical features of several fluid accumulation syndromes are described in this chapter in great detail. Below we will list some interventions that can be performed to prevent and treat FAS.

Avoid fluid accumulation: Key is to prevent fluid accumulation without allowing tissue hypoperfusion. We suggest the following strategies to achieve this goal.

- Avoid large fluid boluses. Fluid bolus as small as 4 ml/kg body weight has shown to be adequate for intravascular volume expansion [1].
- Further fluid boluses should be guided by patient phenotype e.g. history of large fluid loss or poor fluid intake in preceding days, obvious harm of further fluid administration e.g. pulmonary edema or B-profile in the anterior chest).
- Fluid responsiveness must be checked before additional fluid boluses and fluid should not be administered if the patient is not fluid responsiveness. However, the converse may not be true [2].

- Early initiation of vasopressors has been shown to reduce cumulative fluid balance in vasodilatory shock like septic shock [3]. Vasopressors (especially norepinephrine) should be administered along with fluid boluses in patients with diastolic blood pressure <50 mmHg or diastolic shock index >2.3 and after initial fluid volume of not more than 1–2 l of crystalloid [4–6].
- Hyperoncotic albumin boluses have shown to reduce cumulative fluid volume during fluid resuscitation [7, 8]. However, additional data and cost-benefit ratio must be considered before the widespread adoption of this strategy.
- Patients should be reassessed frequently during fluid resuscitation to look for improvement in tissue perfusion, as well as for any harmful consequences of administered fluid. In both situations, further fluid boluses must be stopped. In the ANDROMEDA-SHOCK trial, resuscitation targeting capillary refill time (CRT) as the end-point of tissue perfusion goal was shown to lower resuscitation volume compared to lactate guided resuscitation [9].
- Maintenance fluid and fluid creep contribute to over 60% of administered fluid in critically ill patients [10]. Whenever possible maintenance fluid infusion should be either avoided or limited to the minimal volume. Similarly, 'fluid creep' should be actively looked into and whenever feasible patient can be switched to an oral (enteral) formulation or the drug should be diluted in a smaller volume.
- Moderately hypotonic (sodium concentration 54 mmol/L) maintenance fluid infusion produces lower cumulative fluid balance compared to isotonic (sodium concentration 154 mmol/L) maintenance fluid [11]. Hence, if maintenance fluid is deemed to be necessary, the choice of fluid should be moderately hypotonic.

De-resuscitate when necessary: De-resuscitation is a strategy to remove accumulated fluid forcefully, in an otherwise hemodynamically stable patient with clinical evidence of fluid overload. The aim of de-resuscitation is to treat and/or prevent end-organ damage resulting from fluid overload without producing hypovolemia and organ ischemia. The following questions need to be raised and answered during the process of de-resuscitation [12].

- **When to start?** Patient must be hemodynamically stable on no or minimal dose of vasopressors before considering de-resuscitation. He or she should not be requiring additional boluses or fluid or there should not be any ongoing fluid loss requiring replacement. Clinical and objective evidence of fluid overload should be present with reasonable suspicion of organ damage (or impending one) directly resulting from the fluid accumulation. Evidence of fluid overload has been described in great detail in the chapter.

- **How to initiate?** Active removal of fluid can be achieved either by judicious use of diuretics or by ultrafiltration [continuous renal replacement therapy (CRRT) or slow low efficiency hemodialysis (SLED)]. Mechanisms of action and pharmacological effects of different diuretic agents have been discussed in the chapter. Discussion on CRRT and SLED techniques are beyond the scope of this book. Some relevant points on the subject are given below.
  - Berthelsen and colleagues suggested is to start de-resuscitation process with a 40 mg IV bolus of furosemide followed by an infusion titrated to a maximum dose of 40 mg/h [13]. Other loop diuretics such as torsemide may be considered in place of furosemide. Interestingly, in a large study on diuretic strategies in patients with acute decompensated heart failure, continuous infusion of furosemide was not shown to be of any additional advantage compared to bolus doses [14].
  - In a recent study, addition of intravenous acetazolamide 500 mg once daily in addition to standard loop diuretic regimen, was shown to achieve better decongestion and produce more diuresis and natriuresis compared to loop diuretic alone, in patients with acute decompensated heart failure [15]. Broader application of this combination strategy in general intensive care unit patients needs further evaluation.
  - Ultrafiltration using CRRT or SLED may be considered as alternative options in patients with inadequate response to diuretics or in anuric patients or in patients requiring renal replacement therapy for some other reason or in patients who developed serious adverse effects to furosemide or torsemide [12].
  - Adding hyperoncotic (20 or 25%) albumin to the diuretic and/or ultrafiltration regimen, in addition to maintaining intravascular volume, has been shown to produce synergistic effect [16]. In an elegant study, Greg Martin et al. randomized hemodynamically stable, hypoproteinemic patients who are on mechanical ventilator for ARDS to either furosemide with albumin (100 ml boluses of 20% albumin every 8-h) or furosemide with placebo for 72 h [16]. Addition of albumin was shown to produce larger negative fluid balance and lesser episodes of hypotension, in addition to a significant improvement in oxygenation. Alternatively, hyperoncotic albumin may be administered as a continuous infusion at 10–20 ml/h [12].
  - Addition of positive end-expiratory pressure (PEEP) matching intra-abdominal pressure (IAP), in addition to albumin plus diuretics (or ultrafiltration) (PAL strategy—PEEP, albumin and lasix or furosemide), had shown to be associated with greater negative fluid balance and greater reduction in extravascular lung water index (EVLWI) and IAP compared to control subjects [17]. PAL strategy also showed improved clinical outcomes (improved oxygenation, shorter ICU length of stay) without compromising cardiovascular or renal function.

- **How to monitor?** Patients should be monitored closely for evidence of hypovolemia and/or hypoperfusion and adequacy of fluid removal [12].
  - One suggested goal is to achieve a net negative fluid balance of at least 1 mL/kg IBW/hour [13].
  - Patients should also be monitored for serious adverse effects of diuretics e.g. thrombocytopenia, agranulocytosis, pancreatitis, Steven Johnsons syndrome, toxic epidermal necrolysis, etc.
  - Patients should also be monitored for any electrolyte abnormalities (e.g. hypokalemia, dysnatremia, hypomagnesemia or hypophosphatemia) and cardiac arrhythmias related to it.
- **When to stop?** De-resuscitation should be stopped, if the patient fulfills any of the following conditions.
  - Hemodynamic instability or obvious evidence of hypovolemia; in which case, fluid removal must be suspended and fluid may be re-administered judiciously. Fluid removal may be re-initiated at a lower rate, once hypovolemia or hypoperfusion is mitigated [12].
  - On achievement of de-resuscitation goal—negative or zero fluid balance.

Suggested Reading
1. Aya H, Rhodes A, Grounds RM, Cecconi M. Minimal volume for a fluid challenge in postoperative patients. Crit Care. 2015;19(Suppl 1):P189.
2. Ghosh S. Concept of fluid responsiveness. Fluid challenge. In: Handbook of intravenous fluids. Springer, Singapore, 2022. https://doi.org/10.1007/978-981-19-0500-1_9.
3. Macdonald SPJ, Keijzers G, Taylor DM, Kinnear F, Arendts G, Fatovich DM et al. Restricted fluid resuscitation in suspected sepsis associated hypotension (REFRESH): a pilot randomised controlled trial. Intensive Care Med. 2018;44:2070–8.
4. Karpati PCJ, Rossignol M, Pirot M, Cholley B, Vicaut E, Henry P et al. High incidence of myocardial ischemia during postpartum hemorrhage. Anesthesiology. 2004;100:30–6.
5. Ospina-Tascón GA, Teboul JL, Hernandez G, Alvarez I, Sánchez-Ortiz AI, Calderón-Tapia LE et al. Diastolic shock index and clinical outcomes in patients with septic shock. Ann Intensive Care. 2020;10:41.
6. Roberts RJ, Miano TA, Hammond DA, Patel GP, Chen JT, Phillips KM et al. Evaluation of vasopressor exposure and mortality in patients with septic shock. Crit Care Med. 2020;48:1445–53.
7. Margarson MP, Soni NC. Changes in serum albumin concentration and volume expanding effects following a bolus of albumin 20% in septic patients. Br J Anaesth. 2004;92:821–6.

8. Mårtensson J, Bihari S, Bannard-Smith J, Glassford NJ, Lloyd-Donald P, Cioccari L et al. Small volume resuscitation with 20% albumin in intensive care: physiological effects: The SWIPE randomised clinical trial. Intensive Care Med. 2018;44:1797–1806.

9. Hernández G, Ospina-Tascón GA, Damiani LP, Estenssoro E, Dubin A, Hurtado J et al. Effect of a resuscitation strategy targeting peripheral perfusion status vs serum lactate levels on 28-day mortality among patients with septic shock: the ANDROMEDA-SHOCK randomized clinical trial. JAMA. 2019;321:654–64.

10. Van Regenmortel N, Verbrugghe W, Roelant E, Van den Wyngaert T, Jorens PG. Maintenance fluid therapy and fluid creep impose more significant fluid, sodium, and chloride burdens than resuscitation fluids in critically ill patients: a retrospective study in a tertiary mixed ICU population. Intensive Care Med. 2018;44:409–17.

11. Van Regenmortel N, Hendrickx S, Roelant E, Baar I, Dams K, Van Vlimmeren K et al. 154 compared to 54 mmol per liter of sodium in intravenous maintenance fluid therapy for adult patients undergoing major thoracic surgery (TOPMAST): a single-center randomized controlled double-blind trial. Intensive Care Med. 2019;45:1422–32.

12. Ghosh S. Four phases of fluid resuscitation. In: Handbook of intravenous fluids. Springer, Singapore, 2022. https://doi.org/10.1007/978-981-19-0500-1_10.

13. Berthelsen RE, Perner A, Jensen AK, Rasmussen BS, Jensen JU, Wiis J, Behzadi MT, Bestle MH. Forced fluid removal in intensive care patients with acute kidney injury: the randomised FFAKI feasibility trial. Acta Anaesthesiol Scand. 2018;62:936–44.

14. Felker GM, Lee KL, Bull DA, Redfield MM, Stevenson LW, Goldsmith SR et al. Diuretic strategies in patients with acute decompensated heart failure. N Engl J Med. 2011;364:797–805.

15. Mullens W, Dauw J, Martens P, Verbrugge FH, Nijst P, Meekers E et al. Acetazolamide in acute decompensated heart failure with volume overload. N Engl J Med. 2022;387:1185–95.

16. Martin GS, Moss M, Wheeler AP, Mealer M, Morris JA, Bernard GR. A randomized, controlled trial of furosemide with or without albumin in hypoproteinemic patients with acute lung injury. Crit Care Med. 2005;33:1681–7.

17. Cordemans C, De Laet I, Van Regenmortel N, Schoonheydt K, Dits H, Martin G, Huber W, Malbrain ML. Aiming for a negative fluid balance in patients with acute lung injury and increased intra-abdominal pressure: a pilot study looking at the effects of PAL-treatment. Ann Intensive Care. 2012;2(Suppl 1):S15.

Learning Objectives

This chapter will discuss the harms of excessive IV fluids administration and over-hydration. Various strategies can be employed to avoid and monitor overhydration. Fluid restriction during resuscitation and active removal of excessive fluid, also known as deresuscitation, are the strategies employed to manage overhydration. We will review the recent evidence on fluid restriction and deresuscitation. With the help of a case, we will review the judicious fluid administration, methods of monitoring overhydration, and safe deresuscitation strategy in case of overhydration.

Case Vignette

A 26-year-old man was admitted to the ICU after general seizures, syncope, non-palpable blood pressure, and a suspicion of ventricular tachycardia whilst in the Emergency Room. The emergency room physician (successfully) applied a DC shock to convert to regular sinus rhythm. Afterward the patient was alert and cooperative and he was transferred to the ICU for overnight monitoring. The next day his need for supplemental oxygen increased from 2 l via nasal cannula to 15 l administered with a non-rebreathing mask. The patient was in respiratory distress with a respiratory rate of 34 breaths/min. After the failure of non-invasive ventilation, he was intubated and mechanically ventilated within 24 h after ICU admission, illustrating the dramatic chain of events. After intubation, the patient was in profound shock and resuscitated with 3 consecutive boluses of 4 ml/kg balanced crystalloids. Despite fluids and low dose pressors, he remained hypotensive with increasing lactate and poor P/F ratio (<100). Transpulmonary thermodilution monitoring was started. The initial hemodynamic profile showed a normal cardiac index (CI) of 3.5 L/min m^2 (normal range 3–5), a relatively low intravascular filling status with a GEDVI of 757 ml/m^2 (normal range 680–800), a very low global ejection fraction GEF of 13% (normal range 25–35) in combination with severe capillary leak and high extravascular lung water index (EVLWI) of 12 ml/kg predicted body weight (normal range 3–7). At the same time; however, the patient seemed to be preload responsive with a high pulse pressure variation (PPV) of 19% (normal range <10). Heart rate was regular at 119 beats/min with a MAP of 55 mmHg. The CVP remained at 16 mmHg. His response to a passive leg raising (PLR) maneuver was positive (15% increase in CI and MAP) confirming that he was volume responsive despite the fact that he was in pulmonary edema (EVLWI 12) with a critical oxygenation status at the time (P/F ratio of 57, at IPAP of 34 cmH$_2$O and PEEP of 15 cmH$_2$O).

Questions

Q1. What does this case scenario illustrate?

The patient was given a further small volume dose of fluids in combination with an increasing dose of vasopressors. The following day, his CI increased to 5.7 L/min m², GEDVI increased to 900 ml/m² but also EVLWI had increased to 19 ml/kg PBW. The high EVLWI was suggestive of hyperpermeability edema in view of the high pulmonary vascular permeability index (PVPI) of 2.9 (normal range 1–2.5).

Q2. What is the best treatment at this stage?

Introduction

The administration of intravenous (IV) crystalloid solutions is widely regarded as the initial step in resuscitating the hypotensive critically ill 'septic' patient, with evidence of inadequate organ perfusion. Recent evidence suggests that overzealous administration of IV fluids, especially in the setting of sepsis with poor source control and capillary leak, may lead to fluid overload and subsequent fluid accumulation syndrome (FAS) [1].

Tissue edema is not just of cosmetic concern, it impairs oxygen and metabolite diffusion, disrupts the endothelial glycocalyx architecture, impedes capillary blood flow and lymphatic drainage and disturbs intercellular interactions. All these effects may contribute to the progression of organ dysfunction and failure. These effects are particularly pronounced in encapsulated organs, such as the liver and kidneys, which lack the capacity to accommodate additional volume without an increase in interstitial pressure, resulting in compromised organ blood flow. Furthermore, large-volume resuscitation increases intraabdominal pressure (IAP) which further compromises end-organ (e.g. renal and hepatic) perfusion. This has led to new insights into polycompartment syndrome and more specifically, the cardio-abdominal-renal syndrome (CARS), hepato-abdominal pulmonary syndrome (HAPS) and the hepato-abdominal-renal syndrome (HARS) [2, 3].

Kelm et al. demonstrated that the majority (67%) of patients resuscitated with an early goal directed protocol, had clinical evidence of fluid accumulation after day 1, with 48% showing persistent signs of fluid overload by day 3 [4]. Multiple studies have demonstrated that a positive fluid balance is independently associated with impaired organ function and an increased risk of death [1].

This was neatly demonstrated in a retrospective study performed by Murphy and coworkers in septic patients [5]. It demonstrated that achieving just 2 consecutive negative fluid balance targets within the first week of an ICU stay (late conservative fluid management), was associated with improved organ function and survival. This has also been replicated in other reports [6, 7]. This dynamic time effect and impact of fluids was also

8. Fluid overload: poor cosmetics or bad medicine?

Edema and derailed cumulative fluid balances: are they just collateral damage or do they put the patient in additional danger? Restrictive versus liberal fluid strategies? Is there an additional effect of early removal of fluids or should we go from early adequate over late conservative fluid management towards late goal directed fluid removal? What is the Ebb and Flow phase of shock? Is anasarc edema just of cosmetic concern or is it harmful for the organs and eventually the patient? Maybe we need to rethink the 2 hit ischemia-reperfusion model and replace it by a 3 hit model, where unresolved shock will lead to the third hit, the global increased permeability syndrome? Capillary leak is an inflammatory condition with diverse triggers that results from a common pathway that includes ischemia-reperfusion, toxic oxygen metabolite generation, cell wall and enzyme injury leading to a loss of capillary endothelial barrier function. In such a state, plasma volume expansion to correct hypoperfusion predictably results in extravascular movement of water, electrolytes and proteins. Peripheral tissue edema, visceral edema and ascites may be anticipated in proportion to the volume of prescribed resuscitation fluid. A variety of strategies are available to the clinician to reduce the volume of crystalloid resuscitation utilized while restoring macro- and microcirculatory flow. Regardless of the resuscitation strategy, the clinician must maintain a heightened awareness of the dynamic relationship between capillary leak, fluid loading, peripheral edema, intra-abdominal hypertension and the abdominal compartment syndrome and the potential need and beneficial effect of de-resuscitation.

Fig. 25.1 Screenshot taken from the 1st IFAD proceedings in 2011 coining the term de-resuscitation for the first time

illustrated by other data and has been referred to as the ebb and flow phases of shock. In 1932, Cuthbertson characterized the ebb phase as 'ashen facies, a thready pulse and cold clammy extremities…', while during the flow phase 'the patient warms up, cardiac output increases and the surgical team relaxes…' [8]. Recent data suggests that a substantial number of ICU patients will not enter the flow phase spontaneously after initial resuscitation or EGDT. In order to avoid fluid accumulation and the associated organ edema and dysfunction, these patients may require therapeutic interventions in order to trigger the transition from ebb phase to flow phase [9]. However, it remains largely unknown whether strategies that target a neutral or even negative fluid balance after the initial resuscitative phase are associated with improved clinical outcomes in humans.

The use of the correct definitions, as repeated in this chapter, may limit the deleterious effects of inappropriate fluid prescription and fluid accumulation [10]. We will focus on the deleterious effects of hyper- or overhydration (a better term for fluid overload) and fluid accumulation and will discuss restrictive and liberal fluid management strategies, as well as the different monitoring tools we can use to guide late goal-directed fluid removal, also termed deresuscitation [11]. The term deresuscitation was coined in 2011 during the first International Fluid Academy Day (IFAD) meeting in Antwerp (https://www.fluid-academy.org/memberresources/item/extended-overview.html, congress proceedings page A30—Fig. 25.1) and later on in 2014, defined as active fluid removal in patients with fluid overload using drugs and/or ultrafiltration (UF) [1]. Recently a concise overview has been published [12].

Definitions

The introductory chapter contains a full compendium with a list of definitions and terms. Below, we will briefly discuss those terms related to fluid overload [13–15].

Classification of fluid dynamics: With respect to the different phases of fluid resuscitation (early vs. late), one can classify the dynamics of fluid management by combining early adequate (EA) or early conservative (EC) and late conservative (LC) or late liberal (LL) fluid management. Based on this theoretical concept, four distinct strategies can be defined: EALC, EALL, ECLC, ECLL. The EALC and ECLC groups carry the best prognosis.

Cumulative fluid balance: The sum of fluid accumulated by calculating the sum of daily fluid balances over a set period of time. Usually, the first week of a patient's ICU stay is taken into account for prognostication.

Daily Fluid Balance: The difference between all fluids given to a patient during a 24-h period, and their combined output.

De-escalation: Reduction of the dose or speed of administration of fluid therapy following clinical improvement of the patient.

Deresuscitation (see also Late Goal-Directed Fluid Removal): Correction of fluid accumulation or fluid overload, by actively removing excess fluids using pharmacological and non-pharmacological methods.

Ebb phase: The initial phase of septic shock when the patient shows hyperdynamic circulatory shock, with decreased systemic vascular resistance due to vasodilation, increased capillary permeability, and severe absolute or relative intravascular hypovolemia.

Edema: Peripheral and generalized edema (anasarca) is not merely cosmetic, but harmful to the patient *E:I ratio:* the ECW/ICW ratio is normally below 1 (0.7–0.8). An increase in ICW% will result in a decrease in E:I ratio and is seen in heart failure, liver cirrhosis, and chronic renal failure patients, especially in the early stages. A decrease in ICW% will result in a decrease in E:I ratio and is generally due to osmotic factors. Finally, an increase in ECW% will also increase the E:I ratio. This occurs due to fluid shifts from the intra to extracellular space, or from the capillary leak, which results in second (interstitial) and third-space fluid accumulation and/or edema.

Flow phase: This refers to the phase of septic shock after initial stabilization, where the patient will mobilize excess fluid spontaneously; a classic example is when a patient enters a polyuric phase during recovery from acute kidney injury (AKI).

Fluid accumulation: A pathologic state of overhydration/volume overload, associated with clinical impact which may vary by age, comorbidity, and phase of illness. It describes a continuum and may occur with concomitant intravascular hypovolemia, normovolemia, and hypervolemia. It may or may not be associated with clinical or imaging signs of edema. No specific threshold of fluid balance alone can define fluid accumulation across all individuals.

Fluid accumulation syndrome: Any degree of fluid accumulation or fluid overload with a negative impact on end-organ function, which may or may not be associated with global increased permeability syndrome.

Fluid Creep: The unintentional and unmeasured fluid volumes administered in the process of delivering medication and nutrition through enteral and parenteral routes [16]. In patients with severe burns, this includes the administration of fluids in excess of any requirements calculated by the Parkland Formula [17].

Fluid overload (see overhydration): An increase in total body fluid (both water and electrolytes) in excess of physiologic requirements. This term has sometimes been used interchangeably with volume overload [18], which generally refers to expansion of the extracellular fluid volume.

Preload responsiveness: The state in which a patient will respond to fluid administration by an increase in stroke volume of 15%. This term should replace the traditional misnomer of 'fluid responsiveness'.

Global increased permeability syndrome (GIPS): Some patients will not enter the 'flow' phase spontaneously and will remain in a persistent state of increased permeability and a tendency to fluid accumulation. This is referred to as 'the third hit of shock'. It is defined by a positive cumulative fluid balance with organ failure, in the presence of capillary leak (e.g. increased EVLWI, PVPI, CLI, E:I ratio)

Hypervolemia: The opposite of hypovolemia, defined by intravascular overfilling.

Late Conservative Fluid Management (LCFM): Two consecutive days of negative fluid balance within the first week of the ICU stay; this is a strong and independent predictor of survival [5].

Late Goal-Directed Fluid Removal (LGFR): Active fluid removal by means of diuretics or renal replacement therapy with net ultrafiltration.

Overhydration (see also fluid overload and fluid accumulation): A state of positive fluid balance or where there is excess water in the body. Overhydration may be accompanied by a normal, low or high intravascular or interstitial fluid status, with or without (peripheral or lung) edema. An increase in intravascular fluid status will eventually also lead to increased interstitial fluid by hydrostatic pressure (i.e. cardiogenic edema). Dividing the cumulative fluid balance in liters by the patient's baseline body weight and multiplying by 100% defines the percentage of fluid accumulation. Overhydration or hyperhydration at any stage can be classified as mild (5%), moderate (5–10%) or severe (>10%) fluid accumulation. Historically, it is often defined as increase in body weight relative to admission body weight

- (Fluid intake during observation period)—(fluid losses during observation period)/pre-ICU body weight ×100 or
- Actual increase in body weight (Pre-ICU admission body weight/body weight at the timepoint of fluid overload assessment ×100) or
- Increase in fluid balance (cumulative fluid balance (in L)/pre-ICU body weight × 100) or increase in volume excess (calculated by BIA/pre-ICU body weight × 100) [19].

Positive Fluid Balance: A state in which fluid intake exceeds fluid output. An increase in net fluid balance with accumulation of excess fluids in body tissues and weight gain and in some cases, peripheral edema.

Pathophysiology

We often give too much IV fluid and in particular, too much non-physiological salt. Once within the body, such non-physiological excesses are very difficult to remove and can result in many adverse situations for our patients. There are extremes—increased fluid load can cause major electrolyte swings, whereas dehydration, left unchecked, can lead to poor organ perfusion.

Sick patients have 'leaky capillaries' and in this situation, even careful IV fluid administration can lead to fluid overload and resultant complications (ileus, poor mobility following peripheral edema, pressure sores, pulmonary edema, poor wound healing and anastomotic breakdown).

We have a situation whereby fluid has escaped from its beneficial site within the circulating volume, flooding the extracellular compartment, where it offers no physiological value. What these patients require, after sensible fluid challenges and identification of 'non-response' (better described as being 'volume intolerant/preload un-responsive'). This is where the role of early therapy may now be prudent (i.e. noradrenaline).

Fluid administration potentially triggers a vicious cycle, where interstitial edema induces organ dysfunction, which in turn perpetuates fluid accumulation. It is now well-established that fluid overload in septic patients is associated with edema development and worse outcomes. Fluid overload affects all organ functions from head to toe. GIPS can hence be defined as fluid overload in combination with new-onset organ failure, in the setting of persistent capillary leak (Fig. 25.2).

The following list describes the potential detrimental effects of fluid overload on end-organ function:

- Central nervous system: impaired cognition, delirium, increased intracranial, intra-orbital, and intra-ocular pressure, cerebral edemaand diminished cerebral perfusion pressure. A study of 35 brain injured pigs, with and without hemorrhagic shock, were randomized to Liberal (LR) vs restrictive fluid (HLS). Cerebral edema formation, as indicated by cortical water content (gravity), was studied after 24 h. The study showed that the volume of fluid infused and the fluid balance did affect the ICP, but the amount of Na infused did not [21]. In a retrospective study of 28 severe burn and trauma patients, 8 out of 28 patients required orbital decompression because of increased intra-orbital pressure, related to the amount of fluids administered [22].
- Respiratory system: pulmonary edema, pleural effusions, increased chest wall elastance, decreased dynamic and static respiratory compliance, increased extravascular lung water index, increased pulmonary vascular permeability index, hypercarbia, hypoxia, low P/F ratio, decreased lung volumes (mimicking restrictive lung disease cf. increased intra-abdominal pressure), prolonged ventilation, difficult weaning, and increased work of breathing. In the FACTT trial, 1000 patients with acute lung injury were randomized to receive either conservative vs. liberal fluid treatment. Patients in the conservative arm had a significantly less positive cumulative fluid balance after 1-week, improved lung function and shorter duration of mechanical ventilation [6].

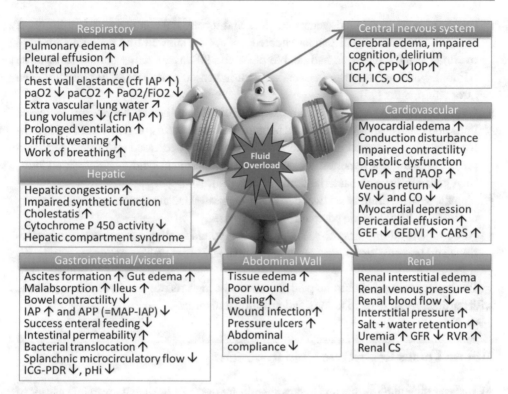

Fig. 25.2 Potential adverse consequences of fluid overload on end-organ function. Adapted from Malbrain et al. with permission [20]. *APP* abdominal perfusion pressure, *IAP* intra-abdominal pressure, *IAH* intra-abdominal hypertension, *ACS* abdominal compartment syndrome, *CARS* cardio-abdominal-renal syndrome, *CO* cardiac output, *CPP* cerebral perfusion pressure, *CS* compartment syndrome, *CVP* central venous pressure, *GEDVI* global enddiastolic volume index, *GEF* global ejection fraction, *GFR* glomerular filtration rate, *ICG-PDR* indocyaninegreen plasma disappearance rate, *ICH* intracranial hypertension, *ICP* intracranial pressure, *ICS* intracranial compartment syndrome, *IOP* intra-ocular pressure, *MAP* mean arterial pressure, *OCS* ocular compartment syndrome, *PAOP* pulmonary artery occlusion pressure, *pHi* gastric tonometry, *RVR* renal vascular resistance, *SV* stroke volume

- Cardiovascular system: myocardial edema, pericardial effusion, conduction disturbance, impaired contractility, diastolic dysfunction, increased filling pressures (central venous and pulmonary artery occlusion pressure), diminished venous return (cf. increased IAP), decreased stroke volume and cardiac output, myocardial depression, decreased stroke volume and pulse pressure variation, venous congestion, low (global) ejection fraction, increased volumetric preload indicators (e.g. global end-diastolic volume index), and cardio-abdominal-renal interactions [23]. A study in 25 dogs examining the effect of induced myocardial edema (via progressive pulmonary artery banding), showed an inversion relationship between interstitial fluid pressure and cardiac compliance [24].
- Renal system: renal interstitial edema, increased renal venous and interstitial pressure, decreased renal blood flow and glomerular filtration rate, increased renal vascular resistance, renal venous congestion, increased or decreased (hemodiluation) creatinine,

increased uremia, salt and water retention, and local renal compartment syndrome. A study in 296 critically ill patients treated with RRT, showed that patients with fluid overload at RRT initiation had double the crude 90-day mortality compared to those without. Fluid overload was associated with increased risk for 90-day mortality even after adjustments [25].

- Gastrointestinal system: gut and bowel edema, diminished bowel contractility, increased ileus and malabsorption, diminished hepatosplanchnic perfusion (low ICG-PDR), ascites formation, increased intra-abdominal pressure and decreased abdominal perfusion pressure, abdominal hypertension, abdominal compartment syndrome, increased intestinal permeability and bacterial translocation [26].
- Hepatic system: diminished liver perfusion, decreased lactate clearance, hepatic venous congestion, local hepatic compartment syndrome.
- Abdominal wall and skin: tissue edema, poor wound healing, increased wound infections and pressure ulcers, decreased abdominal and chest wall compliance.

Particular attention should be paid to patients at high risk of overhydration e.g. those with cardiac, renal, hepatic failure, and nutritional disorders.

Liberal Versus Restrictive Fluid Regimens

As intravascular underfilling and hypovolaemia are the most prevalent reversible causes of shock, a 'liberal' fluid approach with repetitive administration of intravenous fluid boluses until the patient no longer responds with improvement in cardiovascular dynamics (i.e. without increase in mean arterial pressure, central venous pressure, urine output, or cardiac output), is common [27]. This approach is proposed in many international guidelines for the initial management of sepsis such as the NICE, GIFTASUP, ESICM, and SCCM [28, 29]. However, there is no strong rationale for this approach, as the physiological effects of fluid boluses given in ICU appear to be small and short-lived.

Administration of large volumes of intravenous crystalloid fluids often leads to accumulation of a positive fluid and sodium balance. Fluid accumulation and overhydration in critically ill patients, defined by a 10% increase in cumulative fluid balance from baseline body weight, is consistently associated with worse outcomes. This has been shown in broad populations of children and adults with sepsis, acute kidney injury, acute respiratory failure as well as general critical illness. However, this association may not indicate a causal relationship, since severely ill patients are more prone to receiving larger volumes of IV fluids. An interesting question is whether the deleterious effects are related to fluid or sodium accumulation, or both. It is clear that overhydration has extended effects on vascular integrity and permeability, and may trigger ongoing inflammation leading to a vicious cycle (GIPS). Hemodilution, venous congestion, decreased perfusion pressures, increased compartmental pressures (especially in the abdomen and thorax) and interstitial edema further impact on oxygen delivery and diffusion to the tissues. Finally, this may damage the endothelial glycocalyx, a fragile barrier by which fluid is maintained within the intravascular space. Rapid fluid boluses of salt solutions have worse effects on glycocalyx integrity, compared to slow infusion of albumin, the latter having a protective effect.

The FACCT trial, studying 1000 patients with acute lung injury, showed that although there was no significant difference in the primary outcome of 60-day mortality, a conservative strategy of fluid management improved lung function and shortened the duration of mechanical ventilation and intensive care, without increasing non-pulmonary organ failure [6].

As stated above, Murphy and colleagues showed that early adequate fluid therapy in combination with late conservative fluid management, carried the best prognosis in a retrospective study of 212 patients with ALI complicating septic shock [5].

A recent systematic review involving a total of 19577 critically ill patients [1] found that the cumulative fluid balance after 1 week of ICU stay was 4.2 l more positive in non-survivors compared to the survivors (95% CI 2.7–5.6, $p < 0.0001$). A restrictive fluid regimen resulted in a less positive cumulative fluid balance of 5.6 l (95% CI 3.3–7.7, $p < 0.0001$) compared to controls with liberal fluid regimen, after 1 week of ICU stay. Restrictive fluid management was associated with a reduction in ICU mortality from 33.2% to 24.7% when compared to patients treated with a more liberal fluid management strategy (OR of 0.42; 95% CI 0.32–0.55, $p < 0.0001$).

Silversides et al. showed in a recent meta-analysis in adults and children with acute respiratory distress syndrome, sepsis or systemic inflammation (formerly called SIRS), that a conservative or deresuscitative fluid strategy results in an increased number of ventilator-free days and a decreased length of ICU stay compared with a liberal strategy or standard care, although the effect on mortality remained uncertain [30].

The CLASSIC pilot study examined the feasibility of a protocol restricting fluids in 151 patients after initial resuscitation for septic shock [31]. The protocol successfully reduced volumes of resuscitation fluids compared with a standard care protocol. The patient-centred outcomes pointed towards a benefit of fluid restriction, however the trial was underpowered.

In a retrospective cohort study RADAR, investigating the role of active deresuscitation after resuscitation, Silversides et al. found that a negative fluid balance achieved with deresuscitation on day 3 of ICU stay, was associated with improved outcomes [32]. The authors concluded that avoiding and / or minimizing maintenance fluid intake and drug diluents, in combination with deresuscitative measures, represent a potentially beneficial therapeutic strategy that merits investigation in randomized trials.

Although we must also advise caution against the development of hypovolemia (and hypernatremia) and the potential danger of hypoperfusion resulting from aggressive deresuscitation. Indeed, the argument in favour of restrictive fluid therapy is at present mainly based on small physiological observations and studies, and there are, on the other hand, also studies showing the potential harmful effects of restrictive fluid strategy in critically ill patients.

The use of a conservative fluid management approach has been called into question by the long-term follow-up of a subset of survivors of the Fluid and Catheter Treatment Trial (FACTT) [33]. A post-hoc analysis showed that cognitive function was markedly impaired in the conservative fluid group compared with the liberal fluid group, with an adjusted odds ratio of 3.35. Cognitive impairment was defined as impairment in memory, verbal fluency, or executive function. Although all these were more common in the conservative fluid management group, only the deterioration in executive function reached statistical significance ($p = 0.001$) [33].

The best daily target fluid balance needs a balanced view, especially in light of the results of the RELIEF study [34]. In this pragmatic trial, 3000 patients at increased risk for complications during major abdominal surgery, were randomized between a restrictive vs. more liberal fluid strategy. The authors found that whilst a restrictive regimen was not associated with a higher rate of disability-free survival than a liberal fluid regimen, it was associated with a higher rate of acute kidney injury, more RRT and more surgical site infections.

The RADAR-2 pilot study in 180 critically ill patients showed that a strategy of conservative fluid administration and active deresuscitation is feasible, reduces fluid balance compared with usual care but may cause benefit or harm [35]. Deciding when to start and stop deresuscitation is key to improving patient outcomes; research is ongoing to identify the best parameters to guide fluid removal in critically ill patients.

Results of the CLASSIC trial have been published. The study enrolled 1554 critically ill patients (770 were assigned to the restrictive-fluid group and 784 to the standard-fluid group). Primary outcome data were available for 1545 patients (99.4%) [36]. Patients received a median of 3 liters of intravenous fluid before they underwent randomization and were enrolled within 3 h after admission to the ICU. In the ICU, the restrictive-fluid group received a median of 1798 ml of intravenous fluid (interquartile range, 500 to 4366); the standard-fluid group received a median of 3811 ml (interquartile range, 1861–6762). At 90 days, mortality was the same in both groups as were the number of serious adverse events that occurred at least once. Although underpowered, this study supports a strategy of limiting any post-resuscitation fluid to patients who are either preload responsive or volume tolerant, using dynamic indices of preload responsiveness, as was recommended previously by other available data from the FEAST [37] and FACTT trials [33].

More recently the CLOVERS trial showed that among patients with sepsis-induced hypotension, the use of the restrictive fluid strategy did not result in a significant difference in mortality before discharge home by day 90 when compared to the liberal fluid strategy [38]. The CLOVERS study enrolled 1563 patients, with 782 assigned to the restrictive fluid group and 781 to the liberal fluid group. Resuscitation therapies varied between the groups, with less intravenous fluid given to the restrictive fluid group compared to the liberal fluid group (difference of medians, −2134 ml; 95% confidence interval [CI], −2318 to −1949). The restrictive fluid group also had more prevalent and longer duration of vasopressor use. Death from any cause before discharge home by day 90 occurred in 14.0% of patients in the restrictive fluid group and 14.9% in the liberal fluid group (estimated difference, −0.9% points; 95% CI, −4.4 to 2.6; $P = 0.61$). The number of serious adverse events reported was similar in both groups.

While waiting for the results of the full RADAR-2 trial, prevention of fluid accumulation and de-escalation of fluid therapy remain the most effective strategies to avoid deresuscitation [12, 35, 39].

Monitoring Hypervolemia and Guiding Deresuscitation

The renewed concept of 'fluid stewardship' [10], analogous to antibiotic stewardship, focusses on the 4 D's (drug, dose, duration, and de-escalation), the 4 questions (when to start and when to stop fluid therapy, and when to start and when to stop fluid removal), the 4 indications (resuscitation, maintenance, replacement, and nutrition), and the conceptual ROSE model describing 4 fluid phases (resuscitation, optimization, stabilization, and evacuation [13]. Figure 25.3 illustrates the 4 dynamic fluid phases and gives some suggestions regarding triggers and safety limits in each phase.

Clinical Signs of Hypervolemia

The absence of thirst may indicate potential overhydration, but is not very specific. Clinical signs of overhydration should be sought during physical examination, as there is a ubiquitous bias in the direction of hypovolaemia detection. These include vital signs such as increased blood pressure (mean, systolic pressure, diastolic pressure, and pulse pressure), decreased pulse rate, increased central and jugular venous pressure, and absence of orthostatic hypotension and absence of preload responsiveness. Other signs are altered mental status, increased hepatojugular reflux, orthopnea, second and third space fluid accumulation, altered capillary refill time (usually less than 2 s), increased skin turgor, altered peripheral temperature, peripheral pitting edema and anasarca, and a positive daily and cumulative fluid balance. Also, the presence of pulmonary rales or crackles are rather non-specific signs. Many of these signs are subtler, and may not be routinely looked for. Deresuscitation should not solely be based on these non-specific signs. Daily weighing of patients in the ICU is very useful, but unfortunately not routinely used. Increased urine output (regularly checked in ICU patients) can be present (e.g. in polyuric phase after acute tubular necrosis), but depends on many variables and therapeutic interventions. Some advocate the use of a furosemide stress test to identify the risk for acute kidney injury (AKI), or the readiness for deresuscitation. Figure 25.4 summarizes the clinical signs and symptoms related to hypervolemia and fluid accumulation.

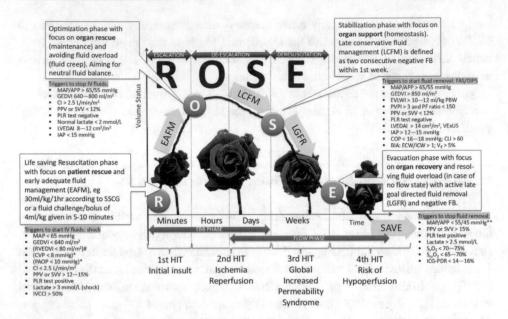

Fig. 25.3 The 4 phases conceptual model and deleterious effects of fluid accumulation syndrome. Graph showing the four-hit model of shock with evolution of patients' cumulative fluid volume status over time during the five distinct phases of resuscitation: Resuscitation (R), Optimization (O), Stabilization (S), and Evacuation (E) (ROSE), followed by a possible risk of Hypoperfusion in case of too aggressive deresuscitation. On admission patients are often hypovolemic, followed by normovolemia after fluid resuscitation (escalation or EAFM, early adequate fluid management), and possible fluid overload, again followed by a phase returning to normovolemia with de-escalation via achieving zero fluid balance or late conservative fluid management (LCFM) and followed by late goal directed fluid removal (LGFR) or deresuscitation. In case of hypovolemia, O_2 cannot get into the tissue because of convective problems, in case of hypervolemia O_2 cannot get into the tissue because of diffusion problems related to interstitial and pulmonary edema, gut edema (ileus and abdominal hypertension). Adapted from Malbrain et al. with permission, according to the Open Access CC BY Licence 4.0 [13]. * volumetric preload indicators such as GEDVI, LVEDAI, or RVEDVI are preferred over barometric ones such as CVP or PAOP. ** vasopressor can be started or increased to maintain MAP/APP above 55/45 during deresuscitation phase. # can only be measured via Swan-Ganz pulmonary artery catheter (PAC) and became obsolete. *APP* abdominal perfusion pressure (APP = MAP-IAP), *BIA* bio-electrical impedance analysis, *CI* cardiac index, *CLI* capillary leak index (serum CRP divided by serum albumin), *COP* colloid oncotic pressure, *CVP* central venous pressure, *EAFM* early adequate fluid management, *ECW/ICW* extracellular/intracellular water, *EVLWI* extravascular lung water index, *FAS* fluid accumulation syndrome, *GEDVI* global end-diastolic volume index, *GIPS* global increased permeability syndrome, *IAP* intra-abdominal pressure, *ICG-PDR* indocyanine green plasma disappearance rate, *IVCCI* inferior vena cava collapsibility index, *LCFM* late conservative fluid management, *LGFR* late goal-directed fluid removal, *LVEDAI* left ventricular end-diastolic area index, *MAP* mean arterial pressure, *PAOP* pulmonary artery occlusion pressure, *PF* P_aO_2 over F_iO_2 ratio, *PLR* passive leg raising, *PPV* pulse pressure variation, *PVPI* pulmonary vascular permeability index, *RVEDVI* right ventricular end-diastolic volume index, $S_{cv}O_2$ central venous oxygen saturation, *SSCG* surviving sepsis campaign guidelines, S_vO_2 mixed venous oxygen saturation, *SVV* stroke volume variation, V_E volume excess (from baseline body weight), *VExUS* venous congestion by ultrasound

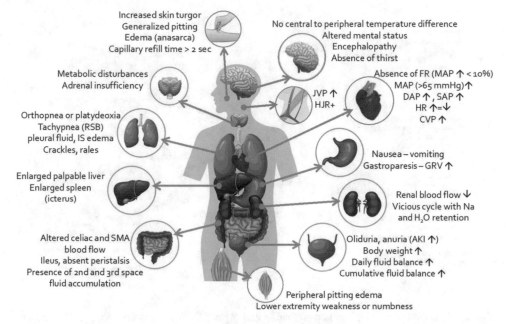

Fig. 25.4 Clinical signs and symptoms related to hypervolemia and fluid accumulation. *CVP* central venous pressure, *DAP* diastolic arterial blood pressure, *FR* preload responsiveness, *GRV* gastric residual volume, *HJR* hepato-jugular reflux, *HR* heart rate, *JVP* jugular venous pressure, *MAP* mean arterial blood pressure, *Na* sodium, *PLR* passive leg raising, *RSB* rapid shallow breathing, *SAP* systolic arterial blood pressure, *SMA* superior mesenteric artery

Laboratory Signs and Biomarkers

Laboratory parameters, although useful, cannot provide independent biomarkers of volume status (Fig. 25.5). Arterial blood gas analysis can be readily obtained and provides a quick estimation of hemoglobin and pO_2. There are reports regarding the relationship between hypervolemia and hemoglobin or hematocrit levels, and it is widely accepted that in states of overhydration, hemoglobin levels will be lower than normal due to the effects of hemodilution [40]. In case of fluid overload, extravascular lung water may also increase. This will be discussed further (related to either hyperpermeability or hydrostatic pulmonary edema), resulting in hypoxia, which in combination with anemia may further contribute to the imbalance between oxygen delivery and consumption. This process of hemodilution is however, subject to confounders (e.g., anemia, blood loss, toxic effect of infection). Renal function can be significantly impaired in states of hypervolemia. The impact of temporary decreased renal perfusion due to venous congestion appears to rely predominantly on the pre-existing physiological condition of the kidneys. Plasma sodium is of specific interest in volume regulation. It is easily measured by point-of-care tests and is strongly associated with volume status. Many patients with hypervolemia and a net fluid gain will develop hyponatremia. However, when the different baroreceptors of the body sense hypervolemia, the secretion of antidiuretic hormone by the pituitary gland is decreased.

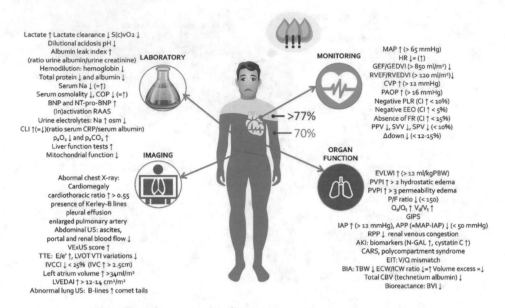

Lactate ↑ Lactate clearance ↓ S(c)vO2 ↓
Dilutional acidosis pH ↓
Albumin leak index ↑
(ratio urine albumin/urine creatinine) **LABORATORY**
Hemodilution: hemoglobin ↓
Total protein ↓ and albumin ↓
Serum Na ↓ (=↑)
Serum osmolality ↓, COP ↓ (=↑)
BNP and NT-pro-BNP ↑
(In)activation RAAS
Urine electrolytes: Na ↑ osm ↓
CLI ↑(=↓)(ratio serum CRP/serum albumin)
p$_a$O$_2$ ↓ and p$_a$CO$_2$ ↑
Liver function tests ↑
Mitochondrial function ↓

IMAGING

Abormal chest X-ray:
Cardiomegaly
cardiothoracic ratio ↑ > 0.55
presence of Kerley-B lines
pleural effusion
enlarged pulmonary artery
Abdominal US: ascites,
portal and renal blood flow ↓
VExUS score ↑
TTE: E/e' ↑, LVOT VTI variations ↓
IVCCI ↓ < 25% (IVC ↑ > 2.5cm)
Left atrium volume ↑ >34ml/m²
LVEDAI ↑ > 12-14 cm²/m²
Abnormal lung US: B-lines ↑ comet tails

MONITORING

MAP ↑ (> 65 mmHg)
HR ↓= (↑)
GEF/GEDVI (> 850 ml/m²) ↓
RVEF/RVEDVI (> 120 ml/m²)↓
CVP ↑ (> 12 mmHg)
PAOP ↑ (> 16 mmHg)
Negative PLR (CI ↑ < 10%)
Negative EEO (CI ↑ < 5%)
Absence of FR (CI ↑ < 15%)
PPV ↓, SVV ↓, SPV ↓ (< 10%)
Δdown ↓ (< 12-15%)

>77%
70%

**ORGAN
FUNCTION**

EVLWI ↑ (> 12 ml/kgPBW)
PVPI ↑ > 2 hydrostatic edema
PVPI ↑ > 3 permeability edema
P/F ratio ↓ (< 150)
Q$_s$/Q$_t$ ↑ V$_d$/V$_t$ ↑
GIPS
IAP ↑ (> 12 mmHg), APP (=MAP-IAP) ↓ (< 50 mmHg)
RPP ↓ renal venous congestion
AKI: biomarkers (N-GAL ↑, cystatin C ↑)
CARS, polycompartment syndrome
EIT: V/Q mismatch
BIA: TBW ↓ ECW/ICW ratio ↓=↑ Volume excess =↓
Total CBV (technetium albumin) ↓
Bioreactance: BVI ↓

Fig. 25.5 Laboratory, imaging, hemodynamic and organ function signs and symptoms related to hypovolemia and hypoperfusion. Total body water accounts for 70% of body weight. Overt signs and symptoms of hypovolemia occur when circulating blood volume is reduced by more than 50%. *AKI* acute kidney injury, *APP* abdominal perfusion pressure, *BIA* bio-electrical impedance analysis, *BNP* brain natriuretic peptide, *BVI* blood volume index, *CARS* cardio-abdominal-renal syndrome, *CBV* circulating blood volume, *CI* cardiac index, *CLI* capillary leak index, *COP* colloid oncotic pressure, *CRP* C-reactive protein, *CVP* central venous pressure, *ECW* extracellular water, *EIT* electrical impedance tomography, *EEO* end-expiratory occlusion, *EVLWI* extravascular lung water index, *FR* preload responsiveness, *GEDVI* global end-diastolic volume index, *GEF* global ejection fraction, *GIPS* global increased permeability syndrome, *HR* heart rate, *IAP* intra-abdominal pressure, *ICW* intracellular water, *IVC* inferior vena cava, *IVCCI* inferior vena cava collapsibility index, *LVOT* left ventricular outflow tract, *MAP* mean arterial blood pressure, *Na* sodium, *P/F ratio* pO$_2$ over FiO$_2$ ratio, *PAOP* pulmonary artery occlusion pressure, *PLR* passive leg raising, *PPV* pulse pressure variation, *PVPI* pulmonary vascular permeability index, *Qs/Qt* shunt fraction, *RAAS* renin angiotensin aldosterone system, *RPP* renal perfusion pressure, *RVEDVI* right ventricular end-diastolic volume index, *RVEF* right ventricular ejection fraction, *ScvO$_2$* mixed central venous oxygen saturation, *SPV* systolic pressure variation, *SVV* stroke volume variation, *TBW* total body water, *TTE* transthoracic echocardiography, *US* ultrasound, *VExUS* venous excess by ultrasonography score, *V/Q* ventilation/perfusion, *VTI* velocity time integral, *Vt/Vd* dead space ventilation

As a consequence, there will be less retention of water, resulting in increase in sodium levels. Sodium values are also confounded by medication (e.g. diuretics), the type of fluids administered (e.g. saline solutions for resuscitation), the phase of fluid therapy (e.g. use of hypertonic lactated saline for deresuscitation), adrenal activity (renin angiotensin aldosterone system), and choice of replacement fluid (isotonic vs hypotonic). Hypervolemic hyponatremia in cirrhosis patients is characterized by a pronounced deficit of free water excretion and leads to inappropriate water retention in comparison with the sodium concentration.

This imbalance results in an expanded extracellular volume and dilutional hyponatremia. Plasma osmolality (normal around 287 mOsm/kg) can be decreased in cases of hypervolemia, although the body will try to regulate osmolality within normal limits. Overhydration may result in extracellular fluid accumulation and also cellular hydration depending on the type of accumulating fluids. Osmolality is mainly influenced by the non-soluble fraction of the extra-cellular fluid compartment, namely elevated concentrations of serum lipids or proteins. Many medications (e.g. diuretics, mannitol) will affect the osmolality. The plasma colloid oncotic pressure (COP) is normally around 20–25 mmHg. In overhydrated patients with sepsis, the COP value may decrease below 16 mmHg. COP values are related to left ventricular filling pressures and may help in the differential diagnosis of pulmonary edema. COP is increased in hydrostatic edema and associated with increased filling pressures, whereas in hyperpermeability edema, COP is usually decreased. As such, COP measurement can be used for the differential diagnosis of pulmonary edema (hydrostatic vs hyperpermeability). Overhydrated patients may also show lower total protein and decreased albumin levels. The measurement of BNP levels can be a useful adjunct when in doubt as to the potential cause of hypervolemia. Low BNP levels have a high negative predictive value for the exclusion of heart failure as a diagnosis. On the other hand, high BNP levels can be non-specific for volume or fluid overload. The ANP-over-BNP ratio may be indicative of chronic congestive heart failure and fluid overload.

We often look at urine output as a marker of fluid requirement, however patients who are unwell, have suffered trauma, or have undergone surgery often have a reduced urine output due to increased sodium retention (and thus water), by the kidneys. This is an evolutionary stress response geared to the preservation of intravascular volume, in order to maintain vital organ perfusion during such stress states. Stress-induced ('inappropriate') anti-diuretic hormone secretion, as well as intrinsic vasopressor hormone secretion, leads to a state of sodium retention and potassium loss in the urine. The patient becomes edematous, hypokalemic and hypernatremia over time, if left unchecked. If normal saline has been given as a resuscitation fluid or maintenance fluid, the potential situation of hyperchloremic metabolic acidosis can ensue, on top of these other electrolyte imbalances.

Radiological and Imaging Signs

Fluid accumulation can be characterized by an abnormal chest X-ray that shows cardiomegaly, dilated upper lobe vessels, interstitial edema, enlarged pulmonary artery, alveolar edema, prominent superior vena cava, increased cardiothoracic ratio (>0.55), presence of Kerley-B lines or pleural effusion (Fig. 25.5). The utility of lung ultrasound offers a greater diagnostic sensitivity and specificity profile over plain radiography of the chest. Moreover, portable chest X-ray, reduces the sensitivity of findings of volume overload, with pleural effusions regularly being missed if the film is performed supine or in intubated patients [41]. Abdominal ultrasound may show 2nd and 3rd space fluid accumulation with edematous abdominal wall, bowel edema, or presence of ascites [42].

Table 25.1 Grading table for assessment of Venous congestion with point-of-care ultrasound

	Grade 0	Grade 1	Grade 2	Grade 3	Grade 4
IVC	<5 mm with respiratory variation	5–9 mm with respiratory variation	10–19 mm with respiratory variation	>20 mm with respiratory variation	20 mm with minimal or no respiratory variation
Hepatic vein	Normal S > D	S < D with antegrade S	S flat or inverted or biphasic trace		
Portal vein	< 0.3 pulsatility index	0.3–0.49 pulsatility index	0.5–1.0 pulsatility index		
Renal doppler	Continuous monophasic/pulsatile flow	Dis-continuous biphasic flow	Dis-continuous monophasic flow (diastole only)		
VEXUS score	IVC grade < 3, HD grade 0, PV grade 0 (RD grade 0)	IVC grade 4, but normal HV/PV/RV patterns.	IVC grade 4 with mild flow pattern abnormalities in two or more of the following HV/PV/RV	IVC grade 4 with severe flow pattern abnormalities in two or more of the following HV/PV/RV	

VEXUS *venous congestion assessment with ultrasound*
Adapted with permission from Rola et al. [48]

Transthoracic cardiac ultrasound may also be highly useful demonstrating increased E/e′ on tissue Doppler imaging and the absence of left ventricular outflow tract (LVOT) velocity time integral (VTI) variations. Care must be taken over reliance upon on the spot IVC measurements to ascertain volaemic status. Extremes of measurement may be more useful. If there is a complete collapse, in conjunction with an empty, hyperdynamic LV, then the patient is likely to be hypovolaemic. The converse is also true, where a plethoric IVC >2.5 cm is present, with little to no collapse at all, pointing to hypervolemia. There may be other causes of an enlarged IVC to exclude however; large PE, cardiac tamponade, severe tricuspid regurgitation, high PEEP, presence of autoPEEP, increased IAP, noninvasive ventilation, assisted spontaneous breathing, right ventricular dysfunction, right ventricular infarction, low tidal volume or respiratory tidal variation, mechanical obstruction [43]. Low IVCCI (<25%) has been quoted as a useful parameter, but only in ventilated patients and the short axis view is the preferred, more reliable measurement modality. Increased left atrium volume (LA >34 ml/m^2) and lung ultrasound, may show B-lines and comet tail artifacts [44, 45]. The importance of venous congestion in the development of organ failure (and especially AKI), in fluid overload, can possibly explain the greatest improvement of renal function after medical treatment for advanced heart failure. This is particularly the case in patients with the echocardiographic signs of right ventricular dysfunction on the inferior vena cava, the portal, hepatic, and renal veins [46, 47] (Table 25.1). To analyse and objectively measure this, the VExUS score (venous excess by ultrasonography) has been suggested (Fig. 25.6) [47].

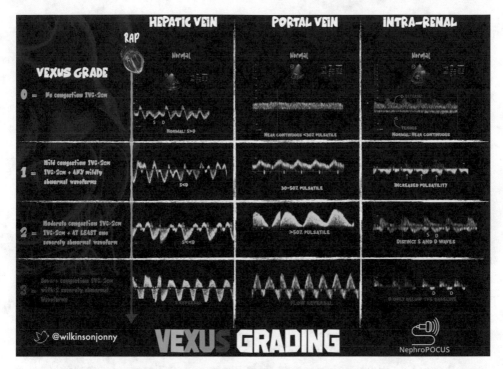

Fig. 25.6 VexUS grading in graphical format (Koratala and Wilkinson)

Advanced Hemodynamic Monitoring

These clinical, biochemical, and radiological parameters are rather non-specific. Hemodynamic assessment of fluid accumulation syndrome includes the absence of preload responsiveness, with a negative passive leg raise test (Fig. 25.7) or end-expiratory occlusion test. Also low functional hemodynamic parameters (PPV, SVV), low systolic pressure variation with normal delta up and delta down, increased MAP, SAP, and DAP, and barometric preload indicators (CVP or PCWP), increased volumetric preload parameters (like global or right ventricular end diastolic volume index; Fig. 25.5).

In critically ill patients treated with renal replacement therapy (RRT), the absence of preload dependence pre-RRT, as assessed by a negative PLR test, was found to be a predictor that fluid removal during RRT would not induce hemodynamic instability [50]. Volumetric preload parameters are superior to barometric parameters, especially if ITP, IAP or PEEP are increased, but correction of these parameters by measures of ejection fraction, can further improve their ability to assess changes in preload over time, as was shown in an heterogeneous group of critically ill patients [51]. The impact of FAS on organ function can be assessed by examining thyroid and adrenal function, looking for signs for polycompartment syndrome (increased IAP, ICP, low APP), gastric distension, gastroparesis or increased GRV, increased EVLWI, PVPI, drop in P/F ratio and ORI, decreased ICG-PDR, and presence of AKI or CARS. With a cut-off value of 3, the

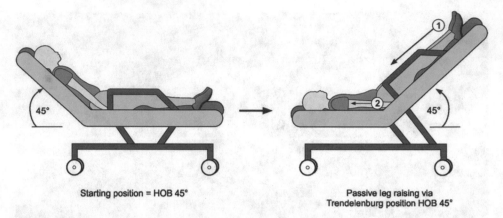

Starting position = HOB 45°

Passive leg raising via
Trendelenburg position HOB 45°

Fig. 25.7 The passive leg raising (PLR) test can also be used to assess the absence of preload responsiveness. In order to perform a correct PLR test, one should not touch the patient in order to avoid sympathetic activation. The PLR is performed by turning the bed from the starting position (head of bed elevation 30–45°) to the Trendelenburg position. The PLR test results in an autotransfusion effect via the increased venous return from the legs and the splanchnic mesenteric pool. Monitoring of stroke volume is required as a positive PLR test is defined by an increase in SV by at least 10%. See text for an explanation. Adapted from Hofer C, Cannesson M. with permission [49]

pulmonary vascular permeability index (PVPI), calculated by transpulmonary thermodilution, allows to discriminate hydrostatic from hyperpermeability pulmonary [52]. In the future, some new and less invasive technologies will become readily available at the bedside. For example bio-electrical impedance analysis with calculation of TBW, ECW/ICW ratio, EVF/IVF ratio, volume excess [19] and BIVA hyperhydration [53], calculation of blood volume index with dye densitometry [54] or total circulating BV with albumin marked isotope dilution [55], or ventilation perfusion (mis)match with EIT [56].

Use of a protocol including BV analysis resulted in a 66% reduction in mortality, a 20% reduction in LOS, 36 h earlier treatment decisions, 44% change in treatment strategy [55]. Fluid overload, defined as a 5% increase in volume excess (measured with BIA) from baseline body weight, was associated with increased mortality in a retrospective study of 101 critically ill patients [19].

How to Perform Deresuscitation?

While more restrictive use of fluid, together with earlier use of vasopressors if needed, may reduce fluid administration, it is unlikely that fluid overload can be entirely avoided using this strategy [27]. Fluid intake in ICU comes from a range of sources, many obligate such as drug diluents and nutrition. A recent study showed that this 'fluid creep' accounts for as much as 33% of all fluid intake compared to around 7% for resuscitation fluids [16]. As well as restriction of fluid resuscitation, avoidance of fluid overload is therefore likely to require deresuscitation, with active fluid removal using diuretics or ultrafiltration [1], an approach that likely shortens the duration of mechanical ventilation and ICU stay [30]. Measures to remove excess fluid include drugs and UF, combined with fluid restriction.

Provided some kidney function is preserved, diuretics are usually tried first, either as monotherapy or in combination. The options include loop diuretics (furosemide, bumetanide), carbonic anhydrase inhibitor (acetazolamide), mineralocorticoid receptor antagonist (spironolactone), thiazides or thiazide-like drugs (indapamide). In case of low serum albumin levels (<30 g/L) or low serum total protein levels (<60 g/L) co-administration of hyperoncotic albumin 20% can be added for synergistic effect along with diuretics and may promote hemodynamic stability [57]. Increased EVLWI and failure to lower EVLWI resulted in poor outcomes in 123 critically ill patients with increased mortality and longer duration of ventilation. A drop in EVLWI was associated with late conservative fluid management and being preload responsive (less positive cumulative fluid balance) [58]. The combination of PEEP (in cmH_2O, set at the level of IAP in mmHg), followed by albumin 20% (up to albumin levels of 30 g/L) and furosemide (or PAL-treatment) resulted in a negative cumulative fluid balance, a reduction of EVLWI and IAP, with improved clinical outcomes in a matched cohort of 114 critically ill patients with hyperpermeability pulmonary edema [59]. In 11 critically ill patients, RRT with 1.9 l net fluid removal was able to lower IAP, EVLWI, and GEDVI significantly [60] (Table 25.2).

Table 25.2 Therapeutic options to avoid and treat fluid accumulation

Treatment options	Description
1. Monitoring (prevention)	– Basic monitoring with arterial and central venous line, pre-alerting to any shock states – Perform baseline transthoracic (or transesophageal) echocardiography – Obtain laboratory results, urea and electrolytes, arterial/venous blood gas analysis, with attention to base excess and lactate – Assess preload responsiveness with functional hemodynamics (PPV or SVV) and perform passive leg raising test or end-expiratory occlusion test – Obtain baseline body weight – Monitor for risk for fluid accumulation (FA): daily body weight, daily and cumulative fluid balance, BIA or BIVA – Assess for impact of FA on end-organ function: IAP, APP, PF ratio, EVLWI, PVPI, daily SOFA (Fig. 25.2)
2. Metabolic optimization (Prevention)	– Limit fluid intake (e.g. de-escalation of IV fluids when oral intake is possible) – Use concentrated enteral formula's with 2 kcal/ml instead of 1 kcal/ml) – Limit sodium intake – KDIGO-derived kidney care and treatment bundle – Limit/avoid maintenance solutions – Limit/avoid fluid creep

(continued)

Table 25.2 (continued)

Treatment options	Description
3. First line diuretics	– Loop diuretic (furosemide, bumetanide): high dose and continuous furosemide (1 mg/kg bolus and 10 mg/h) or bumetanide (0.1 mg/kg bolus and 0.1 mg/h)
4. Vasodilators (calcium antagonists, ACE-I) (care)	– Increase renal blood flow – Reduce filtration fraction – Reduce lymph flow – Improve LV function
5. Inotropes (care)	– Dobutamine: low dose (2.5–5 ug/kg/min) – Milrinone: low dose (0.05–0.1 ug/kg/min), especially in right heart failure or when right heart pressures increased
6. Lower IAP (care)	– Improve abdominal wall compliance – Reduce intraluminal volume (ileus) – Reduce intra-abdominal volume (ascites) – Optimize fluid administration – Optimize systemic regional perfusion
7. Increase APP (care)	– APP = MAP − IAP > 60 mmHg – Vasopressors when needed, low-dose terlipressin (0.5–1 mg over 30 min), vasopressin or norepinephrine (0.05–0.1 ug/kg/min) or norepinephrine
8. Combination therapy of diuretics (cure)	– Loop diuretics: increase dose – Carbonic anhydrase inhibitors (acetazolamide, 250–500 mg IV bolus): inhibition of Na reabsorption in proximal tubule in case of metabolic alkalosis – Thiazide (indapamide, 2.5–5 mg PO): inhibition of Na reabsorption in distal tubule in cases of hypernatremia – Potassium sparing (spironolactone, 25–50 mg PO): aldosterone receptor antagonist, reduction of Na reabsorption at the collector duct (ENaC channel)

	Na^+	K^+	pH	Ca^{2+}	Mg^{2+}
Loop diuretic	↑↓	↓	↑	↓	↓
Carbonic anhydrase inhibitors	–	↓	↓	–	–
Thiazide	↓	↓	↑	↑	↓
Potassium sparing	–	↑	↓	–	↑

Treatment options	Description
8. Active de-resuscitation (cure)	– Increase dose combination therapy diuretics – Application of PEEP – Albumin 20% (where albumin <30 g/L) + diuretics – PAL treatment: PEEP (cmH₂O) = IAP (mmHg) + albumin 20% (200 ml bolus) + Lasix (furosemide 1 mg/kg bolus + drip) – SLEDD with net UF or SCUF – CVVH with net UF

APP abdominal perfusion pressure, *CARS* cardio abdominal renal syndrome, *CVVH* continuous venovenous hemofiltration, *IAP* intra-abdominal pressure, *MAP* mean arterial pressure, *Na* sodium, *PEEP* positive end-expiratory pressure, *SLEDD* slow extended daily dialysis, *UF* ultrafiltration

Case Vignette

Q1. Does this patient have overhydration?

A1. Yes, moderate overhydration.

Overhydration (or hyperhydration) = body weight relative to admission body weight/pre-ICU body weight × 100

(4.9/67) × 100 = 7.3%

Q2. Would you consider fluid removal in this patient (deresuscitation), and how?

A2. Yes, given indicators of overhydration. An initial attempt with diuretics along with hyperoncotic albumin (if serum albumin is <30 g/L) can be attempted to induce diuresis. Using RRT for ultrafiltration can be tried in case of AKI or non-responder to diuretics.

Conclusions

No patient should suffer the effects of cellular dysfunction and ultimately multi-organ dysfunction, as a result of excessive IV fluid administration. Armed with an understanding of fluid physiology, one can see why oliguria is a poor marker of overall volaemic status. Physiological oral fluids should always be first line, unless circumstances absolutely disallow it.

The best fluid is probably the one that has not been given…(unnecessarily) [11]

Back to the case vignette; where we followed a patient, who developed shock within 18 h of ICU admission. Despite initial normal (and thus adequate) filling pressures, further fluid resuscitation was needed to overcome the ebb phase (this was guided by functional hemodynamic parameters, passive leg raising test and volumetric preload indices). However, at the very early stage of shock despite the fact that the patient was preload responsive, lung water was already increased. This is the classic example of a therapeutic dilemma which is a condition in which each therapeutic option (either fluid administration or fluid removal), may cause potential harm. Fluids are a double-edged sword. After initial further fluid resuscitation, diuretics were initiated after 24 h to help the patient transgress to the flow phase because of respiratory failure due to capillary leak, as evidenced by increased extravascular lung water. Based on barometric preload indicators, most physicians would be reluctant to start initial fluid resuscitation, therefore advanced monitoring may be indicated, especially in situations with changes in preload, afterload or contractility. This case nicely demonstrates the biphasic clinical course from ebb to flow during shock as well as the inability of traditional filling pressures, to guide us through these different phases. It also illustrates the four crucial questions that need to be solved in order not to cause harm. Therefore, it is important to know and understand:

1. When to start giving fluids (low GEF/GEDVI, high PPV and positive PLR, increased lactate)
2. When to stop giving fluids (high GEF/GEDVI, low PPV, negative PLR, normalized lactate)
3. When to start removing fluids (high EVLWI, high PVPI, raised IAP, low APP defined as MAP minus IAP, positive cumulative fluid balance, absence of preload responsiveness).
4. When to stop fluid removal (low ICG-PDR, low APP, low ScvO$_2$, neutral to negative cumulative fluid balance, hypovolemia with hypoperfusion).

However, one must realize that the thresholds for the above-mentioned parameters are dynamic targets with dynamic goals (from early adequate goal-directed therapy, over late conservative fluid management towards late goal-directed fluid removal). And above all, one must always bear in mind that unnecessary fluid loading may be harmful. If the patient does not need fluids, don't give them, and remember—the best fluid may be the one that has not been given to the patient!

Take Home Messages
- Tissue edema in ICU patients results from overzealous fluid administration and/ or capillary leaks and may lead to worse outcomes.
- Overhydration affects multiple organs and is independently linked to organ failure and mortality.
- The clinical, laboratory, and radiological signs of overload are non-specific.
- Hemodynamic tools like the absence of fluid responsiveness by negative PLR, EEO, low functional hemodynamic variables (SVV, SPV, PPV), increased volumetric (GEDV, RVEDV) or barometric preload indicators (CVP, PAWP) can be used to diagnose and monitor overhydration.
- Evidence supports the feasibility and safety of restrictive fluid administration during resuscitation.
- Deresuscitation defined as an active removal of excessive fluid using diuretics and/or ultrafiltration, combined with fluid restriction may be considered in selected patients with overhydration.

Acknowledgements Parts of this chapter were published previously as open access under the Creative Commons Attribution 4.0 International Licence (CC BY 4.0) [1, 12, 20]. The European Commission announced it has adopted CC BY 4.0 and CC0 to share published documents, including photos, videos, reports, peer-reviewed studies, and data. The Commission joins other public institutions around the world that use standard, legally interoperable tools such as Creative Commons licenses and public domain tools to share a wide range of content they produce. The decision to use CC aims to increase the legal interoperability and ease of reuse of authors own materials.

References

1. Malbrain ML, Marik PE, Witters I, Cordemans C, Kirkpatrick AW, Roberts DJ, Van Regenmortel N. Fluid overload, de-resuscitation, and outcomes in critically ill or injured patients: a systematic review with suggestions for clinical practice. Anaesthesiol Intensive Ther. 2014;46(5):361–80.
2. Malbrain M, Wilmer A. The polycompartment syndrome: towards an understanding of the inter-actions between different compartments! Intensive Care Med. 2007;33(11):1869–72.
3. Malbrain ML, Roberts DJ, Sugrue M, De Keulenaer BL, Ivatury R, Pelosi P, Verbrugge F, Wise R, Mullens W. The polycompartment syndrome: a concise state-of-the-art review. Anaesthesiol Intensive Ther. 2014;46(5):433–50.
4. Kelm DJ, Perrin JT, Cartin-Ceba R, Gajic O, Schenck L, Kennedy CC. Fluid overload in patients with severe sepsis and septic shock treated with early goal-directed therapy is associ-ated with increased acute need for fluid-related medical interventions and hospital death. Shock. 2015;43(1):68–73.
5. Murphy CV, Schramm GE, Doherty JA, Reichley RM, Gajic O, Afessa B, Micek ST, Kollef MH. The importance of fluid management in acute lung injury secondary to septic shock. Chest. 2009;136(1):102–9.
6. Wiedemann HP, Wheeler AP, Bernard GR, Thompson BT, Hayden D, deBoisblanc B, Connors AF Jr, Hite RD, Harabin AL. Comparison of two fluid-management strategies in acute lung injury. N Engl J Med. 2006;354(24):2564–75.
7. Alsous F, Khamiees M, DeGirolamo A, Amoateng-Adjepong Y, Manthous CA. Negative fluid balance predicts survival in patients with septic shock: a retrospective pilot study. Chest. 2000;117(6):1749–54.
8. Malbrain MLNG, Van Regenmortel N. Fluid overload is not only of cosmetic concern (part I): exploring a new hypothesis. ICU Manage. 2012;12:30–3.
9. Cordemans C, De Laet I, Van Regenmortel N, Schoonheydt K, Dits H, Huber W, Malbrain MLNG. Fluid management in critically ill patients: the role of extravascular lung water, abdomi-nal hypertension, capillary leak and fluid balance. Ann Intensive Care. 2012;2(Suppl 1):S1.
10. Malbrain ML, Mythen M, Rice TW, Wuyts S. It is time for improved fluid stewardship. ICU Manage Pract. 2018;18(3):158–62.
11. Malbrain M, Van Regenmortel N, Owczuk R. It is time to consider the four D's of fluid manage-ment. Anaesthesiol Intensive Ther. 2015;47:S1–5.
12. Malbrain M, Martin G, Ostermann M. Everything you need to know about deresuscitation. Intensive Care Med. 2022;48(12):1781–6.
13. Malbrain M, Van Regenmortel N, Saugel B, De Tavernier B, Van Gaal PJ, Joannes-Boyau O, Teboul JL, Rice TW, Mythen M, Monnet X. Principles of fluid management and stewardship in septic shock: it is time to consider the four D's and the four phases of fluid therapy. Ann Intensive Care. 2018;8(1):66.
14. Chow RS. Terms, definitions, nomenclature, and routes of fluid administration. Front Vet Sci. 2020;7:591218.
15. Malbrain M, Langer T, Annane D, Gattinoni L, Elbers P, Hahn RG, De Laet I, Minini A, Wong A, Ince C, et al. Intravenous fluid therapy in the perioperative and critical care setting: executive summary of the International Fluid Academy (IFA). Ann Intensive Care. 2020;10(1):64.
16. Van Regenmortel N, Verbrugghe W, Roelant E, Van den Wyngaert T, Jorens PG. Maintenance fluid therapy and fluid creep impose more significant fluid, sodium, and chloride burdens than resuscitation fluids in critically ill patients: a retrospective study in a tertiary mixed ICU popula-tion. Intensive Care Med. 2018;44(4):409–17.
17. Cartotto R, Zhou A. Fluid creep: the pendulum hasn't swung back yet! J Burn Care Res. 2010;31(4):551–8.

18. Vincent JL, Pinsky MR. We should avoid the term "fluid overload". Crit Care. 2018;22(1):214.
19. Cleymaet R, Scheinok T, Maes H, Stas A, Malbrain L, De Laet I, Schoonheydt K, Dits H, van Regenmortel N, Mekeirele M, et al. Prognostic value of bioelectrical impedance analysis for assessment of fluid overload in ICU patients: a pilot study. Anaesthesiol Intensive Ther. 2021;53(1):10–7.
20. Malbrain MLNG, Van Regenmortel N, Saugel B, De Tavernier B, Van Gaal P-J, Joannes-Boyau O, Teboul J-L, Rice TW, Mythen M, Monnet X. Principles of fluid management and steward-ship in septic shock: It is time to consider the four D's and the four phases of fluid therapy. Ann Intensive Care. 2018;8(1):66.
21. Ramming S, Shackford SR, Zhuang J, Schmoker JD. The relationship of fluid balance and sodium administration to cerebral edema formation and intracranial pressure in a porcine model of brain injury. J Trauma. 1994;37(5):705–13.
22. Singh CN, Klein MB, Sullivan SR, Sires BS, Hutter CM, Rice K, Jian-Amadi A. Orbital com-partment syndrome in burn patients. Ophthal Plast Reconstr Surg. 2008;24(2):102–6.
23. Verbrugge FH, Dupont M, Steels P, Grieten L, Malbrain M, Tang WH, Mullens W. Abdominal contributions to cardiorenal dysfunction in congestive heart failure. J Am Coll Cardiol. 2013;62(6):485–95.
24. Desai KV, Laine GA, Stewart RH, Cox CS Jr, Quick CM, Allen SJ, Fischer UM. Mechanics of the left ventricular myocardial interstitium: effects of acute and chronic myocardial edema. Am J Physiol Heart Circ Physiol. 2008;294(6):2428–34.
25. Vaara ST, Korhonen AM, Kaukonen KM, Nisula S, Inkinen O, Hoppu S, Laurila JJ, Mildh L, Reinikainen M, Lund V, et al. Fluid overload is associated with an increased risk for 90-day mortality in critically ill patients with renal replacement therapy: data from the prospective FINNAKI study. Crit Care. 2012;16(5):R197.
26. Reintam Blaser A, Starkopf J, Moonen PJ, Malbrain M, Oudemans-van Straaten HM. Perioperative gastrointestinal problems in the ICU. Anaesthesiol Intensive Ther. 2018;50(1):59–71.
27. Silversides JA, Perner A, Malbrain M. Liberal versus restrictive fluid therapy in critically ill patients. Intensive Care Med. 2019;45(10):1440–2.
28. Padhi S, Bullock I, Li L, Stroud M, National Institute for H, Care Excellence Guideline Development G. Intravenous fluid therapy for adults in hospital: summary of NICE guidance. BMJ. 2013;347:f7073.
29. Powell-Tuck J, Gosling P, Lobo D, Allison S, Carlson G, Gore M, Lewington A, Pearse R, Mythen M. Summary of the British consensus guidelines on intravenous fluid therapy for adult surgical patients (GIFTASUP). J Intensive Care Soc. 2009;10(1):13–5.
30. Silversides JA, Major E, Ferguson AJ, Mann EE, McAuley DF, Marshall JC, Blackwood B, Fan E. Conservative fluid management or deresuscitation for patients with sepsis or acute respiratory distress syndrome following the resuscitation phase of critical illness: a systematic review and meta-analysis. Intensive Care Med. 2017;43(2):155–70.
31. Hjortrup PB, Haase N, Bundgaard H, Thomsen SL, Winding R, Pettila V, Aaen A, Lodahl D, Berthelsen RE, Christensen H, et al. Restricting volumes of resuscitation fluid in adults with septic shock after initial management: the CLASSIC randomised, parallel-group, multicentre feasibility trial. Intensive Care Med. 2016;42(11):1695–705.
32. Silversides JA, Fitzgerald E, Manickavasagam US, Lapinsky SE, Nisenbaum R, Hemmings N, Nutt C, Trinder TJ, Pogson DG, Fan E, et al. Deresuscitation of patients with iatrogenic fluid over-load is associated with reduced mortality in critical illness. Crit Care Med. 2018;46(10):1600–7.
33. Mikkelsen ME, Christie JD, Lanken PN, Biester RC, Thompson BT, Bellamy SL, Localio AR, Demissie E, Hopkins RO, Angus DC. The adult respiratory distress syndrome cognitive out-comes study: long-term neuropsychological function in survivors of acute lung injury. Am J Respir Crit Care Med. 2012;185(12):1307–15.

34. Myles PS, Bellomo R, Corcoran T, Forbes A, Peyton P, Story D, Christophi C, Leslie K, McGuinness S, Parke R, et al. Restrictive versus liberal fluid therapy for major abdominal surgery. N Engl J Med. 2018;378(24):2263–74.
35. Silversides JA, McMullan R, Emerson LM, Bradbury I, Bannard-Smith J, Szakmany T, Trinder J, Rostron AJ, Johnston P, Ferguson AJ, et al. Feasibility of conservative fluid administration and deresuscitation compared with usual care in critical illness: the role of active deresuscitation after resuscitation-2 (RADAR-2) randomised clinical trial. Intensive Care Med. 2022;48(2):190–200.
36. Meyhoff TS, Hjortrup PB, Wetterslev J, Sivapalan P, Laake JH, Cronhjort M, Jakob SM, Cecconi M, Nalos M, Ostermann M, et al. Restriction of intravenous fluid in ICU patients with septic shock. N Engl J Med. 2022;386(26):2459–70.
37. Maitland K, Kiguli S, Opoka RO, Engoru C, Olupot-Olupot P, Akech SO, Nyeko R, Mtove G, Reyburn H, Lang T, et al. Mortality after fluid bolus in African children with severe infection. N Engl J Med. 2011;364(26):2483–95.
38. Shapiro NI, Douglas IS, Brower RG, Brown SM, Exline MC, Ginde AA, Gong MN, et al. Early restrictive or liberal fluid management for sepsis-induced hypotension. N Engl J Med. 2023;388(6):499–510.
39. Meyhoff TS, Hjortrup PB, Moller MH, Wetterslev J, Lange T, Kjaer MN, Jonsson AB, Hjortso CJS, Cronhjort M, Laake JH, et al. Conservative vs liberal fluid therapy in septic shock (CLASSIC) trial-protocol and statistical analysis plan. Acta Anaesthesiol Scand. 2019;63(9):1262–71.
40. Perel A. Iatrogenic hemodilution: a possible cause for avoidable blood transfusions? Crit Care. 2017;21(1):291.
41. Claure-Del Granado R, Mehta RL. Fluid overload in the ICU: evaluation and management. BMC Nephrol. 2016;17(1):109.
42. Perez-Calatayud AA, Carrillo-Esper R, Anica-Malagon ED, Briones-Garduno JC, Arch-Tirado E, Wise R, Malbrain M. Point-of-care gastrointestinal and urinary tract sonography in daily evaluation of gastrointestinal dysfunction in critically ill patients (GUTS protocol). Anaesthesiol Intensive Ther. 2018;50(1):40–8.
43. Via G, Tavazzi G, Price S. Ten situations where inferior vena cava ultrasound may fail to accurately predict fluid responsiveness: a physiologically based point of view. Intensive Care Med. 2016;42(7):1164–7.
44. Malbrain M, De Tavernier B, Haverals S, Slama M, Vieillard-Baron A, Wong A, Poelaert J, Monnet X, Stockman W, Elbers P, et al. Executive summary on the use of ultrasound in the critically ill: consensus report from the 3rd course on acute care ultrasound (CACU). Anaesthesiol Intensive Ther. 2017;49(5):393–411.
45. Lichtenstein DA, Malbrain M. Lung ultrasound in the critically ill (LUCI): a translational discipline. Anaesthesiol Intensive Ther. 2017;49(5):430–6.
46. Testani JM, Khera AV, St John Sutton MG, Keane MG, Wiegers SE, Shannon RP, Kirkpatrick JN. Effect of right ventricular function and venous congestion on cardiorenal interactions during the treatment of decompensated heart failure. Am J Cardiol. 2010;105(4):511–6.
47. Beaubien-Souligny W, Rola P, Haycock K, Bouchard J, Lamarche Y, Spiegel R, Denault AY. Quantifying systemic congestion with Point-Of-Care ultrasound: development of the venous excess ultrasound grading system. Ultrasound J. 2020;12(1):16.
48. Rola P, Miralles-Aguiar F, Argaiz E, Beaubien-Souligny W, Haycock K, Karimov T, Dinh VA, Spiegel R. Clinical applications of the venous excess ultrasound (VExUS) score: conceptual review and case series. Ultrasound J. 2021;13(1):32.
49. Hofer CK, Cannesson M. Monitoring fluid responsiveness. Acta Anaesthesiol Taiwanica. 2011;49(2):59–65.
50. Monnet X, Cipriani F, Camous L, Sentenac P, Dres M, Krastinova E, Anguel N, Richard C, Teboul JL. The passive leg raising test to guide fluid removal in critically ill patients. Ann Intensive Care. 2016;6(1):46.

51. Malbrain M, De Potter TJR, Dits H, Reuter DA. Global and right ventricular end-diastolic volumes correlate better with preload after correction for ejection fraction. Acta Anaesthesiol Scand. 2010;54(5):622–31.

52. Monnet X, Anguel N, Osman D, Hamzaoui O, Richard C, Teboul JL. Assessing pulmonary permeability by transpulmonary thermodilution allows differentiation of hydrostatic pulmonary edema from ALI/ARDS. Intensive Care Med. 2007;33(3):448–53.

53. Samoni S, Vigo V, Resendiz LI, Villa G, De Rosa S, Nalesso F, Ferrari F, Meola M, Brendolan A, Malacarne P, et al. Impact of hyperhydration on the mortality risk in critically ill patients admitted in intensive care units: comparison between bioelectrical impedance vector analysis and cumulative fluid balance recording. Crit Care. 2016;20:95.

54. Nishioka M, Ishikawa M, Hanaki N, Kashiwagi Y, Miki H, Miyake H, Tashiro S. Perioperative hemodynamic study of patients undergoing abdominal surgery using pulse dye densitometry. Hepato-Gastroenterology. 2006;53(72):874–8.

55. Yu M, Pei K, Moran S, Edwards KD, Domingo S, Steinemann S, Ghows M, Takiguchi S, Tan A, Lurie F, et al. A prospective randomized trial using blood volume analysis in addition to pulmonary artery catheter, compared with pulmonary artery catheter alone, to guide shock resuscitation in critically ill surgical patients. Shock. 2011;35(3):220–8.

56. de Castro MT, Sato AK, de Moura FS, de Camargo E, Silva OL, Santos TBR, Zhao Z, Moeller K, Amato MBP, Mueller JL, et al. A review of electrical impedance tomography in lung applications: theory and algorithms for absolute images. Annu Rev Control. 2019;48:442–71.

57. Martin GS, Moss M, Wheeler AP, Mealer M, Morris JA, Bernard GR. A randomized, controlled trial of furosemide with or without albumin in hypoproteinemic patients with acute lung injury. Crit Care Med. 2005;33(8):1681–7.

58. Cordemans C, de Iaet I, van Regenmortel N, Schoonheydt K, Dits H, Huber W, Malbrain ML. Fluid management in critically ill patients: the role of extravascualr lung water, abdominal hypertension, capillary leak and fluid balance. Ann Intensive Care. 2012;2(Suppl 1):S1.

59. Cordemans C, De Laet I, Van Regenmortel N, Schoonheydt K, Dits H, Martin G, Huber W, Malbrain ML. Aiming for a negative fluid balance in patients with acute lung injury and increased intra-abdominal pressure: a pilot study looking at the effects of PAL-treatment. Ann Intensive Care. 2012;2(Suppl 1):S15.

60. De Laet I, Deeren D, Schoonheydt K, Van Regenmortel N, Dits H, Malbrain M. Renal replacement therapy with net fluid removal lowers intra-abdominal pressure and volumetric indices in critically ill patients. Ann Intensive Care. 2012;2:S20.

Fluid Management in COVID-19

26

Manu L. N. G. Malbrain (iD), Serene Ho, Prashant Nasa,
and Adrian Wong

Contents

Introduction 530
What Do We Know? 530
What Guidelines Are Available? 531
  Surviving Sepsis Campaign 531
  World Health Organization 532
  UK Joint Anaesthetic and Intensive Care Guidelines 532
Guidance and Recommendations from the International Fluid Academy 533
  Assessment and Monitoring 533
  Resuscitation 534
  Maintenance Fluids 534
    Fluid Creep 535

M. L. N. G. Malbrain (✉)
First Department of Anaesthesiology and Intensive Therapy, Medical University of Lublin,
Lublin, Poland
e-mail: manu.malbrain@telenet.be

S. Ho
Cavendish Clinic, London, UK
e-mail: serene.ho@doctors.org.uk

P. Nasa
Critical Care Medicine, Prevention and Infection Control, NMC Specialty Hospital,
Dubai, United Arab Emirates
e-mail: dr.prashantnasa@hotmail.com

A. Wong
Intensive Care and Anaesthesia, King's College Hospital NHS Foundation Trust, London, UK
e-mail: adrian.wong@nhs.net

© The Author(s) 2024
M. L. N. G. Malbrain et al. (eds.), *Rational Use of Intravenous Fluids in Critically
Ill Patients*, https://doi.org/10.1007/978-3-031-42205-8_26

The Role of Ultrasound 535
Fluid Stewardship: Knowing What We Are Doing 536
Conclusion 538
References 540

IFA Commentary

The outbreak of COVID-19 has contributed to our comprehension of acute respiratory distress syndrome (ARDS). As the lung is the primary target organ of severe acute respiratory syndrome coronavirus 2 (SARS-CoV-2) invasion, there has been a discussion on the optimal respiratory support for such patients since the beginning of the pandemic. Additionally, COVID-19 patients frequently experience acute kidney injury, and adequate intravascular hydration is necessary for their initial care. Worse clinical outcomes have been associated with increased extravascular lung water (EVLW) in patients with ARDS. Fluid therapy is an important aspect of the management of critically ill patients with COVID-19. These patients often present with a range of clinical features that require careful assessment of their fluid status and electrolyte balance. The use of conservative or restrictive fluid management strategies has been reported in some studies, with the aim of avoiding fluid overload and associated complications, such as acute respiratory distress syndrome (ARDS) and multiple organ failure. On the other hand, liberal fluid management has also been reported to maintain organ perfusion and prevent organ failure in critically ill patients with COVID-19. The choice of fluid type is also an important consideration, with balanced crystalloid solutions such as lactated Ringer's or Plasma-Lyte A recommended over normal saline due to their lower chloride content and potential benefits for acid-base balance. In addition, the timing and amount of fluid therapy should be individualized based on the patient's hemodynamic status, fluid losses, and comorbidities, with frequent reassessment and adjustment as necessary. Close monitoring of fluid balance, electrolyte levels, and renal function is also important to prevent adverse events. Overall, the optimal fluid management strategy in critically ill patients with COVID-19 remains an area of active research, and a personalized approach is recommended based on the individual patient's clinical status and response to treatment. In patients with COVID-19, as with other critically ill patients in the ICU, it is recommended to practice fluid stewardship. The conventional approach for patients with ARDS is fluid de-escalation and restriction, and a cautious strategy for intravenous fluid should be employed by considering the 4Ds (drug, dosing, duration, and de-escalation). In some cases of fluid accumulation syndrome where spontaneous egress from the ebb to flow phase does not occur, de-resuscitation using pharmacological or mechanical methods might be considered.

Learning Objectives

Through this chapter, readers will learn about:

1. The available evidence on the impact of extravascular lung water and fluid balance on the outcomes of coronavirus disease (COVID-19) associated acute respiratory distress syndrome (ARDS).
2. The impact of fluid therapy on patient outcomes in critically ill patients with COVID-19.
3. The key principles and importance of fluid stewardship and judicious intravenous (IV) fluid administration in patients of COVID-19.
4. The potential benefits of critical care ultrasound in monitoring and guiding fluid therapy in COVID-19 patients and different ARDS phenotypes.
5. The use of dynamic parameters in assessing fluid responsiveness in COVID-19 patients.
6. The preferred types of fluids for resuscitation of COVID-19 patients.
7. The current guidelines and recommendations for fluid management in COVID-19 patients, and the limitations of the available evidence.
8. Need for future research on the impact of restrictive fluid strategy in the management of COVID-19 patients.

Case Vignette

A 42-year-old male was admitted to the hospital due to cough and shortness of breath. On room air, his peripheral oxygen saturation (SpO_2) was 78%, and an arterial blood gas test revealed severe hypoxemia (PaO_2/FiO_2 = 158). Oxygen was administered via a high-flow nasal cannula at 80% FiO_2 and 60 L/min flow. Lab results showed a positive SARS-CoV-2 PCR, procalcitonin level of 0.2 ng/mL, CRP level of 78 mg/L, and serum creatinine level of 134 µmol/L. The patient's respiratory distress worsened, necessitating invasive mechanical ventilation. After intubation, the patient's hemodynamic status deteriorated, with a mean arterial pressure of 56 mmHg, a heart rate of 121/min, and a lactate level of 3.1 mg/dL.

Questions

Q1. How will you manage the hemodynamic instability of this patient?
Q2. How will you manage intravenous fluid status for this patient post-resuscitation?

Introduction

The global COVID-19 pandemic has sharply focused the attention of the world on critical care as a specialty. At the moment, there are no proven treatments for COVID-19, although several trials and case series extolling the merits of various agents have been published. As always, good intensive care practice is founded on a strong understanding of physiology and doing the basics well.

While issues such as staffing, resources, and ventilation strategies are undoubtedly important when considering a holistic approach to treating COVID-19, fluid management remains a cornerstone of intensive care.

Unsurprisingly, given that it is a novel virus and illness course, published data and guidelines on how best to treat patients with COVID-19 are continually evolving. In this paper, we summarize what has been published on fluid strategies in COVID-19, guidelines available, and provide some reflections on personal practice. Importantly we ask colleagues to rally around this important issue and review their own practice with regards to fluid therapy.

However, a meticulous fluid assessment using volume status, intake and output, and laboratory investigations like serum electrolytes.

What Do We Know?

It is widely recognized that the administration of fluids, whether excessive or inadequate, can have a negative impact on patient outcomes [1]. Although COVID-19 is a new disease, the fundamental principles of fluid management in critical care serve as the basis for fluid therapy in COVID-19. Additionally, insights from colleagues who have treated COVID-19 patients further enhance and refine these principles. As a result, the objectives of resuscitation and management are continually evolving.

As an example, during the early stages of the COVID-19 pandemic, it was common advice to aim for a negative fluid balance. More recently, a higher-than-expected occurrence of acute kidney injury requiring renal replacement therapy has been observed, prompting calls for a more liberal fluid strategy.

The lungs are the primary organ of involvement in patients with COVID-19. Most patients with coronavirus disease 2019 (COVID-19) are haemodynamically stable on initial presentation and do not require resuscitation. However, some patients presenting to the emergency room are dehydrated, because of fever and decreased oral intake of food and fluids at home.

A particular challenge is the fact that patients are presenting at different stages of their illness. Those that are admitted to the hospital later in the illness may be hypovolaemic due to increased losses from fever and tachypnoea. While most cases primarily present with respiratory symptoms, gastrointestinal symptoms such as vomiting and diarrhoea are not uncommon. Hence, it is important to take a concise history (paying particular attention to symptom onset), clinically assess the patient, and individualize therapy. Additionally, SARS-CoV-2 infection can involve kidneys, with the estimated prevalence of acute kidney injury (AKI) varies widely from 1% to 46%. Around 1.5–9.0% of these patients may require renal replacement therapy, with a higher incidence seen in patients with severe disease [2, 3]. The mechanisms proposed for AKI in COVID-19 are multifactorial, like, thromboses, part of systemic inflammation, drug-induced nephrotoxicity, direct viral cyto-toxicity, and hypotension [3, 4]. Hence, initial fluid management in patients should assess signs of dehydration.

Extravascular lung water (EVLW) and pulmonary vascular permeability index (PVPI) are surrogates of lung injury in patients with acute respiratory distress syndrome (ARDS). The PiCCOVID study found a higher amount of EVLW and PVPI and less hemodynamic disturbances in patients with COVID-19-associated ARDS compared to non-COVID-19 ARDS with similar lung mechanics. This translates to greater hypoxemia and a more fre-quent requirement of prone positioning and ECMO [5].

An insight from the PRoVENT-COVID study showed a cumulative fluid balance was associated with a longer duration of mechanical ventilation in patients with COVID-19 ARDS [6]. In another retrospective study, every extra litre of IV fluid administered within the first 24 h is independently associated with the need for RRT [7].

A judicious fluid administration is thus advocated for the management of patients with COVID-19.

In general, a judicious fluid strategy whereby fluid is cautiously administered only after pre-load responsiveness has been assessed is preferable [8]. Given the incidence of myo-cardial dysfunction in a subset of patients [9], early use of vasopressors/inotropes along-side regular assessment via echocardiography would be prudent.

What Guidelines Are Available?

Numerous professional societies and organizations have released guidelines for the man-agement of COVID-19 patients. Regarding fluid therapy, the primary recommendations are derived from the original Surviving Sepsis Campaign guidelines and its COVID-19-specific revision [10]. However, there is currently a lack of direct evidence for patients with COVID-19 and shock, so the guidelines were formulated based on indirect evidence from critically ill patients with sepsis and ARDS. A selection of these guidelines with an emphasis on fluid management is summarized below.

Surviving Sepsis Campaign

The Surviving Sepsis Campaign group has suggested the following in their COVID-19-specific guidelines for acute resuscitation of adults with shock [10]:

- Use dynamic parameters to assess fluid responsiveness (weak recommendation; low quality of evidence (QE)),
- Using a conservative over liberal fluid administration strategy (weak recommendation; very low QE),
- Using crystalloids in preference to colloids (strong recommendation; moderate QE),
- Balanced crystalloids are preferred over unbalanced crystalloids (weak recommendation; moderate QE).

As shown, these recommendations are based on low-quality evidence.

World Health Organization

World Health Organization guidelines recommend that patients with COVID-19 respiratory failure should be treated cautiously with intravenous fluids, especially in settings with limited availability of mechanical ventilation [11].

- Use a conservative fluid management strategy for ARDS patients without tissue hypoperfusion.
- In resuscitation for septic shock in adults, give 250–500 mL crystalloid fluid as a rapid bolus in the first 15–30 min and reassess for signs of fluid overload after each bolus.
- If there is no response to fluid loading or if signs of volume overload appear, reduce, or discontinue fluid administration.
- Consider dynamic indices of volume responsiveness to guide volume administration beyond initial resuscitation based on local resources and experience. These indices include passive leg raises, fluid challenges with serial stroke volume measurements, or variations in systolic pressure, pulse pressure, inferior vena cava size, or stroke volume in response to changes in intrathoracic pressure during mechanical ventilation.
- Starches are associated with an increased risk of death and acute kidney injury compared to crystalloids. The effects of gelatins are less clear, but they are more expensive than crystalloids. Hypotonic (vs isotonic) solutions are less effective at increasing intravascular volume. Surviving Sepsis also suggests albumin for resuscitation when patients require substantial amounts of crystalloids; however, this conditional recommendation is based on low-quality evidence.

UK Joint Anaesthetic and Intensive Care Guidelines

The UK joint anaesthetic and intensive care guidelines advocate the following [12]:

- Conservative fluid management strategy in ARDS.
- In cases of significant hypotension or circulatory shock, standard circulatory assessment (fluid responsiveness, cardiac output assessment) and administration of an appropriate fluid and/or pressor (where appropriate) should occur.
- Balanced electrolyte solutions are preferred to 0.9% saline and colloids.

- While fluid overload should be avoided and more conservative administration may help improve respiratory function, this should be carefully balanced against the risk of inducing acute renal impairment.
- Care should be exercised in 'running patients too dry' in an effort to spare the lungs, as there are increased insensible fluid losses.

Guidance and Recommendations from the International Fluid Academy

The following are some suggestions and best practice recommendations taking into account those mentioned above [13].

Assessment and Monitoring

- The patient's fluid balance is assessed on admission in the hospital and on a daily basis with cumulative fluid balance calculated. Whenever available daily body weight is measured.
- Assessment of fluid as part of every clinical review using a combination of clinical judgement, vital signs, and chart records.
- Recent laboratory results with urea and electrolytes (at least once every 24 h of fluid prescription).
- The use of cardiac output monitors to assess fluid responsiveness, e.g. ultrasound (see below) and bioimpedance monitoring (Fig. 26.1).

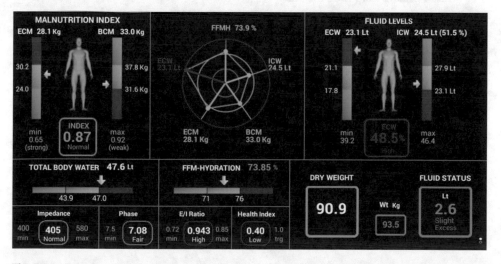

Fig. 26.1 Sample screenshot with results obtained via the full body, multifrequency bioelectrical impedance analysis (BIA) with touch i8 device (Maltron, UK) showing a volume excess of 2.6 L and an increased ECW: ICW ratio of 0.943 indicating capillary leak. The patient's fluid composition is monitored with BIA separating intra- and extracellular water and estimating the volume excess. (Adapted with permission from Myatchin et al. [14])

Resuscitation

- Use balanced crystalloids (e.g. Plasmalyte).
- Do not use starch solutions or gelatins.
- Do not use albumin in the early stages.
- For patients in need of fluid resuscitation:
  - Identify the cause of fluid deficit.
  - Assess for the presence of shock or hypoperfusion.
  - Assess fluid responsiveness (see further).
  - Give a bolus of 4 mL/kg of balanced crystalloids over 10–15 min.
- Fluid responsiveness is assessed before and after fluid administration with functional haemodynamics, e.g. pulse pressure variation (PPV) or other tests, e.g. passive leg raise test or end-expiratory occlusion test, or a combination.
- Mean arterial pressure and cardiac output are continuously monitored.
- Early initiation of vasopressors: noradrenaline at a low dose 0.05 µg/kg/min.
  - Consider the addition of vasopressin/argipressin when noradrenaline dose exceeds 0.5 µg/kg/min.
- Assess for the presence of fluid overload (i.e. 10% increase in body weight or volume excess from baseline).
  - Start de-resuscitation whenever possible.
  - Replace serum albumin to approximately 30 g/L with albumin 20%.
  - Use combination therapy of diuretics: loop + spironolactone + acetazolamide (when BE >5) + indapamide (in cases of hypernatraemia).
  - Consider ultrafiltration (even in the absence of acute kidney injury) when diuretics fail to achieve zero fluid balance.

Maintenance Fluids

- Do not administer maintenance fluids to patients who are eating and drinking sufficiently.
- Use hypotonic balanced solutions (e.g. Glucion 5% or Maintelyte).
- In patients requiring IV fluids for routine maintenance alone, the initial prescription should be restricted to:
  - 25–30 mL/kg/day (1 mL/kg/h) of water.
  - approximately 1 mmol/kg/day of potassium (K^+).
  - approximately 1–1.5 mmol/kg/day of sodium (Na^+).
  - approximately 1 mmol/kg/day of chloride (Cl^-).
  - approximately 50–100 g/day (1–1.5 g/kg/day) of glucose to limit starvation ketosis.

- The amount of fluid intake via other sources should be subtracted from the basic maintenance need of 1 mL/kg/h. e.g. nutrition and fluid creep (see below).

Fluid Creep

- All sources of fluids administered need to be detailed: crystalloids, colloids, blood products, enteral and parenteral nutritional products, intravenous medication, and oral intake (water, tea, soup, etc.)
- Precise data on the concentrated electrolytes added to these fluids or administered separately need to be documented.
- Fluid creep is defined as the sum of the volumes of these electrolytes, the small volumes to keep venous lines open (saline or glucose 5%), and the total volume used as a vehicle for medication.

The Role of Ultrasound

In critical care, there are many different tools available to clinicians for monitoring and diagnosing patients. However, among these tools, ultrasound stands out as one of the most versatile and valuable devices, especially in the context of fluid therapy. Unlike many other monitoring devices, ultrasound is highly portable, which allows clinicians to easily use it at the patient's bedside, even in situations with strict infection control measures in place.

What makes ultrasound particularly valuable for fluid therapy is its ability to non-invasively evaluate and assess the response to therapy for multiple physiological systems, including the cardiovascular, respiratory, and renal systems. No other singular device is able to provide such a comprehensive and integrated approach to patient care.

While critical care ultrasound has always been an important tool for clinicians, the COVID-19 pandemic has made it even more essential. The pandemic has placed tremendous pressure on healthcare systems, making it more important than ever to have access to tools that can provide timely and accurate diagnostic information. Ultrasound's versatility and portability make it an ideal device for use in critical care settings, particularly in the context of fluid therapy. By using ultrasound to guide fluid therapy, clinicians can ensure that their patients are receiving the appropriate treatment to optimize their outcomes.

A non-exhaustive summary of the potential ultrasonographic assessments that can be performed is listed below (Table 26.1).

Table 26.1 Potential ultrasonographic assessments that can be performed are listed below

System	Identifiable structures	Measurable parameters	Potential indication of COVID-19
Airway	Tracheal rings Cricothyroid membrane Thyroid cartilage Hyoid bone	Distance to structures Diameter of trachea Presence of oedema or external compression	Plan for difficult intubation and extubation
Thoracic	A-lines B-lines Consolidation Collapse Effusion Diaphragm	Number of B-lines Volume of effusion, depth to effusion Extent of pneumothorax (lung sliding, lung-point) Diaphragmatic function	Assess the degree of lung involvement Diagnose any concurrent conditions
Cardiac	Right atrium and ventricle Left atrium and ventricle AV valves Pulmonary valves Aortic valves Inferior vena cava	Size and dimension Valvular pathologies Systolic and diastolic dysfunction Presence of mass/vegetation Regional wall motion abnormalities	Assess cardiovascular function Assess response to therapy, e.g. fluid bolus
Abdominal	Free fluid, e.g. ascites, blood Aorta Inferior vena cava Gastric content	Size of organs Size of vascular structures Doppler analysis of vascular flow to organs Volume of free fluid, depth to free fluid Calculation of gastric residual volume (GRV) Inferior vena cava collapsibility index (IVVCI)	Assess the cause of liver dysfunction Part of haemodynamic assessment
Renal	Kidneys Ureter Bladder	Size of kidneys Doppler analysis of vascular flow to kidneys (renal resistive index) volume of bladder	Assess the cause of renal dysfunction
Vascular	Thrombosis (clot visualization) Dissection	Doppler analysis of vasculature compression of veins	Aid vascular catheter placement Diagnose venous thrombosis

Adapted from Malbrain et al. with permission [13]

Fluid Stewardship: Knowing What We Are Doing

As with antibiotic stewardship, fluid stewardship can improve the quality of clinical care. Typically, this would involve a stepwise approach in assessing current practice and outcomes—a clear view of current practice will highlight the areas where we are performing well, and those that are lacking, so as to provide a basis for meaningful change [15].

Table 26.2 Fluid stewardship and the rules of four in practice: the four questions, indications, Ds, stages, and hits

4 Questions	4 Indications	4 Ds	4 Stages	4 Hits
When to start IV fluids	Resuscitation	Drug	Resuscitation	First HIT: Initial insult (e.g. COVID-19 with sepsis)
When to stop IV fluids	Maintenance	Dose	Optimization	Second HIT: Ischemia and reperfusion
When to start removing fluids	Replacement	Duration	Stabilization	Third HIT: Fluid accumulation and GIPS (global increased permeability syndrome)
When to stop removing fluids	Nutrition	De-escalation	Evacuation (de-escalation)	Fourth HIT: Hypoperfusion during de-resuscitation

Adapted from Malbrain et al. with permission [13]

Patients should have an IV fluid management plan, including a fluid and electrolyte prescription over the next 24 h agreed by the intensive care team, taking into account clinical and laboratory findings, supplemented by the appropriate imaging, e.g. ultrasound. These can be summarized by the 'Rules of Fours' in Table 26.2.

It is possible that some colleagues may argue that attempting to collect data on fluid prescriptions during a global pandemic is meaningless or inconvenient. However, we disagree and offer several reasons in support of our stance [16–19].

Firstly, it is undeniable that our clinical practice has undergone significant changes due to modifications in the logistics of critical care delivery. New clinical areas have been established or converted to provide care for critically ill patients, requiring healthcare professionals from non-critical care backgrounds to be redeployed and receive training and education. While collecting data requires time and effort, this time of upheaval underscores the importance of accurate documentation and data analysis to ensure that various aspects of patient care can be evaluated on a larger scale.

In addition, the current situation has made us more aware than ever of the limitations of medical resources, including healthcare professionals, personal protective equipment, machines for mechanical ventilation and haemofiltration, and essential drugs for critical care. Understanding the processes of illness and patient outcomes, as well as how our interventions affect them, will enable us to optimize the use of scarce resources for the benefit of our patients and prevent unnecessary harm.

Moreover, as COVID-19 has spread extensively, many hospitals have seen a predominance of cases. This presents an opportunity to learn valuable lessons quickly about the management of these patients, which can inform treatment plans for future waves of infection and even other epidemics.

Ultimately, when the pandemic subsides, analysing such data would allow us to reflect, review, and improve clinical practice.

Case Vignette

Questions and Answers

Q1. How will you manage the hemodynamic instability of this patient?

A1. This patient needs resuscitation. Balanced crystalloids like Plasmalyte or Ringer's Lactate at 4 mL/kg fluid bolus should be given and followed by need of reassessment for other IV fluid. Dynamic resuscitation measures like SVV/PPV, IVC collapsibility, PLR can be used to assess fluid responsiveness. The goals of resuscitation are to improve tissue perfusion. Resuscitation can target Serum lactates.

Q2. How will you manage intravenous fluid status for this patient post-resuscitation?

A2. The fluid status of this management should be similar to the patients with ARDS. Fluid restriction (target of net negative fluid balance) with close monitoring of organ perfusion Use balanced IV fluids like Glucion 5% for maintenance. Early enteral nutrition after initial resuscitation and haemodynamic stability. Calculation of maintenance IV fluids must consider feeding and fluid creep.

Conclusion

Fluid administration and management represent fundamental practices in intensive care, and their principles are grounded in a thorough comprehension of the underlying pathophysiological processes. However, COVID-19 is a novel illness that presents unique challenges to both clinical practice and the healthcare system as a whole.

In this context, we contend that the principles of fluid stewardship have never been more critical in clinical practice than they are now. The unique challenges presented by this pandemic offer an opportunity to improve the quality of care delivered, not just for the current outbreak, but for future ones as well.

Despite the difficulties inherent in such an undertaking, it is crucial to recognize that this is an unprecedented healthcare event in modern times, with mind-boggling technology and the ability to disseminate information quickly at our disposal. Whether we opt to manage it 'the old way' or embrace all the tools and collaborative opportunities available to us may well determine how this pandemic is remembered in history. We firmly believe in the latter approach, which entails leveraging all available resources and working together to deliver the best possible care to our patients.

Take Home Messages

Fluid administration and management represent critical aspects of care for critically ill COVID-19 patients, particularly those with ARDS. Several key take-home messages can guide optimal fluid therapy and stewardship in these patients, including:

- Increased extravascular lung water and cumulative fluid balance are associated with worse clinical outcomes in COVID-19 patients with ARDS.
- Dynamic parameters should be used over static parameters to assess fluid responsiveness in COVID-19 patients.
- Conservative/restrictive fluid strategies should be used in COVID-19 patients with ARDS.
- Crystalloids are preferred over colloids for resuscitation of COVID-19 patients.
- Balanced/buffered crystalloids are preferred over unbalanced crystalloids for resuscitation of COVID-19 patients.
- When calculating maintenance fluids, consider fluid creep and feeding.

Overall, the general principles of fluid stewardship are critical to improve outcomes and optimize the use of resources in critically ill COVID-19 patients.

About the IFA

The *International Fluid Academy* was founded in 2011 with the goals of foster education and promote research on fluid management and monitoring in critically ill patients, thereby improving the survival of critically ill patients by bringing together physicians, nurses, and others from a variety of clinical disciplines. It aimed to improve and standardize care and outcome of critically ill patients with an emphasis on fluids, fluid management, monitoring, and organ support by collaborative research projects, surveys, guideline development, joint data registration, and international exchange of health care workers and researchers. We invite the reader to follow @ Fluid_Academy and to check this website (www.fluidacademy.org and https://fluid-academy.mn.co) for more information on fluid management and haemodynamic monitoring (under FOAM resources).

Acknowledgements Parts of this chapter were published previously as open access under the creative commons Attribution 4.0 International Licence (CC BY 4.0) [1]. The European Commission announced it has adopted CC BY 4.0 and CC0 to share published documents, including photos, videos, reports, peer-reviewed studies, and data. The Commission joins other public institutions around the world that use standard, legally interoperable tools like Creative Commons licenses and public domain tools to share a wide range of content they produce. The decision to use CC aims to increase the legal interoperability and ease of reuse of author's own materials.

References

1. Malbrain MLNG, Van Regenmortel N, Saugel B, et al. Principles of fluid management and stewardship in septic shock: it is time to consider the four D's and the four phases of fluid therapy. Ann Intensive Care. 2018;8(1):66. https://doi.org/10.1186/s13613-018-0402-x.
2. Farouk SS, Fiaccadori E, Cravedi P, Campbell KN. COVID-19 and the kidney: what we think we know so far and what we don't. J Nephrol. 2020;33(6):1213–8. https://doi.org/10.1007/s40620-020-00789-y.
3. Ostermann M, Lumlertgul N, Forni LG, Hoste E. What every Intensivist should know about COVID-19 associated acute kidney injury. J Crit Care. 2020;60:91–5. https://doi.org/10.1016/j.jcrc.2020.07.023.
4. Nasa P, Shrivastava PK, Kulkarni A, et al. Favipiravir induced nephrotoxicity in two patients of COVID-19. J Assoc Physicians India. 2021;69(6):11–2.
5. Shi R, Lai C, Teboul JL, et al. COVID-19 ARDS is characterized by higher extravascular lung water than non-COVID-19 ARDS: the PiCCOVID study. Crit Care. 2021;25(1):186. https://doi.org/10.1186/s13054-021-03594-6.
6. Ahuja S, de Grooth HJ, Paulus F, et al. Association between early cumulative fluid balance and successful liberation from invasive ventilation in COVID-19 ARDS patients—insights from the PRoVENT-COVID study: a national, multicenter, observational cohort analysis. Crit Care. 2022;26(1):157. https://doi.org/10.1186/s13054-022-04023-y.
7. Holt DB, Lardaro T, Wang AZ, et al. Fluid resuscitation and progression to renal replacement therapy in patients with COVID-19. J Emerg Med. 2022;62(2):145–53. https://doi.org/10.1016/j.jemermed.2021.10.026.
8. Silversides JA, Perner A, Malbrain MLNG. Liberal versus restrictive fluid therapy in critically ill patients. Intensive Care Med. 2019;45:1440–9.
9. Zheng Y, Ma Y, Zhang J, et al. COVID-19 and the cardiovascular system. Nat Rev Cardiol. 2020;17:259–60. https://doi.org/10.1038/s41569-020-0360-5.
10. Alhazzani W, Evans L, Alshamsi F, et al. Surviving sepsis campaign guidelines on the management of adults with coronavirus disease 2019 (COVID-19) in the ICU: first update. Crit Care Med. 2021;49(3):e219–34. https://doi.org/10.1097/CCM.0000000000004899.
11. World Health Organisation Clinical management of severe acute respiratory infection (SARI) when COVID-19 disease is suspected. https://www.who.int/emergencies/diseases/novel-coronavirus-2019/events-as-they-happen.
12. Clinical guide for the management of critical care for adults with COVID-19 during the coronavirus pandemic—AAGBI, RCOA, FICM, ICS. https://www.england.nhs.uk/coronavirus/wp-content/uploads/sites/52/2020/03/C0216_Specialty-guide_AdultCritiCare-and-coronavirus_V2.pdf.
13. Malbrain MLNG, Ho S, Wong A. Thoughts on COVID-19 from the International Fluid Academy. ICU Manag Pract. 2020;20(1):80–5.
14. Myatchin I, Abraham P, Malbrain MLNG. Bio-electrical impedance analysis in critically ill patients: are we ready for prime time? J Clin Monit Comput. 2020;34(3):401–10. https://doi.org/10.1007/s10877-019-00439-0. Epub 2019 Dec 5. PMID: 31808061; PMCID: PMC7223384.
15. Malbrain MLNG, Rice TW, Mythen M, Wuyts S. It is time for improved fluid stewardship. ICU Manag Pract. 2018;18(3):158–62. https://healthmanagement.org/c/icu/issuearticle/it-is-time-for-improved-fluid-stewardship.
16. Poston JT, Patel BK, Davis AM. Management of critically ill adults with COVID-19. JAMA. 2020;323(18):1839–41. https://doi.org/10.1001/jama.2020.4914.
17. Wang D, Hu B, Hu C, et al. Clinical characteristics of 138 hospitalized patients with 2019 novel coronavirus–infected pneumonia in Wuhan, China. JAMA. 2020;323(11):1061–9. https://doi.org/10.1001/jama.2020.1585.

18. Silversides JA, Major E, Ferguson AJ, et al. Conservative fluid management or deresuscitation for patients with sepsis or acute respiratory distress syndrome following the resuscitation phase of critical illness: a systematic review and meta-analysis. Intensive Care Med. 2017;43:155–70. https://doi.org/10.1007/s00134-016-4573-3.

19. Phua J, Weng L, Ling L, et al. Intensive care management of coronavirus disease 2019 (COVID-19): challenges and recommendations. Lancet Resp Med. 2020;8(5):506–17. https://doi.org/10.1016/S2213-2600(20)30161-2.

Part IV

Concepts of Fluid Stewardship and Appropriate Fluid Prescription

Introduction to Fluid Stewardship

27

Adrian Wong, Jonny Wilkinson, Prashant Nasa, Luca Malbrain, and Manu L. N. G. Malbrain ⓘ

Contents

Introduction 547
Definitions 548
  Appropriate Fluid Prescription 548
  The 5 P's of Fluid Prescription 548
Fluid Management in the ICU as a Quality Improvement Project 548
Quality Improvement in Healthcare 549
Stewardship (or Champions in Healthcare) 551
  How to Mandate Change? 551
  Strategy and Policy Development 551
  Designing Overarching Systems 551
  Encouraging Collaboration 552
  Ensuring Robust Governance and Accountability Process 552

A. Wong (✉)
Intensive Care and Anaesthesia, King's College Hospital NHS Foundation Trust, London, UK
e-mail: adrian.wong@nhs.net

J. Wilkinson
Department of Intensive Care and Anaesthesia, Critical Care Northampton, Northampton, UK

P. Nasa
Critical Care Medicine, NMC Specialty Hospital, Dubai, Dubai, UAE
e-mail: dr.prashantnasa@hotmail.com

L. Malbrain
University School of Medicine, Katholieke Universiteit Leuven (KUL), Leuven, Belgium

M. L. N. G. Malbrain
First Department of Anaesthesiology and Intensive Therapy, Medical University of Lublin, Lublin, Poland
e-mail: manu.malbrain@uzbrussel.be

© The Author(s) 2024
M. L. N. G. Malbrain et al. (eds.), *Rational Use of Intravenous Fluids in Critically Ill Patients*, https://doi.org/10.1007/978-3-031-42205-8_27

Fluid Stewardship 553
  Goals 553
  The 4 Questions of Fluid Therapy 554
  The 7 D's of Fluid Therapy 556
Different Phases During Implementation of Fluid Stewardship 558
  Start-up Phase 558
  Knowledge Phase 560
  Strategy Phase 560
  Preparation Phase 561
  Education Phase 561
  Implementation Phase 562
  Post-Implementation Phase 562
Conclusion 563
References 564

IFA Commentary

Intravenous (IV) fluid are the most commonly prescribed drugs in healthcare and needs stewardship. Fluid stewardship is an appropriate use of IV fluids, optimizing clinical outcomes. It requires an in-depth understanding of pharmacokinetics and pharmacodynamics, indications and contraindications (4 D's—drug, dosing, duration and de-escalation), and adverse effects of various IV fluids. It also requires a review of the IV fluid prescription for appropriateness using the 5 P's (prescriber, prescription, pharmacy, preparation and patient). Fluid stewardship should be part of healthcare quality and needs overhauling in the systems to ensure efficiency and effectiveness. To produce a change in the system (implementation of fluid stewardship), one needs to collaborate and engage stakeholders, formulate a plan and policy collectively, training, leadership alignment and robust governance with accountability.

Learning Objectives

After reading this chapter, you will:

1. Learn the processes of stewardship in healthcare under a quality improvement framework.
2. What is fluid stewardship? How can we implement fluid stewardship in the hospital or intensive care unit?
3. The principles (the 5P's) of fluid prescription,
4. The 7 D's (definitions, diagnosis, drug, dose, duration, de-escalation and documentation at discharge) of fluid therapy.
5. How to audit the fluid prescription using hospital- or ICU-based fluid guidelines?

Case Vignette

42-year male with hypertension has undergone emergency laparotomy for perforation peritonitis. The patient was kept nil-per-oral status and prescribed intravenous (IV) 5% dextrose 0.9% normal saline (5% DNS) at 150 ml/h by the surgery trainee. On day 4, the patient's serum sodium was 153 mmol/L, potassium 3.1 mmol/L and chloride 123 mmol/L, serum creatinine 142 μmol/L. His arterial blood gas showed metabolic acidosis with an anion gap of 9. He developed anasarca and acute kidney injury.

Questions

Q1. Was the prescription for IV fluid, correct? Why did the patient develop non-anion gap acidosis or hyperchloremic acidosis?

Q2. How to initiate fluid stewardship in my hospital/ICU?

Introduction

The **primary goal** of fluid stewardship is to optimize clinical outcomes, while minimizing unintended consequences of intravenous fluid (IV) administration. This requires an in-depth understanding of the indications, contra-indications, toxicity, adverse events, fluid dynamics, and kinetics of IV fluids. Put simply, the physician needs to understand fluid physiology (see Chaps 2 and 3). The appropriate use of IV fluids is essential to patient safety and deserves careful oversight and guidance. Given the association between fluid (mis)use and the deleterious effects on patients' morbidity and mortality, the frequency of inappropriate fluid prescription could play a role as a surrogate marker for the avoidable impact on iatrogenic fluid overload, and the subsequent end-organ dysfunction and failure [1].

A **secondary goal** of fluid stewardship is to reduce healthcare costs, without adversely impacting the quality of care. In patients with septic shock, the administration of fluids for resuscitation during initial hemodynamic stabilization remains a major therapeutic challenge, because we are faced with many open questions regarding the type, dose, rate, and timing of fluid administration. In addition, fluids are used for maintenance of intravascular volume, replacement of losses and to cover any unmet daily caloric needs. In this document, we provide definitions of different terms pertaining to fluid therapy in hospitalized patients, the sickest of whom are those with septic shock. We discuss different fluid management strategies, including early adequate goal-directed fluid management, late conservative fluid management, and late goal-directed fluid removal. In addition, we expand on the concept of the "four D's" of fluid therapy (namely drug, dosing, duration and de-escalation) into the 7 D's adding "definitions", "diagnosis" up front and "documentation at discharge" at the very end [2]. In treating patients with shock (of any kind), one should consider the phases of fluid therapy—resuscitation, optimization, stabilization and evacuation. Chap. 28 will discuss A Logical Prescription of Intravenous Fluids

Definitions

Appropriate Fluid Prescription

The process of IV fluid therapy is divided into several stages, based on an audit framework developed by NICE.

1. The physician must assess the patient's IV fluid needs and decide on the right treatment (indication). Only the three major indications need to be examined thoroughly for the purpose of a clinical audit: resuscitation, maintenance and replacement or redistribution.
2. Every IV fluid prescription has to be detailed in order to ensure safe administration, with a fluid management plan to aid continuity of care.
3. The information in the hospital's fluid guidelines should be focussed upon to develop quality standards.
4. These standards represent the necessary elements for a complete and qualitative check of appropriateness.

If all standards are met, the IV fluid therapy will be deemed as appropriate for that patient. A key factor in appropriate empiric fluid therapy, is the consideration of patient risk factors (fluid balance, fluid overload, capillary leak, source control, acid-base status, comorbidity, electrolyte status, kidney function and organ function).

The 5 P's of Fluid Prescription

- **Prescriber:** makes a clinical decision regarding fluid management
- **Prescription:** is written, accounting for drug, dose and duration
- **Pharmacist:** checks the prescription for inconsistencies
- **Preparation:** prescribed fluid is prepared with any necessary additions (e.g. electrolytes)
- **Patient:** fluid is administered to the patient; the process, response and follow-up management are handled by fluid stewards

Fluid Management in the ICU as a Quality Improvement Project

IV fluids are some of the most commonly prescribed day-to-day therapies in modern healthcare. Like any drug, they have their indications, contra-indications, benefits, risks, toxicity, adverse side effects and complications. Often, the task of fluid prescribing is delegated to the most junior members of the healthcare team. Evidence suggests that even when clear guidelines are available, fluid prescriptions can be inappropriate or incorrect [3–5].

Given the association between fluid (mis)use with patient morbidity and mortality, the frequency of inappropriate fluid prescription could be used as a surrogate marker for the quality of care delivered.

The combination of effective fluid management (led with multi-disciplinary involvement), comprehensive fluid guidelines, continuous staff education and an allied quality improvement programme, may limit the deleterious effects of inappropriate fluid prescription and fluid overload [6, 7].

Quality Improvement in Healthcare

In healthcare systems worldwide, patients are exposed to risks of avoidable harm and unwarranted variations in practice and hence outcomes.

In 1999, the Institute of Medicine (IOM) in Washington, DC, USA, released To Err Is Human: Building a Safer Health System [8], a report that brought much public attention to the crisis of patient safety in the United States. In 2001, the IOM issued a second report, Crossing the Quality Chasm: A New Health System for the twenty-first century [9], introducing the **STEEEP** acronym, which outlines six overarching "Aims for Improvement" for healthcare:

- **Safe**: Avoid injuries to patients from the care that is intended to help them.
- **Timely**: Reduce waiting for both patients and carers
- **Effective**: Match care to science; avoid overuse of ineffective care and underuse of effective care
- **Efficient**: Reduce waste
- **Equitable**: Close racial and ethnic gaps in health status
- **Patient-Centred**: Prioritize the individual and respect choice

Quality improvement (QI) is a systematic, formal approach, to analyzing practice, performance and efforts to improve performance, beginning with a clear and agreed aim [10]. Many organizations use the six IOM aims above to help them develop their individualized aims. These should be time-specific and measurable; the specific population of patients that will be affected should also be defined.

There are several existing QI models which include:

- Model for Improvement (Plan-Do-Study-Act [PDSA] cycles (www.ihi.org) (Fig. 27.1): The Institute for Healthcare Improvement's Model for Improvement combines two popular QI models: Total Quality Management (TQM) and Rapid-Cycle Improvement (RCI).
- Six Sigma (asq.org): Six Sigma is a method of improvement that strives to decrease variation and defects in practice.
- Lean (www.ihi.org) is an approach that drives out waste and improves efficiency in work processes so that all work adds value.

Fig. 27.1 Model for qualitty improvement using Plan-Do-Study-Act (PDSA) cycle (adapted from [8])

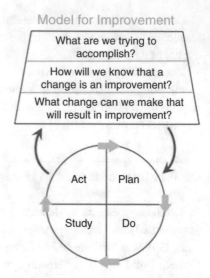

QI can also involve specific interventions intended to improve processes and systems, ranging from checklists and "care bundles" of interventions (a set of evidence-based practices applied consistently) to invasive procedures and clinical care pathways.

Regardless of the specifics, all QI models share common values and themes [11]:

- **Establish** a culture of quality in the team that is aligned with the organization's values, processes and procedures.
- **Determine** and prioritize potential areas for improvement, including identification of the potential barriers to change.
- **Collect** and analyze data. Data collection and analysis lie at the heart of quality improvement. Improvements can only be made if the current situation is known and understood.
- **Communicate** results. QI efforts require the involvement and support of the entire team. Transparent and regular lines of communication should be encouraged. The team's efforts and hard work should be acknowledged.
- **Commit** to ongoing evaluation. Quality improvement is an ongoing process. A high-functioning practice will continually strive to improve performance, revisit the effectiveness of interventions, and regularly seek feedback from patients and staff.
- **Share** and celebrate successes. Share lessons learned with others to support wide-scale, rapid improvement, that benefits all patients and healthcare.

Despite the theoretical benefits provided by the various QI models, there are no randomized controlled trials demonstrating the value of QI processes in improving outcomes [12]; equally, no single QI model has been demonstrated to be superior to others [13]. Hence an in-depth understanding and proper implementation of the chosen technique, as well as a commitment to the cause, is probably more important than a specific QI model.

Stewardship (or Champions in Healthcare)

How to Mandate Change?

Change in healthcare is a time- and resource-consuming process. Stewards (or champions), in healthcare systems, can increase the likelihood of success through:

- Strategy and policy development
- Designing overarching systems
- Encouraging collaboration
- Ensuring robust governance and accountability processes

Strategy and Policy Development

Strategy formulation means setting a clear vision for quality, specifying activities that would lead to achieving that goal, and assigning responsibilities to execute those activities. It provides an overarching framework for other roles. The goal should be 'SMART'—specific, measurable, achievable, relevant and timely. Specific and clearly defined goals are more likely to be achieved.

Once the goals have been determined, the various workstreams required to support the goal can be identified, and a strategy developed. Formal designation and implementation of policies to tackle the various pathways are important. These provide a clear, transparent, robust framework for operational issues and outline the necessary monitoring and governance requirements.

Such policies may require the development of tools such as checklists and protocols to support colleagues in day-to-day tasks. Recommendations in clinical practice guidelines are often lengthy, complex, and easy to forget. Tools such as checklists, flowsheets, protocols and reminders simplify the adoption of guidelines into a step-by-step approach. For example, a well-designed prescription chart with cognitive aids, can promote adherence to prescribing guidelines.

Designing Overarching Systems

A high-quality health system depends on the availability of staff, equipment, infrastructure and supplies in the right location. Also, smooth coordination of care as the patient moves through different stages of illness and encounters different parts of the health system is paramount. A system to ensure best practices are applied consistently and organizational cultures prioritizing quality of care, including patient safety and patient experience, are also essential.

With such a complex set of requirements, it is necessary to view each project across all of the teams and processes involved. Mapping out the various pathways can be helpful, as they may not be apparent initially. For example, in changing a policy of drug administration, the clinician and nursing teams are not the only parties involved—pharmacists, the procurement department and even the personnel responsible for restocking the drugs also need to be considered.

Encouraging Collaboration

Engagement with the relevant stakeholders is crucial; failure to engage and communicate the vision effectively leads to a lack of buy-in and hence resistance/indifference to the project. A project is more likely to succeed if the team shares a **common vision** and a sense of purpose. This way, attrition can be minimized.

As with most QI projects in the healthcare system, a **collaboration** between teams is vital. Collaboration relies on formal mechanisms to bring stakeholders together, with mutually agreed objectives, clear roles and responsibilities. Poorly defined individual and team responsibilities result in misunderstandings about the assigned tasks, redundant efforts and gaps in the work done. Clear agreements between the steward and the collaborating organizations can minimize these risks.

The individual (and skill-set) should be matched to the role and task requirements. It is naïve to think that any individual can simply slot into a role without considering their strengths and weaknesses. Effective **leadership** will maximize the potential of the individuals and foster seamless working of the entire team. Part of achieving and maintaining this goal is to ensure adequate and continuous training is available for individuals and the team.

Building the team requires careful consideration. The **team composition** will vary according to the task, but team members must be familiar with all aspects of the project. An effective team usually consists of team members representing the three different tiers of expertise within the organization: system leadership, technical expertise and day-to-day leadership. This can take the form of individuals each possessing expertise in one area or perhaps individuals skilled in overlapping areas of expertise.

Ensuring Robust Governance and Accountability Process

Measurement is critical to testing and implementing changes; such indicators or outcomes inform a team if the changes are actually bringing any improvement. Regular indicators to monitor implementation, processes and outcomes, ensure that all steps are measured and addressed. It is important that attention is not fixated upon final outcomes alone—it is crucial that all steps in the process are measured, with analysis and learning from any detected inefficiencies. Where more complex systems are in operation, new ways of providing constructive oversight, guidance and monitoring must be developed. Robust accountability processes are crucial tools for the standardization of governance tasks—especially true for ensuring patient safety.

The setting of the project's vision should be followed by the designation of outcome measures. Ideally, stewards should measure quality across multiple dimensions (safety, effectiveness, patient experience, efficiency, equity, and timeliness), using a mix of structure, process, and outcome variables. Measurement activities should include monitoring changes over time, drawing comparisons between institutions, regions, and countries and setting benchmarks or targets for performance.

Activities to map, measure and improve processes, overcome resistance to change, and build strong organizational cultures require strong leadership and technical skills. Failure to invest in the development of these skills may lead to the failed implementation of any of the ideas above.

Fluid Stewardship

Goals

As stated previously, fluid stewardship can be defined as a series of coordinated interventions. These are introduced to select the optimal type of fluid, as well as the dose and duration of therapy, that will result in the best clinical outcome, prevent adverse events, and reduce costs.

The primary goal of fluid stewardship is to optimize clinical outcomes while minimizing unintended consequences of intravenous fluid administration. Ensuring the appropriate use of IV fluids is complex. It requires good theoretical and practical knowledge on the part of the prescriber, alongside clear operating procedures and oversight to ensure that various outcomes are measured, with recognition and learning from any adverse events.

A secondary goal of fluid stewardship is to reduce healthcare spending, without adversely impacting on the quality of care.

These goals can be broken down into several overlapping workstreams:

- Improvement of fluid prescribing practice
- Development of robust guidelines on fluid prescription and management, with regular updates when new scientific knowledge becomes available
- Rolling programme of education across the multidisciplinary team
- Regular quality assurance exercises—defining the key performance index (KPI) or outcomes measured

Like other healthcare QI projects, fluid stewardship is a team effort. Examples of the composition of a fluid stewardship team are shown in Table 27.1.

The roles and desired qualities of stewards can be summarized in Table 27.2.

Table 27.1 Roles and responsibilities of a fluid team

Role	Responsibility
IV fluid steward (champion)	• Oversee prescription safety • Audit practice • Ensure adherence to national/International guidelines on IV fluid safety • Liaise with IV fluid teams • Maintain and deliver an education program on IV fluid safety • Overall responsibility for coordination of care. Liaison with the patient's primary team. Understand the underlying diseases, comorbidities and prognosis amongst patients receiving IV fluids. Suggestion and follow-up of IV fluid prescriptions. Provision of feedback on practice; both poor and good. Provides annual summary report on KPI's
IV fluid lead nurse	• Maintain and assess ward-based practice • Deliver point-of-care education sessions • Teach and supervise appropriateness of fluid prescription • Recognize and manage complications • Train and teache other HCPs regarding calculation of fluid balance, etc.
Prescribers	• Assess patient's fluid requirements • Prescribe safely • Re-assess appropriately • Regularly take and review blood samples
Nurse	• Administer fluids as prescribed • Update fluid balance charts • Weigh patients as per the hospital policy (Should be weekly)
Dietician	• Parenteral nutrition is also fluid • Perform nutritional assessment, calculate daily requirements, design feeding regimens, monitor nutritional and fluid status
Clinical pharmacist	• Responsible for follow-up of prescriptions, delivery and analysis of fluid usage. Optimization of composition and advice on compatibility/stability of IV fluids
IT specialist	• Responsible for data collection and calculation of KPI's

Previous chapters have already discussed the 4 Questions and the 7Ds of Fluid Therapy. Taking each in terms, aims and hence KPIs can be defined as follows.

The 4 Questions of Fluid Therapy

When to start IV fluids (pertaining to the benefits of fluid administration)

- Aim: To guide fluid resuscitation based on macro-hemodynamics e.g. thorough history and examination to determine the volaemic status of the patient. Additional use of dynamic measures to assess volume tolerance–e.g. passive leg raises, POCUS.
- KPI: Understanding clinical signs and symptoms of true hypovolemia and the function/utility of different monitoring tools

Table 27.2 Role and qualities of a fluid steward

Role of stewards/champions
• Understand, demonstrate and promote the values and behaviors expected of all employees, to improve the quality of patient care and the patient and staff experience throughout the organization
• Understand and promote awareness of the organization's quality goals and how they apply to different areas of work
• Work within the multi-disciplinary team to embed a 'culture of quality' across the organization
• Ensure that communication from management, to the workforce, is appropriate and effective and that messages are being delivered to all staff in a timely and consistent manner
• To liaise with other stewards for purposes of promoting the quality agenda in a consistent and coordinated manner
• To escalate concerns through appropriate routes, in relation to activities having an impact on the delivery of quality services, and to signpost colleagues to appropriate escalation processes
Desired qualities of a Stewards
• Stewards should be able to demonstrate passion and commitment to improving quality of patient care in their own role
• Possession of excellent communication skills
• Enthusiasm, with the ability to motivate and inspire others through a positive approach to providing high-quality services.
• A 'can do' attitude
• Ability to offer solutions to identified problems
• Confidence to challenge practice which does not appear to contribute to the organization's quality goals

When to stop IV Fluids (pertaining to the potential risks of ongoing fluid administration)

- Aim: Guidance based on the absence of volume tolerance.
- KPI: Understanding the signs of absence of volume tolerance and resolution of shock

When to start Fluid removal (pertaining to the benefits of active fluid removal, using diuretics or renal replacement therapy with net ultrafiltration)

- Aim: Monitoring hypervolemia based on impact of fluid overload on organ function
- KPI: Understanding the deleterious effects of GIPS and consequences of fluid overload on organ function

When to stop fluid removal (pertaining to the risks of removing excessive volumes of fluid)

- Aim: Avoiding hypoperfusion
- KPI: Understanding different techniques for mobilizing and evacuating fluid and signs of hypoperfusion

The 7 D's of Fluid Therapy

Definitions Comparison of fluid prescription habits and practices is only possible when universal definitions are applied regarding maintenance, replacement or resuscitataion fluids, hypovolemia or hypervolemia etc.

Diagnosis Correct fluid therapy starts with an adequate assessment of the patient's fluid or volume status.

- Aim: Standardizing and driving adoption of hypovolemia screening and assessment tools, including hemodynamic monitoring
- KPI: Systematic process in place for evaluating volume status in 100% of applicable patients

Drug Inappropriate fluid therapy should be avoided. Clear and careful documentation of the choice, dose and duration of fluid therapy are expected, ideally including the indication for fluid therapy.

- Key considerations:
  - Approach an IV fluid the same way as any other drug
  - Select the type of IV fluid with the most suitable composition for the patient
  - Think about the indication of why you are using the fluid
  - Consider contraindications, comorbidities and side effects
- Aim: Appropriate indication, choice and route of fluid administration
- KPI: Correct fluid administered, on time, to the correct patient according to institutional guidelines

Dose As Paracelsus nicely stated: "All things are poison, and nothing is without poison; only the dose permits something not to be poisonous."

- Key considerations:
  - Consider timing, the starting dose, the rate of administration and cumulative dose:
    Fluid bolus: 4 ml/kg/15 min
    Mini-fluid challenge: 1 ml/kg/5 min
    SSCG: 30 ml/kg/1–3 h
  - Determine the daily need for
    Water: 1 ml/kg/u or 25 ml/kg/day
    Glucose: 1–1.5 g/kg/day (to prevent starvation ketosis)
    Sodium: 1–1.5 mmol/kg/day
    Potassium: 1 mmol/kg/day
    Chlorine: 1 mmol/kg/day

  – Consider pharmacodynamics and pharmacokinetics
    Infusion: Same volume effect of crystalloids vs colloids as long as infusion is running
    Distribution: decreased in shock, hypotension, during surgery, after induction and sedation
    Elimination: decreased in shock, hypotension, during surgery, after induction and sedation
- Aim: Meeting daily fluid volume targets, fluid under/overload and considerations for special patient populations
- KPI: Volume, water, glucose and electrolyte targets achieved in accordance with guidelines

Duration The duration of fluid therapy is important. There is an imbalance in clinical research. The mainstay of focus remains on the type of fluid administered, Vs. the far less studied therapeutic maneuver of withholding/removing fluid.

- Key considerations:
  – Always ask yourself the 4 basic questions
    When to start with IV fluid?
    When to stop giving IV fluid?
    When to start fluid removal?
    When to stop fluid removal?
  – Stop IV infusion if the patient no longer responds to fluid administration due to an increase in stroke volume (or blood pressure)
  – Monitor for hypo- and hypervolemia
  – Use dynamic indices of fluid responsiveness
  – Perform passive leg raising test
- Aim: Correct timing of fluid therapy, including initiation, speed, rate, length and transition of each modality
- KPI: Average cumulative fluid status no greater than 2.5–5% at day 7

De-escalation The final step in fluid therapy is to consider withholding or withdrawing resuscitation fluids when they are no longer required.

- Key considerations:
  – Limit IV fluids as soon as the patient can drink again
  – Give concentrated enteral nutrition
  – Start fluid removal in case of fluid accumulation syndrome
  – Fluid accumulation causes increased morbidity and mortality
- Aim: Avoiding and mitigating complications (e.g. hypervolemia, fluid overload, electrolyte/metabolic disturbances, CLABSI) and stopping
- KPI: Zero complications from IV Fluid Management

Documentation
- Aim: Correct discontinuation of fluid therapy
- KPI: Post-discharge fluid intervention plan actioned

Different Phases During Implementation of Fluid Stewardship

A multidisciplinary panel of leading practitioners and experts recently published best practices for ongoing staff education, intravenous fluid therapy, new training technologies, and strategies to track the success of institutional fluid stewardship efforts. Fluid leads should be identified in every hospital to ensure consistency in fluid administration and monitoring. The different phases during implementation of fluid stewardship is summarized in the following steps [14]:"

Start-up Phase

Step 1: Composition of the Fluid Stewardship Core Team

In order to achieve, implement and maintain the best results, the hospital needs a multidisciplinary fluid team. The composition is discussed with the medical and nursing management as well as the head pharmacist and the members of the medical pharmaceutical committee. Ideally, the fluid stewardship (FS) core team consists of:

- ER physician
- Intensivist
- Internist (endocrinologist, cardiologist, nephrologist)
- Surgeon or OR manager (anaesthetist)
- Pharmacist
- Nurse
- Member of quality team

Step 2: Determination of the Targets for Baseline Measurement

The collection of data at the start of the FS program can be used as a benchmark to set strategic goals. A number of questions can be discussed here:

- What is the infusion-related incidence of electrolyte disturbance and acute renal failure?
- Is the body weight and fluid balance tracked correctly?
- Are the international NICE guidelines followed?
- Where can we have the fastest and biggest impact?
- Is there a problem with moisture overload?

All this is to gain a better understanding of the current situation in the hospital as well as to record the benchmarks (peers compare) for improvements.

Step 3: Baseline Measurement

It should be ensured that the baseline measurement contains all the information necessary to achieve and support the intended goal. This is related to the data that will be collected in the future during periodic assessments (tracers). Consultation and coordination is done with the fluid team.

- Snapshot/baseline measurement of the current consumption of the different infusion fluids
  - Data available from pharmacy
  - Compare data with those available via lump sum medication.
- Thinking about and determining future data collection:
  - Population-level biochemical lab data as surrogate markers for change: mean sodium, mean creatinine, and chloride
  - Follow-up logistical problems in prescribing and administering IV fluids such as the lack of infusion pumps or difficulties in weighing patients or monitoring daily fluid balance
  - Follow-up of the number of infusion-related incident reports
  - Analysis of morbidity and mortality

Step 4: Calculation Consumption and KPI

- Action analysis: Excel file with determination of indicators (KPIs) (Query via pharmacy and compare with government data):
  - Total number of litres of consumption on an annual basis per infusion fluid
  - Ratio of total litres of balanced fluid to number of litres of physiological NaCl
  - Ratio of liters of balanced (or buffered) maintenance fluid to number of liters of Gluc
  - Number of litres of infusion fluid per admission/stay
  - Number of liters of infusion fluid per day hospitalization (bed occupancy day)
  - Calculation of total cost of infusion fluids and percentage of lump sum
  - If possible: split between acute vs. chronic services (rehabilitation)
  - If possible: split between OR vs. ICU vs. ER
  - If possible: split between pediatric vs. Adult patients
  - If possible: split between physical vs. Mental illness

Step 5: Benchmarking Snapshot

- Mutual comparison of the figures from different hospitals (peers compare)
- Comparison with international literature data, e.g. from Fife (Scotland – conducted by Marcia McDougall and colleagues)[15].
- Simulation of cost-economic impact based on standard amounts per liter (or real amounts per infusion bag)
- Calculation of possible savings (cf. percentage decrease as observed in Fife and other hospitals)

Knowledge Phase

Step 6: Knowledge Survey of Doctors and Nurses
- Have a separate questionnaire completed by doctors and nurses
- Separate survey of pediatricians and pediatric nurses
- Call for interested doctors and nurses to choose 2 "fluid stewards" per department or ward

Step 7: Performing Medical Audit (Optional)
File analysis of the appropriateness of the infusion prescribing behavior.
- Through retrospective research of about 100 files (50 internist and 50 surgical).
- Possibility of participating in multicentric research

Strategy Phase

Step 8: Determining the Change Objectives
Identification of the short- and long-term changes required using the results of the baseline measurement and determination of clear targets for this change. Breaking down the targets into a series of small chunks to make them more manageable.

Examples may include:

- We want a measured body weight in X% of all admitted patients
- We want a correct fluid balance in X% of the admitted patients
- We want a complete fluid prescription in X%
- We want to decrease in laboratory with kidney function and electrolytes within 24 h of an infusion administration at X%
- We want an increase in incident reports around IV fluids by X%

Step 9: Identification of Stimulators and Blockers of Change
Starting a fluid stewardship implies a change in the current way of working. This often encounters resistance and that has to do with culture. The need for change must be demonstrated by a clear vision and leadership.

Stimulus:

- Responsibility: assigning clearly defined roles. It is best to appoint 2 fluid stewards for each (nursing) department (a doctor and a nurse)
- Information: Provide on the definition of an incident and encourage reporting
- Education: via information sessions
- Restructuring the medication prescribing process with the introduction of mandatory steps that make prescribing the right fluids easier
- Limitation of choice and compliance guidelines: encouraging reporting of all errors

- Getting important services on board: dialogue with doctors who have experience with change
- Fluid stewards (and other key figures) lead by example

  Resistance to change:
- Culture/customs/habits
- Time and pressure
- Lack of knowledge
- Other priorities
- Organizational problem
- Financial misconceptions: IV fluid bags are relatively inexpensive, so the perception may be that there is no financial need for FS
- Fragmented care: no clear policy

Step 10: Target Audience Identification

Identifying the target audience and how the message is best conveyed is an important step in achieving the objectives. We strive for unambiguous transparent communication.

Preparation Phase

Step 11: Coordination by Clinical Pharmacist

It is important that there is a single point of contact (best the clinical pharmacist) who follows up on the FS program. Check which products are available and where. Provide additional education in training. Follow-up core team. Finalizing one's own directive. Increasing visibility and publicity.

Step 12: Feedback results baseline measurement

First to fluid core team (fluid stewards)
- Use this to develop fluid bundles and guidelines for hospital
     Clear regulations on which fluid can be used in which phases (feeding, maintenance, resuscitation and replacement).
Followed by explanation to all doctors
- Results and fluid bundle/guidelines

Step 13: Increase awareness

By means of posters, screensavers, educational lectures, flyers, etc.

Education Phase

Step 14: Preparation of Training and Education Tool

- Introduction to IV fluid management, including a practical test for nurses such as filling in a fluid balance and for doctors such as correctly prescribing an IV fluid
- Presentation overview of errors in prescribing IV fluids from medical record analysis
- Bedside teaching in the departments
- Weekly workshops
- Train pharmacists and quality team staff to perform routine fluid prescription checks
- Adjusting guidelines for specific patient populations

Implementation Phase

Step 15: Roll out new guidelines

Post-Implementation Phase

Step 16: Follow-up
- Performing quick scans/tracers in the various departments regarding the correctness of infusion prescription.
- Follow up on KPIs (as defined above)
- PDCA or PDSA cycle

Case Vignette

Q1. Was the prescription for IV fluid, correct? Why did the patient develop non-anion gap acidosis or hyperchloremic acidosis?

A: The patient developed hyperchloremic acidosis because of the IV fluid prescription of 5%DNS.The prescription of IV fluid 5% DNS at 150 ml/hour does not meet the 6D's of fluid management. The right diagnosis helps decide the need for fluid administration, resuscitation, replacement and maintenance. In the initial phase, a balanced crystalloid would be required for resuscitation. However, the fluid prescription should be reviewed daily, based on the patient's need and hospital guidance on IV fluids. The duration and de-escalation of IV fluids at the earliest when they are no longer required to avoid fluid creep and its deleterious effects.

Q2. How to initiate fluid stewardship in my hospital/ICU?

A: The implementation of fluid stewardship is divided into four stages,
Firstly, the development of the hospital's fluid guideline or bundle based on the recent evidence to create quality standards.

> Secondly, various stakeholders (5 P's) should be involved in the program and education of the staff about the program.
>
> Thirdly, the prescription of every IV fluid in the hospital has to be detailed (based on the 6 D's) to ensure proper administration and warrant the continuity of care.
>
> Finally, audit prescriptions to the quality standards for a qualitative check of appropriateness.

Conclusion

In summary, improved fluid management in healthcare requires engagement and commitment from the multi-disciplinary team to maintain the ethos of continued change and improvement. Such a culture embraces the principles of quality improvement and creates the mindset required to ensure the best possible care within IV fluid management. Fluid stewards provide the necessary vision and leadership to coordinate such a project across the multidisciplinary team, working in separate but overlapping pathways.

Take Home Messages
- Fluid stewardship can optimize patient outcomes by reducing the unintended consequences of IV fluid administration and healthcare costs.
- Components of fluid stewardship include the development of comprehensive hospital-based fluid guidelines, a fluid stewardship team, continuous staff education and an audit or quality improvement framework.
- The optimum fluid prescription includes considering the 6 D's (diagnosis, drug, dose, duration, de-escalation and discharge) of IV fluid administration.
- The audit framework for fluid prescription should include the 6 P's (physician, prescription, pharmacy, preparation and patient).
- Use a validated model of improvement (e.g., PDSA: plan-do-study-act) to assess the quality of the fluid stewardship program.

References

1. Malbrain MLNG, Van Regenmortel N, Saugel B, et al. Principles of fluid management and stewardship in septic shock: It is time to consider the four D's and the four phases of fluid therapy. Ann Intensive Care. 2018;8(1):66.
2. Malbrain ML, Van Regenmortel N, Owczuk R. It is time to consider the four D's of fluid management. Anaesthesiol Intensive Ther. 2015;47:1–5.
3. National Institute of Health and Care Excellence. Clinical guidelines: intravenous fluid therapy in adults in hospitals. https://www.nice.org.uk/guidance/cg174. Assessed 23 December 2019.
4. Sansom LT, Duggleby L. Intravenous fluid prescribing: improving prescribing practices and documentation in line with NICE CG174 guidance. BMJ Qual Improv Rep. 2014;3(1):2409.
5. Padhi S, Bullock I, Li L, Stroud M. National Institute for Healthcare Excellence Guideline Development: intravenous fluid therapy for adults in hospital: summary of NICE guidance. BMJ. 2013;347:f7073.
6. Malbrain ML, Rice T, Mythen M, Wuyts S. It is time for improved fluid stewardship. ICU Manage Pract. 2018;18(3):158–62.
7. Malbrain ML, Marik PE, Witters I, et al. Fluid overload, de-resuscitation, and outcomes in critically ill or injured patients: a systematic review with suggestions for clinical practice. Anaesthesiol Intensive Ther. 2014;46(5):361–80.
8. Kohn LT, Corrigan JM, Donaldson MS, Institute of Medicine (US) Committee on Quality of Health Care in America. To err is human: building a safer health system. Washington: National Academies Press; 2000.
9. Institute of Medicine (US) Committee on Quality of Health Care in America. Crossing the quality chasm: a new health system for the 21st century. Washington: National Academies Press; 2001.
10. Berwick DM. Continuous improvement as an ideal in health care. N Engl J Med. 1989;320:53–6. https://doi.org/10.1056/NEJM198901053200110.
11. Dixon-Woods M. How to improve healthcare improvement—an essay by Mary Dixon-Woods. BMJ. 2019;367:15514.
12. Ioannidis JPA, Prasad V. Evaluating health system processes with randomized controlled trials. JAMA Intern Med. 2013;173:1279–80. https://doi.org/10.1001/jamainternmed.2013.044.
13. Dixon-Woods M, Martin GP. Does quality improvement improve quality? Future Hosp J. 2016;3:191–4. https://doi.org/10.7861/futurehosp.3-3-191.
14. Malbrain MLNG, Caironi P, Hahn RG, Llau JV, McDougall M, Patrão L, Ridley E, Timmins A. Multidisciplinary expert panel report on fluid stewardship: perspectives and practice. Ann Intensive Care. 2023;13(1):89. https://doi.org/10.1186/s13613-023-01177-y. PMID: 37747558; PMCID: PMC10519908.
15. McDougall M, Guthrie B, Doyle A, Timmins A, Bateson M, Ridley E, Drummond G, Vadiveloo T. Introducing NICE guidelines for intravenous fluid therapy into a district general hospital. BMJ Open Qual. 2022;11(1):e001636. https://doi.org/10.1136/bmjoq-2021-001636. PMID: 35115322; PMCID: PMC8814811.

A Logical Prescription of Intravenous Fluids

28

Jonny Wilkinson, Lisa Yates, Prashant Nasa,
Manu L. N. G. Malbrain ⓘ, and Ashley Miller

Contents

Introduction... 570
The Problem... 570
Application of these Clinical Guidelines... 573
   Target Group... 573
   Exclusions... 573
   Professional Groups.. 574
Clarification of Terms.. 574
   Dehydration... 574
   Background Clinical Physiology... 574
Considerations Prior to All IV Fluid Prescriptions.. 576
   Assessment.. 576
   General Principles... 576

J. Wilkinson
Department of Intensive Care and Anaesthesia, Northampton, UK

L. Yates
Department of Intensive Care and Anaesthesia, Critical Care, Northampton, UK

P. Nasa
Critical Care Medicine, Prevention and Infection Control, NMC Specialty Hospital,
Dubai, United Arab Emirates
e-mail: dr.prashantnasa@hotmail.com

Manu L. N. G. Malbrain (✉)
First Department of Anaesthesiology and Intensive Therapy, Medical University of Lublin,
Lublin, Poland
e-mail: manu.malbrain@telenet.be

A. Miller
Department of Intensive Care and Anaesthesia, Shrewsbury, UK
e-mail: ashleymiller@nhs.net

© The Author(s) 2024
M. L. N. G. Malbrain et al. (eds.), *Rational Use of Intravenous Fluids in Critically
Ill Patients*, https://doi.org/10.1007/978-3-031-42205-8_28

Step 1: Assess Fluid Status... 576
Step 2: Check Body Weight... 578
Step 3: Check U&E Levels in the Last 24 h.. 578
Step 4: Calculate Fluid Balance in the Last 24 h.. 578
Step 5: Prescribe the Appropriate IV Fluid on a Daily Basis...................................... 579
Fluid Prescription: Work Out What You Need!.. 580
    Maintenance Fluid.. 580
    Replacement Solutions... 582
    Resuscitation Fluid... 583
Appropriateness of IV Fluid Therapy.. 585
Which IV Fluid?... 587
Difficult Situations and Tips.. 588
Conclusion.. 592
References... 593

IFA Commentary

Fluid prescribing has been shown in the UK to be associated with significant morbidity and mortality. It has been estimated that up to 20% of patients who receive intravenous fluids suffer iatrogenic harm as a result. It is therefore an area in which investing some effort in improvement is likely to prevent a great deal of patient harm. The National Institute for Health and Care Excellence (NICE) has published national guidance in the UK for intravenous fluid therapy in adults. These guidelines, issued in 2013, advised less use of 0.9% sodium chloride than current practice, provided a logical system for prescribing, and suggested further study of electrolyte abnormalities. Recently, Marcia McDougall and colleagues working in a district general hospital in Fife, Scotland, developed a local version of these guidelines and have implemented them over a number of years [1]. Their conclusions were that effective implementation required substantial time, effort, and resources. NICE suggestions of fluid types for maintenance appear appropriate, but prescribed volumes continue to require careful clinical judgement. A stepwise approach should therefore be undertaken:

- Establish a team and decide on its members.
- Perform baseline audits to assess the current situation within an establishment.
- Identify the drivers for change and any barriers to them. This needs to cover issues arising within medicine and nursing.
- Identify the target audience and establish the best ways to engage medical and nursing leaders in the need for change.
- Implementation of the guideline into practice.

- Assess the changes with quality improvement PDCA cycles, roll out new charts, plus additional material forwards (e.g. posters, learning aids).
- Keep the programme up-to-date and ensure it is maintained and monitored going forward.

This chapter outlines common problems with fluid administration, background physiology, volume assessment, prescribing, and troubleshooting along with how to put appropriate measures in place in a hospital setting.

The pitfalls and challenges of introducing large-scale changes such as the ones suggested in this chapter will need to be examined in the future. Suggestions should be made as to how clinicians may be able to effect sustainable change within this rewarding and immensely important area of health care.

Learning Objectives

After reading this chapter, the reader will understand

1. How to assess patients requiring IV fluid therapy.
2. How to manage patients requiring IV fluid therapy.
3. How to assess the patient's volume status and fluid responsiveness.
4. How to manage electrolyte disturbances.
5. How to avoid complications.
6. How to prescribe fluids appropriately.

Case Vignette

A 42-year-old male, post-operative day 3 in the ICU after radical hemicolectomy and primary anastomosis for carcinoma of the ascending colon. The drain output in the last 24 h is serosanguinous. Nasogastric aspirate is 750 mL in the last 24 h. He is afebrile, haemodynamically stable, and his body weight is 81 kg (before surgery, 77 kg).

Laboratory investigation includes haemoglobin 8.1 gm%, platelets 99,000, sodium 131 meq/L, chloride 100 meq/L, potassium 3.1 meq/L, bicarbonate 26 mmol/L, serum creatinine 107 μmol/L.

Questions

Q1. What information do you need to manage IV fluids for this patient?
Q2. How will you write a prescription for IV fluid for this patient?

Introduction

This chapter guides clinicians through the assessment and management of patients requiring intravenous (IV) fluids. It aims to aid in determining the patient's actual fluid or volume status and guides the appropriate prescription and management of electrolyte and fluid therapy to prevent complications like electrolyte disturbances, fluid accumulation, and organ failure or a combination. This is referred to as IV Fluid Stewardship, and it incorporates much of the National Institute for Health and Care Excellence (NICE) guidance published and the British Consensus Guidelines on Intravenous Fluid Therapy for Adult Surgical Patients (GIFTASUP) [2, 3].

Hereafter, we will set the stage for a conceptual framework for developing institutional programs and guidelines to enhance fluid stewardship (especially in the operating room (OR), emergency room (ER), and intensive care unit (ICU) environment), an activity that includes appropriate selection, indication, dosing, duration, de-escalation, and monitoring of fluid therapy. Analogous to the use of antibiotics, the multifaceted nature of fluid stewardship will need collaboration between different disciplines like emergency medicine, critical care, anaesthesiology, as well as general medicine, surgery, and clinical pharmacy [4].

Intravenous (IV) fluids are some of the most commonly prescribed day-to-day therapeutics [5, 6]. They should, however, be considered as any other drug, and they have their indications, contra-indications, benefits, risks, adverse side effects, and complications. Often, the task of IV fluid prescription is delegated to the most junior members of the team. Or even worse, in many circumstances, there is no IV fluid prescription available and the decision to start and choose the right fluid is left to the attending nurse. Evidence suggests that when available, these prescriptions are rarely ever done correctly despite the presence of clear guidelines (NICE CG174: NICE Intravenous Therapy in Adults in Hospital, https://www.nice.org.uk/guidance/cg174).

This is thought to be due to a lack of knowledge and experience, which often leads to confusion. Consequently, this puts many patients at increased risk of serious harm and may incur unnecessary costs.

It is therefore imperative to carefully assess individual patients, their fluid requirements, and the clinical picture (with comorbidities and complications), in order to tailor IV fluid plans safely. Ideally, fluids should be prescribed on the ward-round by the team who knows the patient and their history. Non-parent team prescriptions, particularly out-of-hours, require extra care, and should not be done as a duplication of the last prescription to save time. Clearly, there are emergent situations whereby fluids need to be prescribed outside of this policy. An introduction to fluid stewardship is discussed in Chap. 27.

The Problem

Previous retrospective reviews of prescriptions have identified poor control of the process. There were considerable variations in IV fluid prescriptions, none of which adhered to NICE guidelines. At times, some prescriptions were placing patients at increased risk of associated complications. The knowledge base among medical staff regarding IV fluids was extremely variable, sometimes poor, as shown by the results of the knowledge on different domains listed hereafter [7].

- Fluid volumes.
  - 84% had incorrect volumes prescribed for maintenance fluids.
- Electrolytes and glucose.
  - Patients received excessive amounts of sodium within their IV fluid prescriptions, yet minimal potassium.
  - Only 25% contained the correct amount of glucose.
- Production of a new IV fluid bundle led to significant improvements in the measured outcomes and balancing measures.
  - All patients had a documented review of both fluid status and balance.
  - The incidence of deranged urea and electrolytes (U&Es) decreased from 48% to 35%.
  - The incidence of acute kidney injury (AKI) decreased from 14% to 10%.
  - The average number of days between the latest U&Es and a fluid prescription decreased from 2.2 days to 1.0 day.

More recently, an online survey was conducted and shared with the participants of the ninth International Fluid Academy Days (IFAD) held in Valencia (Spain) at the end of October 2019. The same was conducted amongst delegates preparing for the first Virtual eIFAD (Nov 2020), assessing their views on fluid choices in their daily clinical practice [8]. The survey consisted of 57 multiple-choice or open questions, 26 covering knowledge of fluid management and stewardship. A total of 1045 surveys were received with respondents coming from 97 different countries. The interim results after 645 respondents were presented at the first virtual eIFAD meeting on 27 November 2020. A total of 862 (83.5%) of the respondents reported being qualified specialist (of which 431 (42%) were intensivists) and 131 were still in training. The years of experience ranged from 0 to 52 with a mean of 15 ± 10 years. The average score on the knowledge questions was $47 \pm 14\%$ (range 4–100). The most difficult questions were: "What is the most important clinical parameter to estimate volaemic status?" and "How much free sodium is there in 1 L of saline?" (Table 28.1). Intensivists had the best score $48.6 \pm 13.8\%$, followed by anaesthetists with $45\ 0.8 \pm 14.3\%$, internists $45.1 \pm 16\%$, and emergency physicians $41.7 \pm 10.9\%$ (95% CI 37.8–48.2). About 26% of respondents reported having a hospital fluid guideline and 36% reported to have an ICU fluid guideline. Fluid balance was regularly measured by 88% of respondents and patients' body weight by only 58% [9].

Table 28.1 Overview of knowledge questions with difficulty level and average scores

Knowledge question	Correct answers	Difficulty	Average score (%)
Q39—What is the most important clinical parameter to estimate volemic status?	None of the options listed	1	9
Q15—How much free sodium is there in 1 L of saline?	3.5 g/L	2	11
Q42—You decide to give a fluid challenge, how many mls would you use?	1 mL/kg/5 min	3	12
Q50—Which infusion do you choose as maintenance fluid?	Hypotonic balanced (ready from the shelf) maintenance solution	4	14
Q40—You decide to give a fluid bolus, how many mls would you use?	4 mL/kg	5	20
Q51—What rate of maintenance infusion would you prescribe for this patient?	1250 mL/day	6	29
Q49—What is the strong ion difference of Plasmalyte?	50 mmol/L	7	31
Q17—Which is closest to the sodium content of a ready from the shelve balanced maintenance solution, e.g. maintelyte or glucion 5% (in mEq/L)	50 mmol/L	8	34
Q45—What comes closest to the volume expansion effect of 1 L gluc 5% after 1 h?	100 mL	9	35
Q54—What is the daily glucose requirement for this patient?	1–1.5 g/kg/day	10	38
Q19—When would you use albumin 4%?	Never	11	44
Q18—Which is closest to the glucose content of a balanced solution in g/L (e.g. Plasmalyte)	0 mmol/L	12	47
Q53—What do you think is the daily potassium requirement for this patient?	1 mmol/kg/day	13	50
Q13—Do you think it is safe to give a balanced infusion fluid with a potassium content of 5 mEq/L to a patient with renal insufficiency and clearance of 25 mL/min?	Yes	14	50
Q16—What is the maximum recommended daily sodium intake?	2.3 g/day	15	54
Q43—What is the most important clinical parameter for you to estimate fluid responsiveness?	Passive leg raising test	16	55
Q48—What comes closest to the volume expansion effect of 1 L saline (NaCl 0.9%) after 1 h?	250 mL	17	59
Q47—What is the strong ion difference of saline?	0 mmol/L	18	60

Table 27.1 (continued)

Knowledge question	Correct answers	Difficulty	Average score (%)
Q20—When to use albumin 20%?	Late phase of severe sepsis and septic shock for deresuscitation	19	60
Q52—What is the daily sodium requirement for this patient?	1–1.5 mmol/kg/day	20	61
Q41—Over what period of time do you give the fluid bolus?	Over 10–15 min	21	63
Q46—What is the problem with saline?	All options listed	22	66
Q14—Which is closest to the sodium content of saline or NaCl 0.9% (in mEq or mmol/L)	155 mmol/L	23	72
Q44—Which infusion do you prefer here as a fluid bolus?	Balanced crystalloid	24	81
Q27—If you prescribe an IV fluid infusion, how often do you re-evaluate the prescription?	One to several times a day	25	91
Q12—When do you use starch solutions?	Never, in trauma, in perioperative hypovolaemic hypotension	26	95

Application of these Clinical Guidelines

Target Group

- All critically ill and ICU patients are considered potential candidates for resuscitation fluids.
- Patients are considered for maintenance or replacement IV fluids:
  - Those with existing or developing deficits that cannot be compensated by oral intake.
  - When fluids are lost via drains or stomata, fistulas, fever, open wounds (including evaporation during surgery), polyuria (salt wasting nephropathy or diabetes insipidus).
- The overall aim is to match the amount of fluid and electrolytes as closely as possible, to the fluid that is needed or is being or has been lost, on a daily basis.

Exclusions

- Patients under the age of 16—need a consult by the paediatric team.
- Diabetes and especially diabetic ketoacidosis (DKA)—use current diabetes guidance or diabetic emergency guidance.
- Burns—existing burns calculations should be used.

- Obstetrics—need to discuss with the senior obstetric team for more complex patients.
- Head injury—avoid hypotonic fluids containing glucose and liaise with a neurotrauma centre.
- Renal/Liver patients—discuss with senior gastro/renal team.
- Elective and emergency theatre cases—managed by the anaesthetist caring for the patient in theatre. The relevance of this policy comes in post-operative ward management.

Professional Groups

This guideline is relevant to all doctors, physician associates, advanced nurse practitioners, and nurses working in all areas of the hospital, other than paediatrics.

Clarification of Terms

The used terms often cause confusion in clinicians. There is a plethora of different terms that are used interchangeably. A multidisciplinary consensus statement on dehydration: definitions, diagnostic methods and clinical implications published in 2019 has sought to clarify these terms (DOI: https://doi.org/10.1080/07853890.2019.1628352 or https://bit.ly/2RvAiEF) [10].

Dehydration

Hypertonic dehydration—water deficit causing hyperosmolality. Such a patient will have a high sodium. It results from inadequate water intake or increased losses (e.g. sweating). Intravascular volume is preserved while intracellular volume is reduced.

Isotonic dehydration—water and salt loss causing a deficit of extracellular fluid with normal osmolality. Haemoconcentration will be manifested by a high haemoglobin/haematocrit. Large volume GI losses from vomiting, NG-free drainage, diarrhoea, and large stoma output cause such fluid loss with relatively preserved sodium levels as GI fluid contains varying amounts of sodium. The two types of dehydration often co-exist (e.g. not drinking and vomiting).

Hypovolaemia is caused by loss of blood or ECF and specifically describes intravascular volume depletion.

Background Clinical Physiology

Patients are often given too much IV fluid—particularly non-physiological 0.9% sodium chloride). Once within the body, such sodium excesses are very difficult to remove and can result in harm. The cumulative sodium balance may be more important than the fluid balance per se, as even normal kidneys may take days, if not weeks, to get rid of the excess [11, 12].

There are extremes—increased fluid load can cause major electrolyte swings, whereas dehydration, can lead to poor organ perfusion. Sick patients (particularly those with systemic inflammatory response syndrome (SIRS) and those with sepsis), have "leaky" capillaries. This has been recently referred to as the globally increased permeability syndrome or "GIPS," defined as the absence of a spontaneous transition from the Ebb to Flow phase of shock with a persistent positive cumulative fluid balance and new-onset organ dysfunction or failure [5, 6]. In this situation, even careful IV fluid administration can lead to fluid overload and resultant complications (pulmonary oedema, venous congestion, ileus, poor mobility following peripheral oedema, pressure sores, poor wound healing, and anastomotic breakdown). This is because the administered fluid escapes from the intravascular compartment, flooding the interstitial compartment, where it offers no physiological benefit.

These patients are sometimes incorrectly labelled as being hypovolaemic, when in fact they are vasodilated. We have a situation whereby excess administered fluid has escaped into another body compartment away from its beneficial site within the circulating volume (first space). After sensible fluid challenges and identification of "non-response," these patients require early consideration of vasopressor therapy (i.e. noradrenaline) [13]. Therefore, in sepsis and states of critical illness, poor IV fluid prescribing practice can ultimately lead to morbidity, and even worse, mortality.

We often look at urine output as a marker of fluid requirement; however, patients who are unwell, have suffered trauma, or have undergone surgery often have a reduced urine output due to increased sodium retention (and thus water), by the kidneys. This is a natural stress response and is geared to hold on to intravascular volume to maintain vital organ perfusion during such stress states. Stress-induced ("inappropriate") anti-diuretic hormone secretion, as well as intrinsic vasopressor hormone secretion, leads to a state of sodium and water retention and potassium loss in the urine. The patient becomes oedematous, hypokalaemic, and hypernatraemic over time, if left unchecked. Suppose normal saline has been given as a resuscitation fluid or maintenance fluid. In that case, a potential hyperchloraemic metabolic acidosis can ensue, on top of these other electrolyte imbalances, further leading to AKI.

The arterioles in the kidneys auto-regulate blood flow above a minimum mean pressure (around 60 mmHg). If blood pressure is not very low, then IV fluids can be of no benefit to renal perfusion. They may even lead to high venous pressures which will reduce perfusion (venous congestion).

No patient should suffer the effects of cellular dysfunction and ultimately multi-organ dysfunction, as a result of excessive and/or inappropriate IV fluid prescription and provision. Armed with an understanding of fluid physiology, one can see why oliguria is a poor marker of fluid requirement. Physiological oral fluids should always be the first line unless circumstances absolutely disallow it.

The best fluid may be the one that has not been given ... (unnecessarily) [14].

In the next paragraphs, we will list some practical considerations to IV fluid prescription [15].

Considerations Prior to All IV Fluid Prescriptions

Assessment

- **Patient's fluid status** (hypo/eu/hypervolaemia)—Assess at the time of fluid prescription using: clinical judgement, presence of oedema, vital signs, and fluid balance including urine output.
- Patient's **weight**—Within the last 24 h (ICU) or 3 days (regular ward).
- Patient's **Urea and Electrolytes**—Within the last 24 h assessed as part of every ward review.
- Patient's **fluid balance** charts (input and output)—Over the last 24 h.

General Principles

Prescription safety can be summarised by the "4 D's" principle [14]:

- **D**rug—which fluid [type, colloid vs crystalloid, isotonic vs hypotonic vs hypertonic, balanced or buffered vs unbalanced (saline)].
- **D**ose—calculate how much and how fast (rate) to give via a pump.
- **D**uration—duration of the IV fluid therapy.
- **D**e-escalation—taper or stop IV fluids as soon as possible or start fluid removal (de-resuscitation).

Give the Right fluid in the Right Dose to the Right patient at the Right time.

Step 1: Assess Fluid Status

- Basic history and examination of the patient will give pointers as to what their volaemic status is (see Table 28.2).
- The best fluid to give in case of **hypovolaemia** is physiological fluid, i.e. oral fluid. Always consider this first.

Table 28.2 Volaemic Status assessment [16]. *BP* blood pressure, *HR* heart rate, *JVP* jugular venous pressure, *MAP* mean arterial pressure, *PLR* passive leg raising test, *RR* respiratory rate *UO* urine output

Hypovolaemia	Hypervolaemia
History—Diarrhoea, vomiting, bleeding, dehydration	History: Increased body weight over short period of time while in hospital/ICU
Large negative fluid balance	Large positive fluid balance
No oedema	Oedema
Thirst	No thirst
Confusion	
Postural hypotension	–
Hypotension (systolic BP <100 mmHg or MAP <65 mmHg)	Hypertension
Positive PLR test (increase in blood pressure)—Indicates preload responsiveness	Negative PLR, absence of preload responsiveness
Tachycardia (HR >100 bpm)	Normal HR
Tachypnoea (RR >24)	Pulmonary oedema
Delayed capillary refill time (> 3 s)	Altered capillary refill time
Decreased UO—Oliguria (<0.5 mL/kg/h)	Decreased UO—Oliguria (<0.5 mL/kg/h) if venous congestion
Altered laboratory results: Hemoconcentration, increased plasma osmolality, sodium, total protein, haematocrit, urea over creatinine ratio (>50)	Altered laboratory results: Hemodilution: Low osmolality, low total protein, low albumin, low haematocrit
Urine analysis: Low urinary sodium, high urinary osmolality (density)	Urine analysis: High urinary sodium, low urinary osmolality (density)
Acid-base disturbance: Contraction alkalosis	Acid-base disturbance: Dilutional acidosis
Cold peripheries	Peripheral (pitting) oedema (anasarca)
Veins collapsed—Decreased skin turgor	Raised JVP, positive hepatojugular reflux (distention of the neck veins when pressure is applied over the liver)

- In the case of **euvolemia,** no fluids need to be given except if there are expected losses that cannot be compensated orally, the patient cannot meet basic needs, or electrolyte disturbances are present requiring IV correction and oral supplementation is not possible.
- In the case of **hypervolaemia,** the first step is to check proactively whether the patient is receiving an IV infusion that must be stopped. In the case of the GIPS, defined as fluid accumulation with an impact on organ function, fluids must be removed actively using diuretics or ultrafiltration (see Chap. 25).
- Advanced users may utilize non-invasive cardiac output monitoring, transpulmonary thermodilution with volumetric preload indicators, or point-of-care ultrasound to assess the fluid status of patients. This is out of the scope of this guideline.

Step 2: Check Body Weight

- It is important to record and measure (do not guess) patient weight on admission and at least once or twice weekly.
- Weight gain over a short period of time during hospitalization is usually due to excessive IV fluid loading (as muscles and fat tissue take more time to build up).
- Assess for fluid overload (or better accumulation).
  - Dividing the cumulative fluid balance in litres by the patient's baseline body weight x 100% defines the percentage of fluid accumulation.
  - Fluid overload is defined by a cut-off value of 10% of fluid accumulation, and this is associated with worse outcomes.
    - Check body and fluid composition with bio-electrical impedance analysis (when available) to obtain TBW, ECW/ICW ratio and volume excess.

Step 3: Check U&E Levels in the Last 24 h

- Patients who are being considered for IV fluid therapy should have documented U&E results within the last 24 h. If not, levels should be taken as soon as possible.
- The presence of acute kidney injury (AKI) using KDIGO criteria should be checked.
- This is to gauge both the effects of the exogenous fluid over time on the patient's electrolyte levels and to ensure inappropriate fluid is not administered to them (potassium-containing fluid if already hyperkalaemic or sodium-containing fluid if hypernatraemic, etc.).

Step 4: Calculate Fluid Balance in the Last 24 h

- Fluid balance is key. All patients should have accurate input/output charting. Clearly, it is more challenging to do this precisely in those who are not catheterized.
- Review recent history for:
  - Losses:
    Fasting, operations, sepsis, excessive sweating in febrile states, diarrhoea, and vomiting
    Upper G.I losses in excess, i.e. vomiting, tend to lead to states of alkalosis, potential electrolyte disturbance, and "true" dehydration.
    Lower G.I losses in excess i.e. diarrhoea, tend to lead to states of acidosis, potential electrolyte disturbance including hypokalaemia, and true dehydration.
  - Gains:
    Fluid overload states (oedema and excessive positive balance).

- Assessment for normal intake.
  - Is the patient eating and drinking adequately? The best fluid is physiological fluid, i.e. oral intake.
  - If patients are not nil by mouth and are not suffering from excessive losses, requests to prescribe IV fluids should be challenged.
  - Fluids are drugs, and they should be held in equal esteem.
  - All fluids administered need to be considered: oral, IV, catheter flush (A-line).
- Check recorded losses.
  - Has the patient lost fluid, are they currently losing fluid, or are they not drinking appropriately? Examples include stoma output, vomiting, diarrhoea.
  - Think also of insensible fluid loss (evaporation of water along the skin and respiratory tract). This loss is higher in patients with fever (approximately 10 mL/kg/day) than in ventilated patients with active or passive humidification (approximately 5 mL/kg/day).

Consider adding excessive losses to your calculated daily maintenance fluid. Amount lost in 24 h divided by 24 to give the amount to add to maintenance per hour.

Step 5: Prescribe the Appropriate IV Fluid on a Daily Basis

The IV fluid prescription is adapted to the patient's basal and current needs, deficiencies, as well as any fluid/electrolyte losses. Check for electrolyte disturbances, glycaemia, heart function, liver, and kidney function. Always document the type and indication of the IV infusion in patient's medical records. Make a fluid prescription every 24 h and adapt it according to the patient's needs. Patients should have an IV fluid management plan, including a fluid and electrolyte prescription for the proceeding 24 h. The prescription for a maintenance IV fluid should only change after a clinical exam, a change in dietary intake or after the evaluation of laboratory results. The following information should be included in the IV fluid prescription: the type of fluid, the rate and volume of fluid infusion, the objective, and the safety limits. (Fig. 28.1 illustrates the TROL mnemonic) [5, 6].

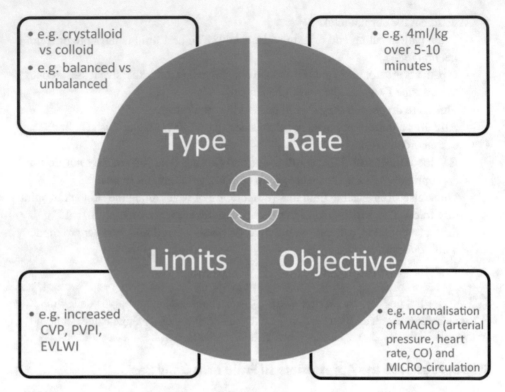

Fig. 28.1 The TROL mnemonic of fluid prescription: considerations for administration of a fluid bolus in critically ill patients. *CO* cardiac output, *CVP* central venous pressure, *EVLWI* extra vascular lung water index, *PVPI* pulmonary vascular permeability index. (Adapted with permission from Malbrain et al. [6])

Fluid Prescription: Work Out What You Need!

Maintenance Fluid

Maintenance fluids are given specifically to cover the patient's daily basal requirements of water and electrolytes. The basic daily needs are summarized in Table 28.3, and a worked example based on body weight is shown in Table 28.4. Some specific maintenance solutions are commercially available, but they are far from ideal. There is a lot of debate whether isotonic or hypotonic maintenance solutions should be used. Data in children showed that hypotonic solutions carry the risk for hyponatremia and neurologic complications. However, studies in adults are scarce and indicate that administration of isotonic solutions will result in a more positive fluid balance as compared to hypotonic solutions. This was confirmed in a recent pilot study in healthy volunteers showing that isotonic

Table 28.3 Maintenance fluid requirements. *IV* intravenous

Maintenance	
IV water required	1 mL/kg/24 h or 25–30 mL/kg/24 h
Na^+	1 mmol/kg/24 h
K^+/Cl^-	1 mmol/kg/24 h
Glucose	1 g/kg/day (50–100 g)
Urine output	1 mL/kg/h
Review output on fluid chart and if excessive (>50 mL/kg/day), divide the total by 24 and consider an addition to daily maintenance	
If on IV fluid for >24 h, then the patient will need U&E monitoring daily	
If nil per mouth glucose needs to be covered to avoid starvation ketosis	

Table 28.4 Body weights and worked examples

Weight (kg)	Fluid needed mL/24 h	Rate mL/h
35–44	1200	50
45–54	1500	65
55–64	1800	75
65–74	2100	85
>75	2400	100 (max)

solutions caused lower urine output, characterized by decreased aldosterone concentrations indicating (unintentional) volume expansion, than hypotonic solutions and were associated with hyperchloraemia. Despite their lower sodium and potassium content, hypotonic fluids were not associated with hyponatremia or hypokalaemia [17]. This was later also confirmed in critically ill patients undergoing major thoracic surgery [18]. When comparing these studies, administration of an isotonic maintenance solution led to 600 mL fluid gain after 48 h in healthy volunteers compared to 900 mL in ICU patients and a 150 mmol sodium gain after 48 h in healthy volunteers compared to 300 mmol in ICU patients (Fig. 28.2) [11].

Important points that need to be considered are.

- Enteral and parenteral feed.
  - The patient may not need the entire calculated maintenance dose per hour if receiving enteral feed and in particular total parenteral nutrition (TPN).
- Time fasting or NBM (nil-by-mouth).
  - Consideration should be given to maintenance fluid in any patient who fasted for over 8 h.
- Drugs = additional fluid!
  - Many IV drugs are administered with large amounts of fluid. These can add large amounts to calculated maintenance rates if forgotten about. Maintenance fluids should be adapted for other fluid sources. Fluid creep must be avoided [12].

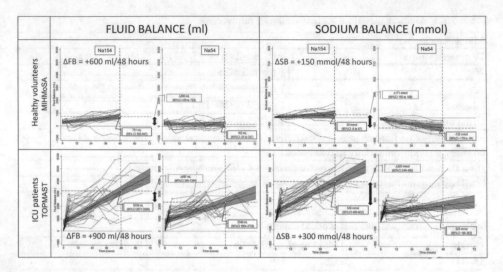

Fig. 28.2 Estimated cumulative fluid and sodium balances of the MIHMoSA and TOPMAST trials. (Adapted with permission from Van Regenmortel et al. [11]). *FB* fluid balance, *SB* sodium balance

- If patients are hypervolaemic.
  - They may require fluid restriction or diuresis. One can try a furosemide stress test (0.1 mg Lasix/kg—patient is responder when UO >200 mL after 2 h).
- Definition of inappropriate fluid prescription in case of electrolyte disturbances.
  - Solutions not containing an adequate amount of sodium in case of hyponatremia from GI losses (Na <135 mmol/L).
  - Solutions not containing an adequate amount of potassium in case of hypokalaemia (K <3.5 mmol/L).
  - Solutions containing too much sodium in case of hypernatremia (Na >145 mmol/L).
  - Solutions containing too much potassium in case of hyperkalaemia (K >5 mmol/L).

Replacement Solutions

If patients have on-going abnormal losses or a complex redistribution problem, the fluid therapy should be adjusted for all other sources of fluid and electrolyte losses (e.g. 0.9% saline may be indicated in patients with hypochloraemic metabolic alkalosis due to gastrointestinal losses). In general, replacement fluids should mimic the fluid that is lost and should be administered to correct fluid deficits that cannot be compensated for by oral intake. Such fluid deficits might exist, or develop in patients with drains or stomata, fistulas, fever, open wounds (evaporation during surgery, severe burn injury, etc.), and polyuria (salt wasting nephropathy or diabetes insipidus). Data on replacement fluids are also scarce. Several recent guidelines advise matching the amount of fluid and electrolytes as closely as possible to the fluid being lost. An overview of the composition of the different body fluids can be found in the NICE guidelines [2]. Replacement fluids are usually isotonic balanced solutions. In patients with a fluid deficit due to a loss of chloride-rich gastric fluid (leading to metabolic alkalosis), high chloride solutions, like saline (NaCl 0.9%), might be used as replacement fluid.

- Other excessive losses.
  - Some may be more occult, like febrile states leading to excessive evaporative losses in sweat. *Consider* adding these to your hourly maintenance rate.
  - Gastric losses may be the only indication for 0.9% saline.
- Replacing urinary losses.
  - Urine does not need to be replaced unless excessive in volume (i.e. with diabetes insipidus or the diuretic phase of resolving renal failure).
- Surgical stress response.
  - In post-op patients, polyuria may be multi-factorial. It may be due to excessive intra-operative fluid provision, or secondary to the surgical stress response. Here, increased anti-diuretic hormone release leads to retention of sodium and water but diuresis of potassium-containing urine.
- Prescription inaccuracy.
  - Try and avoid prescribing fluid bags over × number of hours, instead prescribe in mL/h. All patients receiving IV fluids for over 6 h, or those receiving potassium replacement, should all have fluid delivered via a volumetric pump.
  - Adjust administration rates when extra fluid volume is given for the administration of drugs (antibiotics, painkillers, sedatives, etc.)
- Do not increase maintenance fluid rates!
  - Avoid "speeding up" infusions if patients are deemed "non-responders." This is where IV fluid challenges come in.

Never adjust IV maintenance rates in order to provide a fluid challenge. These are often left running at the challenge rate, resulting in severe fluid overload. Use a prescribed isotonic fluid challenge separately.

Do not use dextrose 5% without electrolytes, or NaCl 0.45% in dextrose 5% as a maintenance fluid; 0.18% NaCl/4% glucose is a good alternative; however, care is needed as this does not contain potassium. This may need to be added if the U&E profile suggests it.

Resuscitation Fluid

Resuscitation fluids refer to fluids given to correct an intravascular volume deficit in cases of absolute or relative hypovolaemia (Table 28.5). Resuscitation fluids have received considerable scientific attention, especially in the light of the recent colloid-crystalloid debate.

Table 28.5 Resuscitation fluid guidance

Resuscitation
1. Prescribe a "STAT" bolus of 200–250 mL balanced/buffered crystalloid (or 4 mL/kg over 5 min)
2. Reassess the patient with the "A, B,C,D,E" approach
3. Monitor blood pressure (BP), pulse pressure variation, heart rate, and urine output response to the challenge
4. If no response repeat challenge and re-assess if adequate response, continue maintenance fluid and continue monitoring
5. If there is an inadequate response after 2000 mL (30 mL/kg) fluid challenge, escalate to a senior team member

However, a large part of the total infused volume during a patient's stay in the hospital does not fall into this category.

- Sepsis and septic shock.
  - Evidence is mounting against excessive fluid resuscitation in this group, favouring a more restrictive (conservative) vs liberal fluid regimen [19].
  - What many of these patients require is earlier vasopressor support in a critical care environment, or certainly early advice from a senior member of the team/critical care, failing this.
  - For patients in need of fluid resuscitation:
    The cause of the fluid deficit should be identified.
    An assessment of shock or hypoperfusion should be made.
    Patients who have received initial fluid resuscitation should be carefully reassessed.
  - If an excess of 2000 mL (30 mL/kg) IV fluid challenge has been provided, consideration of escalation of the level of care should be made, rather than continuing fluid resuscitation. The more fluid a "septic" patient receives, the higher the morbidity and mortality are likely to be [12, 20]. It may be prudent to liaise with critical care if the situation is deemed complex.
  - Patients who have not had >2000 mL of crystalloids, who still need fluid resuscitation after reassessment, can receive another 200–250 mL of crystalloids and be reassessed again.
  - We recommend caution over the usage of 30 mL/kg resuscitation fluid dosage (as recommended by the Surviving Sepsis Campaign), for all patients [21]. This has been debated worldwide, and the prevailing expert opinion is that this may be excessive. It may be applicable to those who are profoundly shocked with sepsis/SIRS, but should always be paralleled with appropriate escalation and advice from more senior clinicians.
  - We recommend starting with 4 mL/kg over 5 min, with an assessment of the response (check the haemodynamic status and preload tolerance, before and after).

- Some facts to remember:
    Less than 50% of haemodynamically unstable patients are "fluid responders".
    It is unproven in humans that fluid boluses in septic shock improve cardiac output or organ perfusion.
    85% of an infused bolus of crystalloid crosses into interstitial space after 4 h in health. This increases to 95% in sepsis in under 90 min
- For urgent resuscitation:
  - We recommend the use of balanced crystalloid solutions.
  - Hartmann's solution (compound sodium lactate/Ringer's lactate) or PlasmaLyte are recommended.
- We do not recommend.
  - The use of 0.9% sodium chloride. This is a very poor choice of IV fluid in shock states with acidosis or AKI, as this fluid potentiates further imbalance (hyperchloraemic metabolic acidosis). It contains a supra-physiological amount of sodium and chloride (both 154 mmol/L) and is therefore not isotonic.
  - Dextrose 5% or any other hypotonic solution as a resuscitation fluid.
- Colloid controversy.
  - There are controversies behind the usage of colloids, as they are not without their problems (high sodium load, incidence of allergic reactions, etc.).
  - Crystalloids are likely to be a safer first choice.
  - Hypertonic albumin 20% can be considered during the later de-resuscitation phase, although there may be a beneficial effect in a small subgroup of patients with severe septic shock.
  - Do not use starch solutions in septic shock, burns, or patients with AKI. Starch solutions can still be used in trauma and perioperative hypotension.
  - Do not use albumin 4%.
  - Do not use gelatins; there is limited evidence supporting their use in critically ill patients.
- Bleeding.
  - The priority is to locate and stop the bleeding.
  - The best replacement for this is blood and any accompanying blood products.
  - Consider initiating the massive haemorrhage protocol through a switchboard.
  - Do not forget calcium, tranexamic acid, and fibrinogen substitution when needed.

Appropriateness of IV Fluid Therapy

The appropriateness of IV fluid therapy should always be checked by looking at the clinical assessment of fluid status, checking the indication for IV fluid therapy, correct prescription, and management. This is summarized in Table 28.6.

Table 28.6 Four stages to check for the appropriateness of IV fluid therapy

Stage of evaluation	Audit standard
1. Assessment	• Patients' fluid status is assessed and documented on admission • The patient's fluid and electrolyte needs are assessed as part of every ward review • The assessment includes the use of an appropriate clinical parameter for the evaluation of the fluid balance • Recent lab result with urea and electrolytes (within 24 h of fluid prescription)

2. Indication	(a) Resuscitation
	 • For patients in need of fluid resuscitation:
	  − The cause of the fluid deficit is identified
	  − An assessment of shock or hypoperfusion was made
	  − A fluid bolus of 500 mL of crystalloids is given
	 • Patients who have received initial fluid resuscitation are reassessed
	 • Care is upgraded in patients who have already been given >2000 mL of crystalloids and are still hypotensive
	 • Patients who have not had >2000 mL of crystalloids and who may benefit from fluid resuscitation after reassessment receive 250–500 mL of crystalloids and have a further reassessment
	
	(b) Maintenance
	 • If patients need IV fluids for routine maintenance alone, the initial prescription is restricted to:
	  − 25–30 mL/kg/day (1 mL/kg/h) of water and
	  − Approximately 1 mmol/kg/day of potassium (K^+) and
	  − Approximately 1–1.5 mmol/kg/day of sodium (Na^+) and
	  − Approximately 1 mmol/kg/day of chloride and
	  − Approximately 50–100 g/day (1–1.5 g/kg/day) of glucose to limit starvation ketosis
	 • Definition of inappropriateness in case of electrolyte disturbances
	  − Solutions not containing an adequate amount of sodium in case of hyponatremia (Na < 135 mmol/L)
	  − Solutions not containing an adequate amount of potassium in case of hypokalaemia (K < 3.5 mmol/L)
	  − Solutions containing too much sodium in case of hypernatremia (Na > 145 mmol/L)
	  − Solutions containing too much potassium in case of hypokalaemia (K > 5 mmol/L)
	
	(c) Replacement and redistribution
	 • If patients have on-going abnormal losses or a complex redistribution problem, the fluid therapy is adjusted for all other sources of fluid and electrolyte losses (e.g. normal saline may be indicated in patients with metabolic alkalosis due to gastro-intestinal losses)

Table 28.6 (continued)

Stage of evaluation	Audit standard

3. Prescription	• The following information is included in the IV fluid prescription:
	  – The type of fluid
	  – The rate of fluid infusion
	  – The volume of fluid
	  – Duration of fluid therapy
	• The IV fluid prescription is adapted to current electrolyte disorders

4. Management	• Patients have an IV fluid management plan, including a fluid and electrolyte prescription over the next 24 h • The prescription for a maintenance IV fluid only changes after a clinical exam, a change in dietary intake, or evaluation of laboratory results

Adapted with permission from Malbrain et al. [4]

Which IV Fluid?

• Knowledge of IV fluid constituents:
  – Be wary of what each bag of fluid contains. Many IV fluids contain a lot of sodium! (See Table 28.7).
• Fluid of choice.
  – Maintenance: 0.18% saline with 4% dextrose with/without potassium or any ready off-the-shelf balanced solution (Glucion, Maintelyte).
      At the correct rate, this should give a balanced solution. Be mindful of the fact there is no potassium in this solution, and it must be added if the patient is hypokalaemic. Excessive amounts can cause hyponatraemia/hypokalaemia.
  – Resuscitation: Hartmann's solution/Ringer's lactate or compound sodium lactate or PlasmaLyte.
      Again, a balanced safe solution. If the patient already has a sodium of less than 132 mmol/L, the use of Hartmann's or PlasmaLyte may be the preferred option. Contains potassium.
      Intuitively one would argue not to use these fluids if the patient has hyperkalaemia; however, there is no contraindication to their use, and in the end, they may even lower serum potassium levels in mild AKI as compared to saline (leading to metabolic acidosis and secondary increase in potassium even if saline does not contain potassium). Also remember that adding an IV solution containing potassium at 5 mmol/L will not increase K in a patient with mild AKI and a potassium level of 6 mmol/L. On the contrary, potassium will be diluted as well.
• Potassium supplementation.
  – Can be added to 0.18% saline with 4% dextrose and normal saline.
  – Can be added to 5% dextrose (though we strongly discourage this fluid's usage in maintenance/resuscitation).

Table 28.7 IV fluid constituents

Fluid	Na	K	Cl	Mg	Ca	Other	Osm
0.9% NaCl	154	0	154	0	0	0	308
0.18%NaCl/4%glucose	30	0	30	0	0	Gluc 40 g/L	284
0.45%NaCl/5%glucose	77	0	77	0	0	Gluc 50 g/L	406
Hartmann's	131	5	111	0	2	Lactate 29	274
Plasmalyte 148	140	5	98	1.5	0	Acetate 27 Gluconate 23	297
5% Dextrose	0	0	0	0	0	Glucose 50 g/L	278

- Do not add to Hartmanns for reason of stability!
- If the potassium is already greater than 5 mmol/L, do not add extra potassium to any IV fluid.
- All potassium-containing fluids should be administered via an appropriate volumetric pump.
- Re-feeding syndrome.
  - Signs: hypophosphatemia, hypomagnesemia.
  - Consider Pabrinex Intravenous High Potency, Concentrate for Solution for Infusion (supplied in pairs of amber glass ampoules of 5 mL) if the patient is at risk of refeeding syndrome, (take this volume into account when calculating their maintenance).

- DO NOT USE 5% dextrose as a maintenance nor resuscitation fluid.
- DO NOT USE colloids as a maintenance fluid.
  - Associated complications and high sodium loads!
- DO NOT USE 0.9% (ab)normal saline for any prolonged period.
  - It has a high sodium and chloride load!
- DO NOT USE maintenance solutions for resuscitation.
- DO NOT USE resuscitation fluids for maintenance use.

Difficult Situations and Tips

- Consider assessment of haemodynamic response to 45° passive leg raise test (See Fig. 28.3).
  - Did the BP increase (10–15%) and pulse rate slow down after 30–50 s?
    If yes, they are likely to be a fluid responder.
    If no, consider the fact they may not be hypovolaemic and there is something else going on.
- Consider urinary catheter in all sick patients.
- Signs of hypovolaemia may be unreliable in:

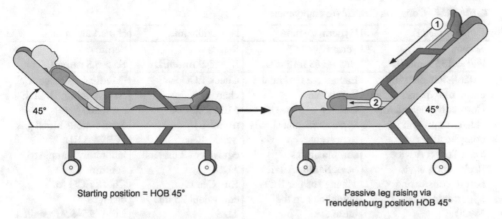

Starting position = HOB 45°   Passive leg raising via Trendelenburg position HOB 45°

Fig. 28.3 Trolley assisted passive leg raise. The passive leg raising (PLR) test. In order to perform a correct PLR test, one should not touch the patient in order to avoid sympathetic activation. The PLR is performed by turning the bed from the starting position (head of bed elevation 30–45°) to the Trendelenburg position. The PLR test results in an autotransfusion effect via the increased venous return from the legs and the splanchnic mesenteric pool. Monitoring of stroke volume is required as a positive PLR test is defined by an increase in SV by at least 10%. See the text for explanation. (Adapted from Hofer et al. with permission [22])

- Elderly patients.
  Often concomitant drugs slow heart rate, e.g. Beta blockers, digitalis, certain calcium-blockers. This may attenuate any pulse rate responses.
  Normal target blood pressures (MAP >65 mmHg) in the elderly may be too low for them if they are normally hypertensive. Diastolic blood pressure may be low in elderly with systolic hypertension and diastolic heart failure (be aware of false-positive PLR).
  Cardiac pathologies and dysautonomic states can cloud responses to fluid challenges and hypovolaemic states.
- Young fit patients.
  High physiological reserve capacity.
  Rapid adrenergic compensatory pressure response to intravascular volume loss. Therefore, much delayed vital sign deterioration.
• Excessive losses.
  – Calculate the losses over the previous 24 h.
  – Consider replacement using Hartmanns or PlasmaLyte in combination with maintenance,
  – If upper GI loss, with low chloride, use 0.9% NaCl.
• See Table 28.8 for electrolyte emergencies.
  – **Hyponatraemia:** The causes of this are varied and complex. A sodium less than 125 mmol/L can be dangerous and senior input should be sought. The treatment for low Na is nearly always fluid restriction; not 0.9% sodium chloride.
  – **Potassium**: Just because the potassium level is normal, does not necessarily mean that there isn't a deficit, therefore consider adding it to replacement fluid.

Table 28.8 Common electrolyte emergencies

Hyponatraemia	Hypernatraemia	Hypokalaemia	Hyperkalaemia
Serum Na$^+$ < **135 mmol/L**	Serum Na$^+$ > **145 mmol/L**	Serum K$^+$ < **3.5 mmol/L**	Serum K$^+$ > **5.5 mmol/L**
Establish underlying cause of hyponatraemia Correct hyponatraemia slowly to prevent complications Seek Senior Advice Seek expert advice before considering hypertonic saline (1.8% NaCl)	Encourage oral intake if possible Correct hypernatraemia slowly to prevent complications **Seek Senior Advice** Manage as per NGH guidelines on the intranet **Do Not Use Fluids Containing Sodium**	Check ECG for changes **Mild (3.0–3.4 mmol/L)** Sando-K or equivalent 2 tablets TDS Kay Cee L or equivalent 25 mL TDS Check level in 3 days **Moderate (2.5–2.9 mmol/L)** Sando-K or equivalent 2 tablets QDS Kay Cee L or equivalent 25 mL QDS Check level in 3 days **Severe (<2.5 mmol/L)** IV replacement using 40 mmol KCl in fluids BD or TDS Check level the next days Check serum Mg^{2+} level	*Medical Emergency* Assess using ABCDE approach Send venous blood gas (VBG) AND laboratory sample to confirm Check ECG for changes **Mild (5.5–5.9 mmol/L)** Repeat in 6 h in unwell patients or daily if stable Review medications & diet **Moderate/Severe (>6 mmol/L)** Give 10 mL calcium Gluconate 10% IV over 3–5 mins via large vein Give 10 units Actrapid IV in 100 mL of 20% glucose over 15–30 min Give 10–20 mg nebulised salbutamol **Seek Senior Advice** Manage as per NGH guidelines on the intranet

- Escalation of the non-responder and consider critical care review if:
  - GCS ≤8 or falling from a higher level.
  - O_2 saturation lower than 90% on 60% oxygen or higher.
  - $PaCO_2$ >7 kPa (or 52 mmHg) unresponsive to noninvasive ventilation (NIV) or CPAP.
  - Persistent hypotension and/or oliguria unresponsive to 2 L fluid and/or concern of cardiac function.
  - Metabolic acidosis: base deficit < −8 or worse, bicarbonate <18 mmol/L, lactate >3 mmol/L and not improving in 2 h with treatment.

- Aggressive or agitated patients whose treatment is compromised due to their agitation.
- Complex pathologies/disease states require closer monitoring than a ward-based level 0 setting can offer.

An overall fluid management infographic example is given in Fig. 28.4.

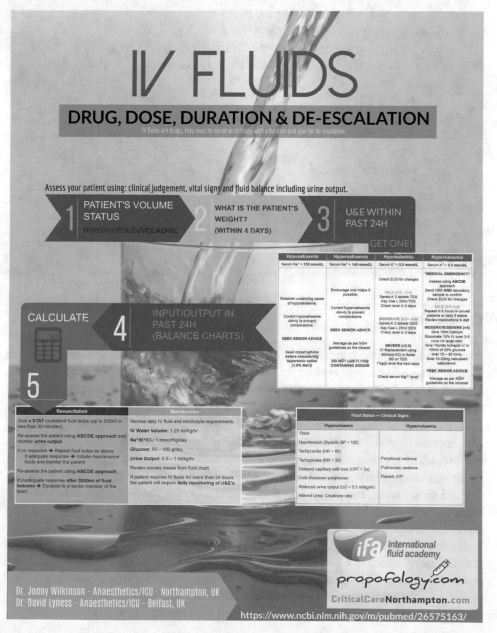

Fig. 28.4 Overall fluid management infographic. (Courtesy from Wilkinson JN, Lyness D, endorsed by the International Fluid Academy)

Case Vignette

Questions and Answers

Q1. What information do you need to safely prescribe IV fluids to the patient?

A1. The following information should be sought, prior to prescription.

1. Fluid status—(hypo/eu/hypervolaemia)
2. Weight change in the last 24 h
3. Urea and Electrolytes in the last 24 h
4. Fluid balance—(Input and output) over the last 24 h

Q2. How will you write a prescription for IV fluid for this patient?

A2. The prescription should contain the following elements

1. Drug—what fluid.
2. Dose—mL/h, via a volumetric pump.
3. Duration—for example, 24 h only or until drinking.
4. De-escalation—there should be a clear stop point, or tapering instruction.

Rare example of appropriate use of 0.9% saline!

Persistent and unrelenting vomiting, for example, causes both hypovolaemia AND a state of hyponatraemic, hypokalaemic metabolic alkalosis. This can also occur due to extensive upper GI NG losses.

0.9% sodium chloride will be a suitable drug to replace these losses but over a limited and controlled, well-monitored period.

Conclusion

In conclusion, the management of intravenous fluid therapy is a critical aspect of patient care, with significant implications for patient safety and outcomes. As highlighted in this chapter, improper fluid prescribing can lead to morbidity and mortality, making it essential to invest in efforts to improve this practice. National guidelines, such as those from the National Institute for Health and Care Excellence (NICE), provide a valuable framework for improving fluid prescription, but effective implementation requires dedication, resources, and ongoing monitoring.

To address the challenges and pitfalls associated with implementing large-scale changes in fluid prescription, healthcare providers should follow a stepwise approach, including team establishment, baseline audits, identifying barriers, engaging medical and nursing leaders, and continuous monitoring and improvement.

By following these principles, healthcare professionals can enhance patient safety and provide more effective care in various clinical settings, including the operating room, emergency room, and intensive care unit. Ultimately, ongoing efforts to improve fluid prescription practices are essential to ensure the well-being of patients and reduce unnecessary risks and costs associated with suboptimal fluid management.

Take Home Messages

There are key points for the implementation of a safe IV fluid policy [23]:

- Establish a feeling of urgency and focus on the three existing problems:
  - Clinical harm.
  - Poor education among prescribers.
  - Lack of accurate fluid balance charting.
- Build a coalition team of willing participants and transgress the usual boundaries by involving the multi-disciplinary team.
- Develop a strategy to be able to give the right amount of the right fluid, at the right time, to the right patient.
- Enlist and present results and plans to stakeholders.
- Generate goals.
- Engage the team with plenty of on-going education sessions for nurses, junior doctors, nurse prescribers, and consultants.
- Embrace modern technology and the digital revolution with E-learning modules or Apps.
- Sustain and capitalize on wins and gains to produce even bigger results.
- Institute and incorporate the programme into the culture of the organization.
- Spread the message—standardize practice and education to improve patient care and propagate a hopeful decrease in morbidity and mortality.

Acknowledgements Parts of this chapter were published previously, as open access under the creative commons Attribution 4.0 International Licence (CC BY 4.0) [5]. Other parts are an in-depth elaboration of another book chapter entitled: *"Intravenous Fluids: Do Not Drown in Confusion!"* by the same authors [15] and have been made available via the critical care Northampton educational website (https://criticalcarenorthampton.com/2019/06/21/iv-fluid-guidance-dont-drown-in-confusion/). The European Commission announced it has adopted CC BY 4.0 and CC0 to share published documents, including photos, videos, reports, peer-reviewed studies, and data. The Commission joins other public institutions around the world that use standard, legally interoperable tools like Creative Commons licenses and public domain tools to share a wide range of content they produce. The decision to use CC aims to increase the legal interoperability and ease of reuse of author's own materials.

References

1. McDougall M, Guthrie B, Doyle A, Timmins A, Bateson M, Ridley E, Drummond G, Vadiveloo T. Introducing NICE guidelines for intravenous fluid therapy into a district general hospital BMJ Open Qual. 2022;11(1).
2. Padhi S, Bullock I, Li L, Stroud M, National Institute for Health, Care Excellence Guideline Development Group. Intravenous fluid therapy for adults in hospital: summary of NICE guidance. BMJ. 2013;347:f7073.

3. Powell-Tuck J, Gosling P, Lobo D, Allison S, Carlson G, Gore M, Lewington A, Pearse R, Mythen M. Summary of the British consensus guidelines on intravenous fluid therapy for adult surgical patients (GIFTASUP). J Intensive Care Soc. 2009;10(1):13–5.

4. Malbrain MLNG, Rice TW, Mythen M, Wuyts S. It is time for improved fluid stewardship. ICU Manag Pract. 2018;18(3):158–62.

5. Malbrain MLNG, Van Regenmortel N, Saugel B, De Tavernier B, Van Gaal P-J, Joannes-Boyau O, Teboul J-L, Rice TW, Mythen M, Monnet X. Principles of fluid management and steward-ship in septic shock: it is time to consider the four D's and the four phases of fluid therapy. Ann Intensive Care. 2018;8(1):66.

6. Malbrain M, Langer T, Annane D, Gattinoni L, Elbers P, Hahn RG, De Laet I, Minini A, Wong A, Ince C, et al. Intravenous fluid therapy in the perioperative and critical care setting: executive summary of the International Fluid Academy (IFA). Ann Intensive Care. 2020;10(1):64.

7. Gomaa AR, Wilkinson JN. Improving i.v. fluid prescribing. Anaesthesiol Intensive Ther. 2019;47:22–4.

8. Malbrain MLNG, Van Regenmortel N, Elbers P, Monnet X, Wong A. Results of a survey on the knowledge of fluid management and fluid stewardship. In: Proceedings first virtual international fluid academy days 2020, Poster presentation Nov 26, Belgium:P26.

9. Nasa P, Wise R, Elbers PWG, Wong A, Dabrowski W, Regenmortel NV, Monnet X, Myatra SN, Malbrain MLNG. Intravenous fluid therapy in perioperative and critical care setting-knowledge test and practice: an international cross-sectional survey. J Crit Care. 2022;71:154122.

10. Jonathan Lacey, Jo Corbett, Lui Forni, Lee Hooper, Fintan Hughes, Gary Minto, Charlotte Moss, Susanna Price, Greg Whyte, Tom Woodcock, Michael Mythen & Hugh Montgomery (2019) A multidisciplinary consensus on dehydration: definitions, diagnostic methods and clinical impli-cations, Annals of Medicine, 51:3-4, 232-251, DOI: 10.1080/07853890.2019.1628352

11. Van Regenmortel N, Langer T, De Weerdt T, Roelant E, Malbrain M, Van den Wyngaert T, Jorens P. Effect of sodium administration on fluid balance and sodium balance in health and the periop-erative setting. Extended summary with additional insights from the MIHMoSA and TOPMAST studies. J Crit Care. 2022;67:157–65.

12. Van Regenmortel N, Moers L, Langer T, Roelant E, De Weerdt T, Caironi P, Malbrain M, Elbers P, Van den Wyngaert T, Jorens PG. Fluid-induced harm in the hospital: look beyond volume and start considering sodium. From physiology towards recommendations for daily practice in hos-pitalized adults. Ann Intensive Care. 2021;11(1):79.

13. Jacobs R, Lochy S, Malbrain M. Phenylephrine-induced recruitable preload from the venous side. J Clin Monit Comput. 2019;33(3):373–6.

14. Malbrain ML, Van Regenmortel N, Owczuk R. It is time to consider the four D's of fluid man-agement. Anaesthesiol Intensive Ther. 2015;47 Spec No:1–5.

15. Wilkinson JN, van Haren FMP, Malbrain MLNG. Intravenous fluids: do not drown in confusion! In: Vincent J-L, editor. Annual update in intensive care and emergency medicine 2020. Cham: Springer; 2020. p. 153–72.

16. Van der Mullen J, Wise R, Vermeulen G, Moonen PJ, Malbrain M. Assessment of hypovolaemia in the critically ill. Anaesthesiol Intensive Ther. 2018;50(2):141–9.

17. Van Regenmortel N, De Weerdt T, Van Craenenbroeck AH, Roelant E, Verbrugghe W, Dams K, Malbrain M, Van den Wyngaert T, Jorens PG. Effect of isotonic versus hypotonic maintenance fluid therapy on urine output, fluid balance, and electrolyte homeostasis: a crossover study in fasting adult volunteers. Br J Anaesth. 2017;118(6):892–900.

18. Van Regenmortel N, Hendrickx S, Roelant E, Baar I, Dams K, Van Vlimmeren K, Embrecht B, Wittock A, Hendriks JM, Lauwers P, et al. 154 compared to 54 mmol per liter of sodium in intravenous maintenance fluid therapy for adult patients undergoing major thoracic surgery (TOPMAST): a single-center randomized controlled double-blind trial. Intensive Care Med. 2019;45(10):1422–32.

19. Silversides JA, Perner A, Malbrain M. Liberal versus restrictive fluid therapy in critically ill patients. Intensive Care Med. 2019;45(10):1440–2.
20. Malbrain ML, Marik PE, Witters I, Cordemans C, Kirkpatrick AW, Roberts DJ, Van Regenmortel N. Fluid overload, de-resuscitation, and outcomes in critically ill or injured patients: a systematic review with suggestions for clinical practice. Anaesthesiol Intensive Ther. 2014;46(5):361–80.
21. Marik PE, Malbrain M. The SEP-1 quality mandate may be harmful: how to drown a patient with 30 mL per kg fluid! Anaesthesiol Intensive Ther. 2017;49(5):323–8.
22. Hofer CK, Cannesson M. Monitoring fluid responsiveness. Acta Anaesthesiol Taiwanica: Off J Taiwan Soc Anesthesiol. 2011;49(2):59–65.
23. Malbrain, MLNG, Caironi P, Hahn R.G. et al. Multidisciplinary expert panel report on fluid stewardship: perspectives and practice. Ann. Intensive Care 13, 89 (2023). https://doi.org/10.1186/s13613-023-01177-y.

Printed in the United States
by Baker & Taylor Publisher Services